Association of Medicine and Psychiatry

Primary Care
Psychiatry

SECOND EDITION

Association of Medicine and Psychiatry

Primary Care Psychiatry

SECOND EDITION

Editors

Robert M. McCarron, DO, DFAPA
Professor and Vice Chair of Education and
Integrated Care
Program Director, Psychiatry Residency Program
Director, Train New Trainers Primary Care
Psychiatry Fellowship
Department of Psychiatry and Human Behavior
University of California, Irvine School of
Medicine
President, California Psychiatric Association
Past President, Association of Medicine and
Psychiatry

Glen L. Xiong, MD
Clinical Professor (VCP)
Department of Psychiatry & Behavioral Sciences
University of California at Davis
Alzheimer's Disease Center
Department of Neurology

Shannon Suo, MD
Past President, Central California Psychiatric Society
Health Sciences Clinical Professor
Program Director, Family Medicine/Psychiatry
Residency
Co-Director, Train New Trainers Primary Care
Psychiatry Fellowship
Department of Psychiatry and Behavioral
Sciences
University of California, Davis School of
Medicine
Sacramento, CA

Paul Summergrad, MD
Past President, American Psychiatric Association
Dr. Frances S. Arkin Professor and Chairman
Department of Psychiatry
Professor of Medicine
Tufts University School of Medicine
Psychiatrist-in-Chief
Tufts Medical Center
Boston, MA

Philip R. Muskin, MD, MA, DLFAPA
Professor of Psychiatry and Senior Consultant in
Consultation-Liaison Psychiatry at Columbia
University Medical Center
Department of Psychiatry: Columbia University
and the New York State Psychiatric
Institute
Faculty: Columbia University Psychoanalytic
Center for Training and Research
New York, NY

Sarah Rivelli, MD, FACP
Past President, Association of Medicine and
Psychiatry
Assistant Professor
Program Director, Internal Medicine-Psychiatry
Residency
Medical Director, Psychiatry Clinical Services,
Duke University Hospital
Director, Medicine-Psychiatry and Hospital
Psychiatry Clinical Professional Unit
Department of Psychiatry and Behavioral Sciences
Department of Medicine
Duke University School of Medicine
Durham, NC

Assistant Editors

Matthew Reed, MD, MSPH
Assistant Dean for Student Affairs
Assistant Professor
Department of Psychiatry
University of California
Irvine, California

Stephanie Mansour, MD

Leigh Goodrich, MD
Resident Physician, Department of Psychiatry
University of California, Irvine

Shawn Hersevoort, MD, MPH
Clinical Professor (VCP)
Department of Psychiatry & Behavioral Sciences
University of California at Davis
Sacramento, California

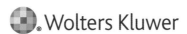

Wolters Kluwer

Philadelphia • Baltimore • New York • London
Buenos Aires • Hong Kong • Sydney • Tokyo

Executive Editor: Rebecca Gaertner
Development Editor: Elizabeth Schaeffer
Editorial Coordinator: Emily Buccieri
Marketing Manager: Rachel Mante Leung
Production Manager: David Saltzberg
Design Coordinator: Elaine Kasmer
Manufacturing Coordinator: Beth Welsh
Prepress Vendor: TNQ Technologies

2nd edition

Library of Congress Cataloging-in-Publication Data

ISBN-13: 978-1-4963-4921-7

Cataloging-in-Publication data available on request from the Publisher.

FOREWORD

There are three indisputable facts about mental health in this country. First, it's an issue that touches all of us and our families. Everyone knows someone who suffers from a brain illness, although it is rarely discussed. Second, it's an issue that underlies virtually every major public policy issue we're trying to tackle—and often aren't very good at tackling: homelessness, criminal justice, family dysfunction; the plight of veterans; children who fall behind in school because of undiagnosed conditions.

And third, despite facts 1 and 2, mental health is not a political priority across our nation. Few governors, legislators, or other elected leaders choose to embrace and elevate this critical cause. It remains the underattended public policy issue of our time.

Over nearly three decades in elected office in California, I have worked alongside other committed advocates to raise the profile of mental health care as an issue central to the well-being of our communities. In 2004, as a member of the State Assembly, I proudly authored California's Mental Health Services Act, legislation that levied a tax on millionaires to fund a vast expansion in treatment and services. The act now generates more than $2.2 billion a year and has helped drive major advances in both early intervention and crisis care for people living with mental illness. It is making a difference—which underscores a fourth essential fact about mental health: We know what to do, but lack the unified vision and political will necessary to do more of it, to scale up and standardize best practices across the nation.

For years now, given the leaps forward in medical research and the evolution of public awareness, we have been hoping to reach a tipping point in mental health care—that magical moment when we have cast aside the stigma, prioritized prevention and early intervention, and established a system of care for brain health as urgent and robust as the one we have built for physical health. We're getting closer. But we're not there yet, for a variety of reasons. Among the most crucial: Even as our understanding of and ability to treat mental illness has matured, our health care workforce can't come close to meeting demand for psychiatric services.

The way forward requires leadership not only from elected officials but also from our medical community. It requires new ways of thinking about how and where we deliver mental health services. It means knocking through the silos and ensuring that the primary care providers who see the majority of patients have the basic training they need to address both body and mind. And it means weaving those front-line providers into a seamless continuum of care so people with serious mental illness have access to more specialized services.

I am grateful for the leadership of Dr. Robert McCarron and his distinguished writing partners as we work to innovate our health care workforce to address the broad gaps in mental health services. What they have produced here—the 2nd edition to their seminal text on primary care psychiatry—reflects an impressive breadth of expertise and an abiding commitment to treating the whole person. I am grateful, as well, to the generations of physicians who will draw on this training to inform their practice. Together, we can forge a new paradigm for care, one built on the concept that there is no health without brain health.

-- Darrell Steinberg

Founder, Steinberg Institute

Darrell Steinberg is Mayor of Sacramento, former President Pro Tem of the California State Senate, and founder of the Steinberg Institute, a nonprofit organization dedicated to advancing the cause of brain health.

PREFACE

Dear Colleague,

Psychiatric disorders such as mood, anxiety, and substance use disorders are among the leading causes of morbidity worldwide. People with these common disorders most frequently present to and are treated by nonpsychiatrists, or primary care providers. Although primary care practitioners deliver the majority of behavioral healthcare in the United States, most only get a brief exposure to the basics of psychiatry during limited formal training. As awareness, recognition, and acceptance of psychiatric disorders increase, the gap between the number of patients who need psychiatric care and the supply of mental health practitioners will continue to grow exponentially. The resultant strain on the public and private mental health systems can, in part, be addressed with a practical, easy-to-use educational tool that will help primary care and mental health trainees and providers feel more comfortable and confident when assessing and treating the most commonly encountered conditions in primary care psychiatry.

Since the first edition publication of the *Primary Care Psychiatry*, the psychiatric workforce has further diminished, with projections to only worsen over the next decade. This second edition of *Primary Care Psychiatry*, now affiliated with the Association of Medicine and Psychiatry, aims to educate nonpsychiatric health care professionals in the diagnosis, treatment, and general conceptualization of adult psychiatric disorders. Most of the authors are dually trained in psychiatry *and* either family medicine, internal medicine, or psychosomatic medicine. This book illustrates a practical approach to primary care psychiatry because it is principally written by practicing primary care physicians who are also psychiatrists. Because we know first-hand what it is like to work in the primary care setting, we have distilled a large volume of information into a practical and focused overview of primary care psychiatry.

Primary Care Psychiatry, 2nd Edition covers the essential psychiatric conditions found in the primary care setting and can therefore be easily used as part of a psychiatric and behavioral health curriculum for trainees of various clinical disciplines. In Section I, we include a framework by which "primary care psychiatry" can most effectively be practiced. This includes an overview on collaborative care, preventive care for those who have severe mental illness, and a guide to cultural considerations in medicine. We continue to emphasize the *AMPS* screening tool as a core educational foundation, as it can easily be used to diagnose the most commonly encountered psychiatric conditions: *A*nxiety, *M*ood, *P*sychotic, and *S*ubstance-related disorders. Section II provides a clinically relevant overview on the most common psychiatric disorders, with helpful diagnostic and therapeutic practice pointers. In Section III, we present a user-friendly approach to the fundamentals of primary care psychiatric treatment. Special topics such as geriatric psychiatry, child psychiatry, suicide risk assessment, somatic symptom disorders, insomnia, sexual dysfunction, and technology in medicine are all presented in Section IV. The e-book companion includes additional resources such as CME multiple choice questions with answers. These tools promote optimal learning and teaching.

We strongly believe in a biopsychosocial treatment approach that enables patients to learn and utilize life-long skills that will result in decreased morbidity and often recovery from mental illness. It is our sincere hope that this book gives you the tools needed to provide exceptional psychiatric patient care, while in a busy nonpsychiatric clinical setting. If you have any suggestions on how we can improve future editions, please let us know.

Robert M. McCarron, DO, DFAPA

Glen L. Xiong, MD

Shannon Suo, MD

Paul Summergrad, MD

Philip R. Muskin, MD, MA, DLFAPA

Sarah Rivelli, MD, FACP

ACKNOWLEDGMENTS

We would like to thank the Association of Medicine and Psychiatry for their endorsement of *Primary Care Psychiatry*, 2nd Edition. We are also grateful to the many authors who took the time to share their knowledge. This book would not be in print without their passion to provide empathic, high-quality patient care and teaching. We are extremely appreciative of the talented and highly professional Wolters Kluwer editorial staff, particularly Emily Buccieri and Rebecca S. Gaertner.

We would like to acknowledge Ruth Benca, MD, PhD, and Robert E. Hales, Chairs of Psychiatry at the University of California, Irvine and the University of California, Davis, respectively. We also dedicate this book to two mentors, friends, and innovative leaders in the field of psychiatry: Captane Thomson MD, Founding President, California Psychiatric Association and Roger Kathol, MD, Founding President, Association of Medicine and Psychiatry. This educational guide could not have been done without the support of Matthew Reed, MD, MSPH (Assistant Editor) and Shawn Hersevoort, MD (Assistant Editor). We are also most grateful for the administrative support from Wendy Cant, MBA.

Robert M. McCarron, DO, DFAPA

Glen L. Xiong, MD

CONTRIBUTING AUTHORS

Lawrence Adler, MD
Assistant Professor
Department of Psychiatry (Geriatric)
University of Maryland School of Medicine
Baltimore, Maryland

Rachel J. Ammirati, PhD
Assistant Professor
Department of Psychiatry and Behavioral Sciences
Emory University School of Medicine
Atlanta, Georgia

Mary Elizabeth Alvarez, MD, MPH
Assistant
Department of Psychiatry
Medical College of Wisconsin
Milwaukee, Wisconsin

Amy Barnhorst, MD
Vice Chair for Community Mental Health
Department of Psychiatry and Behavioral Sciences
University of California
Davis, California

Jessica A. Beauchene, MD
Staff Psychiatrist
Department of Center for Discovery
Granite Bay, California

Gregory D. Brown, MD
Department of Psychiatry and Behavioral Science
Department of Medicine
Duke University
Durham, North Carolina

Vincent F. Capaldi, II, ScM, MD
Associate Professor
Department of Psychiatry and Internal Medicine
Uniformed Services University of the Health Sciences
Bethesda, Maryland

Puja L. Chadha, MD
Assistant Professor
Psychiatry and Behavioral Sciences
University of California
Davis, California

Jeremy DeMartini, MD
Assistant Clinical Professor
Department of Psychiatry
University of California
Davis, California

Lindsey Enoch, MD
Assistant Professor
Department of Psychiatry
Department of Internal Medicine
University of Washington
Seattle, Washington

Jane P. Gagliardi, MD, MHS
Associate Professor
Department of Psychiatry and Behavioral Sciences
Department of Medicine
Duke University School of Medicine
Durham, North Carolina

Mary Margaret Gleason, MD
Associate Professor
Department of Psychiatry and Behavioral Sciences
Tulane University School of Medicine
New Orleans, Los Angeles

Ana Hategan, MD
Associate Clinical
Department of Psychiatry and Behavioural
Neurosciences
Division of Geriatric Psychiatry
McMaster University
Hamilton, Ontario, Canada

Jaesu Han, MD
Clinical Professor
Department of Psychiatry and Human Behavior
University of California at Irvine Orange, California

D. Brian Haver, MS
Doctoral Candidate
Department of Clinical Psychology
Mercer University
Atlanta, Georgia

Shelly L. Henderson, PhD
Associate Clinical Professor
Department of Family and Community Medicine
University of California
Davis, California

Jennifer A. Hersevoort, MD
Staff Psychiatrist
Department of Psychiatry
Pacific Coast Psychiatric Associates
San Francisco, California

Shawn Hersevoort, MD, MPH
Clinical Professor (VCP)
Department of Psychiatry & Behavioral Sciences
University of California at Davis
Sacramento, California

Calvin H. Hirsch, MD
Professor of Clinical Internal Medicine and Public Health Sciences
Division of General Medicine (Geriatrics)
Department of Internal Medicine
University of California
Davis Medical Center
Davis, California

Poh Choo How, MD, PhD
Health Sciences Assistant Professor
Department of Psychiatry and Behavioral Sciences
University of California
Davis, California

Kimberly Kavanagh, MD
Triple Board Resident
Departments of Psychiatry & Behavioral Sciences and Pediatrics
Tulane University School of Medicine
New Orleans, Los Angeles

Craig R. Keenan, MD
Professor
Department of Medicine
University of California
Davis School of Medicine
Davis, California

Chandan Khandai, MD
Consultation Liaison Psychiatry Fellow
University of Washington - School of Medicine
Seattle, Washington

Christine E. Kho, MD
Resident Physician
Internal Medicine and Psychiatry
UC Davis Medical Center
Sacramento, California

Jea-Hyoun Kim, MD
Psychiatrist
Department of Behavioral Health
Santa Clara Valley Medical Center
San Jose, California

Alan Koike, MD, MSHS
Heath Sciences Clinical Professor
Department of Psychiatry and Behavioral Sciences
University of California
Davis School of Medicine
Davis, California

Rohail Kumar, MD
Triple Board Resident
Departments of Psychiatry & Behavioral Sciences and Pediatrics
Tulane University School of Medicine
New Orleans, Los Angeles

Martin H. Leamon, MD
Clinical Professor
Department of Psychiatry and Behavioral Sciences
University of California
Davis, California

Anna Lembke, MD
Associate Professor
Department of Psychiatry and Behavioral Sciences
Stanford University
Stanford, California

Philippe T. Lévy, MD
Resident Physician
Department of Internal Medicine, Psychiatry and Behavioral Sciences
University of California, Davis
Sacramento, California

Simone T. Lew, MD, MS
Internal Medicine/Psychiatry Resident
Department of Internal Medicine
Department of Psychiatry and Behavioral Sciences
University of California
Davis, California

Molly Lubin, MD
Assistant Clinical Professor
Department of Psychiatry
University of Wisconsin
Madison, Wisconsin

Anne B. McBride, MD
Assistant Clinical Professor
Psychiatry and Behavioral Sciences
University of California
Davis, California

Robert M. McCarron, DO, DFAPA
Professor and Vice Chair of Education and Integrated
Care
Program Director, Psychiatry Residency Program
Director, Train New Trainers Primary Care Psychiatry
Fellowship
Department of Psychiatry and Human Behavior
University of California, Irvine School of Medicine
President, California Psychiatric Association
Past President, Association of Medicine and Psychiatry

Myo Thwin Myint, MD
Assistant Professor
Department of Psychiatry and Behavioral Sciences and
Department of Pediatrics
Tulane University
New Orleans, Louisiana

Keeban C. Nam, MD
Chief Fellow Physician
Department of Psychiatry, Child and Adolescent
Fellowship
University of California
Irvine, Orange, California

Amy Newhouse, MD
Assistant Professor
Department of Psychiatry and Behavioral Sciences
Department of Medicine
Duke University School of Medicine
Durham, North Carolina

Chinyere I. Ogbonna, MD, MPH
Adjunct Faculty
Department of Psychiatry and Behavioral Sciences
Stanford University
Stanford, California

John C. Onate, MD
Professor
Department of Psychiatry
UC Davis

Jeremy A. Parker, MD
Clinical Faculty
Department of Psychiatry
California Pacific Medical Center
San Francisco, California

Cameron Quanbeck, MD
Associate Medical Director
Department of Behavioral Health and Recovery
Services
San Mateo County Health System
Cordilleras Mental Health Rehabilitation Center
Redwood City, California

Jeffrey T. Rado, MD, MPH
Associate Professor
Department of Psychiatry and Behavioral Sciences
Northwestern University Feinberg School of Medicine
Chicago, IL

Shaun P. Rafael, DO
Resident Physician
Department of Psychiatry and Behavioral Sciences
University of California
Davis, California

Y. Pritham Raj, MD
Associate Professor
Departments of Internal Medicine and Psychiatry
Oregon Health & Science University
Portland, Oregon

Anna Ratzliff, MD, PhD
Associate Professor
Department of Psychiatry and Behavioral Sciences
University of Washington
Seattle, Washington

Matthew Reed, MD, MSPH
Assistant Dean for Student Affairs
Assistant Professor
Department of Psychiatry
University of California
Irvine, California

Kate M. Richards, MD
Psychiatry-Family Medicine Resident
Department of Psychiatry and Behavioral Sciences
Department of Family and Community Medicine
University of California,
Davis, California

Sarah Rivelli, MD, FACP
Past President, Association of Medicine and Psychiatry
Assistant Professor
Program Director, Internal Medicine-Psychiatry
Residency
Medical Director, Psychiatry Clinical Services, Duke
University Hospital
Director, Medicine-Psychiatry and Hospital Psychiatry
Clinical Professional Unit
Department of Psychiatry and Behavioral Sciences
Department of Medicine
Duke University School of Medicine
Durham, NC

David Safani, MD, MBA
Assistant Professor
Department of Psychiatry and Human Behavior
UC Irvine School of Medicine
Irvine, California

Bharat R. Sampathi, BA
Medical Student
University of California
Irvine School of Medicine
Irvine, California

Eleasa A. Sokolski, MD
Resident Physician
Department of Psychiatry and Behavioral Sciences
Department of Internal Medicine
UC Davis Medical Center
Davis, California

Shannon Suo, MD
Past President, Central California Psychiatric Society
Health Sciences Clinical Professor
Program Director, Family Medicine/Psychiatry
Residency
Co-Director, Train New Trainers Primary Care
Psychiatry Fellowship
Department of Psychiatry and Behavioral Sciences
University of California, Davis School of Medicine
Sacramento, CA

Maria L. Tiamson-Kassab, MD, DFAPA, FACLP
Clinical Professor
Department of Psychiatry
University of California
San Diego, La Jolla, California

Hendry Ton, MD, MS
Professor
Department of Psychiatry and Behavioral Sciences
University of California
Davis, California

Ramanpreet Toor, MD
Assistant Professor
Department of Psychiatry and Behavioral Sciences
University of Washington
Seattle, Washington

Martha C. Ward, MD
Assistant Professor
Department of Psychiatry & Behavioral Sciences
Emory University School of Medicine
Atlanta, Georgia

Scott G. Williams, MD, FACP, FAPA, FAASM
Director for Medicine
Fort Belvoir Community Hospital
Associate Professor of Medicine and Psychiatry
Uniformed Services
University of the Health Sciences
Bethesda, Maryland

Glen L. Xiong, MD
Clinical Professor (VCP)
Department of Psychiatry & Behavioral Sciences
University of California at Davis
Alzheimer's Disease Center
Department of Neurology

ABBREVIATIONS

AA	Alcoholics Anonymous
AAI	Appearance Anxiety Inventory
ACBT	Abbreviated cognitive behavioral therapy
ACT	Assertive community treatment
AD	Alzheimer disease
ADHD	Attention deficit hyperactivity disorder
ADLs	Activities of daily living
AFP	Alpha-fetal protein
AIMS	Abnormal Involuntary Movement Scale
AMPS	Anxiety, Mood, Psychosis, and Substance use disorders
ANA	Antinuclear antibody
APA	American Psychiatric Association
AUDs	Alcohol use disorders
AUDIT	The Alcohol Use Disorders Identification Test
ARFID	Avoidant/restrictive food intake disorder
ASD	Acute stress disorder
BA	Behavioral activation
BDI	Beck Depression Inventory
BDD	Body dysmorphic disorder
BED	Binge eating disorder
BPD	Borderline personality disorder
BZDs	Benzodiazepines
CAD	Coronary artery disease
CBC	Complete blood count
CBT	Cognitive behavioral therapy
CDT	Carbohydrate-deficient transferrin
CES-D	Center for Epidemiological Studies Depression Scale
ChEIs	Cholinesterase inhibitors
CIR	Clutter Image Rating Scale
CIWA-A	Clinical Institute Withdrawal Assessment for Alcohol
COPD	Chronic obstructive pulmonary disease
CT	Computerized tomography
CVAs	Cerebrovascular accidents
DA-2	Dopamine type 2
DBSA	Depressive and Bipolar Support Alliance
DBT	Dialectical behavior therapy
DCSAD	Diagnostic Classification of Sleep and Arousal Disorders
DLB	Dementia with Lewy bodies
DRIs	Dopamine reuptake inhibitors
DSD	Dementia syndrome of depression
DSM-IV-TR	Diagnostic and Statistical Manual of Mental Disorders, 4th edition, text revision
DSM-5	Diagnostic and Statistical Manual of Mental Disorder, 5th edition
DTs	Delirium tremens
DTR	Dysfunctional thought record
ECG	Electrocardiogram
ECT	Electroconvulsive therapy
ED	Emergency department
EDO	Eating disorder
EPDS	Edinburgh Postnatal Depression Scale
EPS	Extrapyramidal symptoms
ERP	Exposure response prevention
FDA	Food and Drug Administration
FGA	First-generation antipsychotics
FTD	Frontotemporal dementia
FTLD	Frontotemporal lobar degeneration
GABA$_A$	Gamma-aminobutyric acid type A
GAD	Generalized anxiety disorder
GAD-7	Generalized Anxiety Disorder Scale
GDS	Geriatric Depression Scale
GERD	Gastroesophageal reflux disease
GGT	Gamma-glutamyltransferase
GI	Gastrointestinal
HADS	Hospital Anxiety and Depression Scale
HAM-D	Hamilton Rating Scale for Depression
HD	Huntington disease
HIV	Human immunodeficiency virus
HPI	History of present illness
HRS	Hoarding Rating Scale
HRT	Habit reversal treatment
ICD	International Classification of Diseases
ICSD	International Classification of Sleep Disorders
IM	Intramuscular

IOM	Institute of Medicine
IPT	Interpersonal psychotherapy
LAI	Long-acting injectable
LEP	Limited English proficiency
LGBTQ	Lesbian, gay, bisexual, transgender, queer
LSD	Lysergic acid
MADRS	Montgomery–Asberg Depression Rating Scale
MAOIs	Monoamine oxidase inhibitors
MCI	Mild cognitive impairment
MDD	Major depressive disorder
MDMA	Methylenedioxymethamphetamine
MDQ	Mood Disorder Questionnaire
MET	Motivational enhancement therapy
MGH-HS	Massachusetts General Hospital Hair Pulling Scale
MI	Motivational interviewing
MMSE	Mini-Mental State Examination
MoCA	Montreal Cognitive Assessment
MRI	Magnetic resonance imaging
MSE	Mental Status Examination
NAMI	National Alliance for Mental Illness
NaSSA	Noradrenergic and specific serotonergic antidepressant
NIAAA	National Institute on Alcohol Abuse and Alcoholism
NDRI	Norepinephrine–dopamine reuptake inhibitor
NMDA	N-methyl-D-aspartate
NMS	Neuroleptic malignant syndrome
NNRTIs	Nonnucleoside reverse transcriptase inhibitors
NOS	Not otherwise specified
NPI	Neuropsychiatric Inventory
NPSs	Neuropsychiatric symptoms
OCD	Obsessive–compulsive disorder
OCF	Outline for Cultural Formulation
OCPD	Obsessive–compulsive personality disorder
OSAH	Obstructive sleep apnea–hypopnea
PANDAS	Pediatric autoimmune neuropsychiatric disorder associated with group A streptococci
PCP	Phencyclidine; Primary care provider
PD	Panic disorder
PET	Positron emission tomography
PHQ	Patient Health Questionnaire
PLMD	Periodic limb movement disorder
PORT	Patient Outcomes Research Team
PSP	Progressive supranuclear palsy
PTSD	Posttraumatic stress disorder
RLS	Restless leg syndrome
SAD	Seasonal affective disorder
SAMe	S-adenosyl methionine
SGA	Second-generation antipsychotic
SIDs	Substance-induced disorders
SNRIs	Serotonin–norepinephrine reuptake inhibitors
SP	Social phobia
SPECT	Single photon emission computed tomography
SPS-R	Skin Picking Scale—Revised
SRDs	Substance-related disorders
SSRIs	Selective serotonin reuptake inhibitors
STAR*D	Sequenced Treatment Alternatives to Relieve Depression
SUDs	Substance use disorders
TCAs	Tricyclic antidepressants
TD	Tardive dyskinesia
TMS	Transcranial magnetic stimulation
TSC	Trichotillomania Scale for Children
TSF	Twelve-step facilitation
TSH	Thyroid-stimulating hormone
UPS	Unexplained physical symptoms
VaD	Vascular dementia
WHO	World Health Organization
Y-BOCS	Yale–Brown Obsessive–Compulsive Scale
ZBI	Zarit Burden Interview
ZDS	Zung Depression Scale

CONTENTS

SECTION I

Behavioral Health in the Primary Care Setting

SECTION II

Psychiatric Disorders

SECTION III

Fundamentals of Primary Care Psychiatric Treatment

SECTION IV

Special Clinical Topics

APPENDICES

BEHAVIORAL HEALTH IN THE PRIMARY CARE SETTING

1

THE PRIMARY CARE PSYCHIATRIC INTERVIEW

Robert M. McCarron, DO, DFAPA, Jeremy DeMartini, MD , Glen L. Xiong, MD, and John C. Onate, MD

A 30-year-old woman with a history of chronic low-back pain and tobacco use presents to transfer care from another provider with the following opening statement, "That horrible doctor ignored my pain and wanted me to suffer! I heard you are the best doctor in town. I can already tell we are going to be great friends!" The woman's speech is loud and somewhat fast. When the provider suggests she try physical therapy instead of an opioid medication, she yells, "Why don't you just kill me now?" The provider wonders if the patient is bipolar and whether she needs to be psychiatrically hospitalized.

CLINICAL HIGHLIGHTS

- The Mental Status Examination (MSE) for a psychiatric evaluation is analogous to the physical examination for a general medical assessment.
- The AMPS screening tool (*Figure 1-1*) includes four primary clinical dimensions of the psychiatric review of systems: **A**nxiety, **M**ood, **P**sychosis, **S**ubstance use. This approach can be easily used in the primary care setting as a starting point to develop a reasonable differential diagnosis for common psychiatric disorders.
- The psychiatric interview places an emphasis on psychosocial function and should give a personalized description of the patient from a biopsychosocial perspective.
- One helpful time-saving strategy is the use of the Supplemental Psychiatric History Form to help gather a preliminary psychiatric history. A patient should complete this form either before the first clinic visit or during later visits, if a psychiatric illness is suspected.

CLINICAL SIGNIFICANCE

Up to 75% of all mental health care is delivered in the primary care setting.[1] Unfortunately, reimbursement constraints and limited psychiatric training in most primary care curricula often discourage full exploration and thorough workup of mental illness.[2] Owing to the stigma of psychiatric conditions, patients are often reluctant to present to mental health settings and may not seek treatment.[3] However, most nonemergent or severe psychiatric conditions can be treated successfully in primary care settings. The ability of the primary care clinician to carefully screen for and evaluate psychiatric symptoms is paramount to accurately diagnose and effectively treat the underlying psychiatric disorder.[4] Also, management of chronic general medical conditions is usually much easier if psychiatric conditions are addressed.

Clinical assessment relies heavily on both obtaining the medical history and completing a physical examination for general medical conditions. A similar approach is taken for psychiatric disorders with two main differences. First, the psychiatric interview places additional emphasis on psychosocial stressors and overall level of functioning. Second, the MSE is analogous to the physical examination for a general medical workup and is the cornerstone for the psychiatric evaluation. Both these tasks may be accomplished effectively with improved organization and practice. This chapter divides the psychiatric assessment into three sections: (1) the psychiatric interview, (2) the MSE, and (3) time-saving strategies.

THE PSYCHIATRIC INTERVIEW

The initial interview is important, as it sets the tone for future visits and will influence the initial treatment.[5,6] While the information obtained from the interview is critical to establish a diagnosis, a collaborative,

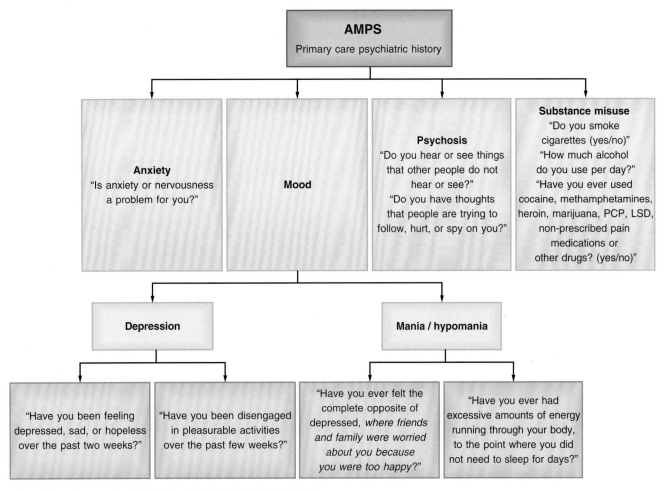

FIGURE 1-1 Psychiatric review of systems: AMPS screening tool.

therapeutic relationship is a key component to a successful treatment plan. Therefore, the clinician should try to balance the urgency to obtain information with the need to establish a positive, trusting therapeutic alliance with the patient. Similar in style and complementary to the general medical history, the psychiatric interview is outlined in *Table 1-1*.

CHIEF COMPLAINT AND HISTORY OF PRESENT ILLNESS

The vast majority of physicians interrupt before patients can share their opening concerns.[7] By starting with open-ended questions and allowing the patient to share his or her perspective, the interviewer can establish rapport and start the patient's MSE. Of course, this investment of time may temporarily take away from discussion of other medical conditions, but it is generally well worth the time. Reflective statements may be used to clarify and summarize particular problems (e.g., "You are telling me that you feel your previous physician did not care

about your pain as he stopped your opiate medication."). Clarification may also be used (e.g., "Can you explain to me why you think your previous physician stopped the opiate medication?"). Gentle confrontation can be used to point out inconsistencies or bring topics to the forefront that a patient is avoiding or expressing ambivalence about (e.g., "When I started asking you about physical therapy you said you want me to kill you, but later you insisted that you are not suicidal, can you explain this to me?")

It is important to organize the sequence of events with each problem individually, giving the most time to the problem with the highest priority. For patients with multiple chronic problems, setting an agenda at the beginning of the encounter will also help them to understand and conceptualize their medical problems. The history of present illness (HPI) should include the duration, severity, and extent of each symptom along with exacerbating and ameliorating factors. Patients vary greatly in their recall of historical material and often vague or contradictory material surfaces. Once consent is obtained

TABLE 1-1 Outline of the Primary Care Psychiatric Interview

Chief complaint and history of present illness (HPI)	• For the first few minutes, just listen to better understand the chief complaint(s) and start the mental status examination • Make note of changes in social or occupational function • Use the AMPS screening tool for psychiatric symptoms
Psychiatric history	• Ask about past mental health providers, past diagnoses and hospitalizations • Inquire about whether the patient has ever thought of or attempted suicide
Medication history	• Ask about medication dosages, duration of treatment, effectiveness, and side effects
Family history	• The clinician might ask, "Did your grandparents, parents, or siblings ever have severe problems with depression, bipolar disorder, anxiety, schizophrenia, or any other emotional problems?"
Social history	***Socioeconomic status*** "How are you doing financially and are you currently employed?" "What is your current living situation and how are things at home?" ***Interpersonal relationships*** "Who are the most important people in your life and do you rely on them for support?" "How are these relationships going?" ***Legal history*** "Have you ever had problems with the law?" "Have you even been arrested or imprisoned?" ***Developmental history*** "How would you describe your childhood in one sentence?" "What was the highest grade you completed in school?" "Have you ever been physically, verbally, or sexually abused?"

from the patient, it is important to follow up on any inconsistencies with the patient and gather collateral information by speaking with family members and other treatment providers.

PSYCHIATRIC REVIEW OF SYSTEMS: AMPS SCREENING TOOL

A thorough review of the major psychiatric dimensions (or "review of systems") should be completed for patients who present with even a single psychiatric symptom. In the time-limited primary care setting, this can be a difficult but critically important task. The most commonly encountered primary care psychiatric disorders involve four major clinical dimensions and can be remembered by the **AMPS** mnemonic: **A**nxiety, **M**ood, **P**sychosis, **S**ubstance use disorders (*Figure 1-1*). We recommend incorporating the AMPS screening tool into your daily practice, especially when a patient has an established psychiatric disorder (including personality and eating disorders) or presents with psychiatric complaints such as depression, anxiety, insomnia, and unexplained physical complaints. When a particular dimension is present and causing distress, further exploration is indicated (*Table 1-2*).

Anxiety

Anxiety is common in the primary care setting and often comorbid with mood, psychotic, and substance misuse disorders. It is sometimes the main catalyst for a depressive

or substance use disorder and the secondary condition(s) will not remit unless the primary anxiety disorder is treated. Anxiety is also a significant acute risk factor for suicide that is commonly underappreciated and poorly screened (see Chapter 14). The quickest and most effective way to screen for an anxiety disorder during the interview is to simply ask, "Is anxiety or nervousness a problem for you?" If the patient reports feeling anxious, it is advisable to say, "Please describe how your anxiety affects you on an everyday basis." Depending on the answer, follow-up questions (e.g., "What types of situations or events trigger your anxiety?") will help develop a reasonable differential diagnosis. Also, if anxiety is a problem, it may be helpful to ask the patient if it is a "big problem, small problem or somewhere in-between." A numerical scale may also be used to quantify the level of anxiety.

Mood

The best way to understand a patient's mood is to ask, "How would you describe your mood or emotions over the past few weeks?" The self-reported mood is also an important part of the MSE and should be rated as either congruent or incongruent with the corresponding affect. The two main components of mood (depression and mania) should be fully assessed during each primary care psychiatric interview.

Depression is often secondary to and comorbid with primary anxiety, sleep, substance use, and other psychiatric disorders. Depressive symptoms should always be discussed with the patient when treating another psychiatric

TABLE 1-2 The AMPS Screening Tool for Common Psychiatric Conditions

	SCREENING QUESTIONS	FOLLOW-UP QUESTIONS	DIAGNOSTIC AND TREATMENT INSTRUMENTS[a]
Anxiety	"Is anxiety or nervousness a problem for you?"	• "Please describe how your anxiety affects you on an everyday basis." • "What triggers your anxiety?" • "What makes your anxiety get better?"	Generalized Anxiety Disorders Scale (GAD-7)
Mood	**Depression[b]** 1. "Have you been feeling depressed, sad, or hopeless over the past 2 weeks?" 2. "What do you usually like to do for fun and have you stopped doing this over the past few weeks?" **Mania/hypomania** 1. "Have you ever felt the complete opposite of depressed, *when friends and family were worried about you because you were too happy*?" 2. "Have you ever had excessive amounts of energy running through your body, to the point where you did not need to sleep for days?"	• "What is your depression like on an everyday basis?" • "How does your depression affect your daily life?" • "When did this last happen, and please tell me what was going on at that time." • "How long did this last?" • "Were you using any drugs or alcohol at the time?" • "Did you require treatment or hospitalization?"	Patient Health Questionnaire (PHQ-9) Mood Disorder Questionnaire (MDQ)
Psychosis	1. "Do you hear or see things that other people do not hear or see?" 2. "Do you have thoughts that people are trying to follow, hurt, or spy on you?" 3. "Do you ever get messages from the television or radio?"	• "When did these symptoms start?" • "What triggers your symptoms?" • "What makes your symptoms get better?"	None recommended for the primary care setting
Substance use	1. "How much alcohol do you drink per day?" 2. "Have you been using any cocaine, methamphetamines, heroin, marijuana, PCP, LSD, ecstasy, or other drugs?"	If yes: • "How often do you use?" • "Do you think use of this substance is a problem in your life?" • "As a result of the use, did you experience any problems with relationships, work, finances, or the law?" • "Have you ever used any drugs by injection?" If no: • "Have you ever used any of these drugs in the past?"	• CAGE[c] • CAGE-AID (adapted to include drugs) • Alcohol Use Disorders Identification Test (AUDIT-C)
Suicide[d]	1. "Do you ever wish you could go to sleep and not wake up?" 2. "Do you have any thoughts of wanting to hurt or kill yourself or somebody else?"	• "Have you ever tried to hurt or kill yourself in the past?" • "What is the chance you will try to hurt or kill yourself within the next 2-4 weeks?" • "Do you have guns or other items you could use to harm yourself?"	

[a]*These are suggested instruments that could be considered. More details about relevant instruments are available in the corresponding chapters.*
[b]*If either of these two questions is answered affirmatively, follow-up questions should be asked and a PHQ-9 should be administered.*
[c]*See Chapters 6 and 7 for details.*
[d]*Suggest asking about suicide if one of the AMPS questions is positive.*

condition(s)—even if the chief complaint is not depression. The two screening questions for a current major depressive episode are (1) "Have you been feeling depressed, sad, or hopeless over the past two weeks?" and (2) "Have you had a decreased energy level in pleasurable activities over the past few weeks?" An alternative way to ask this second screening question is, "What do you normally like to do for fun and have you been doing that over the last few weeks." The sensitivity and specificity for the detection of a major depressive episode using these screening questions are 96% and 57%, respectively.[6] If the answer to either of these two questions is positive, the clinician should have a high index of suspicion for a depressive disorder and probe further. An open-ended approach would be to ask, "What is your depression like on an everyday basis?" or "How does your depression affect your daily life?" In most cases, depressed patients will discuss their troubling symptoms, and there will be no need to go through the entire "checklist" for depression (e.g., changes in appetite, energy, sleep, concentration). The Patient Health Questionnaire (PHQ-9) is a nine-item patient self-report form that can be used in the primary care setting to screen for depression or quantify changes in the severity of depression over the course of treatment. *All depressed patients should be asked about suicidal thoughts, plans, and intent, and a clear assessment of acute suicide risk should be included in the progress note.*

Not all depression is related to a major depressive episode. After screening for depression, one should search for evidence suggestive of a past or current manic or hypomanic episode, as discrete depressive episodes may be related to bipolar spectrum illness. It is important to screen for bipolar disorder, as the comorbidity with some psychiatric disorders is more than 50% to 80% (e.g., attention deficit hyperactivity disorder and substance use disorders). Hypomanic and manic episodes should be considered in most patients with depression, anxiety, irritability, and insomnia. Also, it is important to screen for bipolar disorder when starting an antidepressant, as unopposed antidepressants may increase the risk of inducing a manic episode and will often be ineffective in treating bipolar depression. Once a patient has had one clearly defined hypomanic or manic episode, the lifelong diagnosis of his or her mood disorder becomes a bipolar spectrum disorder with the appropriate specifier for each mood episode (e.g., "bipolar disorder, most recent episode depressed," rather than "major depressive disorder").

On examination, it may be obvious when a manic episode is present. However, it can be quite a challenge to elicit manic symptoms from the past. Asking questions such as "Have there been times when you have had a lot of sex or shopped excessively?" or "Have you ever felt on top of the world?" may confuse the patient and can lead to diagnostic uncertainty. It is preferable to include the opinions of the patients' family and friends, as they may have different perspectives. If collateral history from friends and family is not available, the practitioner can ask, "Have you ever felt the opposite of sad or depressed, *where friends and family were worried your mood was too elevated or irritable for days to the point of needing medical attention?*" or "Have you ever had excessive amounts of energy running through your body, to the point where you did not need to sleep for days?" With the last question, it is important to differentiate primary insomnia from a lack of need for sleep due to a manic episode. If the patient answers yes to either question, the follow-up questions should be, "When did this last happen?" "What was going on at that time?" and "Were you

using any substances such as amphetamines or cocaine?" Most patients will be able to relive that event with you and provide specific information, which will narrow the differential diagnosis.

Psychosis

Psychotic symptoms such as disorganized speech and behavior, paranoid delusions, and hallucinations do not commonly present in the primary care setting. These symptoms are, however, important to assess, as they are often associated with mood disorders and substance misuse disorders or are secondary to a general systemic medical condition. The following questions can be used to evaluate psychosis: (1) "Do you hear or see things that other people do not hear or see?" and (2) Do you have thoughts that people are trying to follow, hurt, or spy on you?" These questions will identify a history of hallucinations or delusions (also known as positive symptoms), while disorganized speech or behavior will usually be evident during the MSE and during collection of the collateral history. In general, persistent psychotic symptoms of unclear etiology warrant further psychiatric consultation and evaluation for schizophrenia.

Substance Use

Comorbid substance use, abuse, and dependence are common in primary care patients presenting with psychiatric symptoms. Alcohol misuse disorders are particularly common in the United States. Substance use disorders mimic nearly all psychiatric symptoms, especially anxiety, depression, insomnia, hyperactivity, irritability, and hallucinations. Clues to substance use may include social factors such as inability to maintain employment, interpersonal and financial problems, repeated legal offenses, and poor adherence to treatment. Key aspects of a substance abuse history include specific substance(s) used; quantity; frequency; total duration; means of getting the drug; impact of drug use on personal, family, and work functioning; and previous sobriety and treatment history. Priority should be placed on active drug use, especially that which negatively affects medical treatment and adherence.

Because nonpathologic use and misuse of alcohol are both widely encountered, we recommend assuming that most patients may use alcohol on a daily basis and screen with this in mind. When asking about use of other substances, it will likely be perceived as less judgment to avoid words such as "recreational," "illicit," or "illegal" when asking the patient about use of nonprescription substances. We recommend listing each substance when inquiring about use (e.g., "Do you use cocaine, heroin, acid, speed, ecstasy, marijuana, or nonprescribed pain medications?").

Suicidal Ideation

Almost half of those patients dying by suicide have seen their primary care provider within 1 month before their death, while fewer than one quarter have seen a mental health professional.[8] Many practitioners are uncomfortable with discussing suicide, but there is no evidence that discussing suicide increases risk.[9] Asking about suicide should not be limited to patients with major depressive disorder, as substance use disorders and schizophrenia have a similar risk of suicide, and anorexia nervosa has a substantially higher risk of suicide.[10] As this can be a sensitive topic for both providers and patients, it is important to both establish rapport and provide empathic rationale for asking questions related to suicide (e.g., "Sometimes when patients are in severe pain, they start to think about going to sleep and not waking up, or even killing themselves; has this happened to you?"). If a patient responds yes to a screening question, ask follow-up questions about intent (e.g., "How likely on a scale from 0 to 10 are you to kill yourself"), plan (e.g., "Have you thought about how you would kill yourself?"), prior attempts, and access to guns or other lethal means of suicide. A provider should document suicide risk, differentiating between acute and chronic risk, whether there are any modifiable risk factors (such as removing guns from the home or stopping alcohol), and if the patient is at moderate or high acute risk to get an emergency mental health professional consult or call 911 before the patient leaves the office.

PSYCHIATRIC AND MEDICATION HISTORY

The structure and content of the psychiatric history is essentially the same as the medical history. Past diagnoses, treatments, hospitalizations, and mental health providers comprise the main categories. Frequency of psychiatric hospitalization may reveal severity and chronicity of the psychiatric condition. It is important to describe medication dosage, duration, response, side effects, and adherence. Obtaining prior medical records is helpful when developing a differential diagnosis and treatment plan.

FAMILY HISTORY

Psychiatric disorders are based on both genetic and environmental factors. Patients with a family history of a first-degree relative with major depressive disorder, bipolar disorder, substance dependence, or schizophrenia have up to a 10-fold increased chance of having a mental illness.[11] Patients who have family members with psychiatric illness often have some understanding of these conditions and may have a better knowledge about treatment and available resources.

SOCIAL HISTORY

The social history lends important information on how the patient functions outside of the clinical setting. Although the information may be detailed and complex, it is most helpful to focus on the patient's level of psychosocial functioning. The social history can be divided into four areas: socioeconomic status, interpersonal relationships, legal history, and developmental history. The four areas with sample questions to prompt dialog in these areas are explained below.

Socioeconomic Status

A quick way to determine one's socioeconomic status is to ask the following questions: "How are you doing financially and are you currently employed?" "What is your current living situation and how are things at home?" A patient's ability to secure such basic necessities as food and shelter is an important priority. For a homeless patient, gathering more detail on the factors that led to homelessness often reveals important diagnostic information. Frequent job changes or loss of employment can be clues to occult substance use or mood disorders. A patient who is seeking disability compensation versus one who must return to school or work immediately may have different urgencies about improving his or her situation.

Interpersonal Relationships and Sexual History

To explore a patient's ability to initiate and maintain relationships with family, friends, and coworkers, the clinician might ask, "Who are important people in your life and do you rely on them for support?" or "How are these relationships going?" This is also a good time to ask about sexual history. Sexual history includes gender identity, sexual orientation, current and past sexual activity, sexual performance, history of sexually transmitted infections, and the use of contraceptives. Perspectives of the patient's family, friends, and cultural group on mental illness should also be considered, because stigma about treatment and nontraditional approaches may influence treatment attitude and outcomes.

Legal History

Open-ended questions such as "Have you ever had problems with the law?" or "Have you ever been arrested or imprisoned?" are easy ways to broach the topic of legal history. Legal history provides information about psychosocial functioning as well as previous experience with violence and crime. Patients who are recently released from prison and are still on parole or have a felony record may have difficulty finding employment and suffer from stigma. Moreover, those who have been imprisoned for many years often find it difficult to reassimilate into a less structured lifestyle upon release from prison. These stressors can increase the risk for substance abuse and exacerbate psychiatric symptoms, which can be a cause for nonadherence to medical care.

Developmental History

The developmental history has multiple components, and it can be a challenge to obtain in one encounter. Suggested questions include (1) "How would you describe your childhood in one sentence?" (2) "What was the highest grade you completed in school?" and (3) "Have you ever been physically, verbally, or sexually abused?" These questions may bring out long-standing stressors and illustrate the patient's most developed (and underdeveloped) coping strategies. Chaotic and unstable childhood development and a history of abuse are often important issues to address as part of a comprehensive psychosocial treatment plan.

MENTAL STATUS EXAMINATION

The Mental Status Examination (MSE) is an observation and report of the present cognitive, emotional, and behavioral state. The MSE is the "physical examination" of psychiatry and is meant to paint a picture of the patient. Much of the MSE is gathered as the interview unfolds. An accurate and concise description of the MSE also facilitates consultation with mental health professionals. Similar to a comprehensive neurologic examination, an in-depth cognitive assessment is not feasible (or necessary) for most clinical encounters in the primary care setting. The following summarizes high-yield, salient components of the MSE (*Table 1-3*).

APPEARANCE

Appearance is a description of the overall hygiene, grooming, and dress of the patients and whether they appear their biologic age. For example, a patient who is malodorous, or wearing clothing inappropriate to weather (three jackets in summer or a tank top in the winter), may be gravely disabled (unable to secure adequate food, clothing, or shelter) due to a severe mental illness such as schizophrenia, major depressive disorder, or bipolar disorder. A patient who is wearing revealing clothing and excessive jewelry or makeup could have mania or a personality disorder. Likewise, a patient who appears much older than expected by age may have had a long history of homelessness, severe mental illness, and/or substance abuse.

ATTITUDE

Attitude is the manner in which the patient responds to or interacts with the interviewer. The attitude can be cooperative in a typical patient; avoidant in a patient with history of trauma; intrusive, hostile, or passive-aggressive in a patient with a personality disorder; or guarded and distrustful in a patient who is paranoid. A patient's attitude and level of engagement help also in evaluating the reliability of the patient.

SPEECH

Speech is described by rate (e.g., slow, rapid, or pressured), volume, articulation (e.g., dysarthric, garbled), and rhythm (e.g., stuttering, stammering). Normal

TABLE 1-3 Key Features of the Mental Status Examination (MSE)

Appearance	• What is the status of the hygiene and grooming and are there any recent changes in appearance?
Attitude	• How does the patient relate to the clinician? • Is the patient cooperative, guarded, irritable, etc., during the interview?
Speech	• What are the rate, rhythm, and volume of speech?
Mood	• How does the patient describe his or her mood? • This should be reported as described by the patient.
Affect	• Does the patient's facial expressions have full range and reactivity? • How quickly does the affect change (lability)? • Is the affect congruent with the stated mood and is it appropriate to topics under discussion?
Thought process	• *How* is the patient thinking? • Does the patient change subjects quickly or is the train of thought difficult to follow?
Thought content	• *What* is the patient thinking? • What is the main theme or subject matter when the patient talks? • Does the patient have any delusions, obsessions, compulsions, suicidal, or homicidal thoughts?
Perceptions	• Does the patient have auditory, visual, or tactile hallucinations?
Cognition	• Is the patient alert? • Is the patient oriented to person, place, time, and the purpose of the interview?
Insight	• Does the patient recognize that there is an illness or disorder present? • Is there a clear understanding of the treatment plan and prognosis?
Judgment	• How will the patient secure food, clothing, and shelter in a safe environment? • Is the patient able to make decisions that support a safe and reasonable treatment plan?
Reliability	• Is the patient able to provide information that is consistent and accurate with other sources?

speech is general described as "regular rate, rhythm and volume." Dysarthric speech may be due to a cerebral vascular accident, medication side effects, and alcohol or substance intoxication. Rapid or pressured speech may indicate intoxication, corticosteroid-induced mania, anxiety, or bipolar mania. Increased speech latency may point to schizophrenia, dementia, or depression with related psychomotor retardation.

MOOD

Mood is a description of the overall pervasive, subjective, and sustained emotional state and can be assessed by simply asking, "How would you describe your mood?" Mood should be ideally noted in the patient's own words, using quotation marks. Mood generally ranges from *depressed* to *euphoric*, with a normal or *euthymic* mood as the reference point. Other common states include empty, guilty, anxious, angry, and irritable mood.

AFFECT

Affect is the expressed emotional state or degree of emotional responsiveness and is inferred from the patient's collective facial expressions. Components of affect include congruency, range, reactivity, rate of change (lability), and intensity. Under normal circumstances, there should be congruency between the patient's mood and affect. If the affect and mood are incongruent and difficult to reconcile, the clinician should consider an active psychotic disorder, malingering, or factitious disorder. For example, a psychotic patient who is depressed may laugh rather than showing a mood-congruent affect. A *restricted* range of affect describes limited expression of emotional states. Reactivity describes the degree of affective change in response to external cues. For example, a depressed patient may have an affect that is restricted to depressive expressions and decreased reactivity to the interviewer. A patient who is manic or intoxicated with a stimulant may exhibit a *labile* and expansive affect. A *blunted* affect is defined as a low-intensity affect with decreased reactivity, often seen in patients who have major depressive disorder or schizophrenia. A *flat* affect is not commonly encountered, has little to no emotional or facial expression, and is often found in those who have advanced Parkinson disease or catatonia.

THOUGHT PROCESS

Thought process describes the organization of thoughts or *how* one thinks. A normal thought process is described as *logical, goal directed,* or *linear*, which means the patient is able to complete a train of thought in reasonable depth. Although no single abnormality of thought process (also referred to as formal thought disorders) is pathognomonic for a specific disorder, this information is critical to the development of an accurate differential diagnosis. A *concrete* thought process may be logical but lacks depth. *Circumstantial* thinking refers to the painstaking movement of thoughts from the origin (point A) to the goal (point B) with excessive focus on insignificant

details. A patient who exhibits *tangential* thinking will quickly change the focus of the conversation in a way that ultimately deviates from the main topic (e.g., "I know it is important to take my medications so my schizophrenia can get better. My neighbor is on a medication for his headaches; do you know which one it might be?"). *Looseness of association* is an abrupt change of focus where the thoughts are numerous and disconnected. A *disorganized* thought process refers to disconnected topics or irrelevant answers to questions posed. *Limited* (or *paucity of*) thoughts occur in patients with severe depression, those with profound negative symptoms (e.g., catatonia), or those who are internally preoccupied with delusions or hallucinations.

THOUGHT CONTENT

Thought content is a description of the main themes and preoccupations expressed by the patient. Simply put, the thought content is *what* the patient is thinking. Depressed patients will usually present with themes of poor self-esteem, worthlessness, or hopelessness. Patients with a somatoform disorder often focus almost exclusively on physical symptoms. *Obsessions* are intrusive thoughts that are the focus of constant and nearly involuntary attention but are, by definition, nonpsychotic in nature (e.g., "What if I accidently left the oven on and my house burns down?"). *Delusions* are fixed, false beliefs and are characterized by a lack of insight. Common delusional themes are paranoid (e.g., "The FBI is trying to kill me."); grandiose (e.g., "I own oil companies and rule five states!"); erotic (e.g., "I know the governor loves me."); and bizarre (e.g., "The Martians have tattooed me and that is why the police always bother me in the park."). *Illusions* are misinterpretations of sensory information (e.g., mistaking a chair for a person). *Hallucinations* are sensory perceptions in the absence of any stimuli and typically are auditory, visual, or tactile. Hallucinations are found in many psychiatric disorders not limited to schizophrenia. Suicidal or violent content should be explored in all patients with severe mental illness, especially those with *command hallucinations* (wherein the hallucination directs the patient's behavior).

COGNITION

Cognitions are higher-order brain functions and include orientation, concentration, calculation, memory, and executive function. Orientation to person, location, date, and purpose should be queried. If the clinician has a high index of suspicion for a cognitive deficit, further assessment can be initiated in the primary care setting. Asking the patient to repeatedly subtract 7 starting from 100 (serial 7's) or spell "world" backward can assess concentration or attention span. Impairment in the level of alertness or consciousness is characteristic of delirium, alternatively termed "encephalopathy" (by neurologists) or less specifically called "altered mental status" (by most health professionals). Long- and short-term memory problems may become evident if the patient is unable to provide clear and organized historical data. Whenever there is a concern for cognitive deficits, the Mini-Mental State Examination (MMSE) or Montreal Cognitive Assessment (MoCA), familiar to most primary care providers, should be performed to screen for dementia and other neurocognitive disorders.

INSIGHT

Insight describes the degree by which the patient understands his or her diagnosis, treatment, and prognosis. A patient who denies a problem that clearly exists or minimizes the severity of symptoms has poor insight. Chronic illness and suboptimal insight often lead to poor outcomes. Restoration of insight is usually a key component to the long-term treatment plan.

JUDGMENT

Judgment is the ability to make reasonable decisions that result in safe, desirable, and socially acceptable outcomes. The ability to weigh benefits versus risks and recognize consequences of behavior is a core part of judgment. Examples of questions that assess "real-time" capacity for judgment include "How might napping during the day affect your sleep at night?" and "What steps can you take to decrease the chance you will binge drink?"

RELIABILITY

Reliability is an assessment of the accuracy of the history that the patient provides. Sometimes the patient recounts events with such inconsistency that they cannot be readily trusted. For example, a depressed patient may be asking to be discharged after being brought to the ER for a tranquilizer overdose. She may initially recall swallowing breath mints and later may report taking sleeping pills but didn't realize she took more than one. In other instances, the interviewer will need to verify the patient's story by obtaining collateral information (with permission) from the patient's family, friends, or health records.

PHYSICAL EXAMINATION

The physical examination gives the clinician another opportunity to build rapport and obtain historical information. Unexplained tachycardia, diaphoresis, tremors, or hyperreflexia should alert the provider about possible stimulant intoxication or alcohol-sedative withdrawal. A careful inspection of the extremities and skin revealing tattoos, burns, bruises, scars, or other injuries should be followed up with inquiries about their origins. For patients with severe mental illnesses (e.g., schizophrenia) and unstable housing, inspection of hair and skin for parasites and teeth for decay or abscesses is important, because these patients may not have routine access to medical care or may place other needs at a higher priority. Similarly, a diabetic patient with severe mental illness may not have the insight to self-monitor for foot ulcers. Therefore, the primary care provider may use the physical examination as another

opportunity to gauge an individual's functional status by his or her ability to maintain activities of daily living (ADLs) independently and to manage his or her medical disorders.

NOT TO BE MISSED

- A complete primary care psychiatric assessment should always include the AMPS screening tool. It is also good to consider asking about thoughts of suicide in the context of assessing mood, anxiety, psychosis, and substance misuse.
- The mood and affect should be assessed and recorded as important parts of the MSE. Mood is the overall internal emotional state, whereas affect is the expressed emotional state that is manifested by changes in facial expression.
- Disorders of speech and behavior are often found in those with severe mental illness and should be monitored carefully. Thought process describes *how* one thinks and thought content describes *what* one thinks.
- A social history should be obtained on all patients who are being treated for a psychiatric illness. The main components of a primary care psychiatric social history include socioeconomic status, interpersonal relationships, legal history, and developmental history.

TIME-SAVING STRATEGIES

We recommend the following time-saving strategies when completing a primary care psychiatric biopsychosocial assessment.

OBTAIN A SOCIAL HISTORY

Obtaining the social history is one of the most important pieces of the primary psychiatric interview. There is much to cover, and it can certainly be time intensive if not done properly. Although it is not all-encompassing, we suggest the following "starter questions" to help the clinician collect the necessary information for a social history.

Socioeconomic Status

- "How are you doing financially? Are you currently employed?"
- "What is your current living situation and how are things at home?"

Interpersonal Relationships

- "Who are the most important people in your life and do you rely on them for support?"
- "How are these relationships going?"

Legal History

- "Have you ever had problems with the law?"
- "Have you even been arrested or imprisoned?"

Developmental History

- "How would you describe your childhood in one sentence?"
- "What was the highest grade you completed in school?"
- "Have you ever been physically, verbally, or sexually abused?"

ASK THESE THREE QUESTIONS

If you could only pick three questions during a primary care psychiatry interview, the following are suggested:

- "What is your number one biggest problem that we can work on together?"
- "Currently, how are you dealing with your problem?"
- "Is there someone in your life who you can go to if you need help?"

USE THE SUPPLEMENTAL PSYCHIATRIC HISTORY FORM

We highly recommend using the Supplemental Psychiatric History Form (*Figure 1-2*) for all new patients or for those who you feel have significant psychiatric symptoms. This form is easy for a patient or clinician to complete and covers the pertinent psychosocial history as well as the AMPS screening questions. The clinician can quickly glance at this form and tailor further assessment accordingly. All "yes" answers should raise concern and prompt further questioning. More in-depth disorder-specific assessments are discussed in the chapters to follow.

PRACTICE CASE

CASE 1: The Primary Care Psychiatric Interview

A 30-year-old woman with a history of chronic low-back pain and tobacco use presents to transfer care to your practice with the chief complaint, "That horrible doctor ignored my pain and wanted me to suffer! I heard you are the best doctor in town. I can already tell we are going to be great friends!" The woman's speech is loud and somewhat fast. When the provider suggests she try physical therapy instead of an opioid medication, she yells, "Why don't you just kill me now?" The provider wonders if she is manic and needs to be psychiatrically hospitalized.

The AMPS screening questions reveal that the patient has struggled with "mood swings" since her childhood. It is clarified that she does not stay in any one mood state for several days or weeks on end but rather fluctuates from happy to sad to anxious to irritable to irate in a matter of a few hours. The triggers for these episodes

tend to be interpersonal conflicts, especially when she feels a threat of being abandoned. When she is stressed she will occasionally have an out-of-body experience or hear a voice that is derogatory and self-critical, but these disturbances do not occur when she is calm and happy. She has a history of binge-drinking alcohol as well as misusing several different prescription painkillers and tranquilizers (trading pills with friends, using the medications more frequently than prescribed, and seeking prescriptions from multiple providers), but she has never been hospitalized or suffered legal consequences because of substance use. She does not endorse any current desire to harm herself and denies access to firearms. She is looking forward to going to her mother's 60th birthday party next week.

The patient has tried several antidepressant medications, but she has never taken any one for more than a few days due to vague and atypical side effects. She has never been prescribed a traditional mood stabilizer such as lithium or valproic acid. As a teenager, she saw a counselor for a couple months, and she briefly tried going to AA (Alcoholics Anonymous), but she has never tried an evidence-based psychotherapy such as Dialectical Behavior Therapy (DBT). She has had numerous ER visits and a couple short inpatient psychiatric hospitalizations for suicidal ideation and intentional overdoses. Her mother struggled with depression and her father died from complications related to alcohol abuse. The patient experienced significant trauma including physical abuse and neglect. She has had numerous romantic relationships in which she has cohabitated with her partner. She is currently living with her mother, whom she feels well supported by, and her fiancé of 3 months, whom she states is her soulmate.

After consent is obtained, a phone call is made to the to the patient's mother. The mother confirms the patient's psychiatric history and agrees that she tends to wear a large amount of jewelry when she leaves the house and that she has had fast and loud speech since she was a child. She also denies that the patient has had periods of hypomania or mania that lasted days or weeks or has any access to firearms.

On MSE, the patient appears her chronological age and she has a plethora of brightly colored jewelry and noticeable makeup. She is generally cooperative but quickly changes to hostile when alternatives to opiates are suggested. Speech is loud with an increased rate, but she is interruptible. Her mood is overall irritable and her affect range is wide but appropriate to thought content. Her thought process is linear and thought content is negative for suicidal or homicidal ideation but includes themes of chronic emptiness and suffering, fears of abandonment, and splitting. She has no perceptual disturbances and is fully alert and oriented without obvious cognitive deficits. Her insight into her substance misuse is poor and judgment is fair at best. Her reliability is fair to good.

AMPS Behavioral Health History Form

Name: _____ Date: _____

Reason for Appointment: _____

Past Psychiatric Diagnoses (circle if applicable):

- Anxiety
- Depression
- Bipolar disorder
- Schizophrenia
- Schizoaffective disorder

- Alcohol misuse
- Drug misuse
- Borderline personality disorder
- Insomnia
- Other Mental health diagnosis

Have you ever been treated by a psychiatrist or other mental health provider?	Yes / No
Have you ever been a patient in a psychiatric hospital?	Yes / No
Have you ever tried to hurt or kill yourself?	Yes / No
Have you ever taken a medication for psychiatric reasons?	Yes / No

If yes, please list the most recent medication(s) below:

#1: _____	Did you have any problems with this medication?	Yes / No
#2: _____	Did you have any problems with this medication?	Yes / No
#3: _____	Did you have any problems with this medication?	Yes / No
#4: _____	Did you have any problems with this medication?	Yes / No
#5: _____	Did you have any problems with this medication?	Yes / No

Family Psychiatric History: Did your grandparents, parents, or siblings ever have severe problems with depression, bipolar disorder, anxiety, schizophrenia, or any other emotional problems?   Yes / No

Social and Developmental History:

Socioeconomic Status

Are you currently unemployed?	Yes / No
Are you having any problems at home?	Yes / No

Interpersonal Relationships

Are you having any problems with close personal relationships?	Yes / No

Legal History

Have you ever had problems with the law?	Yes / No

Developmental History

Have you ever been physically, verbally, or sexually abused?	Yes / No
What was the highest grade you completed in school?	_____

Anxiety Symptoms, Mood Symptoms, Psychotic Symptoms, Substance Use

Is anxiety or nervousness a problem for you?	Yes / No

Mood Symptoms

• Have you been feeling depressed, sad, or hopeless over the past two weeks?	Yes / No
• Have you had a decreased interest level in pleasurable activities over the past few weeks?	Yes / No
• Have you ever felt the complete opposite of depressed, *when friends and family were worried about you because you were too happy?*	Yes / No
• Have you ever had excessive amounts of energy running through your body, to the point where you did not need to sleep for days?	Yes / No
• Do you have any thoughts of wanting to hurt or kill yourself or someone else?	Yes / No

Psychotic Symptoms

Do you hear or see things that other people do not hear or see?	Yes / No
Do you have thoughts that people are trying to follow, hurt, or spy on you?	Yes / No

Substance Use

How many packs of cigarettes do you smoke per day?	_____
How much alcohol do you drink per day?	_____
Have you ever used cocaine, methamphetamines, heroin, marijuana, PCP, LSD, Ecstacy, or other drugs?	Yes / No

FIGURE 1-2 Supplemental Psychiatric History Form.

Discussion

This case illustrates a challenging scenario to many providers. In addition to chronic pain, the patient most likely has an opioid use disorder as well as borderline personality disorder. However, caution is advised before making a personality disorder diagnosis based on an initial evaluation in a busy primary care setting. The provider likely does not have time to obtain collateral information during every intake appointment, and it would be best to observe for a persistent pattern of maladaptive traits over a series of appointments. The provider should consider bipolar disorder based on the patient's extravagant jewelry, loud fast speech, and affective instability; however, in this case these are chronic and persistent, not episodic in nature. When in doubt, the provider may want to consider a psychiatric consultation before starting an antidepressant medication.

While the patient does make a flagrant comment to the provider, "Why don't you just kill me now?," this appears to be a manipulative attempt to obtain opioids. The patient is at higher chronic risk of suicide due to her history of impulsive behavior and prior attempts; however, she is not at an elevated acute risk as she is future-oriented, feels well supported, denies any intent or plan to die, and does not have access to firearms.

The complete biopsychosocial assessment helps the clinician to provide a comprehensive treatment plan. In addition to initiating a multimodal treatment for chronic pain, a plan for psychotherapy such as DBT (which has been shown to decrease suicidal thoughts and impulsive behaviors) should be considered. The clinician might say, "Chronic pain can cause high levels of stress on the body and mind, which may make it harder to deal with mood swings as well as increase the chance that you act impulsively or even harm yourself. DBT has been shown to help patients manage stress and it does not have the risk of side effects that medications may have." The patient should also be encouraged to revisit the idea of attending AA meetings, because impulsivity and chronic pain are associated with higher risk of relapse. An antidepressant that also works on descending spinal pain pathways such as duloxetine or amitriptyline may be useful, although the clinician should take care to start at a low dose given the patients history of multiple antidepressant intolerances as well as provide psychoeducation and a follow-up plan for if the patient experiences any hypomania or mania.

Finally, it is important to understand why the patient has recently changed primary care providers. The therapeutic connection between the patient and the clinician is paramount. In this case, the provider might be compelled to focus exclusively on "opioid-seeking behavior." However, the provider could take this as an opportunity to focus on building rapport and better understand the patient's defenses including catastrophizing and splitting, which may contribute to fragmented care and worse outcomes. Short and somewhat frequent office visits may be indicated over the next few months to address her many concerns and maintain a biopsychosocial treatment approach.

PRACTICAL RESOURCES

- The MacAuthur Inititative on Depression and Primary Care: http://www.depression-primarycare.org/
- Substance Abuse and Mental Health Services Administration: http://www.samhsa.gov/index.aspx
- American Psychiatric Association Practice Guidelines: http://www.psych.org/MainMenu/PsychiatricPractice/PracticeGuidelines_1.aspx
- National Institute of Mental Health: http://www.nimh.nih.gov/health/publications/depression-a-treatable-illness.shtml
- National Alliance on Mental Illness: www.nami.org

REFERENCES

1. Reiger DA, Boyd JH, Burke JD, et al. One month prevalence of mental disorders in the United States. *Arch Gen Psychiatry*. 1988;45:977-986.
2. Onate J. Psychiatric consultation in outpatient primary care settings: should consultation change to collaboration? *Primary Psychiatry*. 2006;13(6):41-45.
3. Kessler RC, Demler O, Frank RG, et al. Prevalence and treatment of mental disorders, 1990 to 2003. *N Engl J Med*. 2005;352(24):2515-2523.
4. Katon W, Roinson P, Von Korff M, et al. A multifaceted intervention to improve treatment of depression in primary care. *Arch Gen Psychiatry*. 1996;53(10):924-932.
5. Vergare MJ, Binder RL, Cook IA, et al. American Psychiatric Association practice guidelines for the psychiatric evaluation of adults second edition. *Am J Psychiatry*. 2006;163(suppl 6):3-36.
6. Whooley MA, Simon GE. Managing depression in medical outpatients. *N Engl J Med*. 2000;343(26):1942-1950.
7. Beckman HB, Frankel RM. The effect of physician behavior on the collection of data. *Ann Internal Med*. 1984;101(5):692-696.
8. Luoma JB, Martin CE, Pearson JL. Contact with mental health and primary care providers before suicide: a review of the evidence. *AM J Psychiatry*. 2002;159:909-916.
9. Dazzi T, Gribble R, Wessely S, Fear NT. Does asking about suicide and related behaviours induce suicidal ideation? What is the evidence? *Psychol Med*. 2014;44(16):3361-3363.
10. Chesney E, Goodwin GM, Fazel S. Risks of all-cause and suicide mortality in mental disorders: a meta-review. *World Psychiatry*. 2014;13(2):153-160.
11. Hales RE, Yudofsky SC, Gabbard GO. *The American Psychiatric Publishing Textbook of Psychiatry*. 5th ed. Washington, DC: American Psychiatric Association; 2008.

2

PRIMARY CARE AND PSYCHIATRY: AN OVERVIEW OF THE COLLABORATIVE CARE MODEL

Anna Ratzliff, MD, PhD and Ramanpreet Toor, MD

INTRODUCTION TO COLLABORATIVE CARE

Common mental disorders, such as depression, are now the leading cause of health disability worldwide, greater than cancer and cardiovascular disease.[1] Mental health disorders often co-occur with chronic medical diseases and can substantially worsen associated health outcomes, decrease work productivity, and increase overall health care costs.[2] Despite the significant impact of mental health disorders, most adults with diagnosable mental health disorders do not receive mental health care, and if patients do access care, they are more likely to receive treatment from a primary care provider (PCP).[3] Although primary care is providing much of treatment for common mental health disorders, there are significant opportunities for improvement in both processes and outcomes of this care. For example, as few as 20% of patients treated in "usual" primary care show substantial clinical improvement.[4,5]

Various strategies to improve the treatment of common mental disorders in primary care have focused on screening for common mental disorders, education of PCPs, development of treatment guidelines, and referral to mental health specialty care.[6] Although these approaches can be helpful, they are not sufficient to improve mental health care delivery, and PCPs continue to report serious limitations in the support available from mental health specialists.[7] Integrated care, developing systems of care that can bring primary care and mental health specialist together, has emerged as the most effective strategy to leverage scarce mental health resources and improve patient outcomes. The Psychiatric Collaborative Care Model (CoCM) of integrated care uses a team of providers and systematic approach to deliver mental health care in primary care settings. The largest randomized control trial of collaborative care to date was the Improving Mood-Promoting Access to Collaborative Treatment (IMPACT), which demonstrated that collaborative care was twice as effective as usual care for treating depression in older adults in primary care settings.[5] To date in over 80 randomized controlled trials, collaborative care has shown to be more effective than care as usual for depression and anxiety disorders, by far the strongest evidence base for any integrated care approach.[8] There is now a growing evidence base that collaborative care is effective for other mental health disorders, such as ADHD and bipolar disorder,[9] and to be effective diverse health care settings and in diverse ethnic minority groups.[10,11] Collaborative care has now been delivered in large-scale implementation efforts such as Depression Improvement Across Minnesota, Offering a New Direction (DIAMOND), including all major health plans in the state of Minnesota, with 1,500 enrolled patients and 85 clinics, and the Mental Health Improvement Program (MHIP), in over 130 federally qualified primary care clinics across Washington State.[9] Studies have demonstrated that collaborative care can achieve the Quadruple Aim[12] of health care system optimization: improved patient satisfaction,[5] improved patient outcomes,[8] cost-effectiveness of care,[13] and improved provider experience.[14,15] Therefore, the CoCM is aligned with other health care system reform approaches such as patient-centered medical homes (PCMHs) and accountable care organizations. This chapter reviews collaborative care team roles and principles, provides guidance to the PCPs about the important role they have to play in delivering of collaborative care, and discusses practical strategies for implementation of collaborative care.

THE COLLABORATIVE CARE TEAM

The core CoCM team includes a PCP, behavioral health provider (BHP)/care manager, and psychiatric consultant. Each team member has a clearly defined role (*Figure 2-1*) to successfully collaborate as a team to achieve shared treatment goals for the patient. Some teams may include other team members, such as therapists or health navigators, depending on the resources in your clinic.

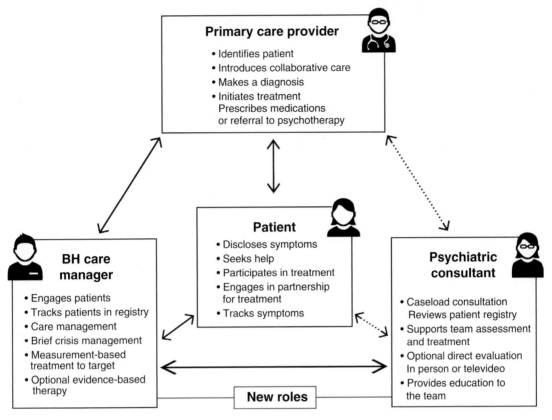

FIGURE 2-1 The Collaborative Care Model (CoCM) team members and their roles. The solid arrows represent regular communication. The dashed arrows represent needed communication. (Used with permission from the University of Washington.)

PRIMARY CARE PROVIDER

A PCP, whether a family physician, internist, pediatrician, advanced practice nurse, or physician assistant, oversees and owns the overall care of the patient and typically have the most established relationship with the patient. They have several important roles including identifying the need for behavioral treatment, introducing the patients to the concept of collaborative care, and then referring them to CoCM for further assessment. PCPs also make the ultimate decision on whether or not to accept the psychiatric consultant's recommendations, such as assigning a psychiatric diagnosis and initiating treatment, including prescribing any psychotropic medications. Over time they continue to manage and adjust treatment in consultation with the BHP/care manager and psychiatric consultant. The CoCM powerfully leverages the PCP–patient relationship, engaging the patient in treatment and encouraging the patient to work closely with the BHP/care manager.

BEHAVIORAL HEALTH PROVIDERS OR CARE MANAGERS

BHPs/care managers typically come from training backgrounds in nursing, psychology, or social work. Most CoCM teams locate the BHP/care manager in the primary care clinic, although in rural areas this model can be adapted to

take advantage of televideo options.[16] The BHP/care manager role in collaborative care consists of providing a combination of care management and brief behavioral health or psychosocial interventions. Once the patient is referred by the PCP, the BHP/care manager assesses the patient and adds them to a collaborative care registry. BHPs/care managers meet with the patient on regular intervals, usually every 2 weeks in person or by phone, to assess progress toward goals, as well as to provide evidence-based counseling/psychotherapy interventions such as problem-solving therapy (PST), cognitive behavioral therapy (CBT), or behavioral activation (BA). BHPs/care managers play important roles in engaging the patient, administering behavioral health measures, tracking the treatment response, and coordinating care being provided to the patient. They meet with the psychiatric consultant weekly to discuss patients who are not responding to initial treatment and, if needed, assist with scheduling in person or televideo consultation with psychiatric consultant.

PSYCHIATRIC CONSULTANT

Although the psychiatric consultant typically has the least direct contact with the patient, this team member can leverage psychiatric expertise through a diverse array of responsibilities. A psychiatric consultant's role in CoCM is different from the direct care provided in traditional specialty service or a colocated consultation model. The main role of the psychiatric consultant is to provide indirect consultation by caseload reviews in weekly meetings with BHPs/care managers without seeing the patient in person. During these sessions, the psychiatric consult and BHP/care manager work together, reviewing the registry and electronic health record (EHR) data on patients without seeing the patient directly to make a brief comprehensive treatment plan. In these case reviews, the psychiatric consultant can support clarification of diagnosis, provide initial treatment recommendations, address treatment resistant presentations, and develop relapse prevention plans. In a weekly hour-long meeting with BHP/care manager, the psychiatric consultant is able to discuss on average five to eight patients depending on complexity. This allows a psychiatric consultant to leverage his or her mental health expertise more effectively compared with the traditional model of consultation in which only one patient would have been evaluated in that time. Additional roles for the psychiatric consultant may include limited direct or formal consultation (in person or televideo) for challenging patients, education of the team, and consistently working on improving the quality of care provided.

DELIVERING CARE USING THE COLLABORATIVE CARE PRINCIPLES

Delivering effective collaborative care requires more than just having the right team members; this team has to learn to work together in new ways. Experts have identified five key CoCM principles (*Table 2-1*) that are necessary to provide patient care, which is consistent with the collaborative care evidence base.[17] These principles are patient-centered collaboration, population-based care, measurement-based treatment to target, evidence-based care, and accountability in care. To deliver accountable care, practices will need to implement the other four principles.

- **Patient-centered collaboration**: Collaborative care starts with the patient, as does all strong primary care. In the CoCM, primary care and BHPs work together in a team to provide care, which is patient centered by using a shared treatment plan each with clearly defined roles (*Figure 2-1*). In most teams, the PCP and BHP/care manager have direct contact with the patient, whereas the psychiatric consultant typically leverages his or her expertise through indirect case reviews with information gathered from the rest of the team.
- **Population-based care**: The concept of population-based care should be familiar to PCPs as it is aligned with the concept of empanelment. In mental health, however, this represents a significant departure from traditional practice. For collaborative care, the population of patients is typically defined as a caseload of patients with identified mental health needs that are in active treatment with the CoCM team. Identifying a population of patients allows the collaborative care team to proactively manage care for these patients and shift away from reactionary care provided only to the patients

TABLE 2-1 Principles of the Collaborative Care Model and Example Clinical Implementation		
PRINCIPLE	**DEFINITION**	**EXAMPLE**
Patient-centered collaboration	A team works to deliver care with the patient goals and preferences guiding collaboration.	The primary care provider (PCP), behavioral health provider/care manager, and psychiatric consultant work to develop a care plan that addresses the biopsychosocial needs of the patient.
Population-based care	Defining a population that needs care and using strategies like a registry to make sure all patients get care. This population is the denominator for evaluating population-level outcomes.	All patients who are identified needing mental health treatment are tracked in a registry to make sure no one "falls through the cracks." This registry is used to identify patient who need treatment intensification.
Measurement-based treatment to target	Regular use of validated screeners to make sure that the treatments being delivered are resulting in meeting patient goals, patient improvement, and ideally remission of symptoms.	Use of the Patient Health Questionnaire (PHQ-9) at most visits to make sure depression symptoms improve and ultimately remit. If symptoms are not improving, treatment is changed.
Evidence-based care	A provisional diagnosis is established, and evidence-based treatments are delivered to support treatment to target.	PCP prescribes evidence-based psychopharmacology with input from the psychiatric consultant as needed. Behavioral health provider/care manager provides evidence-based brief psychosocial interventions. Both providers reinforce the concept of a comprehensive evidence-based treatment plan.
Accountable care	The team is assessing both practice processes and outcomes at both individual patient and population levels. Team engages in continuous quality improvement to provide quality of care at both an individual patient level and a population level.	Both individual patient goals, such as remission of depression, and population targets, such as 50% of the patients identified with depression symptoms achieve remission, are monitored and systems of care and care processes are improved until these goals are achieved.

coming in for care. This is an especially important concept for mental health care, as many of the patients with common mental health disorders, such as depression and anxiety, struggle with symptoms, such as difficulty with activation, that directly affect their ability to attend appointments and engage in care. In collaborative care, population-based care requires a comprehensive list of identified patients needing behavioral health treatment or registry of patients in active treatment. This function can be accomplished simply, using a spreadsheet stored in a secure location. The University of Washington AIMS Center offers a free Excel registry template that can be used for this purpose (*Figure 2-2*). Some organizations use stand-alone registries or have built this registry capacity into their EHR. The registry includes information about the patient, appropriate behavioral health screenings (for example, Patient Health Questionnaire [PHQ]-9 for depression), notes of visits with BHP/care manager and PCP, and consultation notes from the psychiatric consultant. The registry makes it easier to identify patients who are not improving by using measurement scores to see which patients continue to be symptomatic (see column Last Available PHQ-9 Score in *Figure 2-2*). Care is intensified or changed if patients are not responding to initial treatments or not achieving treatment goals. Another population easily identified on the registry are patients who are not actively engaged in treatment, for example by the team can quickly scan the date patients were last seen for a visit and identifying patients not seen in the last month (see column Date of Most Recent Contact in *Figure 2-2*). Patients suffering from mental illness tend to isolate themselves, have high "no show" rates and can be nonadherent with treatment. The registry can help to engage these patients in treatment and avoid anyone "falling through the cracks." The list is continuously updated and maintained by the BHP/care manager by adding new patients identified by the PCP and removing the patients who have achieved remission of mental health symptoms and moved back to the primary care panel.

- **Measurement-based treatment to target**: Before starting the treatment of each identified patient, the collaborative care team works together with the patient to identify a treatment goal. A goal should be behaviorally and functionally defined, measurable, and must be informed by the patient's perspective. Progress toward this goal is monitored over time by using a combination of clinical presentation and behavioral health measures, such as PHQ-9 for depression. Patients complete these measures on regular intervals, typically at each visit, which helps the team to assess symptoms and answer the question "Has this patient improved and accomplished his or her treatment goal?" If the patient has not reached goal, then the team can provide a timely adjustment in treatment. For some patients, only minor adjustments can lead to a remission of symptoms, and for others, multiple adjustments and changes are done before the target is achieved. This process of regularly tracking response to treatment and making adjustments if not at target is likely a key factor in the success of the collaborative care because studies, such as the STAR-D trial for depression, have shown that it can take making up to four changes in treatment before ~70% of the population will have a response to treatment.[18] The CoCM supports the PCP to be able to make these systematic adjustments as part of routine care.

- **Evidence-based care**: After a patient who needs behavioral health care is identified and assessed by PCP and BHP/care manager, he or she is offered evidence-based treatment interventions to deliver a biopsychosocial approach to a provisional diagnosis. One of the advantages of CoCM is to be able to offer a range of evidence-based psychopharmacology and evidence-based brief psychotherapy interventions right in the primary care setting where a patient is often more comfortable. Team members work collaboratively to provide high-quality evidence-based treatments. The PCP initiates medication treatment, the BHP/care manager delivers behavioral or psychotherapeutic interventions, and the psychiatric consultant supports the PCP and BHP/care manager to provide the evidence-based treatment appropriate

View Record	Treatment Status	Name	Treatment Status *Indicates the most recent contact was over 2 months (60 days) ago*				PHQ-9 ✓ Indicates last available PHQ-9 score is at target (<5 or 50% decrease from initial score) ! Indicates the last available PHQ-9 score is more than 30 days old				GAD-7 ✓ The last available GAD-7 score is at target (<10 or 50% decrease from initial score) ! Indicates the last available GAD-7 score is more than 30 days old				Psychiatric Consultation	
			Date of Initial Assessment	Date of Most Recent Contact	Number of Follow-up Contacts	Weeks in Treatment	Initial PHQ-9 Score	Last Available PHQ-9 Score	% Change in PHQ-9 Score	Date of Last PHQ-9 Score	Initial GAD-7 Score	Last Available GAD-7 Score	% Change in GAD-7 Score	Date of Last GAD-7 Score	Flag	Most Recent Psychiatric Case Review
View	Active	Susan Test	9/5/2015	2/23/2016	10	26	22	14	-36%	2/23/2016	18	17	-6%	! 1/23/2016	Flag for discussion & safety risk	1/27/2016
View	Active	Albert Smith	8/13/2015	! 12/2/2015	7	29	18	17	-6%	! 12/2/2015	14	10	-29%	! 12/2/2015	Flag for discussion	
View	Active	Joe Smith	11/30/2015	2/28/2016	6	14	14	10	-29%	2/28/2016	10	✓ 6	-40%	2/28/2016	Flag for discussion	2/26/2016
View	Active	Albert Smith	1/5/2016	3/1/2016	3	9	21	19	-10%	3/1/2016	12	10	-17%	3/1/2016	Flag as safety risk	2/18/2016
View	Active	Bob Dolittle	2/4/2016	2/4/2016	0	4	_	No Score			_	No Score				
View	RP	John Doe	9/15/2015	3/6/2016	10	25	20	✓ 2	✓ -90%	3/6/2016	14	✓ 3	✓ -79%	3/6/2016		2/20/2016

FIGURE 2-2 Example Collaborative Care Model registry. The free UW AIMS Excel Registry is shown (https://aims.uw.edu/resource-library/patient-tracking-spreadsheet-example-data). (Used with permission from the University of Washington.)

for the provisional diagnosis. Although each team member has a clearly defined role, ideally all team members should be familiar with all treatments to reinforce treatment participation to the patient. For example, although medications will be prescribed by the PCP, the BHP/care manager will support medication adherence and may be the first person to hear about side effects. Conversely, although the BHP/care manager will set behavioral goals with the patient, a PCP checking in with the patient about these goals can reemphasize the importance of this part of the treatment plan. The resources provided by this text will support the PCP in delivering this important principle.

- **Accountable care:** This principle is consistent with the concept of commitment to continuous quality improvement, which is now practiced in many primary care settings. The US health care system is increasingly focusing on the concept that a care team is not only accountable for the individual patients that come into the clinic but for the whole identified population on the registry. Just like with all care processes, to achieve excellence in care, the whole team needs to make the commitment to continuously work on improving the quality of care provided to the patients. This process starts with the team identifying goals and targets for the collaborative care program. Regular review of the program data is done to assess the effectiveness of the collaborative care being delivered. Typical quality measures include processes of care (e.g., caseload size or number of patients engaged with two contacts per month), outcomes (e.g., the percentage of patient achieving remission of depression symptoms at 6 months), and other important targets identified by the clinic (e.g., provider and patient satisfaction). Once goal is identified, the next step is to decide ways of measuring this goal and then the intervention to reach this goal. Regular reviews are done to monitor progress and adjust the interventions if needed using standard quality improvement strategies. High-quality CoCM delivery includes this process as a standard practice to make sure this leveraged approach is effectively meeting patient and clinic needs.

THE ENGAGED PRIMARY CARE PROVIDER: CRITICAL TO THE SUCCESS OF THE COLLABORATIVE CARE MODEL TEAM

PCPs are critical for the success of implementation and delivery of CoCM given their central role in the CoCM team. The case presented in *Box 2-1* provides an example of how a CoCM team works together to deliver care to a patient using the CoCM principles. In this case, you can see how the three key PCP functions outlined below support the delivery of effective mental health in a primary care setting.

BOX 2-1 CASE EXAMPLE EPISODE OF COLLABORATIVE CARE MODEL PATIENT CARE[a]

Ms. R is a 43-year-old woman who presents to her primary care provider (PCP) asking for "something to sleep." Her PCP takes a history and finds out she has not been sleeping well for about 6 weeks, she has been struggling to get her kids to school on time and missed a few days of work, she has difficulty concentrating and getting household chores completed, and her husband is worried because she "just doesn't seem like herself." Her PCP completes an initial assessment, generating an initial diagnosis of depression after excluding obvious medical comorbidity, such as sleep apnea. Ms. R's PCP spends time **introducing the Collaborative Care Model** using a flyer the clinic has created for this purpose and the idea that a team of providers will care for her and treat her depression in the primary care clinic. The PCP reinforces that when the patient is meeting with the BHP/care manager, they are engaging in recommended treatment and that the team will communicate closely about a treatment plan.

That first day she meets her BHP/care manager who continues the mental health assessment, including a safety evaluation. The BHP/case manager makes sure she completes a depression measure (in this case, the Patient Health Questionnaire [PHQ-9]) to measure her symptoms. The BHP/care manager also assesses for bipolar disorder, anxiety disorders, and substance use disorders; none of which is found and notes not safety concerns. The BHP/care manager focuses on understanding current functional impairments and Ms. R's goals for treatment. Ms. R's main focus is on sleeping and she is interested in taking medications. Ms. R's BHP/care manager enters her into the clinic patient registry. Ms. R is also scheduled for a close follow-up appointment to make sure she is quickly engaged in care.

Both the PCP and BHP/care manager feel confident in a diagnosis of moderate major depressive disorder, but that input from the psychiatric consultant would be helpful to find a good medication treatment. Ms. R's BHP/care manager discusses her case with the psychiatric consultant by presenting her case over the telephone, and after obtaining a basic history, the psychiatric consultant recommends mirtazapine, an antidepressant that is mildly sedating. Within a week, the PCP prescribes this medication and the BHP/care manager provides psychoeducation about this choice with a special emphasis on why this is a good choice for the patient goal of improving sleep and how depression treatment will also support this goal. The BHP/care manager again schedules close follow-up by telephone (to assess tolerability of the medication in a week) and a future visit in person in 3 weeks.

Ms. R reports having tolerated mirtazapine when contacted by phone a week after her initial appointment by the BHP/care manager. She reports improved sleep but no change in depressed mood. The BHP/care manager provides reassuring psychoeducation that it was a good sign that she was tolerating the medication and experienced improved sleep.

The BHP/care manager also explains that typical response for antidepressant treatment occurs at 6 to 8 weeks. The BHP/care manager introduces the idea of sleep hygiene and helps Ms. R to set a goal to consistently go to bed every night and get up in the morning at the same time, as Ms. R is most concerned about getting her kids to school on time. Ms. R is reminded to attend her follow-up appointment. At her follow-up appointment, Ms. R reports a little less depression when her PHQ-9 behavioral rating scale is administered and some improvement on getting up on time but still notes difficulty with concentration (observe response to treatment). Consistent with the practice of **iterative treatment**, her PCP continues to feel confident in the diagnosis of moderate major depressive disorder (refine assessment and establish a diagnosis), with now a partial response, and decides to increase her dose of mirtazapine to the middle of the dosing range as previously suggested by the psychiatric consultant note (provide evidence-based treatment). The BHP/care manager continues to set goals for sleep hygiene and introduces cognitive behavioral therapy for insomnia (CBTi). This proactive treatment approach continues for 8 weeks until patient has experienced a significant reduction in depression symptoms and improved sleep.

Ms. R achieves remission of her depression in 12 weeks. At that time the BHP/care manager works with Ms. R to develop a relapse prevention plan. This plan includes early warning signs, effective treatments, and clear instructions for follow-up. The psychiatric consultant includes final medication recommendations. The BHP/care manager continues to meet with Ms. R monthly for 3 months. As Ms. R continues to experience minimal depression symptoms, she returns to care as part of her PCP's general patient panel, allowing for new patients to be seen by the BHP/care manager and receive collaborative care treatment. The PCP continue to check in on her relapse prevention plan at future visits and screens her annually for depression symptoms with a PHQ-9 as part of annual wellness visits as part of **continuity of care**.

---

^aThe bolded words highlight three of the most important roles of the PCP in supporting collaborative care.

INTRODUCING COLLABORATIVE CARE

One of the most important roles for the PCP is to effectively introduce collaborative care to the patient. The relationship between a PCP and patient is a trusted partner in health care, and the introduction to the BHP/care manager can make a big difference in patient engagement. The PCP can become more effective in this role through developing a script to introduce the CoCM (*Box 2-2*). Some practices also develop a brochure or flyer to introduce the CoCM team and roles. It can be helpful to add the patient role these communication approaches, so that the active involvement of the patient is clear when engaging in CoCM (example flyer: https://aims.uw.edu/resource-library/introducing-your-care-team).

BOX 2-2   EXAMPLE SCRIPT FOR PRIMARY CARE PROVIDER TO INTRODUCE THE COLLABORATIVE CARE MODEL

Opening the dialog about treatment: "I think you're experiencing depression and I really want to work with you to get better."

Introducing the care team idea: "Our behavioral health provider/care manager could help you understand more about depression and help you find some strategies to turn things around."

Encouraging your patient to consider psychotherapy as part of treatment: "Our behavioral health provider/care manager can work with you around stress in your life and other things that may be contributing to your symptoms using brief therapy if you would like learn more about that."

Encouraging your patient to consider help with medication: "We also have a team psychiatric consultant to make sure we're doing everything possible to help medication work most effectively for you."

Checking if your patient's interested in engaging: "I'm confident that you can feel better. Are you willing to give us a chance to help?"

Wrapping up with a plan for next steps: "Do you have time to meet our behavioral health provider/care manager today? I can see if she's available right now."

SUPPORTING ITERATIVE TREATMENT

In collaborative care, the team supports the PCP to provide systematic treatment to target. The function of tracking treatment response over time is to have the team systematically refine the diagnosis and treatment plan through an iterative process (*Figure 2-3*). This process starts with establishing a provisional diagnosis. Typically the team has information from behavioral health measures, the observations of the PCP and BHP/care manager, and the input from a psychiatric case review to develop this provisional diagnosis. Although in a fast-paced primary care program, there can be some uncertainty in making an initial diagnosis; the team is able to start a treatment plan with the confidence that the patient will be observed and response to treatment monitored over time.

The next step is to provide evidence-based treatment. This will ideally include the option for both brief behavioral interventions and medications. Successful treatment of depression typically requires several adjustments to find an effective medication and dose or psychotherapy, even in the specialty mental health setting. Teams many need to wait 6 to 8 weeks before deciding that an intervention is not working. Lastly, the team can use the information, from both the patient's clinical presentation and the response to interventions, to refine assessment. The process can then start again with a revision to the provisional diagnosis if needed.

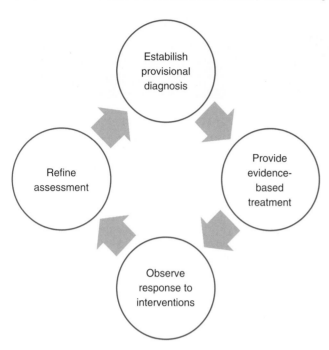

FIGURE 2-3 The Collaborative Care Model allows for systematic iterative diagnosis and treatment to achieve improved outcomes.

Having a strong workflow to support this approach to treatment is a critical part of effective collaborative care. The ability of the team to monitor the patient over time allows for more accurate diagnoses and therefore more targeted treatment interventions. PCPs play a crucial role in this process with both their observations and ability to provide timely adjustments to treatment, especially the prescribing and adjustment of medications.

CONTINUITY OF CARE

During a typical episode of care, a patient will stay in active treatment until one of two outcomes occurs: (1) the patient improves sufficiently to return to routine monitoring on a general panel or (2) the patient's mental health needs exceed the capacity of the PCPs to intervene and the patient needs to be referred to specialty mental health care for more intensive services. The PCP has an important responsibility to provide continuity of care for patients in both these paths. If the patient returns to routine primary care, the PCP should reassess patients for mental health symptoms with scheduled follow-up and a discussion of the relapse prevention plan that was developed during their graduation from the CoCM team. For patients requiring transition to care with external specialty BHPs, the PCP has the responsibility to develop a coordinated care plan that includes exchange of clinical information. Many primary care practices are using care coordination services to deliver strong bidirectional communication to support patients.

PRACTICAL CONSIDERATIONS FOR COLLABORATIVE CARE IMPLEMENTATION

Like any complex clinical workflow, implementation of the CoCM requires the PCP and the primary care practice to engage in significant practice change to deliver effective treatment. Studies have identified key facilitators to effective implementation including an engaged psychiatrist, PCP buy-in, a strong care manager, warm handoffs, strong top leadership support, a strong PCP champion, care manager role well-defined and implemented, and care manager onsite and accessible.[19] Key roles for the PCP in implementation are outlined below.

PRACTICE CHANGE TAKES REAL WORK

Implementation of the CoCM is best accomplished using a structured approach. There are several free resources to help support practices in the important work (*Box 2-3*). It is important to note that even in settings with scarce resources, implementation of the CoCM can be successful with a dedicated team. Most approaches start with identifying goals and creating a vision for the collaborative care team. PCP champion participation in this process is vital to make sure the CoCM goals align with the clinical presentations that could benefit from the most support. Once a set of shared goals have been identified and measures to track impact on these domains decided, developing a workflow that makes it easy to consistently deliver CoCM is the next step.

BOX 2-3   RESOURCES FOR COLLABORATIVE CARE MODEL IMPLEMENTATIONS

- AMA Steps Forward Behavioral Health Integration: https://www.stepsforward.org/modules/integrated-behavioral-health
- APA Integrated Care: https://www.psychiatry.org/psychiatrists/practice/professional-interests/integrated-care
- AHRQ Integration Playbook: https://integrationacademy.ahrq.gov/playbook/using-playbook
- Qualis Safety-Net Medical Home Initiative: http://www.safetynetmedicalhome.org/change-concepts/organized-evidence-based-care/behavioral-health
- UW AIMS Center: http://aims.uw.edu/
  - Financial Modeling Resources: https://aims.uw.edu/collaborative-care/financing-strategies/financial-modeling-workbook

---

In many practices, formal structures such as a clinical protocol development or continuous quality improvement team can be leveraged to support this work if available. Training for each member of the team to learn their role and the opportunity to train together as a team are important milestones to accomplish before starting to deliver patient care. Once the CoCM team has begun to see patients, the collaborative care team will need to consider how to continue to review progress toward goals and adjust clinical processes to accomplish goals. The PCP can champion accountable care delivery by anticipating that delivering collaborative care will require ongoing investment in continuous quality improvement, which will ultimately lead to the most successful implementations.

LIABILITY

To date there is no case law that has examined the liability of each provider in a CoCM team. However, analysis of the potential liability for the CoCM has been explored,[20] and the general consensus is that the liability for each provider is proportional to the amount of direct patient contact and scope of practice for each team member. Because the PCP in most collaborative care teams continues to play the primary role for diagnosis and prescribing, the PCP would be responsible and at risk for this clinical care. However, as the CoCM is itself the gold standard for mental health care in primary care settings, one can make a compelling argument that high-quality care had been provided to any patient treated by a collaborative care team.

FUNDING

As outlined in the evolving literature about implementation of the CoCM, identifying sustainable sources of funding for collaborative care is crucial for successful implementation. Much of the work of the CoCM team, such as the time that a BHP care manager spends on outreach and care coordination and the indirect case reviews performed by the psychiatric consultant, is not reimbursable through traditional fee for service billing. However, there are several exciting developments in this area, as health care is moving toward more value-based models of care delivery focusing on quality and outcomes, which are core principles of collaborative care. Although it is important to think first about creating or improving a strong, high-quality, measurement-based integrated health care delivery model and then determine how to sustain your effort, these new funding sources can help primary care practices cover the costs of providing the CoCM.

Collaborative care can be an important strategy for the many primary care practices that are seeking National Committee for Quality Assurance (NCQA) certification to become a PCMH 2017.[21] For example, elective credits toward certification can be earned by having at least one care manager qualified to identify and coordinate behavioral health needs or integrating behavioral health care providers into the care delivery system of the practice site, both of which are core features of collaborative care. Delivering the CoCM can also help a practice meet the PCMH 2017 standards for monitoring at least one of the core Performance Measurement and Quality Improvement (QI) measures in behavioral health. NCQA defines Healthcare Effectiveness Data and Information Set (HEDIS) measures, and both the measures for Utilization of the PHQ-9 to Monitor Depression Symptoms for Adolescents and Adults and Depression Remission and the Response for Adolescents and Adults are routinely monitored in collaborative care. Becoming a PCMH can have important benefits for a primary care

practice including higher reimbursement for routine primary care visits, and these reimbursements can help cover the costs for the time that BHP/care manager and psychiatric consultant spend to support care delivery by a PCP.

Another new funding approach is to bill new Psychiatric Collaborative Care Model Centers for Medicare & Medicaid Services G codes that were introduced in 2017.[22] These monthly codes can be billed by the PCP for each patient participating in a CoCM program for which a defined amount of time is spent in collaborative care with a team (including BHP/care manager, psychiatric consultant, and PCP) with the following required elements provided by that team:

- Outreach to and engagement in treatment
- Administration of validated rating scales, with the development of an individualized treatment plan
- Review by the psychiatric consultant with modifications of the plan if recommended
- Tracking each patient in a registry and tracking patient follow-up and progress using the registry
- BHP/care manager participation in weekly caseload consultation with the psychiatric consultant
- Provision of brief interventions using evidence-based techniques

These new codes offer a new payment model to help finance the costs associated with providing the value-based services provided in the CoCM, such as for regular monitoring of patients using validated clinical rating scales or for regular psychiatric caseload review and consultation that does not involve face-to-face contact with the patient because they are intended to incorporate the services of all members of the CoCM team as incident to services of the treating provider. It is anticipated that these codes will become standard CPT codes in 2018. Defining these codes has also made it possible for other payers to have a mechanism to reimburse for the CoCM, which could provide additional sources of funding for sustainability of collaborative care. Resources to explore how to model the financial impact of billing for CoCM are available for free from the University of Washington AIMS Center using the APA-AIMS Center financial modeling tool (*Box 2-3*).

CONCLUSION

PCPs have a critical role to play in supporting the delivery of evidence-based mental health treatments as the first-line providers to address this critical heath issue. The CoCM offers a core set of five principles that can be used to improve the quality of mental health care delivered for patients in any primary care setting. Using a team-based chronic care approach that is familiar to many PCPs can be an important strategy to making sure mental health disorders are identified and treated to remission. Collaborative care can also help a primary care setting effectively leverage scare psychiatric resources. This work is aligned with the core ideas in the health care movement toward value-based payment models, and using this alignment with new value-based funding sources may help with implementation and sustainability.

CASES AND QUESTIONS

1. Dr. Smith, MD, a practicing psychiatrist, communicates weekly with a care manager, Mr. Johnson, MA, LMHCA, to discuss their shared caseload of patients. Dr. Smith reviews patients who are not improving and makes treatment recommendations on the caseload of patients. Based on the description, which model of care does this most closely represent?

   A. Behavioral health consultant
   B. Collaborative Care Model
   C. Colocation
   D. Traditional consultation
   E. Inpatient consultation

   Correct answer: B. *The Collaborative Care Model is made up of a team of a PCP, a care manager, and a psychiatric consultant who work together to provide care to a caseload of patients.*

2. Which of the following have been demonstrated for the Collaborative Care Model?

   A. Improved patient outcomes
   B. Increased satisfaction for patients
   C. Increased cost-effectiveness in delivering care
   D. Increased provider satisfaction
   E. All of the above

   Correct answer: E. *The Collaborative Care Model has improved patient outcomes, increased satisfaction for patients, increased cost-effectiveness in delivering care, and increased provider satisfaction.*

3. With over 80 randomized controlled trials, meta-analysis of collaborative care for depression in primary care has found that the Collaborative Care Model is _____.

   A. equally as effective as usual care
   B. more effective than usual care
   C. the same as usual care
   D. less effective than usual care
   E. makes no difference compared with usual care

   Correct answer: B. *In a meta-analysis of collaborative care for depression in primary care settings, the Collaborative Care Model is more effective than usual care.*

4. One of the advantages of the Collaborative Care Model is the ability to achieve the Quadruple Aim. What is the Quadruple Aim?

   A. Improved coordination, patient and provider communication, provider training and scheduling
   B. Improved outcomes, patient and provider satisfaction, increased provider satisfaction, and cost-effectiveness
   C. Improved processes, improved productivity, use of an EHR, and use of a registry
   D. Improved productivity, use of an EHR, provider training, and staffing support

   E. Improved care coordination, use of an EHR, quality improvement, and improved patient surveys

   Correct answer: B. *The quadruple aim includes improved outcomes, patient and provider satisfaction, increased provider satisfaction, and cost-effectiveness.*

5. A primary care clinic has a high volume of patients. Additionally, in this clinic patients with depression and anxiety are common and have limited access to community mental health resources. The clinic has a care manager and a psychiatric consultant who work closely with the PCPs. This team uses a registry to track patients and treat to target. Which model of care best represents this scenario?

   A. Behavioral health consultant
   B. Collaborative Care
   C. Colocation
   D. Traditional consultation
   E. Primary Care Behavioral Health

   Correct answer: B. *The Collaborative Care Model utilizes a team-based approach (including PCPs, a care manager, and a psychiatric consultant) to deliver behavioral health care using a registry to track and treat patients in primary care.*

6. One of the guiding principles of the Collaborative Care Model is providing *population-based treatment*. As part of her role as a care manager, Ms. Wolfe reviews her list of active patients to identify those that are not improving and targets them for additional interventions. In the Collaborative Care Model, what tool does the care team use to track patients at this level?

   A. Catalog
   B. Registry
   C. Rubric
   D. Survey
   E. EHR

   Correct answer: B. *The Collaborative Care Model uses a registry to define a track a population of patients.*

7. Mr. Berry, a care manager, considers using brief behavioral interventions such as problem-solving treatment and FDA-approved antidepressants as part of an integrated care plan to target depression. Adding in this therapy represents which guiding principle of the Collaborative Care Model?

   A. Evidence-based treatment
   B. Accountable care
   C. Provider-centered care
   D. Population-based care
   E. Measurement-based treatment to target

   Correct answer: A. *The Collaborative Care Model team works together to provide both evidence-based brief behavioral interventions or psychosocial treatments and evidence-based psychopharmacology treatments as indicated.*

8. Ms. Cabrera, a care manager, routinely administers the PHQ-9 to her patients and enters their results into the patient registry. Ms. Cabrera and the psychiatric consultant are able to identify patterns in PHQ-9 scores over time and use these patterns to better understand what might be helping patients or possibly creating barriers to recovery. Ms. Cabrera utilizes these data as a way to work with patients to both pick a treatment goal and systematically work toward improvement. Based on this scenario, which guiding principle of the Collaborative Care Model does this *best* represent?

   A. Accountable care
   B. Evidence-based treatment
   C. Measurement-based treatment
   D. Patient-centered care
   E. Population-based care

   Correct answer: C. *Measurement-based treatment routinely assess patient response to treatment using validated behavioral health measures and adjusts treatment until patients achieve their goals.*

9. An important objective in treating patients in Collaborative Care is to pick a treatment goal and systematically work toward that goal over the course of treatment. Which guiding principle of the Collaborative Care Model does this *best* represent?

   A. Accountable care
   B. Evidence-based treatment
   C. Measurement-based treatment
   D. Patient-centered care
   E. Population-based care

   Correct answer: C. *Measurement-based treatment routinely assess patient response to treatment using validated behavioral health measures and adjusts treatment until patients achieve their goals.*

10. The Collaborative Care Model is most successful when care teams commit to improving the quality of the care that they deliver and regularly assess if they meet those quality goals. An example of this would be to focus on improved clinical outcomes for patients. Which guiding principle of Collaborative Care does this *best* represent?

    A. Accountable care
    B. Evidence-based treatment
    C. Measurement-based treatment
    D. Patient-centered care
    E. Population-based care

    Correct answer: A. *In the Collaborative Care Model, teams work together to continuously improve the care delivered to make sure the most patients possibly have high quality outcomes as part of delivering accountable care.*

11. A local community health clinic decides to implement quality aims with the goal of improving patient outcomes in depression care. To do this, the clinic establishes certain measures for the care team to meet over specific increments of time. Measures include number of patients discussed with the psychiatric consultant on a weekly basis, timeliness of entering medication information and PHQ-9 scores in the registry, and a minimum number of patient contacts per month. In analyzing patient outcomes, the clinic determines that they've met their established goal of improving patient outcomes by 10%. Based on this scenario, which of the Collaborative Care Model guiding principles does this *best* represent?

    A. Measurement-based treatment
    B. Accountable care
    C. Patient-centered care
    D. Population-based treatment
    E. Evidence-based treatment

    Correct answer: B. *Setting a goal to improve patient outcomes by 10% is an example of Accountable Care or a Collaborative Care Model team working together to continuously improve the care delivered to make sure the most patients possibly have high quality outcomes.*

12. What is a primary responsibility of the psychiatric consultant on a collaborative care team?

    A. Identify and engage patients in Collaborative Care
    B. Administer behavioral health screeners such as the PHQ-9 and GAD-7
    C. Support the team to develop integrated care plans in weekly case reviews with a BHP/care manager
    D. Complete relapse prevention plans with patients who are ready to graduate to the general PCP population
    E. See patients directly

    Correct answer: C. *The main role of the psychiatric consultant on a collaborative care team is to provide clinical input to the team during weekly caseload reviews with the BHP/care manager.*

13. The first phase of the Collaborative Care clinical workflow is *Identify and Engage.* Which care team member(s) is/are *most directly* involved in this phase?

    A. BHP/care manager only
    B. PCP only
    C. Psychiatric consultant only
    D. PCP and BHP/care manager
    E. Psychiatric consultant and PCP

continued

Correct answer: D. *The PCP and BHP/care manager are typically located in the primary care setting and directly involved in identifying and engaging the patient in Collaborative Care.*

14. A *typical* treatment plan for patients in Collaborative Care will include

    _____.

    A. medication only
    B. psychotherapy only
    C. both medications and psychotherapy
    D. a single treatment option
    E. provider-determined options only

    Correct answer: C. *Collaborative care teams should provide both medication and psychotherapy options for patients when indicated.*

15. Mr. J is a patient who has been engaged in treatment with the Collaborative Care Model for 12 weeks. His initial treatment plan included evidence-based brief psychotherapy only. After follow-up visits with the care manager and PHQ-9 scores that remained at around 15, Mr. J and his care team decided to change his treatment plan to include an initial target dose of an antidepressant and to continue with the evidence-based psychotherapy sessions. By week 10, his PHQ-9 scores had steadily dropped to around 10. Now in week 12, Mr. J has completed his brief psychotherapy course of treatment, his PHQ-9 scores have been consistently below 10, and he will continue taking the prescribed therapeutic dose of antidepressant. This scenario is most representative of which concept?

    A. Ad hoc prescribing
    B. Prescriber-driven care
    C. Using the PHQ-9 because it is required by the clinic
    D. Using the PHQ-9 to drive treatment to target
    E. Population-based care

    Correct answer: D. *This scenario represents using the PHQ-9 to drive treatment to target because adjustments in treatment were made by the collaborative care team until the patient's depression was in remission.*

REFERENCES

1. World Health Organization Depression Fact Sheet; 2017. http://www.who.int/mediacentre/factsheets/fs369/en/. Accessed August 15, 2017.
2. Melek S, Norris DT, Paulus J. Economic impact of integrated medical-behavioral healthcare. *Milliman.* 2014.
3. Wang PS, Lane M, Olfson M, Pincus HA, Wells KB, Kessler RC. Twelve-month use of mental health services in the United States: results from the National Comorbidity Survey Replication. *Arch Gen Psychiatry.* 2005;62(6):629-640.
4. Unutzer J, Park M. Strategies to improve the management of depression in primary care. *Prim Care.* 2012;39(2):415-431.
5. Unutzer J, Katon W, Callahan CM, et al. Collaborative care management of late-life depression in the primary care setting: a randomized controlled trial. *JAMA.* 2002;288(22):2836-2845.
6. Gilbody S, Whitty P, Grimshaw J, Thomas R. Educational and organizational interventions to improve the management of depression in primary care: a systematic review. *JAMA.* 2003;289(23):3145-3151.
7. Cunningham PJ. Beyond parity: primary care physicians' perspectives on access to mental health care. *Health Aff (Millwood).* 2009;28(3):w490-w501.
8. Archer J, Bower P, Gilbody S, et al. Collaborative care for depression and anxiety problems. *Cochrane Database Syst Rev.* 2012;10:CD006525.
9. Huffman JC, Niazi SK, Rundell JR, Sharpe M, Katon WJ. Essential articles on collaborative care models for the treatment of psychiatric disorders in medical settings: a publication by the academy of psychosomatic medicine research and evidence-based practice committee. *Psychosomatics.* 2014;55(2):109-122.
10. Miranda J, Duan N, Sherbourne C, et al. Improving care for minorities: can quality improvement interventions improve care and outcomes for depressed minorities? Results of a randomized, controlled trial. *Health Serv Res.* 2003;38(2):613-630.
11. Woltmann E, Grogan-Kaylor A, Perron B, Georges H, Kilbourne AM, Bauer MS. Comparative effectiveness of collaborative chronic care models for mental health conditions across primary, specialty, and behavioral health care settings: systematic review and meta-analysis. *Am J Psychiatry.* 2012;169(8):790-804.
12. Bodenheimer T, Sinsky C. From triple to quadruple aim: care of the patient requires care of the provider. *Ann Fam Med.* 2014;12(6):573-576.
13. Unützer J, Katon WJ, Fan MY, et al. Long-term cost effects of collaborative care for late-life depression. *Am J Manag Care.* 2008;14(2):95-100.
14. Levine S, Unützer J, Yip JY, et al. Physicians' satisfaction with a collaborative disease management program for late-life depression in primary care. *Gen Hosp Psychiat.* 2005;27(6):383-391.
15. Bentham WD, Ratzliff A, Harrison D, Chan YF, Vannoy S, Unutzer J. The experience of primary care providers with an integrated mental health care program in safety-net clinics. *Fam Community Health.* 2015;38(2):158-168.
16. Fortney JC, Pyne JM, Mouden SB, et al. Practice-based versus telemedicine-based collaborative care for depression in rural federally qualified health centers: a pragmatic randomized comparative effectiveness trial. *Am J Psychiatry.* 2013;170(4):414-425.
17. Ratzliff A, Unutzer J, Katon W, Stephens KA. *Integrated Care: Creating Effective Mental and Primary Health Care Teams.* Wiley; 2016.
18. Rush AJ. STAR*D: what have we learned? *Am J Psychiatry.* 2007;164(2):201-204.
19. Whitebird RR, Solberg LI, Jaeckels NA, et al. Effective implementation of collaborative care for depression: what is needed? *Am J Manag Care.* 2014;20(9).

20. Bland A, Lambert K, Raney L. Resource document on risk management and liability issues in integrated care models. *Am J Psychiatry*. 2014;171(5):1-7:data supplement.

21. National Committee for Quality Assurance Standards Review Patient-Centered Medical Home Recognition; 2017. http://www.ncqa.org/Portals/0/Programs/Recognition/PCMH/2017%20PCMH%20Concepts%20Overview.pdf?ver=2017-03-08-220342-490. Accessed August 15, 2017.

22. Centers for Medicare & Medicaid Services Federal Register; 2016. https://www.federalregister.gov/documents/2016/11/15/2016-26668/medicare-program-revisions-to-payment-policies-under-the-physician-fee-schedule-and-other-revisions#h-106. Accessed August 15, 2017.

3

PREVENTIVE MEDICINE AND BEHAVIORAL HEALTH

Gregory D. Brown, MD and Jane P. Gagliardi, MD, MHS

Preventive services are a key component of primary care, but the presence of psychiatric illness may bring challenges in implementing recommended preventive care.

Psychiatric disease confers an increased risk of poor outcomes from commonly preventable and treatable disease. Multiple studies demonstrate worse outcomes among patients with comorbid mental illness and diabetes,[1] coronary heart disease,[2] anticoagulation management,[3] and chronic obstructive pulmonary disease (COPD).[4] In a landmark study by Colton and Manderscheid (2006), the Centers of Disease Control and Prevention (CDC) reported that patients with severe mental illness (SMI)—generally defined to include schizophrenia, schizoaffective disorder, bipolar disorder, and major depression—have an average life expectancy 25 years less than the general population.[5] Schizophrenia carries a lifetime prevalence of about 1%[6]; bipolar mood disorder occurs in 2% to 4% of adults[7,8]; and major depressive disorder is expected to be the worldwide leader of disability by 2020, with a 15% prevalence.[8,9] In addition to major psychotic and mood disorders, anxiety disorders are prevalent in nearly 1/3 of adults and are likely more common among patients who present to primary care settings.[8,10,11] Indeed, the consensus of evidence reveals that patients with SMI have two to three times higher excess mortality translating to 13 to 30 years of potential life lost (YPLL) with 60% of the difference attributable to physical illness.[12-15]

COMPONENTS OF PREVENTIVE CARE

Preventive care typically consists of four interrelated clinical activities: immunizations, counseling on lifestyle changes to reduce unhealthy or high-risk behaviors, screening tests to find diseases early, and preventive medications to prevent further disease or complications. "Prevention" can also be divided into primary, secondary, and tertiary prevention. *Primary prevention* aims to avoid disease or injury before it occurs. Examples can include immunization against infectious disease, smoking cessation to reduce lung cancer risk, or seat belt education to prevent motor vehicle–related mortality. *Secondary*

prevention aims to detect and halt progression of disease or injury while it is still asymptomatic. Screening tests are key to secondary prevention. Examples can include procedures such as colonoscopy to detect and treat colon cancer, imaging such as computed tomography (CT) scan of the chest to detect lung cancer, laboratory tests such as cholesterol levels to help calculate cardiovascular risk and consider cholesterol-lowering drugs, and physical examination findings such as blood pressure to detect hypertension. If a screening test is positive, additional confirmatory testing often is needed; to be effective, screening programs are associated with action, such as implementation of a treatment plan. *Tertiary prevention* aims to reduce complications of the disease or injury after diagnosis and/or to improve quality of life and function. Together, the range of services thus described comprises what is often termed "chronic disease management." Examples can include statin and antiplatelet therapy after myocardial infarction or stroke. It should be noted that secondary prevention is often inappropriately used when tertiary prevention is the appropriate term.

A fundamental component of primary prevention involves behavioral or lifestyle change. For adults, lifestyle changes center on nutrition, physical activity, and limitation of unhealthy substances. At least one study of directly observed dietary patterns in patients with SMI demonstrated high intake of caloric beverages and low intake of fruits and vegetables with preference for high-fat meats and nonnutritious snacks.[16] According to the 2009 to 2011 National Survey on Drug Use and Health (NSDUH), over 36% of adults with any mental illness smoked in the last month compared with 21% with no mental illness.[17] Adults with any mental illness smoked on average 20 more cigarettes per month than their peers without mental illness.[17]

Excess mortality among patients with SMI may be partially explained by lifestyle factors such as unhealthy diet and tobacco smoking, although this is likely only at best a partial explanation and does not absolve the primary care provider from making sure patients undergo appropriate screening. Unfortunately, research demonstrates that patients with SMI receive fewer preventive services and screenings. Patients with SMI are significantly less likely to have appropriate blood pressure monitoring, cholesterol monitoring, mammography, osteoporosis screening, and vaccinations in particular.[18] However, given their increased risk of morbidity and mortality and the possible benefits of early intervention, patients with SMI are exactly the patients who are the most in need of preventive care—and probably at an earlier age than the general population. The prevalence of hypertension, obesity, diabetes mellitus, or the entire syndrome termed "the metabolic syndrome"; diabetic ketoacidosis in type 2 diabetes; cardiovascular disease including coronary artery disease and sudden cardiac death; cerebrovascular disease; infectious disease including those caused by human immunodeficiency virus (HIV), hepatitis B virus, and hepatitis C virus; and respiratory disease including tuberculosis, pneumonia, and COPD all have been shown to be higher in populations with SMI.[12]

Taking the evidence together, patients with SMI have increased prevalence of multiple chronic diseases and worse outcomes with regard to many of these diseases, have higher rates of lifestyle choices that place them at risk for exacerbation and/or acceleration of said diseases, *and* also receive fewer preventive services. At the same time, ensuring that patients with SMI undergo

appropriate screening can be a challenging endeavor, and primary care providers may experience frustration and a sense of futility—particularly considering the worse prognosis conferred by SMI in the first place. Whether patient centered (social, behavioral, or, more specifically, psychiatric) or provider related, barriers to ensuring appropriate preventive care are not isolated to patients with mental illness. Although barriers may be more pronounced among patients with mental illness, behavioral obstacles can pose challenges to accomplishing preventive care even in patients without psychiatric illness. Therefore, strategies to enhance primary care services among the psychiatrically ill will apply to all patients, and such strategies will be vital to primary care providers in optimizing the care of all patients.

This chapter will make use of illustrative case examples to demonstrate barriers and approaches to help improve the ability of primary care providers to apply preventive strategies to their patient panel. Preventive health care activities described in this chapter will be drawn from United States Preventive Services Task Force (USPSTF) guidelines and include primary, secondary, and tertiary prevention. Current guidelines can be found at https://www.uspreventiveservicestaskforce.org/ (*Table 3-1*).

TABLE 3-1 USPSTF A and B Recommendations for Nonpregnant Adults

TOPIC	DESCRIPTION	GRADE	RELEASE DATE OF CURRENT RECOMMENDATION
Abdominal aortic aneurysm screening: men	The USPSTF recommends one-time screening for abdominal aortic aneurysm by ultrasonography in men of ages 65-75 years who have ever smoked. (There is insufficient evidence to recommend screening for women.)	B	June 2014
Alcohol misuse: screening and counseling	The USPSTF recommends screening adults (age 18 years or older) for alcohol misuse and providing brief behavioral counseling interventions to reduce alcohol misuse among persons engaged in risky or hazardous drinking.	B	May 2013
Aspirin preventive medication: adults aged 50-59 years with a ≥10% 10-year cardiovascular risk	The USPSTF recommends initiating low-dose (81 mg) aspirin for the primary prevention of cardiovascular disease and colorectal cancer in adults aged 50-59 years who have a 10% or greater 10-year cardiovascular risk, are not at increased risk for bleeding, have a life expectancy of at least 10 years, and are willing to take low-dose aspirin daily for at least 10 years.	B	April 2016
Blood pressure screening: adults	The USPSTF recommends screening for high blood pressure in adults aged 18 years or older. The USPSTF recommends obtaining measurements outside of the clinical setting for diagnostic confirmation before starting treatment.	A	October 2015

(continued)

TABLE 3-1 USPSTF A and B Recommendations for Nonpregnant Adults (continued)

TOPIC	DESCRIPTION	GRADE	RELEASE DATE OF CURRENT RECOMMENDATION
BRCA risk assessment and genetic counseling/testing	The USPSTF recommends screening women who have family members with breast, ovarian, tubal, or peritoneal cancer using one of several screening tools designed to identify a family history that may be associated with an increased risk for potentially harmful mutations in breast cancer susceptibility genes (*BRCA1* or *BRCA2*). Women with positive screening results should receive genetic counseling and, if indicated after counseling, BRCA testing.	B	December 2013
Breast cancer preventive medications	The USPSTF recommends engaging in shared, informed decision-making about medications to reduce breast cancer risk. For women who are at increased risk for breast cancer and at low risk for adverse medication effects, clinicians should offer to prescribe risk-reducing medications, such as tamoxifen or raloxifene.	B	September 2013
Breast cancer screening[a]	The USPSTF recommends biennial screening mammography for women aged 50-74 years.	B	January 2016
Cervical cancer screening	The USPSTF recommends screening for cervical cancer in women aged 21-65 years with cytology (Pap smear) every 3 years. For women aged 30-65 years who want to lengthen the screening interval, screening with a combination of cytology and human papillomavirus (HPV) testing every 5 years is acceptable.	A	March 2012
Chlamydia screening: women	The USPSTF recommends screening for chlamydia in sexually active women aged 24 years or younger and in older women who are at increased risk for infection.	B	September 2014
Colorectal cancer screening	The USPSTF recommends screening for colorectal cancer starting at age 50 years and continuing until age 75 years.	A	June 2016
Depression screening: adults	The USPSTF recommends screening for depression in the general adult population, including pregnant and postpartum women. Screening should be implemented with adequate systems in place to ensure accurate diagnosis, effective treatment, and appropriate follow-up.	B	January 2016
Diabetes screening	The USPSTF recommends screening for abnormal blood glucose as part of cardiovascular risk assessment in adults aged 40-70 years who are overweight or obese. Clinicians should offer or refer patients with abnormal blood glucose to intensive behavioral counseling interventions to promote a healthful diet and physical activity.	B	October 2015
Falls prevention in older adults: exercise or physical therapy	The USPSTF recommends exercise or physical therapy to prevent falls in community-dwelling adults aged 65 years and older who are at increased risk for falls.	B	May 2012

TABLE 3-1 USPSTF A and B Recommendations for Nonpregnant Adults (continued)

TOPIC	DESCRIPTION	GRADE	RELEASE DATE OF CURRENT RECOMMENDATION
Falls prevention in older adults: vitamin D	The USPSTF recommends vitamin D supplementation to prevent falls in community-dwelling adults aged 65 years and older who are at increased risk for falls.	B	May 2012
Folic acid supplementation	The USPSTF recommends that all women who are planning or capable of pregnancy take a daily supplement containing 0.4-0.8 mg (400-800 µg) of folic acid.	A	January 2017
Gonorrhea screening: women	The USPSTF recommends screening for gonorrhea in sexually active women aged 24 years or younger and in older women who are at increased risk for infection.	B	September 2014
Healthy diet and physical activity counseling to prevent cardiovascular disease: adults with cardiovascular risk factors	The USPSTF recommends offering or referring adults who are overweight or obese and have additional cardiovascular disease (CVD) risk factors to intensive behavioral counseling interventions to promote a healthful diet and physical activity for CVD prevention.	B	August 2014
Hepatitis B screening: nonpregnant adolescents and adults	The USPSTF recommends screening for hepatitis B virus infection in persons at high risk for infection.	B	May 2014
Hepatitis C virus infection screening: adults	The USPSTF recommends screening for hepatitis C virus (HCV) infection in persons at high risk for infection. The USPSTF also recommends offering one-time screening for HCV infection to adults born between 1945 and 1965.	B	June 2013
HIV screening: nonpregnant adolescents and adults	The USPSTF recommends that clinicians screen for HIV infection in adolescents and adults aged 15-65 years. Younger adolescents and older adults who are at increased risk should also be screened.	A	April 2013
Intimate partner violence screening: women of childbearing age[b]	The USPSTF recommends that clinicians screen women of childbearing age for intimate partner violence, such as domestic violence, and provide or refer women who screen positive to intervention services. This recommendation applies to all women regardless of identifiable signs or symptoms of abuse.	B	January 2013
Lung cancer screening	The USPSTF recommends annual screening for lung cancer with low-dose computed tomography in adults aged 55-80 years who have a 30-pack-year smoking history and currently smoke or have quit within the past 15 years. Screening should be discontinued once a person has not smoked for 15 years or develops a health problem that substantially limits life expectancy or the ability or willingness to have curative lung surgery.	B	December 2013

(continued)

TABLE 3-1 USPSTF A and B Recommendations for Nonpregnant Adults (continued)

TOPIC	DESCRIPTION	GRADE	RELEASE DATE OF CURRENT RECOMMENDATION
Obesity screening and counseling: adults	The USPSTF recommends screening all adults for obesity. Clinicians should offer or refer patients with a body mass index of 30 kg/m² or higher to intensive, multicomponent behavioral interventions.	B	June 2012
Osteoporosis screening: women	The USPSTF recommends screening for osteoporosis in women of age 65 years and older and in younger women whose fracture risk is equal to or greater than that of a 65-year-old white woman who has no additional risk factors.	B	January 2012
Sexually transmitted infections counseling	The USPSTF recommends intensive behavioral counseling for all sexually active adolescents and for adults who are at increased risk for sexually transmitted infections.	B	September 2014
Skin cancer behavioral counseling	The USPSTF recommends counseling children, adolescents, and young adults aged 10-24 years who have fair skin about minimizing their exposure to ultraviolet radiation to reduce risk for skin cancer.	B	May 2012
Statin preventive medication: adults aged 40-75 years with no history of CVD, one or more CVD risk factors, and a calculated 10-year CVD event risk of 10% or greater	The USPSTF recommends that adults without a history of CVD (i.e., symptomatic coronary artery disease or ischemic stroke) use a low- to moderate-dose statin for the prevention of CVD events and mortality when all of the following criteria are met: (1) they are of age 40-75 years; (2) they have one or more CVD risk factors (i.e., dyslipidemia, diabetes, hypertension, or smoking); and (3) they have a calculated 10-year risk of a cardiovascular event of 10% or greater. Identification of dyslipidemia and calculation of 10-year CVD event risk requires universal lipids screening in adults aged 40-75 years.	B	November 2016
Tobacco use counseling and interventions: nonpregnant adults	The USPSTF recommends asking all adults about tobacco use, advising them to stop using tobacco, and providing behavioral interventions and U.S. Food and Drug Administration (FDA)–approved pharmacotherapy for cessation to adults who use tobacco.	A	September 2015
Tuberculosis screening: adults	The USPSTF recommends screening for latent tuberculosis infection in populations at increased risk.	B	September 2016
Syphilis screening: nonpregnant persons	The USPSTF recommends screening for syphilis infection in persons who are at increased risk for infection.	A	June 2016

Adapted from USPSTF A and B Recommendations. U.S. Preventive Services Task Force. Rockville, MD; April 2018. https://www.uspreventiveservicestaskforce.org/Page/Name/uspstf-a-and-b-recommendations/.
ᵃOther organizations including the American Cancer Society recommend different starting ages and screening intervals.
ᵇThere is insufficient evidence to suggest screening for intimate partner violence among men, vulnerable adults (mentally or physically disabled), or the elderly.
HIV, human immunodeficiency virus; USPSTF, the United States Preventive Services Task Force.

PRACTICE CASE 1

Mr. A is a 55-year-old man with schizophrenia, hypertension, impaired glucose tolerance, and ongoing tobacco use. Dr. C has been his primary care physician for more than 20 years, yet she still struggles to get Mr. A to follow age-appropriate screening and other preventive services. Mr. A has been stable on long-acting injectable fluphenazine for years; he continues to follow with a local psychiatrist and has not been hospitalized psychiatrically in over 10 years. Like many patients (and exacerbated by the "negative symptoms" and cognitive impairment associated with chronic schizophrenia), Mr. A struggles to remember to take all his oral medications. Dr. C accordingly has tried to limit his medication regimen to the "essentials." At his most recent visit last month, Mr. A's blood pressure was 166/94 mm Hg, he continued to smoke over 1 pack per day, and he had not yet undergone the screening colonoscopy for which referral has taken place annually for five consecutive years.

Today, Mr. A presents to see Dr. C for a follow-up visit. His medication list includes amlodipine 5 mg PO daily, hydrochlorothiazide (HCTZ) 25 mg PO daily, fluphenazine decanoate 25 mg IM q2 weeks, benztropine 1 mg PO BID, and atorvastatin 40 mg PO nightly. Mr. A's blood pressure has improved to 148/88 mm Hg since the addition of amlodipine at last visit (although he also admits to missing doses of his blood pressure medications a few times per week). He says he finds it hard to remember his atorvastatin and nightly dose of benztropine, stating that he often falls asleep before taking them. Dr. C, who is running behind owing to multiple complicated cases from the morning, decides to focus on his smoking and a colonoscopy referral today in clinic.

Motivational Interviewing

Mr. A begins the visit with Dr. C asking about his right knee, which he bumped while walking up the stairs the other day. Together, Dr. C and Mr. A set an agenda for the visit. They will begin the visit by discussing and examining Mr. A's knee. Mr. A agrees to thereafter talk about smoking cessation and completing a colonoscopy. With further history and an unremarkable examination, both are reassured that there is no significant knee injury.

Dr. C, who is adopting strategies of motivational interviewing in her primary care practice, begins the conversation around smoking cessation by assessing Mr. A's current willingness to stop smoking.

Dr. C: What are your plans regarding smoking cigarettes 3 months from now?

Mr. A: Well, I haven't really thought about it. Probably still smoking.

Dr. C: So, I am hearing you don't feel ready to quit smoking right now. What would tell you that you were ready to quit?

Mr. A: Hmm, if I had one of those heart attacks. My brother smokes and has high cholesterol, and he had a heart attack. And a pack of cigarettes costs so much nowadays.

Dr. C: Having a heart attack is something that scares you.

Mr. A: It does.

Dr. C: What have doctors or other people explained about the risk between smoking and heart attacks?

Mr. A: Smoking isn't good for your heart. I know that.

Dr. C: You're right. Smoking significantly increases your risk of having a heart attack. Lowering your risk for a heart attack sounds like a big reason to stop smoking. Your family history, high cholesterol, age, and that you are a man all increase your risk. Stopping smoking would help cut that risk by a lot.

Mr. A: I'm still not sure I could quit right now. It would be nice to save some money.

Dr. C: How much money do you spend on cigarettes per month?

Mr. A: Not sure.

Dr. C: What would it take to keep track of how much you spend each month? How much would knowing those costs impact your decision to quit?

Mr. A: I always buy the same kind of cigarettes. I could write down how much a pack costs. Maybe it could make a difference.

Dr. C: Sure, that seems like a great start. Maybe then you could also keep a tally of each time you buy a new pack.

Mr. A: Yah, that sounds like something I could do.

Dr. C: Great. So, when I see you next time, you will have a tally of how many packs you buy this coming month and how much one pack costs. We can then calculate the total monthly cost. Stopping smoking is a decision only you can make. As your doctor, I recommend quitting, but I hear that you are not ready to stop today. Please know that I and the clinic staff are here to help you quit whenever you are ready.

With regard to smoking cessation, Mr. A is precontemplative at the start of the conversation and moves toward being contemplative (*Figure 3-1* and *Table 3-2*). Dr. C reinforces the smoking cessation discussion by validating Mr. A's lack of current readiness. She clarifies that the decision to continue or to stop smoking is his, and she educates him about his significantly increased personal risk for cardiovascular disease. Mr. A agrees to try to estimate his monthly expenditures on cigarettes.

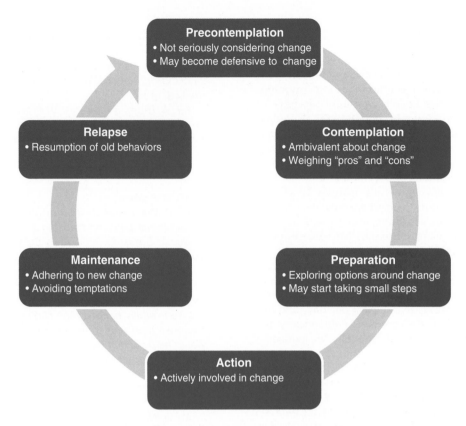

FIGURE 3-1 Transtheoretical model stages of change.

TABLE 3-2 Transtheoretical Model Stages of Change With Stage-Specific Findings and Patient Approaches

STAGE OF CHANGE	COMMON FINDINGS	APPROACHES TO PATIENT
Precontemplation	• Not considering change • May downplay or not understand risk	• Validate that patient is not ready to change • Clarify to patient that it is his or her choice to change • Encourage reevaluation and self-exploration • Personalize risk
Contemplation	• Ambivalent about change • May be weighing pros and cons	• Validate that patient is not ready to change • Encourage weighing of pros and cons • Promote expected positive outcomes with change
Preparation	• Planning to change • May be bypassed for some persons	• Identify and help to problem-solve around obstacles • Ensure patient has the skills/means for change • Encourage small, measurable, and attainable goals
Action	• Practicing new behavior	• Boost self-efficacy for dealing with obstacles • Address any sense of loss and support long-term goals/benefits
Maintenance	• Continued commitment to change	• Reinforce external and internal supports • Discuss coping with relapse
Relapse	• Resumption of old behavior • May be the norm in many situations	• Identify and evaluate trigger(s) for relapse • Reassess motivation and where patient has reentered along the stages of change

Adapted with permission from http://www.cpe.vt.edu/gttc/presentations/8eStagesofChange.pdf.

Discussion

Miller and Rollnick define motivational interviewing as a "collaborative, goal-oriented style of communication with particular attention to the language of change. It is designed to strengthen personal motivation for and commitment to a specific goal by eliciting and exploring the person's own reason for change within an atmosphere of acceptance and compassion."[19] Motivational interviewing involves four related processes: engaging, focusing, evoking, and planning. *Engaging* is the process of building a working relationship. *Focusing* helps set a mutual agenda. *Evoking* the patient's own arguments for change can help crystallize the patient's motivation to change. *Planning* develops commitment and formulates a specific plan of action. Key skills involved with all four processes include using open-ended questions, affirming, reflecting, and summarizing.

In this case example, Dr. C had the benefit of a long-standing therapeutic relationship with the patient, so she was able to quickly engage Mr. A and focus on his cigarette smoking. She evoked reasons for stopping smoking including myocardial infarction risk and cost, and she planned on making an inventory of the financial costs to the patient from buying cigarettes. Dr. C began the entire process with an open-ended question. By the end of the brief conversation, Dr. C could reflect Mr. A's concerns around having a heart attack and spending a lot of money on cigarettes, summarize the plan around assessing monthly costs, and affirm his lack of readiness to stop smoking.

A significant amount of literature exists on the use of motivational interviewing across a wide range of health-related behavioral changes. Systematic reviews have shown promise for motivational interviewing's role both for improving health screening rates[20] as well as for improving adherence to medications for chronic diseases, especially if coaching exists during the intervention implementation.[21] A review of studies looking at motivational interviewing techniques or theory to increase physical activity among patients with SMI demonstrated mixed results.[22] Taken together, the data suggest that motivational interviewing is a practical option for patients with SMI to promote health-related behavioral change.

PRACTICE CASE 1 *(Continued)*

Barriers to Care

Returning to Dr. C's appointment with Mr. A, with the time left in their visit, the doctor and patient now transition to a referral for colonoscopy. Dr. C avoids accusatory language (such as asking, "Why didn't you have the colonoscopy done?") by simply inquiring "What happened with the last colonoscopy referrals?" By avoiding wording that could imply fault, Dr. C allows for an open discussion. In dialogue with the patient, two barriers to the colonoscopy referral become apparent. Although he has gone for preoperative testing and received his colonoscopy preparation prescription at least once before, he did not have anyone who would be able to drive him to and from the procedure itself. He is also apprehensive that the doctors could be working with the FBI and implant a listening device during the procedure. Mr. A always worries about the FBI monitoring him. Today, he is comforted by Dr. C that there would be doctors and nurses involved in the procedure to keep him safe, so he admits that "someone would catch if something fishy was going on."

No one is sure how best to address one of the main barriers to obtaining a colonoscopy: a lack of someone to drive Mr. A home after the procedure, compounded by an institutional policy that forbids public transportation or a cab as the means to return home after conscious sedation. Dr. C is not entirely sure how to address this barrier, but now that she recognizes it she agrees to investigate resources available in the clinic and will ask the clinic social worker to explore options.

Discussion

In conceptualizing barriers to preventive health services, authors have categorized *patient factors, physician (provider) factors,* and *health system factors.*[23] Emerging themes include lack of time, lack of knowledge, lack of access (generally in relation to lack of available testing or treatment), lack of insurance, prohibitive cost, and fragmented systems or inadequate infrastructure. Still missing are the individual and/or local barriers that often go overlooked but may be most difficult to overcome. For instance, Mr. A does not have a strong social support network. He relies on public transportation. Needing a ride to and from a colonoscopy, especially a ride that cannot be public transportation or a taxi cab, is a significant barrier. Some patients may have access to vehicles, but the considerable financial impact of parking fees and gasoline costs can be a deterrent. In similar situations, working with the patient to explore his or her support network can often find a family member or friend willing to help. This person may be someone the patient was hesitant or did not even think to ask. Communities also have varying transportation options associated with paratransit services. These services often require an application and/or fees associated with their use. Other community organizations, churches, or hospital systems may also have additional transportation programs or may be able to assist on a case-by-case basis.

Dr. C asks the social worker who works within the clinic practice about transportation options to and from a colonoscopy for Mr. A. The social worker agrees to explore transportation options. The next day, the social worker calls Mr. A, and together they identify a friend with a car who is willing to drive Mr. A and wait for the

TABLE 3-3 USPSTF A and B Recommendations for Mr. A

USPSTF RECOMMENDATIONS	SCREENING DETAILS	GRADE OF RECOMMENDATION
Alcohol misuse screening	Screen and provide brief behavioral interventions for risk alcohol use	B
Depression screening	Screen adults when systems for evaluation and management are available	B
Hypertension screening	Screen adults and exclude white coat hypertension before starting therapy	A
Obesity screening	Screen adults and offer or refer patients with body mass index ≥ 30 kg/m^2 to intensive behavioral interventions	B
Tobacco use screening	Screen adults and provide behavioral and U.S. Food and Drug Administration–approved intervention therapy for cessation	A
HIV screening	Screen individuals 15-65 years of age	A
Lipid disorder screening	Screen men of age 35 years and older	A
Hepatitis C virus screening	Offer one-time screening of patients born between 1945 and 1965	B
Colorectal cancer screening	Screen patients of age 50-75 years for fecal occult blood (or immunochemical) test, sigmoidoscopy, colonoscopy, CT colonography, or multitargeted stool DNA test	A
Lung cancer screening	Screen annually with low-dose CT for individuals 55-80 years of age with a 30-pack-year history who currently smoke or quit within the past 15 years; consider overall health in decision to screen	B
Aspirin for primary prevention of CVD and colorectal cancer	Recommend low-dose aspirin for patients 50-59 years of age with a 10-year CVD risk of 10% or greater, appropriate bleeding risk, and life expectancy of at least 10 years	B

Adapted from USPSTF A and B Recommendations. U.S. Preventive Services Task Force. Rockville, MD; April 2018. https://www.uspreventiveservicestaskforce.org/Page/Name/uspstf-a-and-b-recommendations/.
CT, computed tomography; CVD, cardiovascular disease; HIV, human immunodeficiency virus; USPSTF, the United States Preventive Services Task Force.

colonoscopy in exchange for the cost of a tank of gas. The social worker also initiates a paratransit application for Mr. A to help in the future with transportation to locations where public bus lines do not easily reach.

Mr. A is fortunate in that he has a consistent relationship with his health care providers, has ongoing mental health with symptoms that are well controlled, has housing, and has sufficient insurance coverage to cover doctor's visits, preventive care, and medication costs. Among a population of patients with SMI in community mental health clinics, male gender and lack of insurance were associated with less use of preventive services.[14] On the other hand, Mr. A's preventive care could also be improved. Based on the U.S. Preventive Services Task Force guidelines as of publishing, Mr. A would meet criteria for consideration of multiple other grade A or B recommendations (*Table 3-3*).

Visit Management and Setting Priorities

Part of the difficulty in adhering to published guidelines for preventive health care services stems from a sense on the part of health care providers that there are so many guidelines that it can be difficult to know where to start, especially in patients who do not seem to follow recommendations. A health care provider may find himself or herself feeling sufficiently overwhelmed that the inertia of inaction takes over. Some health care providers may lack comfort or fail to recognize that patients with SMI can be effectively enlisted in shared decision-making and goal setting. When appointment time is limited and preventive screening seems unwieldy, the best recommendation is to engage in a conversation with the patient to set priorities. A multidisciplinary interprofessional team can provide invaluable support not only to patients with SMI but also can aid in the care of any patient who needs preventive care. At their recent visits, Mr. A and Dr. C addressed multiple concerns with the expert assistance of social work and clinic resources and support staff. In busy clinics without such support, time may be more limited to address preventive care. Therefore, visit management becomes important.

One important visit management technique is setting an agenda, in which the physician and patient agree upon that day's topics for discussion. Dr. C used this technique in the example of the appointment with Mr. A As another example, the patient may have one or two (or more) acute concerns and the physician may choose one preventive care topic to discuss. If there are more topics than can be discussed during that visit, a closer follow-up may be needed with expectations set to discuss preventive care at that subsequent visit. Using supportive though clear language is important. For example, "I (or we) want to address your 'x' and I want to make sure we have the time and opportunity to do so appropriately. So, I want you to make a n-week follow-up appointment when we can discuss 'x.'" Dr. C concludes the visit, "Next time, Mr. A, we will discuss your medications and strategies to make sure you are best able to take them. I will see you back in four weeks." She documents their conversation and ending point so that the discussion can resume at the next visit.

PRACTICE CASE 1 *(Continued)*

Shared Decision-Making

Mr. A returns for his follow-up visit. During the visit, the doctor and patient discuss Mr. A's difficulties remembering all of his medications. Mr. A agrees to try a pill box. Although some pharmacies in the area provide prepackaged medications in daily blister packs, Mr. A has been working for 15 years with a pharmacist he trusts, and prepackaged blister pack service is not available at his usual pharmacy. Dr. C and Mr. A agree that Mr. A will bring a pill box to the next clinic visit along with his medication bottles so that one of the nurses can help him fill it. To simplify his medication regimen to a feasible once-daily dose schedule, Dr. C acknowledges that although atorvastatin is best administered at bedtime, Mr. A could take it in the morning to limit his medication administration times to once daily. Dr. C has been working with Mr. A for a long time, and Dr. C and Mr. A's psychiatrist have been collaborating on his care for years; Dr. C uses 5 minutes of the clinic visit to call the psychiatrist's office and leave a message requesting consideration of moving the benztropine dose to morning, as well, to improve Mr. A's ability to take his medications regularly.

Discussion

Although Dr. C has not completely understood or agreed with some of Mr. A's priorities as it comes to health care in general and preventive care, she has been willing to work with him around his choices. Mr. A opted against daily low-dose aspirin for prevention of cardiovascular disease (CVD) and colorectal cancer, even though he has a 10-year CVD risk of greater than 10%, does not have increased bleeding risk, and has at least 10 years of life expectancy, because he did not want to take another pill. He has, however, been willing to take a high-intensity statin for primary prevention of CVD based on his 10-year CVD risk because he is worried that other family members also have high cholesterol. Shared decision-making has been instrumental in building a lasting rapport between doctor and patient. Balancing patient preference with the most medically necessary preventive health care services increases the likelihood of adherence. The goal is not to overwhelm the patient but to

provide sufficient information for rational decision-making, so the patient will not indiscriminately choose for or against aspects of care.

Risk Assessment

Key to addressing preventive care is having the skills to do so. With Mr. A, barriers to care span a biomedical model and a biopsychosocial model. With shared decision-making and limit setting, visits can be focused. However, more skills are needed to best promote preventive care among patients with mental illness. A systematic review with meta-ethnography by Rubio-Valera et al. identified education and skills training on risk assessment and motivational interviewing as key components to promote implementation of primary prevention and health promotion activities.[24]

Risk assessments in the context of preventive care activities for patients with SMI must account for the higher rates of endocrine/metabolic comorbidities including obesity, metabolic syndrome, and diabetes mellitus; cardiovascular disease; and infectious disease including those caused by HIV, hepatitis B virus, and hepatitis C virus. USPSTF and other guideline recommendations do not necessarily consider the increased risks for patients with SMI. Among a cohort of patients with schizophrenia, schizophreniform, or schizoaffective disorders in Spain, researchers elucidated that metabolic syndrome prevalence and cardiovascular risk using the Framingham score were similar to persons 10 to 15 years older in the general population.[25] Patients with SMI appear to "age" prematurely and, as previously noted, have significantly shorter life expectancies. Clinicians must remain attuned to this and, as an example, might beneficially consider earlier cardiovascular screening.

PRACTICE CASE 1 *(Continued)*

Between Dr. C and Mr. A, his tobacco smoking is an ongoing topic at most, if not all, visits. At a previous visit, they discussed smoking cessation with Dr. A using a motivational interviewing perspective and helping to personalize his risk for CVD as with respect to Mr. A's tobacco smoking. Today, the doctor and patient agree as part of the agenda for the visit to conclude again with a conversation around smoking. Mr. A has brought back his tally of cigarette packs for the month.

Dr. C: Now, I'd like to return to how things have been going with your smoking.

Mr. A: Well, it's about the same.

Dr. C: So, the number of cigarettes you are smoking is about the same. Last time, we planned on you keeping a tally of the number of cigarette packs that you bought? How'd that go?

Mr. A: I got that here. (He pulls out a piece of folded paper.)

Dr. C: Okay, let's see here. (She counts the tallies.) I count 48 packs here or about 1.5 packs per day. Does that sound about right to you?

continued

Mr. A: I think so 'cause some days I buy 1 and some days 2.

Dr. C: And you wrote that you spend about $5.50 per pack. Doing some quick calculation (uses calculator on computer)...that's $264 for the month and would be...$3,168 dollars for the year.

Mr. A: Wow, I never thought of it that way. That would be a lot of money I could put toward rent, or even something nice like a new T.V. Maybe I could at least cut down to 1 pack a day.

Dr. C: What would help you cut down to 1 pack per day? How would you cut down?

Mr. A: Well, I may just cut back to buying 1 per day?

Dr. C: Sure, and what would help you do that?

Mr. A: I think if I told my friends and my sister then they can remind me. I also know I smoke less if I am walking. Maybe, I could go for a few more walks during the week.

Dr. C reinforces his change talk. She asks for permission to introduce another possible reason to stop smoking, and Mr. A assents. Dr. C introduces the link between smoking and lung cancer. They go on to discuss the possibility of doing a low-dose CT scan because he is now 55 years of age, has smoked more than a pack of cigarettes for over 30 years, and continues to smoke. Mr. A is a little concerned about the radiation and unwilling to commit to screening currently, although he remains willing to discuss screening and consider it in the future.

Discussion

Preventive care among those with SMI is especially important not only owing to lifestyle factors including higher rates of smoking[26] but also owing to the increased metabolic risks associated with many psychiatric medications. For lifestyle factors, motivational interviewing can be key as has been discussed. For increased metabolic risks, primary care physicians must be attuned to patients' psychiatric medications, some of which may cause increased metabolic risks. In addition to the underlying biological, environmental, and social risk factors of cardiovascular disease among patients with SMI, certain psychotropic medications prescribed for psychotic as well as mood disorders, namely second-generation antipsychotics, increase the risk of metabolic syndrome. High-level evidence supports an increased risk of weight gain, insulin resistance, and dyslipidemia with most second-generation antipsychotics. Some emerging data suggest that antipsychotics that are considered intermediate risk, including some first-generation antipsychotics, may carry higher risk for major cardiovascular events than previously thought.[27] Although not all antipsychotics worsen metabolic profiles, the antipsychotics considered most efficacious for refractory disease (namely, olanzapine [Zyprexa] and clozapine [Clozaril]) carry the highest risk.[28] Among other psychotropics, valproic acid or sodium valproate, a common antiepileptic and mood

stabilizer, also carries significant risk for weight gain. Less attention has been paid to this risk; however, monitoring may be warranted.

The American Psychiatric Association, American Diabetes Association, American Association of Clinical Endocrinologists, and the North American Association for the Study of Obesity published shared guidelines on metabolic monitoring for all patients on second-generation antipsychotics in 2004[29] (*Table 3-4*). Briefly, at initiation of antipsychotic treatment, weight or body mass index (BMI), waist circumference, blood pressure, fasting plasma glucose, and fasting plasma lipid panel should be checked. Weight should then be checked every 4 weeks up to 12 weeks and quarterly thereafter. Repeat blood pressure and fasting plasma glucose should be measured at 12 weeks and annually thereafter. Also at 12 weeks, a repeat fasting lipid panel is recommended before extending monitoring to every 5 years. Waist circumference measurement is recommended annually. Despite the clarity of the guidelines, which have been available since 2004, full adaptation has been slow. Multiple studies demonstrate low screening rates for diabetes, dyslipidemia, and hypertension among patients prescribed atypical antipsychotic medications,[30] with an even lower rate of baseline testing per recommendations.[31] A systematic review and meta-analysis, by Mitchell et al., of 48 studies between 2000 and 2011 examining routine metabolic screening practices for patient taking antipsychotics in psychiatric care found improved rates of monitoring postguideline implementation but still only approximately 76% for weight, 75% for blood pressure, 56% for fasting glucose, and only 29% for lipids.[32] Detection does not equate to treatment, however. Even in the Clinical Antipsychotic Trials of Intervention Effectiveness (CATIE), the landmark study on treatment for psychotic spectrum disorders, the rates of treatment for diabetes, dyslipidemia, and hypertension were only 70%, 40%, and 12%, respectively.[33]

Although monitoring is the key first step and data on treatment for diabetes, dyslipidemia, and hypertension are robust, less is known on how to alter antipsychotic treatment in response to metabolic side effects. Randomized controlled studies have shown that obesity and metabolic syndrome can be managed within a controlled setting using lifestyle and pharmacologic approaches.[34,35] However, further research is needed to test the long-term effectiveness of these guidelines and to guide how and if to change antipsychotics. Gradual conversion from an antipsychotic with high risk of metabolic adverse effects to one with lower risk may be effective in improving weight and metabolic parameters; however, some patients may experience exacerbation of their underlying illness and convert back to the prior antipsychotic.[36] At present, continued monitoring is warranted and careful attention is given to the risks and benefits of antipsychotic switching for the individual patient in shared decision-making with the patient, psychiatrist, and primary care physician.

TABLE 3-4 Second-Generation Antipsychotic Monitoring							
	BASELINE	**4 WEEKS**	**8 WEEKS**	**12 WEEKS**	**QUARTERLY**	**ANNUALLY**	**EVERY 5 YEARS**
Personal/family history	X					x	
Weight (BMI)	X	x	x	X	x		
Waist circumference	X					X	
Blood pressure	X			X		X	
Fasting plasma glucose	X			X		X	
Fasting lipid panel	x			x			x

From Consensus development conference on antipsychotic drugs and obesity and diabetes. Diabetes Care. 2004;27(2):596-601. Copyright and all rights reserved. Material from this publication has been used with the permission of American Diabetes Association.
BMI, body mass index.

PRACTICE CASE 2

Ms. B is another patient in the primary care clinic. She has symptoms of both depression and anxiety, although has never been formally diagnosed with major depression or a specific anxiety disorder. She has been reluctant to go to the local psychiatry practice because she is worried about what other people would say about her. In general, she finds it difficult to work up the motivation to make it to appointments. If she is not taking care of her grandchildren, Ms. B rarely gets out of her home and sometimes does not even get out of bed. Dr. D is a new physician to the primary care clinic and is meeting Ms. B for the first time today. He had the chance to review the chart briefly before the visit.

Discussion

Screening Tools

The clinic has recently started screening patients at all new visits and at least once annually for depression and anxiety through use of the Patient Health Questionnaire-9 (PHQ-9) and General Anxiety Disorder 7-item (GAD-7), respectively. Both instruments have been validated in a range of clinical settings. A cutoff of 10 on the PHQ-9 has a pooled sensitivity of 0.78 (95% confidence interval [CI], 0.70 to 0.84) and pooled specificity of 0.87 (95% CI, 0.84 to 0.90) based on a meta-analysis of 36 studies by Moriarty et al. for the diagnosis of major depression.[37] The depression screening began after the clinic's health system hired a psychiatrist and case managers to deliver the Improving Mood—Promoting Access to Collaborative Treatment (IMPACT) model of depression care. The IMPACT model was initially described in a landmark 2002 study demonstrating over double the effectiveness for depression treatment among older adults compared with usual care.[38] Subsequent studies have shown effectiveness of the model in younger adults with comorbid diabetes and/or cancer.[39,40]

PRACTICE CASE 2 *(Continued)*

Dr. D recognized a recurrent history of depressive and anxiety symptoms in his chart review for Ms. B, so he asks one of the clinic nurses to provide Ms. B with a PHQ-9 and GAD-7 screening questionnaire. Ms. B completes the screening questions while Dr. D is finishing up with the patient before her. Dr. D is handed the results as he is about to meet Ms. B Her scores are 15/27 on the PHQ-9 and 6/21 on the GAD-7, indicating moderate depression and mild anxiety symptoms.

Ms. B is sitting quietly on the examination table when Dr. D enters. Anticipating that they will be discussing depression and potentially sensitive subjects, he makes a conscious effort to remain seated in a comfortable position, facing Ms. B, although slightly to the side to avoid the potentially intimidating position of sitting directly face to face.

Dr. D: What brings you to clinic today?

Ms. B: I've just been feeling so tired, like I just don't have the energy to do things any more.

Dr. D: So, you are feeling more fatigued than in the past. Tell me more about what has been going on.

Ms. B: It's like I can't fall asleep sometimes and when I do then I wake up early in the morning and all the time never feeling like I got any good sleep.

Dr. D: There were a few forms that you filled out when you first came in.

Ms. B: Yes, it seemed like I had all those things going on.

Dr. D: And I see that you have been feeling pretty down.

Ms. B: Yah, I don't feel like my old self. I've been sad and I don't always understand why.

Dr. D goes on to discuss the likely diagnosis of depression. He assesses for suicidal ideation by asking nonjudgmentally if Ms. B has ever had thoughts that life is not worth living, she would be better off dead, or maybe even that she might think about taking her own life. Ms. B is adamant that she has never thought about

continued

(nor could she ever consider) killing herself because of her close relationship with her family and faith in God. She also shares with Dr. D that she has a lot of trepidation about turning 65 next month because 65 is the age at which her mother died. Dr. D validates her concerns and provides reassurance.

As the interview progresses, Dr. D completes a review of symptoms to satisfactorily lower his pretest probability for hypothyroidism among his differential diagnoses. To improve his interview skills, Dr. D is working to ask fewer "yes" or "no" questions. He wants to screen for alcohol misuse and the use of other illicit drugs, especially in the context of her depression. He begins by screening for alcohol misuse by asking the CAGE questionnaire. She scores zero on the CAGE questionnaire (*Box 3-1*). Ms. B reports only rare alcohol use on holidays. She denies ever using any illicit drugs. The doctor and patient go on to broadly discuss various treatment options for depression from medications to therapy or both. Dr. D introduces the option of the depression collaborative care initiative that the clinic has started. Ms. B says she is interested and agrees to meet with the depression care manager. Before starting an antidepressant, Dr. D has Ms. B complete a self-rating scale, the Mood Disorder Questionnaire (MDQ), to screen for a possible history of mania. Use of the MDQ screening has led to improved detection of bipolar disorder among general practitioners.[41,42] After the negative screen, they agree to start an antidepressant, sertraline 25 mg PO daily. Dr. D sets a goal for next visit to discuss preventive care screenings that Ms. B will be 65 years old in 1 month. He introduces this as a way to ensure she is as healthy as possible now that she will be 65.

Over the course of the next 4 weeks, Ms. B works with the depression care manager on goals to promote physical activity and thereby behavioral activation. The psychiatrist with the depression care collaborative offers suggestions to titrate her sertraline, up to 100 mg PO daily. Ms. B presents back to the clinic now after 4 weeks. Her PHQ-9 is now down to 10. She says she is starting to feel better overall and has noticed an improvement in her mood and energy. Both patient and doctor are content with the progress she has made. They both decide to turn their attention to preventive health care as planned at last visit. Ms. B asks about getting a Pap smear. She has been getting a Pap smear yearly up until a few years ago with her gynecologist. She does not recall ever having an abnormal examination. Dr. D discusses the USPSTF recommendations that she would no longer need screening based on age and especially as she has not had an abnormal examination.

Dr. D and Ms. B move on to discuss vaccinations. Ms. B has generally been apprehensive of needles. She cannot recall her last immunizations, although she is certain she received "all the childhood vaccines." Based on CDC Recommended Immunization Schedule for Adults (available at https://www.cdc.gov/vaccines/schedules/downloads/adult/adult-combined-schedule.pdf), Ms. B is due for influenza, tetanus toxoid, reduced diphtheria toxoid, and acellular pertussis (Tdap), herpes zoster, 13-valent pneumococcal conjugate vaccine (PCV13), and 23-valent pneumococcal polysaccharide vaccine (PPSV23). Ms. B is willing to consider receiving one vaccine today. They agree on influenza and work out a rough schedule for PCV13 and Tdap at the next visit with the zoster and PPSV23 vaccines to follow.

Ms. B has been worried about breast cancer screening. She reports that in her forties she had an abnormal mammogram, the details of which she cannot definitively recall. However, she thinks that all subsequent tests have been normal. Her most recent mammogram was last year. Although she finds it difficult to make it to appointments, her anxiety around the possibility of breast cancer drove her to ensure yearly mammogram follow-up. She has also had a few friends and relatives diagnosed with breast cancer, some now in remission and some who unfortunately have died from the disease. She requests to have another mammogram now.

Dr. D asks for the opportunity to share some more information about mammogram screening. Rather than reflexively reordering a mammogram, he wants to help Ms. B make a more informed decision about proceeding with breast cancer screening. Dr. D takes the rest of the visit to go through risks versus benefits of breast cancer screening with attention to mammography. To assist in the discussion, Dr. D uses a decision aid. In this case, they go over the Physician Data Query (PDQ) from the National Cancer Institute (available at https://www.cancer.gov/types/breast/mammograms-fact-sheet). Dr. D emphasizes the differing recommendations as to optimal timing of mammography: USPSTF recommending every other year mammograms from 50 to 74 years of age versus the American Cancer Society recommending yearly mammograms starting at 45 years of age if the patient is in good health with consideration for every other year screening starting at 55 years but only with patient preference.

Using a decision aid with patient-friendly language, Dr. D generally finds that patients not only get to make a more informed decision but also have improved satisfaction because of the ability to partner in their health care. However, as with the PDQ, some of the decision aids are written at a grade level above some patients' comprehension. So, Dr. D also uses visual aids such as an infographic from a 2014 JAMA Patient Page on the benefits and harms of breast cancer screening.[43] He uses a similar style infographic from the National Cancer Institute website based on the USPSTF statement on prostate cancer screening (available at https://www.cancer.gov/types/prostate/psa-infographic). After their discussion, Dr. D and Ms. B agree to space out screening mammography to once every 2 years. She takes comfort that multiple recommendations concur that every other year screening is an option especially beyond 55 years of age. Owing to time constraints and because of their more thorough discussion around breast cancer screening, they defer discussion of osteoporosis screening to next visit.

Two months elapse before Ms. B returns to clinic. Her PHQ-9 is now down to 6, and she is nearing full remission of her depression. She is getting out of the house more and enjoys spending more time with her grandchildren. She continues to work with her depression care manager. Her sertraline has been stable at 150 mg PO daily for the last month. The higher dose has helped with her symptoms of anxiety.

Ms. B reports experiencing a fall approximately 2 weeks ago. From her description, Dr. D determines that she most likely had a mechanical fall. She denies any injuries and, on physical examination, has no apparent sequelae from the fall. The doctor and patient focus their visit again on preventive care. Given the recent fall, Ms. B wonders if she should be screened for osteoporosis. She has never had a broken bone but knows that her mother had a hip fracture after a fall. They discuss that based on her age and sex alone she is due for osteoporosis screening. Dr. D places an order for a bone densitometry (dual-energy X-ray absorptiometry [DEXA]) scan.

The risk of osteoporosis is higher among individuals with SMI and especially for patients on antipsychotics. The UK General Practice Research Database cohort study showed an increased relative risk of fracture among community-dwelling patients with mental illness,[44] and a Danish case–control study showed a small increased fracture risk with anxiolytics, sedatives, and neuroleptics.[45] Pathophysiology is likely multifactorial and is thought to relate to lifestyle factors, such as reduced calcium and vitamin D intake, reduced physical activity, and increased alcohol and tobacco use, as well as disease-related factors such as hypercortisolemia, and medication-related factors such as hyperprolactinemia with certain antipsychotics leading to secondary sex hormone suppression and decreased bone mineral density.[46] Osteoporosis is yet another example where preventive care for patients with behavioral health diagnoses must consider increased disease risk and earlier screening as appropriate.

Ms. B also wonders if there is anything she can do to help prevent falls, as she never wants to risk breaking her hip. They discuss the importance of regular exercise and talk about how vitamin D supplementation has been shown to decrease fall risk. The USPSTF recommends vitamin D supplementation for fall prevention in community-dwelling adults of age 65 years or older and in those at increased risk of falls, which includes a history of prior falls. Because of the variability among the trials assessing vitamin D supplementation, an optimal dosing regimen of vitamin D for fall prevention is not known. Some studies supplemented only in vitamin D–deficient individuals whereas others included vitamin D–sufficient individuals. The total daily dose was consistently above 400 international units (IU) of vitamin D whether as ergocalciferol (vitamin D2) or cholecalciferol (vitamin D3).[47] After the discussion, Dr. D and Ms. B agree that she will start over-the-counter cholecalciferol 1,000 IU PO daily.

BOX 3-1 THE CAGE QUESTIONNAIRE

- Have you ever felt you should Cut down on your drinking?
- Have people Annoyed you by criticizing your drinking?
- Have you ever felt bad or Guilty about your drinking?
- Have you ever had a drink first thing in the morning to steady your nerves or to get rid of a hangover (Eye opener)?

PRACTICE CASE 3

Ms. E is yet another patient at this busy primary care practice. She is a 40-year-old woman with chronic pelvic pain. She presents to see Dr. D today for a routine annual examination. Dr. D notes that Ms. E is overdue for cervical cancer screening and her weight has increased since last visit about 6 months ago to 110 kg with a BMI over 40 kg/m². Ms. E's medication list is notable for both hydrocodone/APAP 10/325 mg and oxycodone 5 mg.

Dr. D asks one of the nurses who is allocated and approved to review the state-controlled substance database to review Ms. E's recent prescriptions while Dr. D is completing orders and instructions for his previous patient. Review of the controlled substance database shows multiple short-term, small quantity prescriptions generally in the range of 10 to 15 tablets of short-acting narcotics from multiple emergency departments (EDs) in the area. Based on this full history, Dr. D estimates Ms. E has had at least two ED visits per month since her last primary care follow-up. Dr. D met Ms. E for the first time at her last visit, when she established care at the clinic after transferring from another provider. Dr. D recalls the patient being quite anxious at her last visit. The reason for visit today indicates only "routine examination."

On entering the room, Dr. D observes that Ms. E has kept the door slightly ajar. She is sitting facing the door, anxious and uncomfortable but not in acute distress. The visit begins with Dr. D asking what brought her into clinic today.

Ms. E: I want to get tested.

Dr. D: Sure, what were you looking to be tested for?

Ms. E: For everything. I want to make sure he didn't give me anything.

Dr. D: (Dr. D intuits that Ms. E is requesting screening for sexually transmitted infections (STIs) and that this is a difficult topic for her to discuss.) I sense this is difficult thing to talk about. Thank you for coming in today. Are you wanting to be screened for sexually transmitted infections?

Ms. E begins to cry and nods her head "yes." She goes on to share that she recently discovered that her current partner had multiple infidelities during their relationship, and he had inconsistently used condoms. Dr. D provides nonjudgmental support. He also notices

continued

some bruising on her arms. Concerned about the possibility of intimate partner violence (IPV), he asks:

Dr. D: Do you feel safe?

Ms. E: I would never hurt myself. I'm not suicidal.

Dr. D: I am hearing this is a hard time and you are not having thoughts of hurting yourself. [Pause] Has your partner hurt you in anyway?

Ms. E states that her recent boyfriend has gotten physical when they argue. Dr. D and Ms. E discuss talking to social work after the visit to help identify resources that may be available for Ms. E She is willing to meet with social work. Dr. D returns to discussing Ms. E's main concern for the visit: obtaining screening for STI. They go over a plan to test for chlamydia, gonorrhea, syphilis, hepatitis C, and HIV.

The USPSTF defines high-risk sexual behaviors as having multiple current partners, having a new partner, using condoms inconsistently, having sex while under the influence of alcohol or drugs, or having sex in exchange for money or drugs. Syphilis and hepatitis screening is indicated based on these high-risk sexual behaviors whereas the USPSTF recommendations include HIV testing for anyone requesting STI testing.

Ms. E is asked to do a self-swab to obtain the needed samples. Dr. D clarifies that some of the testing is done through blood work as well. Knowing that she is overdue for cervical cancer screening, he inquires if she would be willing to have a pelvic examination to also complete a Pap smear. Ms. E is adamant that she does not want a pelvic examination. Dr. D accepts her decision and invites the opportunity to discuss having a Pap smear in the future. The self-swab and laboratory work are obtained. Ms. E then meets with the clinic social worker for further safety assessment and to provide domestic violence resources.

Discussion

Based on the National Intimate Partner and Sexual Violence Survey, nearly in one in two women experience sexual violence other than rape, while nearly one in five experience rape at some point in their lifetime. For men, the rate is 1 in 5 and 1 in 71, respectively. A history of sexual trauma is associated with long-term physical health problems, especially chronic pain syndromes, as well as increased incidence of mental health diagnoses and high-risk behaviors.[48] There also is an association between a history of sexual violence and decreased rates of preventive health care with multiple studies showing lower rates of cervical cancer screening.[49,50] Of particular concern is the fact that women with a history of sexual trauma have an increased rate of STIs, cervical dysplasia, and invasive cervical cancer.[51] It is important to recognize that patient's reluctance to proceed with examination may be trauma based; gynecologic and breast examinations can trigger retraumatization.

Clinicians must remain attuned to a history of sexual trauma given the markedly high lifetime prevalence, although they must also remain sensitive regarding when and how to ask about sexual and nonsexual violence. Most victims will not share this history without being specifically asked. Before asking about sexual trauma, Taylor et al. recommend that the practitioner "should establish rapport and trust with their patient; monitor their own personal and professional attitudes and beliefs; be nonjudgmental and open to discussing sexual trauma; be prepared to acknowledge and validate the disclosure; make the patient feel safe and protected; ensure confidentiality; provide sufficient consultation time for discussion;" and be able to refer to specialty services when necessary.[48]

PRACTICE CASE 3 *(Continued)*

Promoting Preventive Services to Prevent Emergency Department Visits

Ms. E completed her STI testing, all of which returned negative. She returns to the clinic for a follow-up appointment 2 months later. In the interim, she has had three additional ED visits for abdominal pain or nausea. The workup into etiologies of her symptoms including multiple CT abdomen and pelvis scans has been unremarkable. Dr. D and Ms. E work out an agenda at the start of the visit. Ms. E is worried about continued weight gain, so they place weight gain as item number one. Dr. D also asks to discuss her recent ED visits. As part of their discussion on obesity, Dr. D recommends screening for obesity-related diseases, namely to evaluate for diabetes with a hemoglobin A1c and dyslipidemia with a lipid panel.

Ms. E shares that she finds herself overeating to the point of being uncomfortably full especially when stressed. Dr. D inquires nonjudgmentally, and Ms. E denies any purging behaviors such as self-induced vomiting or use of laxatives, enemas, or diuretics. Ms. E indicates that the past month has been particularly stressful, as one of her two children has been suspended from school.

Ms. E says she has tried many diets and may lose 5 to 10 pounds while following the diet but then regains more weight afterward. Dr. D explains the difference between diets and dietary or lifestyle changes. They discuss making gradual dietary changes over time, moving from unhealthy to increasingly healthy choices. Dr. D offers information for a one-time, free consultation with a nutritionist through the county health department. Ms. E wants to think about this option. They mutually set a dietary goal to cut the number of sodas she drinks per day from four to one before her next visit.

In addition to discussing dietary modifications, Dr. D and Ms. E also discuss the importance of physical activity. Ms. E is largely sedentary throughout the day, watching television when she is not driving her children to school and other activities. Ms. E offers that she could start walking for 60 minutes per day every day. Because she is not physically active, Dr. D makes the conscious effort to set an attainable goal, so he supports that this is a great goal and one for which to aim. However, he suggests starting at an initial goal of waking 5 minutes per day and adding 1 minute every 3 to 4 days so that by 6 months she is walking an hour per day.

Dr. D reflects to the patient that the day her son was suspended from school was also a day she went to the emergency room for abdominal pain. Ms. E does not necessarily see any connection between these two events. Dr. D goes on to explain how intertwined the mind and body are, and when people feel stressed, it often brings out physical symptoms. Ms. E has noticed that she does tend to get headaches when she is stressed, too. Wanting to introduce slowly the likely connection of her probable trauma history and stress to her chronic pain complaints, Dr. D decides to stop there. They go on to problem-solve around what other resources may be available instead of going to the emergency room. Ms. E admits she does not like the long wait. Dr. D shares that the clinic can often work out same day appointments with little wait and can even provide certain pain and nausea medications intramuscularly. They agree to continue to talk about her abdominal pain more at a follow-up appointment in a few weeks.

Discussion

The limited access to primary and preventive care among patients with SMI has been well known and researched for decades.[52,53] From a health system perspective, greater use of preventive services, especially in place of acute care services, can lead to cost savings. Reduced use of preventive services by patients with SMI has been linked with higher use of ED services.[54,55] Higher ED use not only can further fragment care but can be a significant driver to higher costs for health care systems. Although there are many additional factors that complicate or drive high ED use, ensuring appropriate preventive care for patients with psychiatric illness may lead not only to improved patient outcomes but also to lowered health system costs.

At the following visits, Dr. D continues to reinforce the mind–body connection and to reflect to Ms. E how her abdominal pain worsens when she experiences various stressors. Over the span of months, Dr. D builds rapport with Ms. E, and she agrees to see a mental health provider. She is starting to accept how pain, stress, and a history of trauma interrelate. As she learns alternative coping skills, Ms. E visits the ED fewer and fewer times. While she continues to have intermittent ED visits, she has transitioned to having a medical home and focusing on preventive care.

SUMMARY

It is important for the primary care provider to remember that although patients with behavioral health disorders can pose additional challenges in terms of accomplishing

primary, secondary, and tertiary prevention, they are some of the most vulnerable and most in need of preventive services. Patients with anxiety, mood, and psychotic disorders are prevalent in primary care, and SMI confers additional risk of morbidity and mortality from preventable illness. It therefore is incumbent on the primary care provider to adopt strategies to improve the likelihood of success in accomplishing recommended screening including among patients with mental illness. Matching one's approach to the patient's current state of change allows clinicians to partner with patients. Using a nonjudgmental approach and motivational interviewing strategies and adopting a multidisciplinary approach to help troubleshoot logistic barriers to screening can all be effective in improving patient well-being and longevity and, in the long run, can improve provider satisfaction and efficacy.

REFERENCES

1. Frayne SM, Halanych JH, Miller DR, et al. Disparities in diabetes care: impact of mental illness. *Arch Intern Med.* 2005;165(22):2631-2638.
2. Leung YW, Flora DB, Gravely S, Irvine J, Carney RM, Grace SL. The impact of premorbid and postmorbid depression onset on mortality and cardiac morbidity among patients with coronary heart disease: meta-analysis. *Psychosom Med.* 2012;74(8):786-801.
3. Paradise HT, Berlowitz DR, Ozonoff A, et al. Outcomes of anticoagulation therapy in patients with mental health conditions. *J Gen Intern Med.* 2014;29(6):855-861.
4. Felker B, Bush KR, Harel O, Shofer JB, Shores MM, Au DH. Added burden of mental disorders on health status among patients with chronic obstructive pulmonary disease. *Prim Care Companion J Clin Psychiatry.* 2010;12(4).
5. Colton CW, Manderscheid RW. Congruencies in increased mortality rates, years of potential life lost, and causes of death among public mental health clients in eight states. *Prev Chronic Dis.* 2006;3(2):A42.
6. McGrath J, Saha S, Chant D, Welham J. Schizophrenia: a concise overview of incidence, prevalence, and mortality. *Epidemiol Rev.* 2008;30:67-76.
7. Schaffer A, Cairney J, Cheung A, Veldhuizen S, Levitt A. Community survey of bipolar disorder in Canada: lifetime prevalence and illness characteristics. *Can J Psychiatry.* 2006;51(1):9-16.
8. Kessler RC, Berglund P, Demler O, Jin R, Merikangas KR, Walters EE. Lifetime prevalence and age-of-onset distributions of DSM-IV disorders in the National Comorbidity Survey Replication. *Arch Gen Psychiatry.* 2005;62(6):593-602.
9. Treating depression and anxiety in primary care. *Prim Care Companion J Clin Psychiatry.* 2008;10(2):145-152.
10. Viron MJ, Stern TA. The impact of serious mental illness on health and healthcare. *Psychosomatics.* 2010;51(6):458-465.
11. Vermani M, Marcus M, Katzman MA. Rates of detection of mood and anxiety disorders in primary care: a descriptive, cross-sectional study. *Prim Care Companion CNS Disord.* 2011;13(2).
12. DE Hert M, Correll CU, Bobes J, et al. Physical illness in patients with severe mental disorders. I. Prevalence, impact of medications and disparities in health care. *World Psychiatry.* 2011;10(1):52-77.

13. Viron M, Baggett T, Hill M, Freudenreich O. Schizophrenia for primary care providers: how to contribute to the care of a vulnerable patient population. *Am J Med.* 2012;125(3):223-230.

14. Xiong GL, Iosif AM, Bermudes RA, McCarron RM, Hales RE. Preventive medical services use among community mental health patients with severe mental illness: the influence of gender and insurance coverage. *Prim Care Companion J Clin Psychiatry.* 2010;12(5).

15. Parks J, Svendsen D, Singer P, Foti ME. *Morbidity and Mortality in People With Serious Mental Illness.* Alexandria, VA: National Association of State Mental Health Program Directors (NASMHPD) Medical Directors Council; 2006.

16. Casagrande SS, Anderson CA, Dalcin A, et al. Dietary intake of adults with serious mental illness. *Psychiatr Rehabil J.* 2011;35(2):137-140.

17. Center for Behavioral Health Statistics and Quality. *Results From the 2011 National Survey on Drug Use and Health: Summary of National Findings. HHS Publication No. SMA 12-4713 ed.* Rockville, MD: Substance Abuse and Mental Health Services Administration; 2012.

18. Lord O, Malone D, Mitchell AJ. Receipt of preventive medical care and medical screening for patients with mental illness: a comparative analysis. *Gen Hosp Psychiatry.* 2010;32(5):519-543.

19. Miller WR, Rollnick S. *Motivational Interviewing: Helping People Change.* 3rd ed. New York, NY: The Guilford Press; 2013.

20. Miller SJ, Foran-Tuller K, Ledergerber J, Jandorf L. Motivational interviewing to improve health screening uptake: a systematic review. *Patient Educ Couns.* 2017;100(2):190-198.

21. Zomahoun HT, Guenette L, Gregoire JP, et al. Effectiveness of motivational interviewing interventions on medication adherence in adults with chronic diseases: a systematic review and meta-analysis. *Int J Epidemiol.* 2016.

22. Farholm A, Sorensen M. Motivation for physical activity and exercise in severe mental illness: a systematic review of intervention studies. *Int J Ment Health Nurs.* 2016;25(3):194-205.

23. Hensrud DD. Clinical preventive medicine in primary care: background and practice: 1. Rationale and current preventive practices. *Mayo Clin Proc.* 2000;75(2):165-172.

24. Rubio-Valera M, Pons-Vigues M, Martinez-Andres M, Moreno-Peral P, Berenguera A, Fernandez A. Barriers and facilitators for the implementation of primary prevention and health promotion activities in primary care: a synthesis through meta-ethnography. *PLoS One.* 2014;9(2):e89554.

25. Bobes J, Arango C, Aranda P, Carmena R, Garcia-Garcia M, Rejas J. Cardiovascular and metabolic risk in outpatients with schizophrenia treated with antipsychotics: results of the CLAMORS study. *Schizophr Res.* 2007;90(1-3):162-173.

26. Glasheen C, Hedden SL, Forman-Hoffman VL, Colpe LJ. Cigarette smoking behaviors among adults with serious mental illness in a nationally representative sample. *Ann Epidemiol.* 2014;24(10):776-780.

27. Szmulewicz AG, Angriman F, Pedroso FE, Vazquez C, Martino DJ. Long-term antipsychotic use and major cardiovascular events: a retrospective cohort study. *J Clin Psychiatry.* 2017.

28. Simon V, van Winkel R, De Hert M. Are weight gain and metabolic side effects of atypical antipsychotics dose dependent? A literature review. *J Clin Psychiatry.* 2009;70(7):1041-1050.

29. Consensus development conference on antipsychotic drugs and obesity and diabetes. *J Clin Psychiatry.* 2004;65(2):267-272.

30. Jennex A, Gardner DM. Monitoring and management of metabolic risk factors in outpatients taking antipsychotic drugs: a controlled study. *Can J Psychiatry.* 2008; 53(1):34-42.

31. Morrato EH, Newcomer JW, Allen RR, Valuck RJ. Prevalence of baseline serum glucose and lipid testing in users of second-generation antipsychotic drugs: a retrospective, population-based study of Medicaid claims data. *J Clin Psychiatry.* 2008;69(2):316-322.

32. Mitchell AJ, Delaffon V, Vancampfort D, Correll CU, De Hert M. Guideline concordant monitoring of metabolic risk in people treated with antipsychotic medication: systematic review and meta-analysis of screening practices. *Psychol Med.* 2012;42(1):125-147.

33. Nasrallah HA, Meyer JM, Goff DC, et al. Low rates of treatment for hypertension, dyslipidemia and diabetes in schizophrenia: data from the CATIE schizophrenia trial sample at baseline. *Schizophr Res.* 2006;86(1-3):15-22.

34. Alvarez-Jimenez M, Hetrick SE, Gonzalez-Blanch C, Gleeson JF, McGorry PD. Non-pharmacological management of antipsychotic-induced weight gain: systematic review and meta-analysis of randomised controlled trials. *Br J Psychiatry.* 2008;193(2):101-107.

35. Maayan L, Vakhrusheva J, Correll CU. Effectiveness of medications used to attenuate antipsychotic-related weight gain and metabolic abnormalities: a systematic review and meta-analysis. *Neuropsychopharmacology.* 2010;35(7):1520-1530.

36. Newcomer JW, Weiden PJ, Buchanan RW. Switching antipsychotic medications to reduce adverse event burden in schizophrenia: establishing evidence-based practice. *J Clin Psychiatry.* 2013;74(11):1108-1120.

37. Moriarty AS, Gilbody S, McMillan D, Manea L. Screening and case finding for major depressive disorder using the Patient Health Questionnaire (PHQ-9): a meta-analysis. *Gen Hosp Psychiatry.* 2015;37(6):567-576.

38. Unutzer J, Katon W, Callahan CM, et al. Collaborative care management of late-life depression in the primary care setting: a randomized controlled trial. *JAMA.* 2002;288(22):2836-2845.

39. Katon WJ, Von Korff M, Lin EH, et al. The pathways study: a randomized trial of collaborative care in patients with diabetes and depression. *Arch Gen Psychiatry.* 2004;61(10):1042-1049.

40. Ell K, Xie B, Quon B, Quinn DI, Dwight-Johnson M, Lee PJ. Randomized controlled trial of collaborative care management of depression among low-income patients with cancer. *J Clin Oncol.* 2008;26(27):4488-4496.

41. Vohringer PA, Jimenez MI, Igor MA, et al. Detecting mood disorder in resource-limited primary care settings: comparison of a self-administered screening tool to general practitioner assessment. *J Med Screen.* 2013; 20(3):118-124.

42. Sasdelli A, Lia L, Luciano CC, Nespeca C, Berardi D, Menchetti M. Screening for bipolar disorder symptoms in depressed primary care attenders: comparison between mood disorder questionnaire and hypomania checklist (HCL-32). *Psychiatry J.* 2013;2013:548349.

43. Jin J. Breast cancer screening: benefits and harms. *JAMA.* 2014;312(23):2585.

44. Abel KM, Heatlie HF, Howard LM, Webb RT. Sex- and age-specific incidence of fractures in mental illness: a historical, population-based cohort study. *J Clin Psychiatry.* 2008;69(9):1398-1403.

45. Vestergaard P, Rejnmark L, Mosekilde L. Anxiolytics, sedatives, antidepressants, neuroleptics and the risk of fracture. *Osteoporos Int.* 2006;17(6):807-816.

46. Holt RI. Osteoporosis in people with severe mental illness: a forgotten condition. *Maturitas.* 2010;67(1):1-2.

47. Michael YL, Lin JS, Whitlock EP, et al. U.S. Preventive Services Task Force Evidence Syntheses, formerly Systematic Evidence Reviews. *Interventions to Prevent Falls in Older Adults: An Updated Systematic Review.* Rockville, MD: Agency for Healthcare Research and Quality (US); 2010.

48. Taylor SC, Pugh J, Goodwach R, Coles J. Sexual trauma in women—the importance of identifying a history of sexual violence. *Aust Fam Physician.* 2012;41(7):538-541.

49. Coker AL, Hopenhayn C, DeSimone CP, Bush HM, Crofford L. Violence against women raises risk of cervical cancer. *J Women's Health.* 2009;18(8):1179-1185.

50. Farley M, Golding JM, Minkoff JR. Is a history of trauma associated with a reduced likelihood of cervical cancer screening? *J Fam Pract.* 2002;51(10):827-831.

51. Springs FE, Friedrich WN. Health risk behaviors and medical sequelae of childhood sexual abuse. *Mayo Clin Proc.* 1992;67(6):527-532.

52. Druss BG, Rosenheck RA. Mental disorders and access to medical care in the United States. *Am J Psychiatry.* 1998;155(12):1775-1777.

53. Druss BG, Bradford WD, Rosenheck RA, Radford MJ, Krumholz HM. Quality of medical care and excess mortality in older patients with mental disorders. *Arch Gen Psychiatry.* 2001;58(6):565-572.

54. Hackman AL, Goldberg RW, Brown CH, et al. Use of emergency department services for somatic reasons by people with serious mental illness. *Psychiatr Serv (Washington, DC).* 2006;57(4):563-566.

55. Berren MR, Santiago JM, Zent MR, Carbone CP. Health care utilization by persons with severe and persistent mental illness. *Psychiatr Serv (Washington, DC).* 1999;50(4):559-561.

4

THE PATIENT AND YOU: PSYCHOLOGICAL AND CULTURAL CONSIDERATIONS

Alan Koike, MD, MSHS, Shaun P. Rafael, DO, and Hendry Ton, MD, MS

Mr. Y is a 24-year-old Mandarin-speaking Chinese man who arrives with his father 10 minutes late to an appointment at a primary care clinic. With the use of an interpreter, the patient raises concerns about "abdominal pain" and "headaches" for a year. Social history reveals that the patient, his parents, and his siblings immigrated to the United States from rural China 2 years ago. They live in a small apartment in an inner-city neighborhood with his aunt and uncle. Mr. Y has the equivalent of a fifth-grade education and speaks very limited English. He was a factory worker back in China and now works part time in a restaurant making minimum wage. Physical examination, review of systems, and results from a recent diagnostic workup at an urgent care center do not clearly point to any somatic disorders.

CLINICAL HIGHLIGHTS

- Patients experiencing mental health problems may endorse somatic symptoms due to social and cultural factors.
- Language barriers can adversely influence the development of an accurate diagnosis and treatment plan. When possible, interpreters should be used during examinations to decrease the chance for miscommunication.
- Structural barriers may contribute to the patient's presentation and lead to health disparities.
- A structured cultural formulation is a useful tool for assessing cultural and linguistic issues.

CLINICAL SIGNIFICANCE

The good physician treats the disease; the great physician treats the patient who has the disease.

William Osler

Each patient has a story. This story consists of their illness, their experiences, their social situation, and their beliefs. Understanding their story and reflecting on it with compassion and empathy is fundamental to the doctor–patient relationship. Comas-Dias recommends adopting an open and inclusive perspective.[1] This approach starts with the desire to work with patients of diverse cultural backgrounds. It emphasizes understanding the patient's point of view, developing a therapeutic relationship, and adapting one's approach to meet the patient's needs. This is a reciprocal learning experience that requires self-reflection and continuous assessment. Also, this perspective incorporates the concept of "cultural humility," which starts not with the patient's belief system, but rather with the health care provider's beliefs, assumptions, and goals of the encounter.[2] Often in medicine, we tend to view culture as something made up of fixed facts and thus we mistakenly believe it can be completely understood. However, as practitioners, we should be humble when considering our patients' stories. Narratives cannot be reduced to oversimplified stories, as they are dynamic entities that are full of ambiguity and contradiction.[3] We should strive to constantly engage in self-evaluation, working to understand our own story, our expectations of our patients' stories, and how we ultimately affect the patient encounter.

Our patients come from diverse backgrounds, and understanding their narratives is fundamental to providing quality care. Ethnic minority populations are growing at a tremendous rate in the United States, but the growth of health care professionals from some minority groups (e.g., African-Americans, Latinos, and Native Americans) has not kept up with their representation in the general population.[4] The Institute of Medicine's groundbreaking report, *Unequal Treatment*, found that racial and ethnic minorities—even those with equivalent access to health services—receive lower quality of care than nonminorities for several medical conditions.[5]

These disparities in health care are associated with worse outcomes and increased mortality. Inequities give rise to health disparities that adversely affect groups of people who have systematically experienced greater obstacles to health, based on characteristics historically linked to discrimination or exclusion: ethnicity, religion, socioeconomic status, gender, age sexual orientation, etc.[6] For example, studies have shown that lower household income, low level of education, and unemployment are factors leading to common mental health disorders such as depression and anxiety.[7,8]

The Surgeon General's Supplement to the Report on Mental Health entitled, *Mental Health: Culture, Race and Ethnicity* identified striking disparities in mental health care for racial and ethnic minorities.[9] It reported that minorities have less access, availability, and quality of mental health services. Furthermore, a consequence of this disparity is that racial and ethnic minorities bear a disproportionate burden of disability from untreated and inadequately treated mental health problems. Sadly, a recent study found no reduction in racial-ethnic disparities in access to mental health care between 2004 and 2012. More disturbing still, this study found the disparities actually increased for African-Americans and Hispanics during this period.[10]

STRUCTURAL COMPETENCE

Cultural competency emerged two decades ago in response to US medical system's failure to respond the diversity issues of our patients.[11] Yet it is still unclear whether having culturally sensitive clinicians improves health outcomes. Structural competency[12] has emerged as a new paradigm. Health inequity must be conceptualized in relation to the institutional and social conditions that effect health-related resources and, ultimately, health outcomes. A recent Robert Wood Johnson survey found that 85% of primary care providers believed that unmet social needs are leading to worse health for Americans, but they did not "feel confident in their capacity to meet their patients' social needs."[13] Structure includes not only buildings, transportation systems, and communication systems but also the less visible bureaucratic structures and assumptions embedded in the language and attitudes of the health care system that may create barriers to care for some groups.[11]

The paradigm of structural competency is made up of five core competencies.[11] The first is the understanding that structures shape clinical interactions. We must acknowledge that physical, economic, and political factors affect health care decisions. For example, rather than simply focusing on patient education to address medication nonadherence, one may look at the costs of the medications, where the patient fills their medications, and how side effects from the medications may affect the patient's ability to care for their children. The second component of structural competency is the need to develop an extra-clinical language of structure. Taking our cue from economists, historians, political scientists, anthropologists, and sociologists, we should begin talking in terms of urban planning, public policy, urban food deserts, transportation, access to clean water, resource-poor environments, and systems of privilege to truly address the health needs of our patients. Third is the need to rearticulate cultural presentation in structural terms. The idea is not to dismiss the importance of culture, but rather to more deeply examine the ways in which complex cultural structures lead to inequalities and barriers to care. The fourth component is to imagine structural interventions. We must recognize how structures affect our patients' interactions with us and figure out how we can intervene. In *Box 4-1*, we briefly describe how structural competence might improve patient care. The fifth and final component of structural competency is to develop structural humility.[3] We must recognize the limitations of structural competency and humbly acknowledge that we may never fully understand our patients or their circumstances.

BOX 4-1   STRUCTURAL INTERVENTIONS

1. Recognize the potential power inequalities between you and your patient.
2. Think of how traditional hierarchies may silence your most vulnerable patients (race, gender, sexuality, class, immigration status).
3. Pay extra attention to the social history in your assessment.
4. Visit you patients' communities.
5. Partner with community organizations.

We know that social issues affect our patients' health and obtaining a social history has long been part of a thorough clinical interview. Structural competency challenges us to explore the social determinants of health with a new lens. We propose obtaining a more comprehensive social history to properly assess the patient's treatment plans. Primary care providers may need multiple visits to obtain a rich social history, and it is important to revisit these questions over time. For example, a spiritual history might be easily incorporated into the social history. Considering time constraints, a spiritual history should be direct and brief but elicit sufficient information to determine whether more time is needed for a more in-depth discussion. The clinician might ask, "You mentioned earlier how difficult it has been to deal with diabetes and some of the associated pain symptoms. When you're feeling particularly ill, what keeps you going? Do you consider yourself a religious or spiritual person?"

Structural competency also calls on providers to examine the structure, policy, and processes that affect how health care is delivered and received. There is significant evidence that health care disparities are perpetuated not only at the individual provider level but also at the level of the health care organizations. Programs and policies that ensure culturally and linguistically appropriate communication, such as formally trained health care interpreters and language-appropriate patient resources, for example, may improve patient safety and reduce overall cost.[14] Likewise, recruitment programs that specifically diversify the health care workforce can improve health care access and cultural competence of their organizations.[15] These reflect some of the 15 guidelines and mandates put forth in the National Culturally and Linguistically Appropriate Services Standards, developed by the Office of Minority Health in 2001 and updated in 2013[16] to "provide effective, equitable, understandable, and respectful quality care and services that are responsive to diverse cultural health beliefs and practices, preferred languages, health literacy, and other communication needs." These standards are organized into three domains: (1) Governance, Leadership, and Workforce; (2) Communication and Language Assistance; and (3) Engagement, Continuous Improvement, and Accountability. These standards help establish a blueprint for transforming health and health care structures to reduce health care disparities and better serve the needs of diverse communities.

A STRUCTURED CULTURAL FORMULATION

Many providers recognize that cultural issues may play an important role in interactions with patients, yet feel ill-equipped to address these concerns. The complexity of the interplay between culture and illness can make this process overwhelming. Factual knowledge about cultural groups, while essential, can have limited utility without a framework to organize and to make sense of the information. The Outline for Cultural Formulation (OCF), first introduced in the DSM-IV[17] and revised for the DSM-5 in 2013, provides a systematic

approach for assessing the impact of culture on illness and treatment.[18] Although designed for the psychiatric encounter, we believe the OCF may be useful in the primary care setting as well. The OCF is made up of five components: (1) Cultural identity of the patient; (2) Cultural conceptualizations of distress and illness; (3) Psychosocial stressors and cultural features of vulnerability and resilience; (4) Cultural elements of the relationship between the individual and the clinician; and (5) Overall cultural assessment.

CULTURAL IDENTITY

Cultural identity refers to the multifaceted set of identities that contribute to an individual's understanding and interactions with his or her environment. Although ethnicity is an important part of cultural identity, other factors such as religious and spiritual beliefs, country of origin, sexual orientation, and socioeconomic status may be as or more important in any given person.

CULTURAL CONCEPTUALIZATIONS OF DISTRESS

Primary care providers should be aware that patients may have other explanations for their illnesses that differ from Western medical concepts. Asian models of illness, for example, might include explanations that imbalances of hot and cold energy may cause illnesses, which can be cured by eating foods to make up for the imbalance. Latino illness beliefs regarding diabetes might emphasize emotional factors such as feelings of social isolation as causes of the disease and may lead to a more fatalistic view of the course of the illness.[19]

PSYCHOSOCIAL STRESSORS AND CULTURAL FEATURES OF VULNERABILITY AND RESILIENCE

The third component of the OCF can be thought of as stressors and supports for the patient and can be conceptualized as the role that the patient plays in his or her family and community. Examples of roles that patients could play include the primary breadwinner, parental caregiver, childcare provider, dutiful child, cultural broker, interpreter, etc.

CULTURAL FEATURES OF THE RELATIONSHIP BETWEEN THE INDIVIDUAL AND THE CLINICIAN

Stereotypes, cultural misunderstandings, and conflicts in world views that affect social relationships outside of the health care environment play a significant role in the clinical exchange. It is important to be aware of the influence of these cultural factors on the patient–provider relationship.

TABLE 4-1 High-Yield Questions		
SECTION	**QUESTION**	**RELEVANCE**
History of present illness	**1.** People often understand their problems in their own way, which may be similar or different from how doctors explain the problem. How would you describe your problem to someone else? **2.** Sometimes people use particular words or phrases to talk about their problems. Is there a specific term or expression that describes your problem?	Opens dialogue about patient's cultural beliefs and idioms.
Medical history	**1.** Often, people also look for help from people outside of medical clinics and hospitals. What kind of treatment from other sources have you sought for your problem? **2.** How helpful have they been?	Ascertains cultural resources for healing and the perceived effectiveness of such healing practices.
Social history	**1.** Please tell me about the important people, positive and negative, in your life including your intimate or romantic partners. How have they affected or been affected by your problem? **2.** Are there barriers that make it difficult for you to get the help you need, such as financial barriers, insurance issues, discrimination, language barriers, or cultural issues? **3.** Are there considerations about your background, such as culture, race, ethnicity, sexual orientation, or gender identity that you feel I should know about to give you the best care possible?	These questions help patients elaborate on their cultural identity and sociocultural determinants that are relevant to their treatment and health.

OVERALL CULTURAL ASSESSMENT

The overall assessment should include the key issues identified in the previous four sections of the cultural formulation. Treatment planning should incorporate strategies that address culturally based problems or build on cultural strengths. *Table 4-1* suggests some high-yield questions that may be useful in assessing the patient.

PRACTICE CASE

Introduction

Mr. Y is a 24-year-old Mandarin-speaking Chinese man who arrives with his father 10 minutes late to an appointment at a primary care clinic. With the use of an interpreter, the patient is said to complain of "abdominal pain" and "headaches" for a year. History reveals that the patient, his parents, and his siblings immigrated to the United States from rural China 2 years ago. They live in a small apartment in an inner-city neighborhood with his aunt and uncle. Mr. Y has the equivalent of a fifth-grade education, only speaking very limited English. He was a factory worker back in China and now works part time in a restaurant making minimum wage.

Before performing a physical examination, the provider kindly asks the patient's father to leave the room to speak with Mr. Y privately. After his father leaves, Mr. Y is asked if he has any other concerns. He hesitantly shares that it is painful when he urinates. It is revealed that he is having unprotected sexual intercourse with multiple same-sex partners. Additionally, Mr. Y complains that he has trouble concentrating at work and has been experiencing *fan nao* (which the interpreter notes as meaning "feeling vexed"). As a follower of Taoist beliefs, he reports feeling that his *qi* is being blocked.

DISCUSSION

A systematic approach to cultural formulation can be used as a guide to assess a patient's culture and enhance your interaction and understanding of your patient.

Cultural Identity

In this case, the provider recognized that the patient had several intersecting identities with varying levels of significance. The concept of intersectionality can be helpful in forming a more holistic, culturally informed understanding of all patients. Intersectionality theorizes that the various aspects of a person's identity—including, but not limited to, gender, ethnicity, socioeconomic status, age, sexual orientation, religion, education, and disability—are not mutually exclusive.[20] In other words, all aspects of one's identity are intricately interrelated and should be examined collectively rather than in complete isolation. However, it is still important to identify and appreciate each individual aspect so that one can consider how they can influence one another.

Ethnicity

Ethnicity can be defined as the fact or state of belonging to a social group that has a common national or cultural tradition.[21] Language, ancestry, and geographic location are other characteristics that can connect people identifying with a particular ethnic group. Ethnicity is often used synonymously with the terms *culture* and *race*, although one should recognize that there are nuanced, but not unimportant, differences between them.

In the case example, Mr. Y is a young man from China. This alone should elicit the provider's awareness of the variable beliefs, customs, and social mores that are unique to the Chinese people. A general example would be to appreciate the virtues of modesty and politeness commonly shared among those of Asian descent, which might affect the way in which the provider will conduct an interview and examination of the patient.[22] Another example is the notion of stigma surrounding mental illness among the Asian population. As a recent immigrant, Mr. Y is more likely to hold traditional Chinese values and thus may have significantly more reluctance discussing psychiatric symptoms.[23]

In addition to nationality, migration status is another aspect that can shape ethnic identity. Not only is Mr. Y Chinese, but he is also an immigrant. It might be important to explore the context of his migration history (including impetus for immigration, experiences of loss, or trauma) as this can help to identify important factors influencing a patient's relationship with his or her culture and may reveal sources of stress related to underlying mental health problems.

Sexual and Gender Identity

The lesbian, gay, bisexual, and transgender (LGBT) community is a very diverse group of people and much more heterogeneous than the label LGBT would suggest. The term is also commonly used to include individuals who identify with one or more of many other nonheterosexual and gender nonconforming labels, such as queer, intersex, and asexual. Although imperfect and not completely exhaustive, the notion of the "gender unicorn" helps to illustrate the different elements that comprise identity in the context of LGBT community: gender identity, gender expression, sex assigned at birth, physical, and emotional attraction.

Those in the LGBT community are disproportionately affected by stigma and mental health issues.[7] A study showed that those in the LGBT population are 1.5 times more likely to experience depression and anxiety than heterosexual people.[24] Although mood disorders are prevalent, providers should be aware of the increased potential for other diagnoses such as eating disorders and substance use. Suicidality is also more common within the community. Among LGBT youth, research shows about 4% higher rate of suicide attempts than in their straight counterparts with victimization and low social support as notable risk factors.[25]

In this case example, the patient's reticence in sharing his sexual behaviors may indicate concern for being judged, misunderstood, or possibly internal conflict. His sexual orientation and ethnic identity might be at odds, as homosexuality within some Asian cultures does not align with typical societal norms. Such a conflict between sexual and ethnic identities may be a source of significant stress relating to his chief complaints.

Cultural Conceptualizations of Distress

Limited or lack of communication in health care is associated with disparities in access to services, as well as in diagnosis and treatment.[26] Language barriers can impede access, compromise quality of care, and increase the risk of adverse health outcomes among patients with limited English proficiency.[16] Mr. Y does not speak English, so in an effort to communicate effectively and accurately, his provider is using a qualified interpreter, who should be regarded as an integral part of the clinical team. Interpreters should be trained and fluent in both the source and target language lest there be a high risk for adding or omitting information, changing the message, or giving inappropriate opinions. Other helpful tips for using interpreters in the primary care setting are included in *Table 4-2*.

TABLE 4-2 How to Work Effectively With an Interpreter

1. Greet the patient first, then introduce yourself to the interpreter.
2. Look directly at the patient throughout, not at the interpreter.
3. Speak at an even pace and pause after a full thought.
4. Assume that everything you say will be interpreted.
5. If you must address the interpreter about an issue, let the patient know what you are going to discuss.
6. Avoid the use of slang, technical medical terminology, and complicated sentences.
7. Ask the interpreter to point out potential cultural misunderstandings that may occur.
8. Do not hold the interpreter responsible for what the patient says or doesn't say.
9. Be aware that many concepts have no linguistic or conceptual equivalent in other languages.

Adapted from Cynthia E. Roat MPH, 12/2007 "Communicating Effectively through an Interpreter" from the Cross Cultural Health Care Program.

PRACTICE CASE *(Continued)*

With the use of an interpreter, the patient is said to complain of "abdominal pain" and "headaches" for several months. He was told by a doctor in China that he had shenjing shuairuo. Additionally, Mr. Y reports feeling that his qi is being blocked.

DISCUSSION

Individuals, even within the same set of cultures, can have very different ideas about their illnesses. Alternate descriptions can be used by patients to communicate their distress. Clinicians should try to elicit the patient's "explanatory model" of each illness, which the provider should compare with their own model of the patient's illness.[27]

Mr. Y expresses various nonspecific complaints that may or may not be related to one another. He states that his *qi* is also being affected. Further inquiry might reveal that he believes his *qi* is a cause for his headaches and concentration difficulties—or vice versa. He also mentions shenjing shuairuo ("weakness of the nervous system" in Mandarin Chinese),[28] which is a cultural syndrome based in Chinese traditional medicine that might translate in Western culture to anxiety and depression. With this in mind, the provider could ask the interpreter for clarification on the concept or continue to explore the presence of a mood disorder.

Although it is well understood that mental illness can manifest with physical symptoms, somatization is an example of an idiom of distress that is frequently employed by patients. Asian and Latino people, in particular, will often convey psychological issues through somatic complaints. Mr. Y's abdominal pain should be taken seriously and appropriately worked up to rule out medical causes, but in the context of his other symptoms, there should be some suspicion that the pain is psychiatric in nature.

Once the patient's explanatory model is understood, clinicians can develop a collaborative approach that bridges the cultural divide, show an understanding of the patient's perspective, and negotiate a treatment plan which may increase adherence to treatment.

The patient uses different ways to convey and interpret his illness. He endorses physical symptoms that might be somatic manifestations of an underlying psychiatric disorder. He then explains his condition in the context of his spiritual beliefs, citing the imbalance of forces he refers to as his "qi." The provider now recognizes that the patient's explanation of his illness is different than their own, and that the patient may have had very little contact with or understanding of Western medicine. In addition, the patient appears unfamiliar with concepts of mental illness such as depression or anxiety.

Spirituality and Religion

Spirituality is an often-overlooked element of individual cultural identity and understanding of illness. The United States is home to a number of diverse religious faiths.[29] Surveys have found that 95% of people in the United States believe in God and 84% of Americans claim that religion is important in their lives.[30] In the case example, Mr. Y is a follower Taoism, which is a Chinese religious philosophy that views the world as containing opposite and complementary forces yin and yang.[31] He believes that imbalance of these forces is partially resulting in his illness and blockage of his qi, or "vital energy." Mr. Y might be more accepting of his diagnosis if the provider incorporates his beliefs to help explain his illness. At the end of the encounter the provider recommends a holistic treatment plan that includes medications and acupuncture (a treatment that has roots in Chinese medicine and is gaining popularity in Western culture for various ailments).

Psychosocial Stressors and Cultural Features of Vulnerability and Resilience

Social Determinants of Mental Health

The social determinants of health are the circumstances in which people are born, grow up, live, work, and age and the systems put in place to deal with illness.[32] Educational attainment, occupation, food security, access to health care, transportation, social support, adverse childhood experiences, and neighborhood infrastructure are such examples. Mental health is influenced by these environments, which are in turn shaped by a wider set of forces including economics, social policies, and politics.[33]

PRACTICE CASE *(Continued)*

Mr. Y and his family live in a small apartment in an inner-city neighborhood with his aunt and uncle. Mr. Y has the equivalent of a fifth-grade education, only speaking very limited English. He was a factory worker back in China and now works part time in a restaurant making minimum wage.

DISCUSSION

Mr. Y is 10 minutes late to his appointment, but rather than asking him to reschedule, the provider can use this as an opportunity to learn about the patient's environment. Living in an inner city, transportation was likely to have been a large barrier to a timely arrival. The patient and his father may have had to take several buses to get to the clinic, traveling across town because there are no other primary care providers in the area. Perhaps they also had trouble navigating the bus system because of their limited English-reading ability.

Although one provider may not have the power to address these issues at the policy level, there are small interventions that can be helpful. Providers might create or locate a resource guide that can link patients to the available various community-based social services, including alternative housing options. Screening patients for poverty, food insecurity, and housing stability should be part of the initial assessment. Maintaining flexibility to one's practice, allowing for same-day scheduling, and expanding appointment schedules may help to alleviate some of the barriers to accessing care. Ultimately, providers might make an impact by identifying and educating patients about how the various social, economic, and environmental factors affect their health.

Cultural Features of the Relationship Between the Individual and the Clinician

It is key that the provider agrees to see Mr. Y even though he is 10 minutes late to his appointment. Such flexibility no doubt puts stress on the provider, but it conveys a sense of caring that helps build the relationship between the provider and the patients. The patient was evaluated with Mandarin-speaking interpreter. This reassures the patient that the provider will make a concerted effort to understand the patient's perspective of his physical and emotional health. The provider asks the patient, family, and the interpreter to provide some insight about the concept of "shenjing shuairuo" and their understanding about what the treatment might be.

Mr. Y is a follower Taoism. Several studies suggest that many patients prefer a clinician who is accepting and attentive to their religious or spiritual beliefs.[34] Most patients seem to want their providers to inquire into coping and means of social support and, when indicated, be willing to participate in a spiritually oriented discussion. Patients' spiritual or religious faith may play a role in their medical decision-making, such as consideration of blood transfusions, planning an advance directive, or considering do-not-resuscitate status.

Providers should attempt to create a welcoming and safe space that is inclusive of LGBT individuals. This includes a physical environment in which staff are trained to provide sensitive care and are educated on LGBT-specific terminology. Brochures and reading material in multiple languages that are all-encompassing—that are reflective of both straight and LGBT culture can be a small, but powerful sign of acceptance. A safe space also includes one in which the provider avoids assumptions and stereotypes and elicits clarification when needed. Mr. Y did not disclose the

symptoms related to his genitals or share his sexual behavior until his father left the room. The provider should avoid discussing Mr. Y's sexuality once his father returns unless he has explicit permission. He may be experiencing shame surrounding his homosexuality, particularly related to fear about what his parents might think. When caring for LGBT individuals, providers can use normalizing language to validate their feelings and foster a sense of positive self-identity. Providers should also continually reflect on their own biases and consider how they may influence the care they deliver.

Overall Cultural Assessment

Given his cultural identity, recent immigration, and poor education, the provider hypothesized that the patient was not familiar with Western medical concepts. As the only son of a working-class family, he may feel a strong sense of duty to help provide for his parents. However, his identification as a gay man appeared much more tentative. Ethnic, class, and sexual identities emerge as factors that may be compromising his health and affecting his ability to seek treatment. The provider recognized the importance of integrating the patient's spiritual beliefs into the conceptualization and treatment of his illness. The provider also acknowledged significant losses and stresses that the patient experiences as an immigrant living with limited means and as a homosexual with conflicting family values. Expressing commitment to help alleviate some of the physical and emotional suffering, the provider encourages the patient to seek support within his religious community such as Taoist temples and provides information about if possible minority LGBT resources. Because of the prevalence of mental illness within minority and LGBT communities, it is important to understand how sexual/gender identity may be a factor in an underlying psychiatric disorder. Thus, Mr. Y's provider should screen for depression, anxiety, and thoughts of self-harm in this case.

CONCLUSION

Unlike the practice of diagnostic medicine where the explanations of illness are largely governed by the principle of parsimony, performing a cultural formulation should not be an exercise in simplification and reducing assumptions. Rather, every patient should be considered a complex being of many unique identities and needs, which the provider should attempt to understand in a way that is as holistic and inclusive as possible.

PRACTICAL RESOURCES

Resources for Spiritual Issues.

- http://depts.washington.edu/bioethx/topics/spirit.html
- http://www.gwish.org/

Resources for Language and Cultural Issues.

- http://www.jointcommission.org/PatientSafety/HLC/
- http://ethnomed.org
- http://erc.msh.org/
- http://www.thinkculturalhealth.org/

REFERENCES

1. Comas-Dias L. *Multicultural Care: A Clinician's Guide to Cultural Competence.* Washington, DC: American Psychological Association; 2012.
2. Trevalon M, Murray-Garcia J. Cultural humility versus cultural competence: a critical distinction in defining physician training outcomes in multicultural education. *J Health Care Poor Underserved.* 1998;9:117-125.
3. DasGupta S. Narrative humility. *Lancet.* 2008;22:980-981.
4. Smedley BD, Butler AS, Bristow LR, eds. *In the Nation's Compelling Interest: Ensuring Diversity in the Health Care Workforce/Committee on Institutional and Policy-Level Strategies for Increasing the Diversity of the U.S. Health Care Workforce.* Washington, DC: National Academies; 2004.
5. Smedley BD, Stith AY, Nelson AR, eds. *Unequal Treatment: Confronting Racial and Ethnic Disparities in Health Care.* Washington, DC: National Academies; 2002.
6. *Healthy People 2020.* Washington, DC: U.S. Department of Health and Human Services, Office of Disease Prevention and Health Promotion. Available a www.healthypeople.gov. Accessed May 24, 2017.
7. Bostwick WB, Boyd CJ, Hughes TL, Mccabe SE. Dimensions of sexual orientation and the prevalence of mood and anxiety disorders in the United States. *Am J Public Health.* 2010;100(3):468-475.
8. Sareen J, Afifi TO, Mcmillan KA, Asmundson GJ. Relationship between household income and mental disorders. *Arch Gen Psychiatry.* 2011;68(4):419-427.
9. United States Department of Health and Human Services (USDHHS). *Mental Health: Culture, Race, and Ethnicity: A Supplement to Mental Health: A Report of the Surgeon General.* Rockville, MD: US Dept of Health and Human Services, Public Health Service, Office of the Surgeon General; 2001.
10. LeCook B, Trinh M, Li Z, Hou SS, Progovac AM. Trends in racial-ethnic disparities in access to mental health care, 2004-2012. *Psychiatr Serv.* 2017;68(1):9-16.
11. Metzl JM, Hansen H. Structural competency: theorizing a new medical engagement with stigma and inequality. *Soc Sci Med.* 2013;103:126-133.
12. Metzl JM. *The Protest Psychosis: How Schizophrenia Became a Black Disease.* Boston: Becon; 2010.
13. Harris Interactive. *2011 Physicians' daily life report. Electronic document.* http://www.rwjf.org/en/library/research/2011/12/health-care-s-blind-side.html?cid=XEM_2809280. Accessed June 18, 2017.
14. Berstein J, Berstein E, Dave A, et al. Trained medical interpreters in the emergency department: effects on services, subsequent charges, and follow-up. Department of Maternal and child Health. Boston, Massachusetts. *J Immigr Health.* 2002;4(4):171-176.
15. Jackson C, Gracia J. Addressing health and health-care disparities: the role of a diverse workforce and the social determinants of health. *Publ Health Rep.* 2014;129(suppl 2):57-61.
16. Services (CLAS) in Health and Health Care: A Blueprint for Advancing and Sustaining CLAS Policy and Practice; Office of Minority Health (OMH), U.S. Department of Health Office of Minority Health. *National standards for culturally and linguistically appropriate and human services, April, 2013, Vol. 191.* Retrieved from https://www.thinkcultural-health.hhs.gov/pdfs/EnhancedCLASStandardsBlueprint.pdf.
17. American Psychiatric Association. *Outline for cultural formulation and glossary of culture-bound syndromes.* In: *Diagnostic and Statistical Manual, Fourth Edition, Text Revision (DSM-IV-TR).* Washington, DC: American Psychiatric Association; 2000.
18. American Psychiatric Association. *Diagnostic and Statistical Manual of Mental Disorders.* 5th ed. Washington, DC: American Psychiatric Association;2013
19. Santos SJ, Hurtado-Ortiz MT, Sneed CD. Illness beliefs regarding the causes of diabetes among Latino college students. *Hisp J Behav Sci.* 2009;31(3):395-412.
20. KCrenshaw. Demarginalizing the Intersection of Race and Sex: A Black Feminist Critique of Antidiscrimination Doctrine, Feminist Theory and Antiracist Politics. University of Chicago Legal Forum. 1989;140:139-167.
21. *Ethnicity.* OxfordDictionaries.com. Oxford Dictionaries, 2017. Web. 24 May. 2017.
22. Kramer EJ, Kwong K, Lee E, Chung H. Cultural factors influencing the mental health of Asian Americans. *West J Med.* 2002;176(4):227-231.
23. Bhugra D, Becker MA. Migration, cultural bereavement and cultural identity. *World Psychiatry.* 2005;4(1):18-24.
24. King M, Semlyen J, Tai SS, et al. Systematic review of mental disorder, suicide, and deliberate self harm in lesbian, gay and bisexual people. *BMC Psychiatry.* 2008;8(70). doi:10.1186/1471-244X-8-70.
25. CDC (Center for Disease Control). *Sexual Identity, Sex of Sexual Contacts, and Health-risk Behaviors Among Students in Grades 9-12: Youth Risk Behavior Surveillance.* Atlanta, GA: U.S. Department of Health and Human Services; 2016.
26. OCR (Office of Civil Rights). *Guidance to Federal Financial Assistance Recipients Regarding Title VI Prohibition against National Origin Discrimination Affecting Limited English Proficient Persons;* 2002. Available at http://www.lep.gov. Accessed December 23, 2007.
27. Kleinman A. *The Illness Narratives: Suffering, Healing and the Human Conditions.* Basic Books; 1988:43-44.

28. Lee S. Diagnosis postponed: shenjing shuairuo and the transformation of psychiatry in post-Mao China. *Cult Med Psychiatry*. 1999;23:349-380.

29. Koenig HG. *Spirituality and Patient Care: Why, How, When, and What*. Philadelphia: Templeton Foundation Press; 2002.

30. Gallup G. *Religion in America—50 Years, 1935-1985. The Gallup Report*. Princeton, NJ: Princeton Religion Research Center; 1985.

31. Reid DP. *The Complete Book of Chinese Health & Healing*. New York: Barnes & Noble Books; 1998.

32. Allen J, Balfour R, Bell R, et al. Social determinants of mental health. *Int Rev Psychiatr*. 2014;26(4):392-407.

33. World Health Organization Commission on Social Determinants of Health. *Closing the Gap in a Generation: Health Equity Through Action on the Social Determinants of Health. Commission on Social Determinants of Health Final Report*; 2008.

34. Hebert RS, Jenckes MW, Ford DF, et al. Patient perspectives on spirituality and the patient-physician relationship. *J Gen Intern Med*. 2001;16:685-692.

II

PSYCHIATRIC DISORDERS

5

ANXIETY DISORDERS

Jaesu Han, MD, Kate M. Richards, MD, and Jea-Hyoun Kim, MD

A 31-year-old woman presents for follow-up of difficulty sleeping. She reports lying in bed at night for hours ruminating about the day but has noticed that she worries all day as well. She reports feeling like she "can't relax" and always anticipates that "something will go wrong."

CLINICAL HIGHLIGHTS

- Screening requires asking about both physical and psychological symptoms of anxiety.
- The somatic presentation of anxiety disorders, where physical symptoms predominate, is common in the primary care setting.
- Anxiety disorders are defined and categorized by the presence or absence of specific situational triggers.
- More than 70% of patients diagnosed with an anxiety disorder in the primary care setting also have a comorbid psychiatric disorder, most commonly depression or another anxiety disorder. AMPS (Anxiety, Mood, Psychotic, Substance) is a quick and effective tool to screen for anxiety, mood, psychotic, and substance misuse disorders.
- Initial management of anxiety disorders includes establishing a trusting relationship while addressing psychosocial stressors in an empathic way.
- General medical conditions can trigger or masquerade as an anxiety disorder; both need to be treated.
- Cognitive behavioral therapy or medications such as serotonin reuptake inhibitors are both first-line treatment options regardless of the specific anxiety disorder. In general, when treating an anxiety disorder, it is best to start with half the usual "antidepressant starting dose" to decrease irritability and anxiety during the first few weeks of treatment.
- Success with medications relies more on providing good patient information and follow-up than prescribing a specific drug.

CLINICAL SIGNIFICANCE

Anxiety disorders represent the most prevalent group of psychiatric disorders in both the general and primary care patient population, accounting for significantly decreased quality of life for the affected patients and at least $42 billion per year in health care costs and lost productivity.[1] Data from the 12-year longitudinal, naturalistic Harvard/Brown Anxiety Disorders Research Program showed that, with the exception of panic disorder without agoraphobia, the course of anxiety disorders is both chronic and enduring.[2] Twelve years after the original episode, the majority of patients with generalized anxiety disorder (GAD), panic disorder with agoraphobia, or social anxiety disorder never achieved recovery, and of those who did recover, nearly half had a recurrence during the follow-up period.[2]

The economic and social costs of these chronic and recurrent disorders are increased when anxiety disorders in the primary care setting are unrecognized or undertreated. One recent study found that nearly one in five patients had at least one clinically significant anxiety disorder and that 41% of these patients were not receiving treatment of any kind.[3] With many effective treatments readily available for anxiety disorders, proper screening and early diagnosis is crucial to reduce suffering and optimize function.

DIAGNOSIS
DIAGNOSIS CONSIDERATIONS

Anxiety is commonly defined as excessive worrying, nervousness, or feeling "on edge." The prompt and accurate diagnosis of anxiety disorders in the primary care setting can be challenging for several reasons. Anxiety itself is a very normal human emotion, and it can be difficult to decide when it is pathologic. For example, anxiety can be adaptive when it motivates one to complete a task but pathologic when it is excessive and prevents one from completing necessary functions despite possible repercussions or missed opportunities. To ensure an accurate diagnosis and effective treatment plan, it is important to screen for an anxiety disorder, document the disability, consider the differential diagnosis, and identify the specific anxiety disorder.

SCREEN FOR AN ANXIETY DISORDER

The advantage of a screening tool includes the ability to administer and score a validated test before seeing the patient. However, unlike validated tools such as the Patient Health Questionnaire-9 (PHQ-9) for major depression, there is currently no commonly accepted screening tool for anxiety disorders in clinical practice. One commonly used screening tool is the Generalized Anxiety Disorder Scale (GAD-7), which is sensitive for panic disorder, GAD, and social anxiety disorder in the primary care setting (*Table 5-1*).[4] This tool consists of a series of seven questions that incorporates the diagnostic criteria for GAD from the *Diagnostic and Statistical Manual of Mental Disorders*, Fifth Edition (*DSM-5*). The first two items (GAD-2 subscale) can be used as an ultrarapid screening tool. A score of 8 or more on the GAD-7 or 3 or more on the GAD-2 should prompt a more thorough investigation for anxiety disorders.

The GAD-2 highlights the two key components of anxiety that are present regardless of the specific diagnosis: (1) psychiatric symptoms: excessive ruminations or worry, poor concentration, and racing thoughts and (2) physical symptoms: muscle tension, sweating, fatigue, restlessness, and tremors. During the screening interview, it is therefore important to inquire about both components. When one component predominates, the clinical presentation may change drastically.

When psychiatric symptoms such as anxiety predominate, the patient often presents to seek confirmation of an anxiety disorder diagnosis. Sometimes the patient's assessment of an anxiety disorder is correct, but at other times the diagnosis may be another psychiatric disorder or even a general medical condition. Although this presentation may be easier for clinicians to recognize because they are "primed" to consider an anxiety disorder, it is the less common presentation.

When physical symptoms predominate, the patient usually does not consider a psychiatric cause. The somatic presentation is more common than the psychiatric presentation in the primary care setting and is more likely to lead to misdiagnosis.[5] This may occur when a patient attributes the symptoms to such things as lack of sleep, stress, or poor diet, and the clinician halts further workup. Alternatively, there may be an extensive workup in response to multiple medically unexplained physical complaints such as chest pain, dizziness, gastrointestinal symptoms, or dyspnea before an anxiety disorder is considered.

DOCUMENT DISABILITY

Pathologic and clinically relevant anxiety is persistent and excessive, causing impairment in a person's daily functioning. Essentially, "normal" anxiety helps the patient to maintain order, whereas "pathologic" anxiety creates disorder. Clinicians should ask questions such as, "What have you given up because of your symptoms?" or "Have your symptoms prevented you from doing something you wanted or needed to do?" When considering a diagnosis of anxiety, one might ask, "How does the anxiety or nervousness change your everyday life?" In addition to ensuring that the anxiety is clinically significant, the documentation also provides tangible goals for treatment. Diagnosis should include documentation of specific functional impairment, which may include the following:

- Social impairment: withdrawal from family, friends, and hobbies
- Occupational impairment: job avoidance, inefficiency, lack of promotion, or even disciplinary action
- Impairment with activities of daily living: inability to shop for groceries, take the bus, or drive a car

TABLE 5-1 Generalized Anxiety Disorder 7-Item (GAD-7) Scale

HOW OFTEN DURING THE PAST 2 WEEKS HAVE YOU FELT BOTHERED BY:

1. Feeling nervous, anxious, or on edge?	0	1	2	3
2. Not being able to stop or control worrying?	0	1	2	3
3. Worrying too much about different things?	0	1	2	3
4. Trouble relaxing?	0	1	2	3
5. Being so restless that it is hard to sit still?	0	1	2	3
6. Becoming easily annoyed or irritable?	0	1	2	3
7. Feeling afraid as if something awful might happen?	0	1	2	3

Each question is answered on a scale of:
0 = not at all
1 = several days
2 = more than half the days
3 = nearly every day

A score of 8 or more should prompt further diagnostic evaluation for an anxiety disorder.

SPECIFIC ANXIETY DISORDERS

Significant changes were made in the categorization of anxiety disorders in *DSM-5*. Obsessive-compulsive disorder is now described separately within the Chapter 6 because of improved diagnostic validity within the disorders of that group. Posttraumatic stress disorder, acute stress disorder, and adjustment disorders are described separately within the Chapter 7. These changes were made because these disorders share depressive symptoms, anger, and even dissociation in response to trauma. Symptoms of anxiety are common but are not felt to be the key indicator of those disorders.

The following brief descriptions are intended to distill some salient points to differentiate the anxiety disorders. Keep in mind that the symptoms of anxiety often manifest as a waxing and waning "blanket" of symptoms but may also include time-limited "bursts" of symptoms in the form of panic attacks. Panic attacks, sometimes referred to as "anxiety attacks," are a type of fear response and, in themselves, are not an anxiety disorder. Although panic attacks are required as a feature of the diagnosis of panic disorder when they occur spontaneously, they may also occur in other anxiety disorders or mental health disorders. A typical panic attack occurs when patients experience a sudden onset of symptoms that typically peak within 10 minutes and rarely last longer than an hour. During a panic attack, psychological symptoms often include fear of losing control, dying, or "going crazy." Physical symptoms reflecting autonomic activation are equally intense and include sweating, shaking, shortness of breath, nausea, dizziness, fast heart rate, and chest discomfort.

Differentiating among the anxiety disorders relies on distinguishing if these symptoms, including panic attacks, are precipitated by specific situational triggers or are pervasive regardless of the situation (*Figure 5-1*). The three disorders with specific situational triggers are social anxiety disorder, agoraphobia, and specific phobia. The two disorders without consistent specific situational triggers are panic disorder and GAD.

Disorders with a Situational Trigger

Social Anxiety Disorder

Social anxiety disorder, also known as social phobia, is sometimes thought of as pathologic shyness. The hallmark is the fear of embarrassment or humiliation in front of others that is out of proportion for the situation, is persistent (usually lasting at least 6 months), and causes distress and loss of function. This fear may be limited to public speaking or more severe and generalized to almost all social situations. Patients may report fears that they will offend others, will be negatively evaluated or rejected, or will have noticeable blushing, sweating, or shaking. Panic attacks may occur but are situationally bound to the social trigger. Onset is usually in the early teenage years and patients will often have symptoms for over 15 years before seeking treatment. During this time, anxiety and avoidance of social situations can lead to missing important social gatherings, avoiding job promotions, dropping out of school, and overall decreased quality of life.

Agoraphobia

Agoraphobia is the fear and avoidance of places or situations from which escape is difficult, help is unavailable, or where it would be embarrassing to be seen if a panic attack or other incapacitating symptom occurred. Agoraphobia was previously considered a complication of panic disorder, but in *DSM-5* it is understood as a disorder that can arise without discrete panic attacks. Commonly avoided places include buses, trains, stores, theaters, parking lots, crowds, or lines. In severe cases, patients may be unable to work and may become homebound. Some patients may require a companion when leaving the house to feel safe.

Specific Phobia

Specific phobia is severe, disproportionate anxiety related to a particular trigger, such as animals, airplanes, elevators, heights, enclosed spaces, blood, or needles. Fight-or-flight symptoms, panic attacks, or a vasovagal reaction occurs immediately and consistently when the

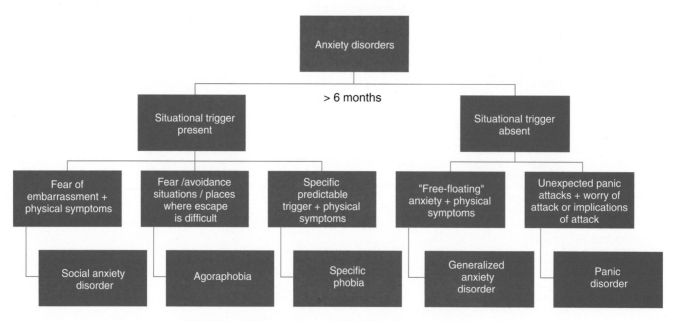

FIGURE 5-1 Diagnostic algorithm for anxiety disorders.

trigger is encountered or imagined, resulting in avoidance of the trigger to the point of impairing daily function. Onset is often in childhood and fears can initially be developmentally appropriate, but become pathologic when they are unremitting, impairing, and excessive.

Disorders without a Situational Trigger

Panic Disorder

Panic disorder is characterized by recurrent panic attacks (sudden surges of fear with multiple physiological symptoms that resolve within minutes), which are experienced at least initially as spontaneous and unexpected. A typical panic attack will peak in severity at about 10 minutes. Careful review with the patient may reveal benign cues such as emotional stress from an argument or a slightly elevated heart rate from caffeine that is interpreted as a symptom of an impending attack. Although panic attacks can be terrifying and temporarily disabling, it is the anticipatory anxiety of when the next attack will come, avoidant behaviors, and persistent worry lasting over a month that perpetuates the disability. Frequency and severity of panic attacks can vary, but the course is usually chronic, especially if untreated. Patients may undergo extensive testing to find the etiology of symptoms, such as chest discomfort, nausea, or dizziness before a diagnosis of panic disorder is made. Panic disorder is twice as common in women as in men and onset peaks in late adolescence to early adulthood. Although the initial panic attack by definition is not caused by an obvious trigger, the majority of patients report some antecedent adverse life event or physical stressor in the months before onset of illness. Panic disorder is often comorbid with other mental disorders and is important to recognize, given that it is associated with increased suicidality and high health care utilization.

Generalized Anxiety Disorder

GAD is another anxiety disorder without a situational trigger. In fact, the hallmark of GAD is the presence of free-floating anxiety consisting of pervasive and excessive ruminations on most days about often trivial matters. Worries often wax and wane, and content can change with age (school, work, family, health, safety, catastrophes), but the anxiety is distressing, impairs efficiency and function, and lasts longer than 6 months. Patients often describe themselves as "chronic worriers." They may also be concerned about physical symptoms such as muscle tension, restlessness, and fatigue. GAD is relatively common among primary care patients who present with chronic insomnia.

Unspecified Anxiety Disorder

Many patients in the primary care setting will not initially fit neatly into any of the anxiety disorders noted earlier. Assuming the symptoms are causing significant clinical distress, a diagnosis of unspecified anxiety disorder can be made. As patients become more comfortable and provide additional history, a more definitive diagnosis may become apparent. At other times, the diagnosis of a specific anxiety disorder is not possible owing to confounding general medical conditions, comorbid substance abuse, or the fact that some patients may never manifest the required number of diagnostic criteria. For example, it would be

reasonable to initially diagnose a patient with unspecified anxiety disorder while medical workup is being done to rule out anxiety disorder due to a general medical condition before the diagnosis of panic disorder is made.

ANXIETY DISORDERS DIAGNOSTIC CRITERIA ADAPTED FROM DSM-5

GENERALIZED ANXIETY DISORDER

Excessive anxiety and worry that is difficult to control and related to a number of different activities or events in multiple contexts on a nearly daily basis for at least six months.

The anxiety and worry are associated with at least three of the following:

- Restlessness
- Fatigue
- Poor concentration
- Irritability
- Muscle tension
- Sleep disturbance

Social Anxiety Disorder

Marked fear or anxiety about acting in a way that is humiliating or embarrassing in social situations for at least six months.

The social situations provoke intense fear and anxiety and are generally avoided if possible.

Symptoms are out of proportion to the actual threat.

Panic Disorder

Recurrent, unexpected panic attacks followed by one month or more of one or both of the following:

- Persistent concern about having additional panic attacks or consequences of having panic attacks.
- Maladaptive change in behavior in response to the panic attacks.

Panic Attack Specifier

Panic attacks alone is not a mental disorder. Panic attacks can occur as part of another mental disorder where it is noted as a specifier (e.g., social anxiety disorder with panic attacks). Panic attacks become panic disorder when the additional criteria for panic disorder are fulfilled.

Abrupt onset of intense fear or discomfort that peaks within minutes and includes at least four of the following symptoms:

- Palpitations
- Sweating
- Trembling or shaking
- Feeling short of breath
- Sensation of choking
- Chest pain
- Nausea or abdominal discomfort
- Dizziness, lightheadedness, or feeling faint

- Chills or flushing
- Paresthesias
- Derealization or depersonalization
- Fear of losing control
- Fear of dying

Agoraphobia

Intense fear or anxiety in response to or in anticipation of entering two or more situations where the person feels stuck, unable to escape, or not able to get help:

- Public transportation
- Open areas
- Closed-off areas
- Lines or in a crowd
- Alone outside of the home

The above situations are actively avoided if possible.

The fear or avoidance is out of proportion to the actual threat and has been present for at least six months.

Specific Phobia

Persistent unreasonable or excessive fear caused by the presence or anticipation of a specific object or situation.

Exposure to the object or situation results in anxiety, often on the form of a panic attack.

The object or situation is generally avoided if possible.

The fear or avoidance is out of proportion to the actual threat and has been present for at least six months.

For all the conditions noted above, the following also apply:

Symptoms are very distressing or impair function in some way.

Symptoms are not due to a substance or medication and not better explained by another mental or general medical disorder.

DIFFERENTIAL DIAGNOSIS

The different presentations of anxiety disorders highlight the need for a comprehensive patient assessment and consideration of a broad differential diagnosis before a definitive diagnosis is made. Patient assessment begins with obtaining the medical history, especially the onset of symptoms because anxiety disorders tend to present in late adolescence and early adulthood. For example, new-onset anxiety symptoms in a previously healthy patient beyond the age of 35 years without a recent significant life event or trauma are suspicious for an underlying medical condition. A family history of mood or anxiety disorders increases the likelihood of a primary anxiety disorder. Assessment should also include reviewing both prescription and over-the-counter medications. Within social history, evaluate relational and occupational factors and screen for potential substance abuse. After an appropriate physical examination with patients presenting with physical symptoms, reasonable initial tests include a complete blood count, thyroid-stimulating hormone, and a comprehensive metabolic panel.

Common general medical conditions and basic laboratory workup for symptoms of anxiety are listed in *Table 5-2*. Many of these conditions will manifest with concurrent symptoms unrelated to anxiety and risk factors that will guide the extent of the diagnostic workup. For example, a nonobese 35-year-old patient who does not have ischemic chest pain and has no risk factors for coronary disease is unlikely to have an acute coronary syndrome and therefore should not undergo invasive diagnostic cardiac procedures.

Medications may cause anxiety-like symptoms (*Table 5-3*).[6] For example, patients taking antipsychotics may complain of akathisia, which consists of an intense sense of internal restlessness that resolves after discontinuation of the medication. Stimulants such as methylphenidate used for attention deficit hyperactivity disorder (ADHD) can cause side effects such as a fine tremor, tachycardia, and irritability that can be confused with anxiety. Overcorrecting hypothyroidism with levothyroxine can cause iatrogenic hyperthyroidism with symptoms of

TABLE 5-2 Medical Conditions With Anxiety-Like Symptoms	
MEDICAL CONDITION	**SUGGESTED BASIC WORKUP**
Cardiovascular: coronary artery disease, congestive heart failure, arrhythmias, pulmonary embolism, mitral valve prolapse, hypertensive emergency	ECG, holter monitor (especially patients >40 years of age with palpitations or chest pain)
Pulmonary: pneumonia, asthma, chronic obstructive pulmonary disease	Pulmonary function test, CXR
Endocrine: thyroid dysfunction, hyperparathyroidism, hypoglycemia, menopause, Cushing disease, insulinoma, pheochromocytoma	TSH, complete metabolic panel
Hematologic: anemia	CBC
Neurologic: seizure disorders, encephalopathies, essential tremor	EEG, brain MRI
Substance abuse/dependence	Urine toxicology

CBC, complete blood count; CXR, chest X-ray; ECG, electrocardiogram; EEG, electroencephalogram; MRI, magnetic resonance imaging; TSH, thyroid-stimulating hormone.

TABLE 5-3 Medications and Substances That Cause Anxiety-Like Symptoms	
Stimulant intoxication	Caffeine, nicotine, cocaine, methamphetamines, phencyclidine (PCP), MDMA (ecstasy)
Sympathomimetics	Pseudoephedrine, methylphenidate, amphetamines, beta-agonists
Dopaminergics	Amantadine, bromocriptine, levodopa, levodopa-carbidopa, metoclopramide
Anticholinergics	Benztropine mesylate, meperidine, oxybutynin, diphenhydramine
Miscellaneous	Anabolic steroids, corticosteroids, indomethacin, ephedra, theophylline
Drug withdrawal	Alcohol, benzodiazepines, opiates, barbiturates, short half-life selective serotonin reuptake inhibitors (SSRIs)/and serotonin norepinephrine reuptake inhibitors (SNRIs)

generalized anxiety. While rare, pheochromocytoma can cause symptoms of headache, palpitations, and diaphoresis and can mimic symptoms of a panic attack.

Primary anxiety disorders are commonly accompanied by other psychiatric disorders. One study found that more than 70% of patients diagnosed with an anxiety disorder in the primary care setting had a comorbid psychiatric disorder. Over 60% had an additional anxiety disorder, over 40% had comorbid major depression, and 14% had a concurrent substance use disorder.[7] Somatic symptom disorder and personality disorders can also be present. Identifying comorbid illness will likely lead to more effective treatment, a quicker recovery, and significantly decrease the likelihood of recurrence.

Unrecognized substance use disorders, including use of marijuana, can trigger or exacerbate an anxiety disorder. Symptoms may present during acute intoxication or withdrawal from substances. The workup for anxiety disorders must include nonjudgmental screening for substance use in the past month. If a substance use disorder is detected, a longitudinal history is necessary to determine if current symptoms represent a substance-induced state or an anxiety disorder with a comorbid substance use disorder. History suggesting two separate concurrent disorders would include (1) onset of symptoms before the first use of the substance and (2) continued symptoms despite sustained abstinence for at least 1 month. Management of comorbid substance use disorders and anxiety disorders includes treatment for the anxiety disorder in addition to the substance use treatment.

NOT TO BE MISSED

- Substance intoxication or withdrawal
- Comorbid major depression
- Obsessive-compulsive disorder
- Posttraumatic stress disorder
- Adjustment disorder with anxiety
- Illness anxiety disorder (formerly hypochondriasis)
- Medication-induced causes
- Systemic medical disorder/delirium
- Suicidal ideation or intent

BIOPSYCHOSOCIAL TREATMENT
GENERAL PRINCIPLES
Overview

Effective management of an anxiety disorder includes a balanced consideration of other nonspecific but equally crucial steps before actually treating anxiety disorders. These include first establishing a trusting, therapeutic relationship and addressing comorbid general medical and psychiatric conditions. Thereafter, specific targeted pharmacotherapy and psychotherapy are incorporated into the treatment.

Establishing Trust

The best plans for medication treatment and referrals to specialists are doomed to fail without a therapeutic alliance between the patient and provider. The establishment of trust begins with empathy. As noted in Chapter 1, empathy requires the clinician to briefly "become the patient." Key steps include recognizing and validating the patient's strong emotions during the interview, pausing to imagine how the patient may be feeling, verbally acknowledging and legitimizing the patient's perceived feelings, and offering support and reassurance. Consider that many patients have suffered for many years before finally presenting for treatment and have probably been told to "just get over it." Employing an empathic approach with patients who have pronounced anxiety is both time-saving and effective despite unjustified concerns that it will take too much time or be too emotionally exhausting to the clinician.

Comorbid Conditions

Comorbid general medical and psychiatric conditions that may contribute to or mimic anxiety symptoms should be treated simultaneously with the anxiety disorder. As noted with the case of panic disorder, it may be tempting to ignore the anxiety disorder and only treat the general medical condition in the hope that the anxiety disorder will resolve spontaneously. Unfortunately, this is not often the case. The same can be said with comorbid substance, personality, and mood disorders, and earlier concurrent treatment of the other conditions should be considered.

PSYCHOPHARMACOLOGY

Several classes of medications are used to treat anxiety disorders. Most of these medications also function as antidepressants, alter serotonergic neurotransmission, and appear to exert their action by attenuating the physiologic cues associated with anxiety disorders over several weeks. Selective serotonin reuptake inhibitors (SSRIs) and serotonin norepinephrine reuptake inhibitors (SNRIs) are FDA approved for treatment of many anxiety disorders. Older medications, such as monoamine oxidase inhibitors (MAOIs), and some tricyclic antidepressants (TCAs) are also effective antianxiety medications but are generally considered second-line treatment options due to complex side effect profiles. There is a large body of evidence that shows various antidepressant classes have roughly equal efficacy in treating anxiety disorders in both the acute and maintenance phases.

However, not all antianxiety medications are considered first-line agents. MAOIs have a number of side effects that limit their tolerability and require dietary restrictions to avoid a hypertensive crisis. The TCAs require more dosage titration and have decreased receptor specificity, including significant anticholinergic side effects such as sedation, constipation, and dry mouth. The two classes of medication most often prescribed for anxiety disorders are the SSRIs and SNRIs. Both have emerged as first-line treatments because of their proven efficacy, safety, and ease of use with few side effects. Additionally, benzodiazepines (BZDs) are still commonly used in current practice. However, owing to concerns about dependence and potential adverse effects, BZDs should be used with caution.

Another medication used to treat anxiety is buspirone. As a 5-HT1A receptor agonist, buspirone has been shown to be effective for GAD but not the other anxiety disorders or depression. While it lacks the abuse potential of the BZDs, the narrow spectrum of efficacy, delay in therapeutic effect of several weeks, and twice-daily dosing tend to limit its popularity.

Serotonin Reuptake Inhibitors

Although SSRIs and SNRIs are more commonly known for the treatment of depression, they have also been shown to be effective for anxiety disorders. While not every SSRI or SNRI is FDA approved for every anxiety disorder, in clinical practice they are generally used interchangeably. Medication choice is therefore not based on efficacy but rather on the potential side effects and drug–drug interactions. Antidepressants with short half-lives (e.g., paroxetine) have a higher likelihood of causing discontinuation syndrome and related anxiety with abrupt cessation. If a first-degree relative has had a good response to a particular drug or a patient has benefited from prior use of a specific medication, this should be strongly considered when deciding on a treatment plan. Finally, the cost of a medication may be an additional factor. Currently, all the SSRIs are available in generic formulations (*Table 5-4*).

Once a medication is chosen, clinical effectiveness depends on the initial information provided to the patient and adherence to treatment. Both understanding of the information provided and medication adherence should be explored and clarified in follow-up visits. This information should include expectations of treatment, a discussion of side effects, and the need for gradual titration.

TABLE 5-4 Selective Serotonin Reuptake Inhibitors (SSRIs) and Serotonin Norepinephrine Reuptake Inhibitors (SNRIs) for Anxiety Disorders

SSRIs	STARTING DOSE (mg/day)	THERAPEUTIC DOSE (mg/day)	HALF-LIFE	DRUG INTERACTIONS
Fluoxetine (Prozac)	10	20-60	Long[a]	2D6 inhibitor
Sertraline (Zoloft)	25	50-200	Medium[a]	(–)
Citalopram (Celexa)	10	20-40	Short	(–)
Escitalopram (Lexapro)	5	10-30	Short	(–)
Paroxetine (Paxil)	10	20-60	Short	2D6 inhibitor
Paroxetine controlled release (Paxil CR)	12.5	12.5-25	Short	2D6 inhibitor
Fluvoxamine (Luvox)	50	150-300	Short	3A4 and 1A2 inhibitor
SNRIs				
Venlafaxine extended release (Effexor XR)	37.5	75-225	Short[a]	(–)
Duloxetine (Cymbalta)	30	60-120	Short	2D6 inhibitor

[a]Including active metabolites.

ALWAYS DISCUSS BEFORE PRESCRIBING SSRIs/SNRIs

- Patient expectations
- Delayed therapeutic effects
- Not an "as-needed" medication
- Long-term treatment is often indicated
- Common class side effects
- Initial activation or transient increased anxiety
- Sexual side effects
- Gastrointestinal side effects
- Slow titration
- Usually start at half the standard starting "antidepressant dose"
- Increase the dose slowly and cautiously in the elderly

Patient Expectations

Most patients have heard of antidepressants such as fluoxetine and may have positive or negative expectations that need to be explored. They may also be asking themselves, "Why am I being prescribed an antidepressant when I have anxiety?" or "Why am I not feeling better when I've been taking this drug for over a week?" These questions should be addressed at the time of initiating therapy rather than 3 months later when the patient continues to suffer from anxiety symptoms due to poor medication adherence. A thorough discussion at the initial visit will help to set patients' expectations and encourage adherence to treatment. Similarly, patients may take the antidepressant on an as-needed basis once symptoms initially respond, leading to subtherapeutic drug levels and a subsequent relapse.

Side Effects

While SSRIs have improved tolerability compared with older antidepressants, there are several side effects common to all SSRIs that warrant discussion:

Initial activation: Some patients may experience increased activation and nervousness after initiation of the SSRI. This effect is usually dose dependent and time limited to the first 1 to 2 weeks. This is a common cause of noncompliance and can be minimized by preparing the patient for the possibility and using gradual dose titration.

Gastrointestinal side effects: Transient nausea represents one of the most common effects of SSRIs and a common cause of early medication discontinuation. This may be minimized by a slower titration and patient education. These symptoms usually resolve within several weeks.

Sexual side effects: This occurs to some degree in approximately 30% to 50% of patients and can affect all phases of the sexual cycle but most commonly leads to delayed ejaculation and absent or delayed orgasm.[8] While the sexual side effects are dose dependent, they do not appear to improve with time. It is important to tell patients sexual side effects are reversible once the medication is decreased or removed. There is good evidence for adding sildenafil for sexual dysfunction in men and limited evidence for adding bupropion for decreased libido in men and women.[9]

Dosage and Slow Titration

The final step to discuss with patients is the need for a slow initial titration. As mentioned earlier, this slow titration will minimize the dose-dependent side effects of initial activation and nausea. A reasonable strategy would include starting at half the dose normally prescribed for major depression and increased to the initial dose for major depression after the first week. The effective therapeutic dosage is usually similar for major depression and anxiety disorders.

Benzodiazepines

While antidepressants are considered the first-line choice for patients with anxiety disorders, BZDs continue to serve an adjunctive role or even as monotherapy for some carefully chosen patients. Although there is evidence to support the use of BZDs as monotherapy for panic disorder and GAD, there are limited data to support use with social phobia.[10]

One advantage that BZDs have over antidepressants is their rapid onset of action. In the adjunctive role, BZDs can provide immediate relief of symptoms and help mitigate the initial activation or jitteriness when initiating an antidepressant. Evidence for this role is strongest for panic disorder, where this strategy can more rapidly stabilize patients during the initial phase compared with an SSRI alone. After several weeks on both medications, the BZD is quickly tapered off without risk of significant withdrawal symptoms. For example, clonazepam (Klonopin) can be initiated 0.5 mg twice daily along with sertraline 25 mg daily. The sertraline can be increased to 50 mg by the end of the first week and increased to a more therapeutic dose of 100 mg after another week. At week 4 to 8 the clonazepam can be gradually discontinued over the next 2 weeks.

As monotherapy for panic disorder, GAD, and social anxiety disorder, the high-potency BZDs (e.g., alprazolam and clonazepam) are the best studied. The lowest effective dose of BZDs should be prescribed in divided doses. When using BZDs, the potential benefits must be balanced with the potential drawbacks of use. These drawbacks include the following:

Side effects: While generally well tolerated, BZDs can produce sedation as well as impairment in working memory and learning new information. There is also an increased risk of falls and confusion with elderly patients.

Increased risk of overdose when used with opioid medications: Concurrent use of opiates and BZDs are associated with a greater risk of opioid overdose compared with patients on opiates alone.[11] In 2016, the FDA added a boxed warning stating BZDs should be used with great caution in these patients, because they can potentiate the sedation and respiratory depression caused by opioids leading to an increased risk of coma and death.

Abuse: Patients who use higher doses of BZDs with faster onset (e.g., diazepam, alprazolam) and those with a history of alcohol and drug abuse have a heightened risk of developing benzodiazepine tolerance and subsequent withdrawal. As it is often difficult to determine whether a patient has a primary anxiety disorder versus a substance-induced anxiety disorder, BZD use may serve as a trigger for substance misuse and should be used with caution in those who have a substance abuse history.

Physical dependence and withdrawal: Chronic use can result in a withdrawal syndrome in 40% to 80% of patients upon BZD discontinuation.[12] A gradual taper is recommended if used longer than 2 weeks.

Comorbidity: Monotherapy is not usually indicated and does not address comorbid major depression. However, BZDs can be used under the following pre-scribing parameters during times of significant and acute life stressors (e.g., death in the family, divorce):

1. Use of *long-acting* BZDs, such as clonazepam
2. Use of *short-term* treatment of usually no more than 8 to 12 weeks
3. Use of *low-dose* BZDs

Despite these drawbacks, a short course of BZDs may be preferable to antidepressants for patients with relatively infrequent symptoms, documented intolerance, or lack of improvement on antidepressants. *Table 5-5* illustrates the balancing of relative risks and benefits when con-sidering the use of BZDs. If a patient requesting a BZD is not a good candidate, it is important that the provider avoid nonspecific statements such as, "You're going to get addicted" or "I don't like to use them." These statements can be received as value judgments and damage the ther-apeutic relationship. Providing the specific and personal-ized risks and relative contraindications is more likely to result in acceptance of treatment recommendations.

PSYCHOTHERAPY

Over the past 30 years, cognitive behavioral therapy (CBT) has emerged as an effective first-line therapy for the treatment of anxiety disorders. Evidence from meta-analysis and large prospective studies has indicated that CBT is at least as effective as medication alone.[13,14] Despite this evidence, CBT continues to be underuti-lized. In the following section, we will discuss the prin-ciples of CBT and the role of the primary care clinician.

Cognitive Behavioral Therapy

CBT is a psychotherapeutic technique delivered by trained mental health professionals in a group or indi-vidual format. Patients are typically seen weekly and the therapy is time limited (generally 10 to 24 sessions). This "brief psychotherapy" is active in that the therapist and patient collaboratively work together to develop and test hypotheses. There is also an expectation that the patient will complete CBT-related "homework" and discuss this work during follow-up sessions.

The general premise of CBT rests on the observa-tion that patients with anxiety disorders hold distorted beliefs and expectations about their world, which lead to symptoms and avoidance behaviors. It incorporates symptom management techniques such as progressive muscle relaxation and deep breathing. The cognitive therapy part of CBT is used to identify and address dis-torted beliefs through a process called cognitive restruc-turing. During this process, patients are asked to identify and logically evaluate thoughts that affect their mood and behavior by writing a dysfunctional thought record. They become aware of cognitive distortions such as mind reading (e.g., "People think I'm a bad parent.") and cata-strophizing (e.g., "If I don't leave I'm going to pass out.") and are challenged to replace them with more accurate, reality-based, and adaptive explanations that decrease anxiety symptoms. See Chapter 16 for more information on Cognitive Behavioral Therapy.

Cognitive restructuring is often coupled with expo-sure interventions to help the patient relearn a sense of safety in previously feared situations. This exposure is performed in a stepwise hierarchical fashion from the least to the most feared (as ranked by the patient). This allows an opportunity to put into practice what has been learned during sessions. For example, the patient with social anxiety might start with simply imagining a brief conversation with a neighbor. Once the patient achieves some mastery over symptoms, the exposure might esca-late to a brief conversation with a neighbor. All the while the patient would be working to cognitively restructure his or her thoughts of embarrassment. Ultimately the patient might invite the neighbor over for lunch.

The role of the primary care clinician for a patient undergoing CBT is largely supportive, although many providers may wish to learn CBT through formal train-ing. In such patients, the provider may briefly review the dysfunctional thought record with the patient and rein-force what is learned from therapy. Also, reminding the patient that symptoms may actually increase initially as fears are challenged rather than avoided may be helpful in preventing premature discontinuation from therapy. CBT is well tolerated, cost-effective, and associated with minimal side effects. Patients routinely experience the benefits of CBT within the same time frame as antide-pressants, as early as the second session.

TABLE 5-5 Relative Considerations for Benzodiazepines Use in Anxiety Disorders

BENEFITS/INDICATIONS	RISKS/CONTRAINDICATIONS
Need for rapid symptom control	Chronic opiate therapy
Lack of effect or intolerance to multiple antidepressants	History or active substance use disorder
Panic disorder, generalized anxiety disorder	Memory impairment, sedation, imbalance
Infrequent symptoms	Risk of delirium, falls in elderly

Social Interventions

As part of the empathic process, the clinician may become aware of obvious social situations exacerbating or complicating a patient's anxiety disorder. While it is often not possible to solve potentially complicated social issues for patients, reasonable interventions may go a long way in developing trust. Interventions may include assessment of safety for a patient in an abusive or unsafe relationship, consideration of short-term disability or time off from work, and consultation with a social worker if available.

Treatment Recommendations (Acute Phase)

The initial treatment for the anxiety disorders is remarkably similar regardless of the specific diagnosis. Options will include some combination of an SSRI, and/or psychotherapy, and in some cases, a BZD. The exact choice will depend on patient preference and to a lesser extent on diagnosis (*Table 5-6*). A notable exception is specific phobia where CBT is the preferred option over medication. In situations where the exposure is infrequent and predictable such as an airplane flight, a short-onset BZD (e.g., lorazepam 0.5 to 1 mg) can be taken 30 minutes before the exposure. For panic disorder, GAD, and social anxiety disorder, starting with either an SSRI or CBT is a reasonable first option, as they are equally effective. Because success is equally likely with either option, choice may depend on factors other than efficacy. While many therapists may be familiar with the principles of CBT, this does not always translate to competency in providing CBT. This is important because outcome is influenced by how closely a therapist adheres to the guiding principles and techniques. Even when available, therapists may not accept health insurance. Another potential logistical challenge is the time commitment required from the patient. Weekly visits may not be possible owing to required time off from work, the need for childcare, or lack of consistent transportation.

If the patient chooses to take an SSRI and does not respond within 2 months of adequately dosed treatment, options would include a trial of another SSRI versus switching to an SNRI such as venlafaxine or duloxetine. For patients with a history of inadequate response to a medication in the past, CBT can still be effective. Despite the theoretical appeal of combined treatment with CBT and an SSRI, the current evidence has not consistently shown a substantial benefit over CBT alone except with the possible exception of panic disorder, particularly if there is moderate to severe agoraphobia present.[15,16] On the other hand, combined treatment was also not associated with diminished effectiveness. Therefore, use of combined medication and psychotherapy may be individually tailored until further information becomes available.

Treatment Recommendations (Maintenance Phase)

The maintenance phase of treatment begins once a patient responds to an antianxiety medication. The goal of maintenance treatment is relapse prevention. Most guidelines suggest a minimum of 6 months to 1 year of treatment. Chances for success with discontinuation of medication treatment may be increased by considering several factors: (1) if there is a history of one or more relapses in the past, long-term, indefinite treatment with an antidepressant may be warranted; (2) a gradual discontinuation of the antidepressant or BZD over several weeks will decrease the likelihood of recurrence as well as prevent the discontinuation syndrome or withdrawal; and (3) the use of CBT in conjunction with the taper from medication to decrease the likelihood of relapse.

WHEN TO REFER

- Diagnostic uncertainty
- Significant comorbid psychiatric illness: substance abuse, suicidal patients, bipolar disorder, personality disorders
- Severe illness in terms of marked socio-occupational disability
- Prior treatment failure with multiple medications and psychotherapy
- Patient prefers initial trial of psychotherapy
- Close follow-up (e.g., every 2 to 3 weeks) during medication initiation phase is not feasible
- Severe agitation or suicidal ideation

TABLE 5-6 Acute Treatment for Anxiety Disorders

	SSRI	CBT	CBT + SSRI[a]	BENZODIAZEPINE MONOTHERAPY	BENZODIAZEPINE ADJUNCTIVE
PD	++	++	+[b]	++	+
GAD	++	++	+/−	++	+/−
SAD	++	++	+/−	+	+/−
SP	−	++	−	+[c]	−

[a]*Additional combined benefit.*
[b]*Especially if moderate to severe agoraphobia is present.*
[c]*If the exposure is infrequent and predictable.*
CBT, cognitive behavioral therapy; GAD, generalized anxiety disorder; PD, panic disorder; SAD, social anxiety disorder; SP, specific phobia; SSRI, selective serotonin reuptake inhibitor.
++, good evidence; +, some evidence; +/−, inadequate/mixed evidence; −, no evidence.

CASES AND QUESTIONS

CASE 1: "Beating Heart"

A 32-year-old healthy, nonobese man presents for follow-up after multiple recent visits to the emergency department. He does not have any cardiac history or risk factors for coronary disease but states "I keep having these episodes where it feels like my heart is beating out of my chest and I can't breathe." He witnessed his 85-year-old grandfather have a heart attack years ago and says, "I don't want the same thing to happen to me." He describes feeling sudden attacks of chest pain, with nausea, dizziness, chills, and sweating that last a few minutes then resolve spontaneously. He first had an attack while exercising 7 to 8 months ago, but now it "just happens whenever." He has been seen by cardiologists in the emergency department several times, and a cardiac workup showed no signs of arrhythmia, EKG changes, or elevated troponins. He has also had Holter monitoring with no abnormalities, but he does not feel reassured. He has stopped driving because "I can't afford to have this happen while I'm on the road" and avoids public transportation because "I might not be able to get to the hospital fast enough." He stays next to the exit in public places and checks to see if there is an automated external defibrillator nearby. He is planning to cancel his business meetings because "I don't want my co-workers to see me like this" and asks what can be done to help him.

1. This patient's presentation is most consistent with
   _____

   A. panic disorder
   B. social phobia
   C. posttraumatic stress disorder
   D. generalized anxiety disorder

   Correct answer: A. *This case highlights the progression of panic disorder and frequent use of medical resources for evaluation of somatic symptoms related to anxiety. While the initial episode was triggered by exercise, subsequent episodes have occurred out of the blue, and the patient is developing early signs of agoraphobia given fear of being in public places where he may have a panic attack. While it may be appropriate to do an initial workup for palpitations, this patient does not have a prior cardiac history and is low risk for acute coronary syndrome. After a reasonable medical workup, panic disorder should be high on the differential.*

2. Initial short-term treatment may include
   _____

   A. low-dose antipsychotic
   B. fluoxetine
   C. gabapentin
   D. clonazepam
   E. zaleplon or zolpidem

Correct answer: D. *Early and appropriate management of panic disorder will be key in his recovery and preventing unnecessary and potentially harmful investigations, such as invasive cardiac diagnostic procedures. In patients with known general medical disorders, psychiatric disorders can coexist (e.g., angina and panic disorder), and both should be treated if comorbid. A trusting patient–provider relationship must be developed with empathic statements noting the patient's fears and frustration. Clearly describing how his panic symptoms are driven by the sympathetic nervous system can also help normalize the symptoms and help the patient open up to treatment options, such as a trial of CBT. For immediate relief, a short-term course of benzodiazepine such as clonazepam may be prescribed. However, this should be avoided in patient with risk factors or history of substance use and personality disorders. A slow titration of an SSRI could be considered instead of CBT for longer term treatment, depending on patient preference.*

CASE 2: "Trouble Sleeping"

A 31-year-old woman presents for follow-up of for difficulty sleeping. She reports lying in bed at night for hours ruminating about the day but has noticed that she worries all day as well. She reports feeling like she "can't relax" and always anticipates that "something will go wrong." She reports feeling this way since she was a teenager. She worries about her children's futures, her job as an accountant, her husband's high cholesterol, her mother who is in assisted living, finances, politics, and the weather. She recently had a well-woman visit with normal laboratory findings, Pap smear, breast examination, and thyroid screening, all of which were normal, but worries that "maybe they missed something." She has started feeling hot and tremulous and asks if laboratory tests can be done to see if she is starting menopause or if she should get workup for a seizure disorder.

1. What screening tool might be useful in evaluating this patient's complaints?
   A. Patient Health Questionnaire (PHQ-9)
   B. Alcohol Use Identification Test (AUDIT-C)
   C. Mood Disorders Questionnaire (MDQ)
   D. Adverse Childhood Experiences (ACES)
   E. None of the above

   Correct answer: E. *The presence of multiple, pervasive, and long-term worries without a unifying trigger suggests a diagnosis of GAD, and screening with GAD-7 can help uncover additional symptoms and assess severity.*

2. This patient presents with somatic concerns in addition to worry. Somatic concerns

_____

A. are unusual for an anxiety disorder
B. suggest co-occurrence of bipolar disorder
C. are typical for an anxiety disorder
D. suggest co-occurrence of obsessive-compulsive disorder
E. suggest posttraumatic stress disorder

Correct answer: C. _Patients with anxiety disorders often present to their primary care provider with somatic complaints, such as insomnia, so anxiety must be considered in each assessment. Her symptoms of insomnia likely would improve with treatment of GAD. Assuming she agrees to initiate treatment, we can see from her propensity to worry that it will be important to provide clear information about expectations and potential side effects of treatment options. Initiation of an SSRI or CBT would be equally reasonable at this point._

CASE 3: "The Struggling Student"

A 20-year-old college student presents for a well-woman visit. When asked about school, she says, "It depends on the course." In courses with traditional lectures and tests she does well. However, she feels she "totally botched" a speech in Spanish class earlier in the year where she "turned red," started sweating, and felt like she was unable to give coherent response to a question. She reports spending most of her classes worrying about whether she will be called on and sitting in the furthest seats from the professor. She has missed classes saying she had a headache and had to make up several tests. She notes that she has struggled since middle school with studying with classmates for fear she may say something stupid or embarrassing.

1. This case describes someone who presents with

_____

A. acute stress disorder
B. panic disorder
C. schizoid personality
D. social anxiety disorder
E. health anxiety

Correct answer: D. _This case highlights the distress many patients have in asking for help due to a sense of shame or embarrassment. Being on the lookout for physical symptoms, patterns of avoidance, and level of impairment in functionality is important. If the triggers are circumscribed around social interactions exclusively, social anxiety disorder would be the diagnosis._

2. This patient is most likely to have comorbid

_____

A. bipolar II disorder
B. fibromyalgia
C. restless leg syndrome
D. generalized anxiety disorder
E. borderline personality disorder

Correct answer: D. _Initial management should begin with recognition that the patient has really struggled with symptoms over at least 6 months. While medications and psychotherapy are again equally effective for social anxiety disorder, many patients are hesitant about seeing a therapist because, by definition, they find new social interactions very uncomfortable. If a reasonably strong therapeutic relationship has developed, the patient may be more open to psychotherapy if a trial of a medication was not effective or was only partially effective._

CASE 4: "Anxious at Work"

A 38-year-old man presents to your office reporting he was placed on probation by his work for drinking alcohol on the job. He reports that he was feeling increased stress and pressure from his job starting one year ago owing to multiple ongoing projects. Around that time, he also began noticing episodes of suddenly feeling shaky, sweaty, and that he was going to lose control. This happened multiple times out of the blue while he was at home or working in the office. He says he couldn't take it anymore and started drinking beer to calm his nerves before going into work. The drinking increased and soon he was drinking 6 to 8 beers every day. After getting in trouble for drinking, he quit drinking 6 weeks ago but says he still feels "on edge" and is having trouble concentrating. "Beer is the only thing that works, doctor. I don't know what else to do!"

1. This patient most likely has _____

A. posttraumatic stress disorder
B. borderline personality disorder
C. panic disorder
D. pheochromocytoma
E. malingering

Correct answer: C. _When a patient presents with both substance use and anxiety symptoms, it is important to clarify the timeline of onset. In this case, the patient had many symptoms of anxiety occurring before his initiation of substance use and has continuing symptoms despite 6 weeks of sustained abstinence from alcohol. Collectively, this seems to suggest a primary anxiety disorder and, although likely worsened by the use of alcohol, it is unlikely a causative factor._

continued

2. Co-occurring substance use that may present with a similar presentation includes

---

  A. opiate use
  B. tobacco use
  C. phencyclidine use
  D. amphetamine use
  E. none of the above

    Correct answer: D. *It may be helpful to conduct urine drug screens and gather collateral information to validate cessation of substances.*

3. Treatment for this patient might include

  A. Suboxone
  B. low-dose risperidone
  C. sertraline
  D. alprazolam
  E. valproic acid

    Correct answer: C. *Patient education regarding symptoms of anxiety and symptoms of alcohol withdrawal is also important. In this case, treatment of substance use disorder is important given the patient's escalation in use. However, management of his probable panic disorder with an SSRI or CBT may help him to cope with his anxiety without using alcohol. Benzodiazepines, such as alprazolam, would be unwise given their abuse liability.*

PRACTICAL RESOURCES

- The Anxiety Disorders Association of America: www. adaa.org
- Nonprofit organization with information on anxiety disorders and help with finding a therapist
- The National Institute of Mental Health: http://www. nimh.nih.gov/healthinformation/anxietymenu.cfm
- Information on diagnosis and treatment as well as on how to participate in clinical trials

REFERENCES

1. Greenberg PE, Sisitsky T, Kessler RC, et al. The economic burden of anxiety disorders in the 1990s. *J Clin Psychiatry.* 1999;60:427-435.
2. Bruce SE, Yonkers KA, Otto M, et al. Influence of psychiatric comorbidity on recovery and recurrence in generalized anxiety disorder, social phobia, and panic disorder: a 12-year prospective study. *Am J Psychiatry.* 2005;162:1179-1187.
3. Kroenke K, Spitzer RL, Williams JB, et al. Anxiety disorders in primary care: prevalence, impairment, comorbidity, and detection. *Ann Intern Med.* 2007;146(5):317-325.
4. Spitzer RL, Kroenke K, Williams JB, et al. A brief measure for assessing generalized anxiety disorder: the GAD-7. *Arch Intern Med.* 2006;166:1092-1097.
5. Kirmayer LJ, Robbins JM, Dworkind M, et al. Somatization and the recognition of depression and anxiety in primary care. *Am J Psychiatry.* 1993;150:734-741.
6. Goldberg RJ. *Practical Guide to the Care of the Psychiatric Patient.* St. Louis: Mosby Year Book; 1995.
7. Rodriguez BF, Weisberg RB, Pagano ME, et al. Frequency and patterns of psychiatric comorbidity in a sample of primary care patients with anxiety disorders. *Compr Psychiatry.* 2004;45(2):129-137.
8. Rosen RC, Lane RM, Menza M. Effects of SSRIs on sexual function: a critical review. *J Clin Psychopharmacol.* 1999;19:67-85.
9. Balon B. SSRI-associated sexual dysfunction. *Am J Psychiatry.* 2006;163:1504-1509.
10. Davidson JRT, Potts N, Richichi E, et al. Treatment of social phobia with clonazepam and placebo. *J Clin Psychopharmacol.* 1993;13:423-428.
11. Sun EC, Dixit A, Humphreys K, Darnall BD, Baker LC, Mackey S. Association between concurrent use of prescription opioids and benzodiazepines and overdose: retrospective analysis. *BMJ.* 2017;356. doi:10.1136/bmj.j760.
12. Rickels K, Rynn M. Pharmacology of generalized anxiety disorder. *J Clin Psychiatry.* 2002;63(suppl 14):9-16.
13. Gelernter CS, Uhde TW, Cimbolic P, et al. Cognitive-behavioral and pharmacological treatments of social phobia: a controlled study. *Arch Gen Psychiatry.* 1991;48:938-945.
14. Mitte K. A meta-analysis of the efficacy of psycho- and pharmacotherapy in panic disorder with and without agoraphobia. *J Affect Disord.* 2005;88:27-45.
15. Black DW. Efficacy of combined pharmacotherapy and psychotherapy versus monotherapy in the treatment of anxiety disorders. *CNS Spectr.* 2006;11(suppl 12-10):29-33.
16. Van Apeldoorn FJ, Van Hout WJ, Timmerman ME, Mersch PP, den Boer JA. Rate of improvement during and across three treatments for panic disorder with or without agoraphobia: cognitive behavioral therapy, selective serotonin reuptake inhibitor or both combined. *J Affect Disord.* 2013;150(2):313-319.

6

OBSESSIVE–COMPULSIVE AND RELATED DISORDERS

Shawn Hersevoort, MD, MPH

A healthy 32-year-old man with a history of anxiety presents to clinic after being turned down for a procedure by a cosmetic surgeon. He has been on fluoxetine 20 mg since you began treating him 2 years ago, and his PHQ-9 and GAD-7 scores have been within normal limits. When you inquire further he becomes emotional and states that he failed some kind of "test" when he met with a surgeon about getting rhinoplasty. "I just want to feel better and I can't do that until I look normal," he says. "It's not just my nose, either. It's my skin and teeth as well." You now recall his fluoxetine, and ask more about the past anxiety symptoms and treatment. He says that it helps with the lock checking and organizing, but not as much as in the past when symptoms were present less than an hour a day.

CLINICAL HIGHLIGHTS

- The obsessive–compulsive and related disorders are a collection of distinct, common, and often debilitating disorders including obsessive–compulsive disorder, hoarding disorder, body dysmorphic disorder, trichotillomania, and excoriation disorder.

- The most common comorbid conditions are anxiety disorder, major depressive disorder, personality disorder, substance use disorder, eating disorder, tic disorder, attention-deficit/hyperactivity disorder, and others.

- Selective serotonin reuptake inhibitors are the first-line pharmacologic treatment, followed by the tricyclic antidepressant clomipramine, and the second-generation antipsychotic risperidone.

- Pharmacologic treatment often requires dosages as much as twice as high and for twice as long as traditionally used for other disorders.

- Cognitive behavioral therapy assignments focus on examining cognitive errors to decrease the intensity of obsessions and make tolerating compulsions less uncomfortable.

- Exposure and response prevention is the treatment of choice for obsessive–compulsive disorder and a modified form for body dysmorphic disorder.

- Habit reversal treatment for trichotillomania and excoriation disorder is made up of four stages including education, relaxation, competing response, and replacement behaviors.

- Other options available for patients with limited benefit to standard therapies include repetitive transcranial magnetic stimulation, electroconvulsive therapy, deep brain stimulation, and ablative neurosurgery.

CLINICAL SIGNIFICANCE

The obsessive–compulsive (OC) and related disorders are distinct, common, and often debilitating. They include obsessive–compulsive disorder (OCD), hoarding disorder, body dysmorphic disorder (BDD), trichotillomania, and excoriation disorder (*Table 6-1*). The lifetime prevalence of OCD is estimated to be between 1% and 3%, and is roughly equal in men and women.[1,2] Point prevalence for the others ranges from 2% to 4%.[3-5] Age of onset is usually in adolescence or early adulthood. Primary care providers may recognize these disorders less than one-third of the time, despite anxiety-related disorders being present in up to 20% of their patients. Additionally, between 25% and 50% of primary care visits include medically unexplained symptoms, many anxiety-related.[6] Patients with body dysmorphia, trichotillomania, or excoriation are far more likely to present to primary care, dermatology, or cosmetic surgery centers than to mental health.

Patients with OC disorders present significant costs in terms of health care use, productivity loss, disability, and reduction in quality of life. A 2005 study estimated

TABLE 6-1 Obsessive–Compulsive and Related Disorders (OCRDs)

Obsessive–compulsive disorder

Includes obsessions and/or compulsions often involving thoughts or behaviors related to contamination, checking, symmetry, and/or upsetting graphic images

Body dysmorphic disorder

Is an intense and persistent preoccupation with perceived physical flaws, leading to repeated attempts to evaluate, hide, or alter appearance through interventions such as makeup or surgery

Hoarding disorder

Is characterized by an intense discomfort in parting with possessions, regardless of their actual value, and usually resulting in a problematic accumulation of objects

Excoriation disorder (skin-picking disorder)

Involves repeated and difficult-to-control skin picking, which usually leads to some amount of ongoing skin injury

Trichotillomania (hair-pulling disorder)

Involves repeated and difficult-to-control hair pulling usually leading to some amount of ongoing hair loss

Substance/medication-induced OCRD

Symptoms develop after exposure to a substance or medication known to cause or worsen symptoms
E.g., cocaine-induced OCRD

OCRD due to another medical condition

Symptoms develop as a direct physiological result of another medical condition (other than delirium)
E.g., OCRD due to hyperthyroidism

Other specified OCRDs

Symptoms that fall short of meeting full criteria
E.g., body dysmorphia-like disorder without repetitive behaviors

Unspecified OCRD

Symptoms with insufficient evidence to make a more specific diagnosis

---

that patients with OCD lose 3 years of wages over their lifetime because of their illness.[6] Rates of spontaneous remission are below 20%. However, the remission rate is greater than 60% with proper treatment. Although up to 40% of childhood cases resolve by adulthood, those that persist often cause significant impairments. Adolescents may avoid socialization, and young adults may find it difficult to relate to others outside of the family. Like anxiety disorders, patients with OCD demonstrate elevated divorce rates, greater unemployment, and increased reliance on public assistance.[6] A 2016 study showed that patients with OCD are 10 times more likely to commit suicide than the general population.[7]

OC symptoms may at times be related to an organic cause including stroke, hypothyroidism, meningitis, encephalitis, traumatic brain injury, dementia, or a genetic disorder.[8] Pediatric autoimmune neuropsychiatric disorder associated with group A streptococci is an autoimmune condition believed to result in rapid onset, or sudden worsening of OCD, tics, and/or attention-deficit/hyperactivity disorder (ADHD) symptoms. Perinatal traumas such as drug exposure, maternal illness, and even use of forceps have been associated with more tic-related OCD, as well as early onset and increased severity of OCD.[2] Patients with BDD will often present repeatedly to

dentists, dermatologists, or cosmetic surgeons, exposing them to pain, infection, disfigurement, or even death. Comorbid eating disorders can pose grave metabolic and cardiac risks. Patients with trichotillomania or excoriation risk infection or injury from repeated hair pulling and skin picking. Health risks to hoarders include injury from falls, fires, or infection secondary to sometimes unsanitary home environments.

DIAGNOSIS
DIAGNOSTIC CONSIDERATIONS

The OC disorders share much in common with both the anxiety and the trauma- and stressor-related disorders with which they were grouped before May 2013. This reclassification was made because of increasing evidence that the OC disorders were distinct from the anxiety disorders in their core symptoms, risk factors, course, comorbidities, neuronal circuitry, and treatment responses. Whereas all three categories include intense mental and emotional distress, both the OC and trauma-related disorders are much more homogenous and specific.

The OC disorders share intense, sometimes panic-level, distress with the anxiety disorders, as well as the intrusive, recurrent thoughts of posttraumatic stress disorder (PTSD). Whereas "being trapped in memory" describes PTSD, "being trapped in thought" (obsession) or "being trapped in behavior" (compulsion) describes the OCDs (*Figure 6-1*). Whereas the fear associated with anxiety can be quite intense, it usually fades quickly as the trigger is removed. Thoughts related to OC disorders not only emerge suddenly, but they can be difficult or impossible to dismiss as well. It is this quality of "stickiness" that patients use to describe obsession. Like trying to drop a paper that you have glued to your fingers, it will not drop no matter how hard you wave your arms. As a matter of fact, the distress usually increases over time. Similarly, the compulsive action has an "itchiness" that gets worse the longer you ignore scratching it.

Disorders Including Obsessions and Compulsions

Obsessive–compulsive disorder. This disorder, for which the class is named, includes recurrent obsessions and/or compulsions that must lead to functional difficulties. Obsessions are frequent and difficult-to-ignore thoughts that provoke intense anxiety. Compulsions are frequent and difficult-to-resist behaviors often performed to decrease the anxiety or distress caused by obsessions. OCD most often includes paired obsessions and compulsions, although it may have only one or the other. Most patients experience more than one type of obsession. The behaviors are usually very specific physical rituals aimed at undoing or preventing the dreaded subject of the obsession. At times, compulsions can take the form of mental rituals such as counting or repeating words in a particular pattern. This "question and answer" pairing is pathognomonic for OCD.

Common examples include the following:

- Contamination: "My hands feel dirty, so I must wash them."
- Checking: "I may not have locked the door, so I must check it."
- Symmetry: "These books don't line up, so I must straighten them."
- Intrusive images: "I might have hit someone with my car, so I must search the roadside."

Other symptoms include fears related to loss of control, responsibility for disasters, unwanted sexual thoughts, religious obsessions, excessive concern with right/wrong or morality, and superstitious ideas about lucky/unlucky numbers or colors. Onset is usually gradual, although acute onset can be seen when related to hormonal factors such as those associated with pregnancy and childbirth, emotional trauma, or even physical illness or infection. Around half of childhood cases resolve to some extent but can reemerge again later in life. Although most patients are aware of the abnormality of the thoughts and behaviors, there is a range of insight from "good" to "absent/delusional."

Screening for OCD should be done for vulnerable populations such as patients with common comorbid conditions such as anxiety or depression, patients who are pregnant or postpartum, or children with ADHD and/or tics. It is often sufficient to ask patients about the presence of the most common symptoms listed above. If suspected, a validated rating scale such as the Yale–Brown Obsessive Compulsive Scale (Y-BOCS) should be used (*Table 6-2*). This includes a symptom checklist to identify current and past obsessions and compulsions as well as a symptom severity scale to judge impairment and follow progress. The Y-BOCS is readily available online for free in either downloadable or printable versions.

Body dysmorphic disorder. BDD is an intense and persistent preoccupation with perceived physical flaws, leading to recurrent attempts to evaluate, hide, or alter appearance. These flaws are said to be "slight or not observed by others," but to the patients take on an exaggerated, distorted, and even delusional intensity. This disorder was previously classified under the somatoform disorders, now somatic symptom disorders, because of being body-focused. It was reclassified because of its close relationship with the OC disorders, including the core symptoms of obsession and compulsion, as well as the close overlap of successful treatment strategies. Unlike OCD, which usually includes obsession and compulsion, a BDD diagnosis requires both. Patients will spend from 3 to 8 hours a day dealing with their preoccupations and will focus on five to seven distinct areas over the course of the illness.[3] The most commonly disliked body parts are the skin, hair, nose, stomach, hips, buttocks, and breasts. A predominantly male specifier is "with muscle dysmorphia." Nearly 90% of patients take part in camouflaging, comparing, or mirror checking. Other common behaviors include skin picking, hair pulling, or excessive shopping, exercising, or weight lifting. Cosmetic treatments, including plastic surgery, are sought by up to 71% of patients and obtained by 64%. Unfortunately, these interventions are successful only 4% of the time, show no change 91% of the time, and lead to worsened symptoms in 5%.[3]

Screening should be done in patients with common comorbid conditions and those seeking cosmetic procedures. Patients can be asked if they are unhappy with how they look and about particular concerns. Screening tools include the Appearance Anxiety Inventory (AAI) and the Yale–Brown Obsessive Compulsive Scale modified for BDD (BDD-YBOCS) (*Table 6-2*). Suicide rates are believed to be up to 23 times that of the general population.[3] When skin picking or hair pulling are involved, it should be determined whether the behaviors are exclusively aimed at modifying appearance, or whether comorbid trichotillomania and/or excoriation disorder are also present.

Hoarding disorder. Hoarding disorder is characterized by an intense discomfort in parting with possessions, regardless of their actual value, because of a belief that they will later be needed. This leads to accumulation that can cause difficulties with housing and relationships. The obsessional focus is on the usefulness or beauty of objects, sentimental attachment, or fear of losing valuable information. At times, the clutter can completely impede use of an area, necessitating adaptations such as cooking in the bedroom or sleeping in the bathroom. Although any item can be hoarded, the most common are newspapers, clothing, bags, books, paperwork, or less frequently, food or animals. Cognitive

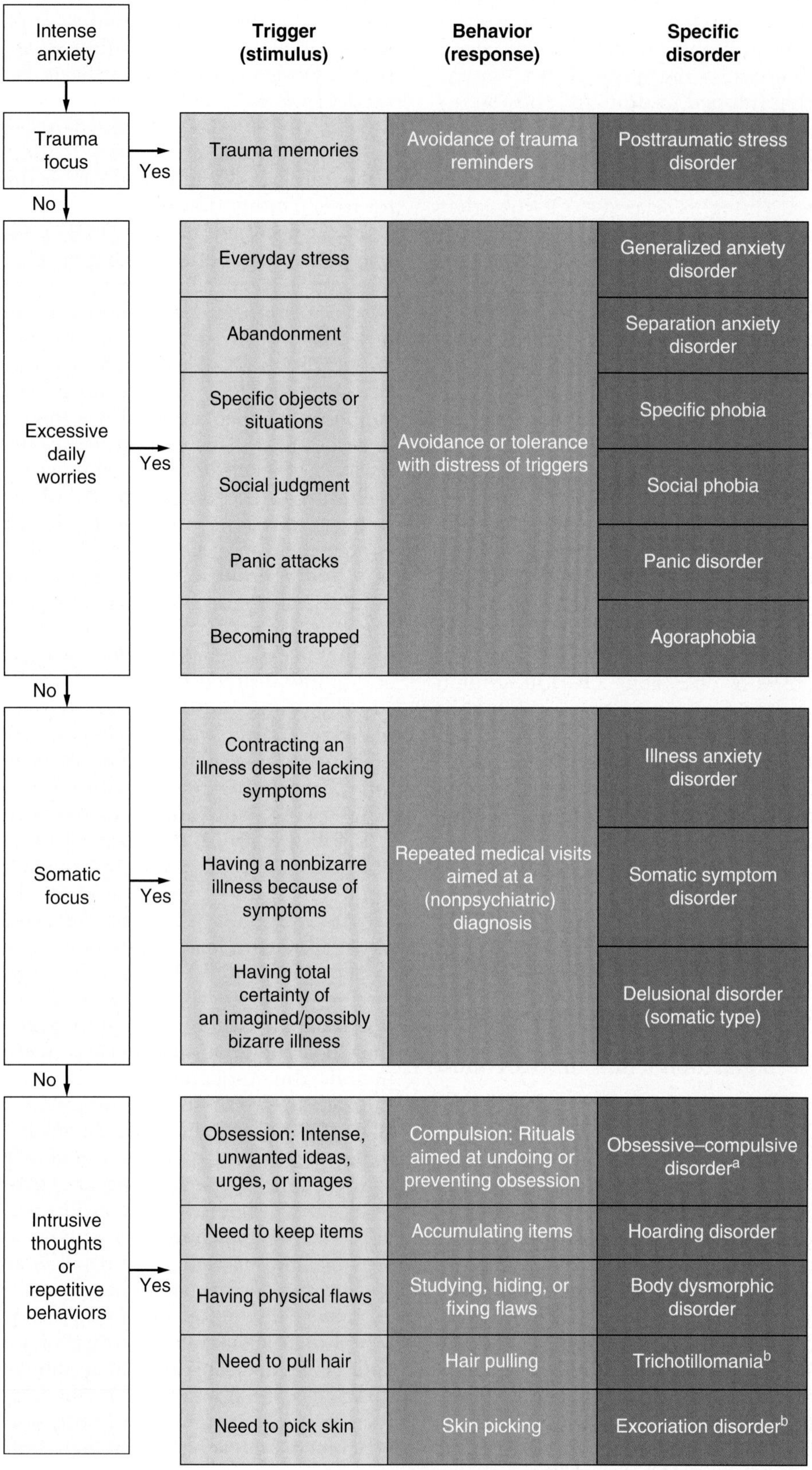

	Trigger (stimulus)	**Behavior (response)**	**Specific disorder**
Intense anxiety → Trauma focus — Yes →	Trauma memories	Avoidance of trauma reminders	Posttraumatic stress disorder

No ↓

	Trigger (stimulus)	**Behavior (response)**	**Specific disorder**
Excessive daily worries — Yes →	Everyday stress	Avoidance or tolerance with distress of triggers	Generalized anxiety disorder
	Abandonment		Separation anxiety disorder
	Specific objects or situations		Specific phobia
	Social judgment		Social phobia
	Panic attacks		Panic disorder
	Becoming trapped		Agoraphobia

No ↓

	Trigger (stimulus)	**Behavior (response)**	**Specific disorder**
Somatic focus — Yes →	Contracting an illness despite lacking symptoms	Repeated medical visits aimed at a (nonpsychiatric) diagnosis	Illness anxiety disorder
	Having a nonbizarre illness because of symptoms		Somatic symptom disorder
	Having total certainty of an imagined/possibly bizarre illness		Delusional disorder (somatic type)

No ↓

	Trigger (stimulus)	**Behavior (response)**	**Specific disorder**
Intrusive thoughts or repetitive behaviors — Yes →	Obsession: Intense, unwanted ideas, urges, or images	Compulsion: Rituals aimed at undoing or preventing obsession	Obsessive–compulsive disorder[a]
	Need to keep items	Accumulating items	Hoarding disorder
	Having physical flaws	Studying, hiding, or fixing flaws	Body dysmorphic disorder
	Need to pull hair	Hair pulling	Trichotillomania[b]
	Need to pick skin	Skin picking	Excoriation disorder[b]

[a]Obsessive–compulsive disorder only requires obsessions or compulsions, but often includes both.
[b]Trichotillomania and excoriation disorders do not require triggers (obsessions) for their compulsions.

FIGURE 6-1 Diagnostic algorithm for obsessive–compulsive and related disorders.

TABLE 6-2 Rating Scales for Obsessive–Compulsive and Related Disorders		
DIAGNOSIS	**RATING SCALE**	**DESCRIPTION**
Obsessive–compulsive disorder	Yale–Brown Obsessive Compulsive Scale II (Y-BOCS) Children's Yale–Brown Obsessive Compulsive Scale[a] (CY-BOCS), Parent Report (CY-BOCS-PR)	Symptom checklist and 14-item severity scale Symptom checklist and 10-item severity scale, parent report version also available
Hoarding disorder	Hoarding Rating Scale (HRS-SR) Clutter Image Rating Scale (CIR)	5-item interview or self-report scale 3-item visual comparison rating scale
Body dysmorphic disorder	Appearance Anxiety Inventory (AAI) Yale–Brown Obsessive Compulsive Scale modified for BDD (BDD-YBOCS)	10-item self-report scale 12-item observer rated scale
Trichotillomania	Massachusetts General Hospital Hair Pulling Scale (MGH-HS) Trichotillomania Scale for Children[a] (TSC)	7-item self-report scale 12-item self-report scale, child and adult versions available
Excoriation disorder	Skin Picking Scale-Revised (SPS-R) Yale–Brown Obsessive Compulsive Scale modified for Neurotic Excoriation (NE-YBOCS)	8-item self-report scale 10-item self-report scale

[a]*Scales validated for use in children.*

difficulties in planning and organizing have also been observed in patients with hoarding disorder, including pathologic indecisiveness, perfectionism, avoidance, procrastination, and circumstantial, overinclusive language.[9]

Screening for hoarding disorder should be done when commonly comorbid disorders are present, and in high-risk populations such as unemployed and elderly women who live alone. Patients can be asked whether they have difficulty parting with objects, and whether they have a large amount of clutter at home. The Hoarding Rating Scale (HRS-SR) or Clutter Image Rating Scale (CIR) can be used to assist in diagnosis (*Table 6-2*). Collateral from family, a photograph of the home, or a home visit may also be helpful.

Disorders Including Only Compulsions

Excoriation disorder. Excoriation (skin-picking) disorder involves repeated and difficult-to-control skin picking, which usually leads to some amount of tissue injury. Patients with this disorder repeatedly pick, scratch, rub, dig at, or squeeze their skin. The most frequently targeted areas are the face, scalp, cuticles, extremities, shoulders, back, perianal, and scrotal regions. A typical episode lasts from 6 to 10 minutes, although they can last several hours. Symptoms tend to worsen in the evening and often occur while either distracted or focusing intently in the mirror. Unlike OCD, BDD, and hoarding, there need not be any obsession leading to the picking behavior. The gender ratio in BDD is the most disproportionate of all OC disorders, with an 8:1 female-to-male ratio.[5]

Excoriation will often present in primary care or dermatology. Although often reluctant to volunteer information spontaneously, patients will often admit to picking behavior when asked directly. Patients should be asked about the timing and emotions around the picking. The Skin Picking Scale-Revised (SPS-R) and the Yale–Brown Obsessive Compulsive Scale modified for Neurotic Excoriation (NE-YBOCS) can be used (*Table 6-2*). Picking secondary to other conditions is discussed in the Differential Diagnosis section and *Table 6-3*.

Trichotillomania. Trichotillomania (hair-pulling disorder) involves repeated and difficult-to-control hair pulling, usually leading to some amount of hair loss. Behaviors can be either automatic, in which patients repeatedly pull out hair when distracted, or focused, which occurs during periods of intense stress, where the behavior helps them to self-soothe. The most common locations are the scalp, face, arms, legs, and pubic regions. Eyebrows and/or eyelashes are often involved. Hair-biting or ingestion (trichophagia) is sometimes seen.[5] Like excoriation disorder, there need not be any obsession leading to the compulsion. Trichotillomania appears earlier than most OC disorders. It is seven times more prevalent in children than in adults, with peak prevalence between 4 and 17 years.[10] Patients may cut their hair short or wear wigs to disguise the hair loss.

Like excoriation, trichotillomania is more likely to present in primary care or dermatology. Patients can be asked if they frequently pull out hair and how they feel while they are doing so. Rating scales include the Massachusetts General Hospital Hair Pulling Scale (MGH-HS) and the Trichotillomania Scale for Children (TSC) (*Table 6-2*).

DIFFERENTIAL DIAGNOSIS

The differential diagnoses for the OC disorders can be very broad (*Table 6-3*). The most closely related conditions are the anxiety, trauma-related, somatic symptom, and psychotic disorders. Each of these has a unique fingerprint made up of defining cognitions, emotions, and behaviors. By focusing on the trigger and the resulting behavior, the other disorders can

TABLE 6-3 Differential Diagnosis for Obsessive-Compulsive and Related Disorders

DISORDER	DISTINGUISHING CHARACTERISTICS
Generalized anxiety disorder	Worry involves practical, real-world problems and lacks compulsions
Social phobia	Fear is limited to social situations and/or performance, and lacks compulsions
Specific phobia	Feared object or situations are very specific and lack compulsions
Panic disorder	Fear is focused on having more panic attacks and lacks compulsions
Agoraphobia	Fear is of being trapped without assistance and lacks compulsions
Major depressive disorder	Recurrent negative thoughts are mood congruent and lack compulsions
Tic disorder	Sudden, simple movements or sounds not in response to obsessions
Illness anxiety disorder (hypochondriasis)	Fear is focused on having, or later being diagnosed with, a specific disease despite little evidence (e.g., cancer or dementia)
Paraphilia	Specific sexual thoughts and urges, which are not usually disturbing or resisted
Impulse control disorder	Patient enjoys repeated behaviors (e.g., gambling, starting fires, stealing)
Substance use disorders	Patient enjoys repeated use even if regretting later
Posttraumatic stress disorder	Intrusive thoughts and images are frightening memories and lack compulsions
Delusional disorder	A fixed belief that cannot be weakened despite evidence to the contrary
Eating disorder	Fear and behaviors are all focused on appearance, weight, and food
Bipolar disorder	Manic delusions are grandiose in nature, and increase in goal-directed behavior is not intended to decrease anxiety
Cluster A personality disorder (e.g., paranoid)	Intrusive thoughts are limited to persistent suspicion of the motives and intentions of individuals, groups, or organizations
Cluster B personality disorder (e.g., borderline)	Repeated self-harm (e.g., cutting) is done to calm overwhelming feelings of abandonment, anger, or emotional distress
Cluster C personality disorder (e.g., obsessive–compulsive)	Patient is not disturbed by perfectionistic, rigid, rule-focused beliefs and behaviors, and repetitive behaviors are not in response to obsessions
Autism spectrum disorders	Stereotyped interests or behaviors are often enjoyed rather than tolerated
Normal development	Some magical thinking or repetitive/ritualistic behaviors can be age appropriate (e.g., superstition, fascination with symmetry)

usually be differentiated and an accurate diagnosis isolated (*Figure 6-1*). Look for trauma, somatic focus, or an exaggeration of usual day-to-day anxieties. The associated behaviors associated with these diagnoses involve simple avoidance of triggers, rather than elaborate and specific compulsions. A family history can be particularly helpful as the OC disorders are believed to have a much higher genetic contribution than anxiety or trauma disorders. It is also important to be aware that comorbid conditions are the rule and not the exception when discussing OC disorders. The most common comorbid conditions are an anxiety disorder (37% to 76%), major depressive disorder (MDD; 31% to 75%), personality disorder (50%), substance use disorder (40%), eating disorder (33%), tic disorder (29%), and/or other OC disorders (5% to 68%).[1-5] Others include ADHD, PTSD, bipolar disorder, psychotic spectrum disorders, and learning disorders.

In children, magical thinking or an intense need for rules might be completely normal for developmental stage. In the elderly, many neurodegenerative disorders can present with both obsessions and compulsions. Intense and repetitive thoughts and behaviors associated with personality disorders are ego syntonic (in line with the self), rather than ego dystonic (at odds with the self). The rigid order demanded by a patient with OCPD is felt as a part of himself or herself, whereas ritual in patients with OCD feel imposed upon them.

Skin picking secondary to BDD can be distinguished by being primarily for aesthetic purposes, rather than stress relieving. In patients with self-injury, pain and distraction are the desired outcomes (vs. picking), lesions are more likely on the arms and legs (vs. face), and cutting or scratching (vs. picking) is far more common. Delusional parasitosis is a form of somatic delusion, which is most often seen in middle-aged women with depression and older patients with dementia. A sudden-onset form is associated with stimulant abuse. In Morgellons disease, patients are convinced that fibers are growing out of their skin and will often present samples or even travel with their own microscope.

BIOPSYCHOSOCIAL TREATMENT
OVERVIEW OF TREATMENT

OC disorders respond to both pharmacologic and psychotherapeutic interventions (*Figure 6-2*). Like anxiety and depression, the treatment of choice for mild to moderate severity is psychotherapy. For more severe symptoms, or those that do not respond to counseling, medications are recommended. In most circumstances, the combination is more effective than either treatment alone. The pharmacologic approach to treatment involves the use of serotonergic medications at higher than antidepressant dosages and for longer duration. Medications used for OCD are also effective, albeit less so, for the related disorders. The various psychotherapies are based on the principles of cognitive behavioral therapy (CBT) with particular focus on confronting distorted thoughts and extinguishing compulsive behaviors. Unfortunately, many patients with BDD and hoarding disorder have very limited insight, and adherence to any

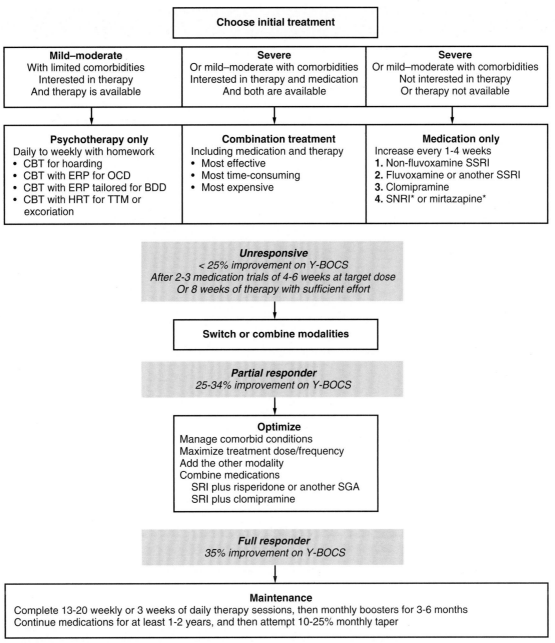

Choose initial treatment

Mild–moderate With limited comorbidities Interested in therapy And therapy is available	**Severe** Or mild–moderate with comorbidities Interested in therapy and medication And both are available	**Severe** Or mild–moderate with comorbidities Not interested in therapy Or therapy not available
Psychotherapy only Daily to weekly with homework • CBT for hoarding • CBT with ERP for OCD • CBT with ERP tailored for BDD • CBT with HRT for TTM or excoriation	**Combination treatment** Including medication and therapy • Most effective • Most time-consuming • Most expensive	**Medication only** Increase every 1-4 weeks 1. Non-fluvoxamine SSRI 2. Fluvoxamine or another SSRI 3. Clomipramine 4. SNRI* or mirtazapine*

Unresponsive
< 25% improvement on Y-BOCS
After 2-3 medication trials of 4-6 weeks at target dose
Or 8 weeks of therapy with sufficient effort

Switch or combine modalities

Partial responder
25-34% improvement on Y-BOCS

Optimize
Manage comorbid conditions
Maximize treatment dose/frequency
Add the other modality
Combine medications
   SRI plus risperidone or another SGA
   SRI plus clomipramine

Full responder
35% improvement on Y-BOCS

Maintenance
Complete 13-20 weekly or 3 weeks of daily therapy sessions, then monthly boosters for 3-6 months
Continue medications for at least 1-2 years, and then attempt 10-25% monthly taper

* Limited evidence

Y-BOCS, Yale–Brown Obsessive Compulsive Scale-II; SSRI, selective serotonin reuptake inhibitor; SNRI, serotonin and norepinephrine reuptake inhibitor; SRI, serotonin reuptake inhibitor including SSRI, SNRI, and mirtazapine; SGA, second-generation antipsychotic; OCD, obsessive–compulsive disorder; BDD, body dysmorphic disorder; TTM, trichotillomania; CBT, cognitive behavioral therapy; ERP, exposure and response prevention; HRT, habit reversal therapy.

FIGURE 6-2 Example of fear level during exposure exercise.

treatment is limited. In children with OCD, or in patients of any age with hoarding disorder, the evidence for psychotherapy is much stronger than for medication.

PSYCHOPHARMACOLOGY

The selective serotonin reuptake inhibitor (SSRI) is the foundation of medication management. All, except for citalopram and escitalopram, have indications for the treatment of OCD. A safe practice is to begin with half of the standard starting dosage (e.g., 10 mg of fluoxetine) to limit initial side effects. After 1 week, an increase is usually well tolerated. As it often takes a much higher dosage relative to the treatment of depression or anxiety, the initial target dose is usually at least half way up the dosage range. Although some providers will give the classic 4 to 6 weeks between dose changes, others have opted for a more aggressive schedule including changes

TABLE 6-4 Medication Dosing in Obsessive–Compulsive Disorder

MEDICATION	LEVEL OF CLINICAL EVIDENCE	STARTING DOSE AND INCREMENTAL DOSE (MG/DAY)	USUAL TARGET DOSE (MG/DAY)	USUAL MAXIMUM DOSE (MG/DAY)
SSRI				
Fluoxetine	Indication	10-20, 20	40-60	80
Paroxetine	Indication	10-20, 20	40-60	60
Paroxetine ER	Case control	12.5-25, 25	50-62.5	75
Sertraline	Indication	25-50, 50	100-200	200
Fluvoxamine	Indication	25-50, 50	100-200	300
Fluvoxamine ER	Indication	25-50, 50	100-200	300
Citalopram	Case control	10-20, 20	40-60[a]	60[a]
Escitalopram	Case control	5-10, 10	20	20
SNRI and mirtazapine				
Venlafaxine	Case control	37.5-75, 75	225-375[a]	375[a]
Venlafaxine ER	Case control	37.5-75, 75	150-225	225
Desvenlafaxine	Case control	25-50, 50	100-200	200
Duloxetine	Case control	20-30, 30	60-120	120
Milnacipran	Case report	12.5-25, 25	50-100	200
Mirtazapine	Case report	7.5-15, 15	30-45[a]	45[a]
TCA				
Clomipramine	Indication	12.5-25, 25	100-250[a,b]	250[a,b]

[a]*Screening electrocardiogram is recommended to rule out long QT syndrome.*
[b]*Monitor blood levels for toxicity, particularly when combining with other antidepressants.*
ER, extended release; mg, milligram; SNRI, serotonin and norepinephrine reuptake inhibitor; SSRI, selective serotonin reuptake inhibitor; TCA, tricyclic antidepressant.

every 1 to 2 weeks. Evidence has also demonstrated that dosages greater than standard guidelines may be necessary (*Table 6-4*). Another difference is that symptom response may take as long as 10 to 12 weeks to present, in contrast to the 4 to 6 weeks often seen in other disorders.[11]

Although screening labs are not required for initiating treatment, special attention should be given to long QT syndrome. This is a concern with citalopram over 40 mg, venlafaxine and mirtazapine at maximum dosages, and with clomipramine at any dose. In these cases, a thorough cardiac history should be taken, and a screening electrocardiogram (ECG) be performed. Paroxetine, fluvoxamine, and clomipramine, in that order, are increasingly anticholinergic and therefore more likely to cause sedation, constipation, dry mouth, and weight gain. Clomipramine levels should be monitored during dose changes because of unpredictable metabolism and toxicity.

Rapid cross-taper to a second SSRI should be done if the first has not demonstrated a significant clinical effect after 10 to 12 weeks, where at least 4 weeks have been at a maximum indicated or tolerable dose (*Table 6-5*). Like initial treatment, transition between agents can be done quickly (weekly) or slowly (monthly), based on symptom severity and comfort concerns. After a trial of two to three high-dose SSRIs, including fluvoxamine, a trial of clomipramine should be attempted. If ineffective, intolerable, or contraindicated, an SNRI (serotonin norepinephrine reuptake inhibitor) can be substituted. Although not formally indicated, multiple case-controlled studies have shown effectiveness for venlafaxine and duloxetine. Case reports have suggested efficacy for SNRI milnacipran, and tetracyclic antidepressant mirtazapine. If not already in place or previously failed, addition of CBT at this point is indicated. The final steps in the medication algorithm include an SSRI, SNRI, or

TABLE 6-5 Examples of Cross-tapering Antidepressants in Obsessive–Compulsive Disorder

MEDICATION	STARTING DOSE	STEP 1	STEP 2	STEP 3	FINAL DOSE
Example 1: Transitioning from fluoxetine to sertraline (in mg)					
Fluoxetine	80	60	40	20	0
Sertraline	0	50	100	150	200
Example 2: Transitioning from fluvoxamine to clomipramine (in mg)					
Fluvoxamine	300	200	100	50	0
Clomipramine	0	50	100	150	200

mg, milligram.

clomipramine in combination with an atypical or second-generation antipsychotic (SGA). Evidence supports the use of risperidone at dosages between 0.5 and 3 mg, particularly when insight is poor, or symptoms verge on delusional. Fewer studies also support use of olanzapine, quetiapine, or aripiprazole. Combining an SSRI or SNRI with clomipramine is another augmentation that may be effective.

Once symptoms are treated successfully, maintenance treatment should continue for at least 1 to 2 years before a slow tapering off medications at 10% to 25% of the dose per month is attempted. For BDD, the recommendation is 3 to 4 years. In cases of severe disease, relapse, or comorbidities, medications may be needed long term.

Psychopharmacology Pearls

- SSRIs are first line, followed by clomipramine.
- Augmentation strategies include combining an SSRI with clomipramine or risperidone.
- Required dosages may be twice as high, and take twice as long to be effective, compared with other disorders.
- Medications for OCD work to a lesser extent for BDD, hoarding, trichotillomania, and excoriation disorder.
- In children, medication alone is less effective than CBT or combination treatment.
- Children should be closely monitored for suicidal thoughts and mania when treated with antidepressants.[12]

PSYCHOLOGICAL APPROACHES

Psychological approaches include CBT, CBT with exposure and response prevention (ERP), CBT tailored to BDD, and habit reversal treatment (HRT) (*Table 6-6*).

CBT-ERP has been shown to be effective in a variety of schedules, with the best evidence for weekly therapy for 13 to 20 weeks or 5 days a week for 3 weeks. Evidence shows that 83% of patients demonstrated 30% or more improvement, and that results persisted for more than 2 years in 76% of patients.[13] Shorter courses have also demonstrated benefit in some studies. Roles for the primary care provider can include choosing the initial treatment, assigning a workbook, providing abbreviated in-office treatment including homework, or referring patients to a therapist with CBT training.

Assessment

A full mental health history augmented by rating scales (*Table 6-2*) will identify both a specific diagnosis as well as baseline severity. Next, explore and list obsessional thoughts, ideas, and impulses and their effect on function. Use motivational interviewing to determine readiness for change, then list personal reasons for wanting treatment, including concrete goals.

Education

Education begins with the core principle that everyone has intrusive or obsessive thoughts. The difference is that a patient with an OC disorder overestimates the danger of these thoughts and uses ritual to quickly experience relief. Giving in to this paired process of worry and ritual reinforces symptoms and hinders recovery. Relaxation techniques can be started at this time, including mindful deep breathing and progressive muscle relaxation.

Cognitive Therapy

This phase helps to decrease false beliefs to directly lower stress as well as allow for greater tolerance of behavioral exercises to follow. CBT assignments are initiated based on the unique needs of the patient[14] (*Table 6-6*). These exercises can be written into scripts and used before behavioral treatments (e.g., "anxiety is normal, temporary, and nonlethal"). In hoarding, support groups such as "The Buried in Treasure Workshop" may also be helpful.[15]

TABLE 6-6 Psychotherapy for Obsessive–Compulsive and Related Disorders

Cognitive Behavioral Therapy

Indications: OCD, BDD, hoarding disorder, trichotillomania, and excoriation disorder

Examining the evidence: Looks at cognitive errors by asking for objective evidence supporting fear beliefs
Continuum technique: Looks at "thought–action fusion" by comparing the "badness" of taboo thoughts with the actions
Pie-chart technique: Looks at exaggerated responsibility by estimating true patient contribution to a feared event
Life-saving wager technique: Looks at the need for certainty by asking the patient to bet his or her life savings on his or her certainty of the outcome of a fear belief
Double-standard technique: Looks at cognitive errors by asking what advice they would give to a friend regarding a fear situation
Cost–benefit analysis: Looks at cognitive errors using a two-column table of what the fear helps and hurts
Experiment techniques: Looks at "thought–action fusion" and the need for control by testing the outcome of a real-world fear experiment

Exposure and Response Prevention

Indications: OCD and hoarding disorder

Exposure hierarchy: For each type of symptom (e.g., hygiene, symmetry), a list is made, ordered from bottom to top, and 30-45-minute weekly exercises begin in the middle (*Figure 6-4*)—each week a higher level is addressed before moving on to another symptom type
Exposure fear level: Should be noted in 10-minute increments during daily sessions (*Figure 6-3*)
Lifestyle exposures: Extra credit for catching and preventing yourself from avoiding a spontaneous fear trigger (e.g., preparing to change lanes to get away from an ambulance that signifies death)
Imagined exposures script: Helpful for difficult-to-treat obsessions or difficult-to-test compulsions (e.g., murder)—write out a worst-case scenario, record, and play in a loop as an exposure

Habit Reversal Treatment

Indications: Trichotillomania and excoriation disorder

1. **Education**: The patient is educated about the diagnosis and therapy, completes a behavior questionnaire, and a daily self-monitoring form is given
2. **Relaxation**: The self-monitoring form is reviewed, and the patient is then taught diaphragmatic breathing and progressive muscular relaxation to be practiced twice daily, and when needed
3. **Competing response**: The patient is taught a muscle tensing activity that is somewhat opposite to, and incompatible with, hair pulling, most commonly a clenched fist held at the hip for 60 seconds—this is paired with relaxation exercises whenever the urge to pick or pull arises
4. **Replacement behaviors**: Preemptory relaxation techniques can be practiced when entering a stressful situation and competing postures are employed, such as keeping hands away from hair by sitting on them—obstacles such as wearing a hat or wearing hair back may also be helpful

BDD, body dysmorphic disorder; OCD, obsessive–compulsive disorder.

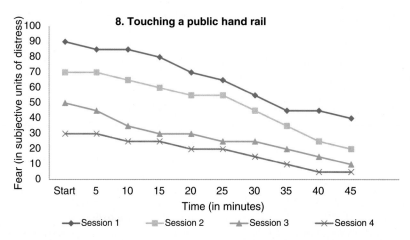

FIGURE 6-3 Treatment algorithm for obsessive–compulsive disorder.

Description of contamination fear	SUD
10. Touching a public urinal	95
9. Touching the floor in a public bathroom	90
8. Touching a public handrail	75
7. Shake hands with a stranger	65
6. Wearing someone else's hat	60
5. Touching public doorknob	55
4. Touching paper money	50
3. Using someone else's pen	40
2. Touching neighbor's mail	35
1. Touching my own mail	20

SUD, subjective units of distress

FIGURE 6-4 Example of an exposure hierarchy.

Behavioral Therapy

These include ERP and HRT. ERP is the treatment of choice for classic OCD and has been modified to successfully treat BDD. The core of this treatment is the exposure hierarchy (*Figure 6-4*). For each type of symptom (e.g., hygiene, symmetry), a list is made with subjective units of distress (SUDs) noted from 1 to 100, with 1 being easily tolerated, and 100 being intolerable for any length of time. They are then ordered from bottom to top, and treatment begins in the middle. Weekly exercises are practiced first with the therapist in the office and then in situ over the week, where SUDs are recorded in 5-minute increments to determine improvement (*Figure 6-3*). HRT is the treatment of choice for trichotillomania and excoriation disorder. The technique can be taught in four brief lessons followed by booster sessions to follow results and refine techniques.[14] The stages include education, relaxation, competing response, and replacement behaviors. See *Table 6-6* for details.

OTHER TREATMENT CONSIDERATIONS

A variety of novel agents known to modify the activity of serotonin, dopamine, glutamate, or gamma-aminobutyric acid have been investigated. Unfortunately, most of these studies are either small or of low quality, and some of the agents in question can be difficult or dangerous to use (stimulants or opioids). Those with good safety profiles and intersecting indications, such as gabapentin, buspirone, topiramate, and naltrexone, are likely better considerations. Medications which may be of use as augmentation include ondansetron and topiramate. As monotherapy, memantine and minocycline may be helpful. Agents found not to be beneficial in the treatment of OCD unless comorbid with other conditions are benzodiazepines, gabapentin, buspirone, L-iodothyronine, desipramine, and lithium. Naltrexone has shown some utility specifically for symptoms of excess grooming. In hoarding, there is some evidence for the use of stimulants.[16] N-acetylcysteine of up to 3,000 mg may have benefits in both trichotillomania and excoriation disorder.

Repetitive transcranial magnetic stimulation has shown mixed results, with both negative and positive study outcomes published. Electroconvulsive therapy has shown promise, but still with mixed findings. Deep brain stimulation is a much more intrusive, although ultimately reversible, surgical treatment. The most commonly used neurosurgic intervention is cingulotomy. Unfortunately, only around one-third of patients respond to the treatment. Short-term side effects include nausea, vomiting, and headaches. Long-term side effects include apathy, memory deficits, urinary incontinence, hydrocephalus, and seizures.[16]

EDUCATION, PREVENTION, TREATMENT ADHERENCE

Extensive self-help materials and advocacy organizations are available. Many of these are described in both the 2007 and 2013 American Psychiatric Association (APA) practice guidelines. There is no known way to specifically prevent these disorders, but general principles of good mental and physical health can help to mitigate effects on quality of life. These include healthy diet, frequent exercise, socialization, a healthy spiritual life, and the avoidance of drugs and alcohol. Listed below are several of the best rated and most recent resources for the various disorders.

- **Getting Over OCD: A 10-Step Workbook for Taking Back Your Life**, by Abramowitz
- **Stuff: Compulsive Hoarding and the Meaning of Things**, by Frost and Steketee
- **Understanding and Treating Body Dysmorphic Disorder**, by Phillips
- **Trichotillomania: An ACT-enhanced Behavior Therapy Approach Workbook**, by Woods and Twohig
- **Skin Picking: The Freedom to Finally Stop**, by Pasternak

Patient adherence can be particularly tricky in the treatment of OC disorders. To some extent, this can be addressed by discussing concerns at the outset of treatment and educating patients. In describing CBT, the clinician should note that it involves confronting feared thoughts and situations, but at a tolerable rate. Family members may be important allies, particularly when colluding with patients regarding rituals, or for younger patients. The fears, doubting, and need for certainty that are characteristic of OCD can be a particular barrier when patients obsess about possible medication side effects and then refuse pharmacotherapy. In addition to a conversation about side effects, it is important to inform patients about the delay between starting medication and experiencing substantial symptom relief, as well as the need for extended periods of medication use uniquely associated with treating OCD. A detailed discussion of managing side effects can be found in the 2013 APA practice guidelines update.[17]

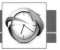

- When initial symptoms are severe or include psychosis or suicidality
- If several steps of treatment have not yielded any meaningful progress
- When patients have other serious comorbid conditions such as bipolar disorder, psychosis, or substance abuse
- In children with more than moderate illness, or with complicating tics, ADHD, or behavioral disorders

CASES AND QUESTIONS

CASE 1: Surgical Refusal and Time-Consuming Behaviors

A healthy 32-year-old man with a history of anxiety presents to clinic after being turned down for a procedure by a cosmetic surgeon. He has been on fluoxetine 20 mg since you began treating him 2 years ago, and his PHQ-9 and GAD-7 scores have been within normal limits. When you inquire further he becomes emotional and states that he failed some kind of "test" when he met with a surgeon about getting rhinoplasty. "I just want to feel better and I can't do that until I look normal," he says. "It's not just my nose, either. It's my skin and teeth as well." You now recall his fluoxetine, and ask more about the past anxiety symptoms and treatment. He says that it helps with the lock checking and organizing, but not as much as in the past when symptoms were present less than an hour a day.

1. What was the test likely screening for?

   A. OCD
   B. MDD
   C. Suicidal ideation
   D. BDD
   E. Anxiety disorder

   Correct answer: D. *Although a cosmetic surgeon may be interested in symptoms of OCD, MDD, suicidality, and anxiety disorder, none of these by themselves are contraindications for surgery. Cosmetic surgeons, dentists, and dermatologists need to rule out BDD before initiating treatment because of the risks involved with treatment and the poor patient satisfaction outcomes.*

2. What is the most likely diagnosis?

   A. MDD
   B. Anxiety disorder
   C. OCD
   D. BDD
   E. OCD and BDD

   Correct answer: E. *Criteria for both disorders are met including thoughts and behaviors focused on physical flaws, as well as symptoms of clinically significant obsessions and/or compulsions. There is no clearly stated trigger consistent with one of the named anxiety disorders.*

3. What treatment should be recommended for this patient?

   A. Surgery
   B. Medication
   C. Psychotherapy
   D. Psychotherapy and medication
   E. None of the above

   Correct answer: D. *In adults, a combination of medications and psychotherapy is virtually always superior to either treatment alone. As stated above, surgery for perceived flaws is very rarely effective and comes with significant health risks.*

CASE 2: A Messy House and Family Difficulties

A 67-year-old woman with hypertension and type 2 diabetes presents for a health maintenance follow-up. On reviewing her vitals and labs you notice that her body mass index has increased steadily over 18 months, her hemoglobin A1c value is 10, and her PHQ-9 score is 17. When you ask her about her blood sugar logs, she begins to weep and pulls dozens of crumpled papers out of her large and overfull purse. On further examination, you notice that she is more unkempt than usual, speaking more slowly, and seeming even more distracted than her usual unfocused self. When you ask what is happening, she reports that her adult children will no longer bring the grandchildren to her house because of the mess and have threatened to call the city on her. "I can't throw away my treasures," she says, "I keep trying to move things around, but my kids say that something could fall and hurt a child." She goes on to tell you that since her husband died 7 years ago, she has had increasing trouble remembering things, sleeping, and sometimes even just feels like giving up.

1. What is the most likely diagnosis?

   A. MDD
   B. Hoarding disorder
   C. OCD
   D. Dementia (major neurocognitive disorder)
   E. MDD and hoarding disorder

   Correct answer: E. *The patient clearly describes at least five out of nine symptoms of depression, as well as difficulty parting with objects leading to clinically significant accumulation. Other paired obsessions and compulsions are not present. Cognitive difficulties are a common feature in patients with hoarding disorder as well as major depression. Although possibly present, criteria for a neurocognitive disorder are not described in adequate detail for a diagnosis.*

2. What treatments should be recommended for this patient?

   A. Medication
   B. Psychotherapy
   C. Psychotherapy and medication

D. Hospitalization

E. None of the above

> **Correct answer: C.** *In cases of comorbid OC and related disorders, medication is recommended to be involved in the initial treatment. In hoarding disorder, psychotherapy is at least as effective as medications alone, thus the combination is recommended for the comorbid disorders described.*

3. What is the role of the primary care provider in this case?

A. Prescriber

B. Educator

C. Therapist

D. None of the above

E. Prescriber and educator

> **Correct answer: E.** *It should be well inside the skill set of a primary care provider to write an antidepressant and to give patient information on hoarding disorder. Limited behavioral therapy may be provided by some primary care providers. More in-depth psychotherapy would be beyond the scope of primary care. Medication unresponsive and more severe patients should be referred to therapists with proper training and experience in managing hoarding disorder. Supportive therapy alone is unlikely to be sufficient in the more severe cases.*

CASE 3: Baldness, Blinking, and Distractibility

A thin, 18-year-old male patient with no significant medical history presents for a new intake to the internal medicine clinic. You are immediately aware that the patient is behaving strangely when you enter, as he is shaking his legs rhythmically, looking around the room, sitting on his hands, and wearing dark glasses and a baseball cap. Already starting to think about a substance use disorder, you ask the patient to remove his hat and glasses to find, unexpectedly, large patches of missing hair, and an extremely high rate of blinking. "I haven't ever been able to sit still or pay attention in class, so I've never been able to do well in school until now," he says. "My parents don't believe in medications, so they never let me get the treatments my doctor told them about. I went online and it said that drinking 2 pots of coffee a day would help me with school if I couldn't get pills. Problem is, now the blinking and the hair-pulling are back from when I was a kid." He denies any drugs or alcohol history and gives a convincing story of academic difficulties as well as a family history of several siblings with symptoms like those he is experiencing.

1. What three often co-occurring disorders appear to be present in this patient?

A. Depression, anxiety, and tic disorders

B. Anxiety, tic, and ADHD

C. Tic, ADHD, and trichotillomania

D. All of the above

E. None of the above

> **Correct answer: C.** *Although depression and anxiety may be present, insufficient information is given to make these diagnoses.*

2. What is the best way to approach the next step in treatment?

A. Medication

B. Psychotherapy

C. Psychotherapy and medication

D. More evaluation

E. None of the above

> **Correct answer: D.** *Although ultimately some combination of medications and psychotherapy are likely to be chosen, we need more information from the patient before we can proceed. When multiple diagnoses are present, it is important to first characterize the severity of each and discuss with the patient which symptoms are the most problematic. In the above example, evidence-based treatment of any one of the diagnoses could lead to worsening of the others. Rating scales should be employed.*

3. What behavioral treatment might be helpful to the patient for his hair pulling?

A. Diaphragmatic breathing

B. CBT including ERP

C. Progressive muscle relaxation

D. HRT

E. All of the above

> **Correct answer: D.** *Diaphragmatic breathing and progressive muscle relaxation are components of HRT. CBT, including ERP, although possibly helpful, is the treatment of choice for OCD, not trichotillomania.*

4. What medication should be considered for the treatment of the two reemerging symptoms?

A. Venlafaxine

B. Fluoxetine

C. Fluvoxamine

D. Clomipramine

E. Risperidone

> **Correct answer: B.** *Fluoxetine, as an SSRI, is a first-line treatment for both trichotillomania and tic disorder. Venlafaxine is considered third-line treatment for trichotillomania and tic disorder because of lack of double-blind placebo-controlled studies. Fluvoxamine is not generally considered first-line for the OC disorders because of a high degree of anticholinergic side effects. Also, because of side effects, clomipramine is recommended for use only after failing at least two to three other agents. Risperidone is an augmentation reserved for use only after multiple failures of single agents for an OC disorder, or second-line for tics. Alpha adrenergic blockers (for tics and ADHD) or stimulants (for ADHD) could be considered later depending on treatment focus.*

PRACTICAL RESOURCES

- American Psychiatric Association: www.psychiatry.org/patients-families/ocd
  APA education portal on OCD for patients and families
- National Institute of Mental Health: www.nimh.nih.gov/health/topics/obsessive-compulsive-disorder-ocd/index.shtml
  OCD specific information from the NIMH
- International OCD Foundation: iocdf.org/, hoarding.iocdf.org/, and bdd.iocdf.org/
  Organization dedicated to fighting stigma, education, and fostering a treatment community
- Body Dysmorphic Disorder Foundation: bddfoundation.org/
  Charitable organization focused on the treatment of BDD
- The TLC Foundation for Body-Focused Repetitive Behaviors: www.bfrb.org/index.php
  Organization dedicated to comprehensive treatment for body-focused repetitive behaviors such as trichotillomania and excoriation disorder

REFERENCES

1. Simpson H. Obsessive-compulsive disorder in adults: epidemiology, pathogenesis, clinical manifestations, course, and diagnosis. In: UpToDate. 2017. Accessed April 27, 2017.
2. Rosenberg D. Obsessive-compulsive disorder in children and adolescents: epidemiology, pathogenesis, clinical manifestations, course, assessment, and diagnosis. In: UpToDate. 2017. Accessed April 27, 2017.
3. Phillips K. Body dysmorphic disorder: epidemiology, pathogenesis, and clinical features. In: UpToDate. 2017. Accessed April 27, 2017.
4. Mataix-Cols D, Fernandez de la Cruz L. Hoarding disorder in adults: epidemiology, pathogenesis, clinical manifestations, course, assessment, and diagnosis. In: UpToDate. 2017. Accessed April 27, 2017.
5. Park K, Koo J. Skin picking (excoriation) disorder and related disorders. In: UpToDate. 2017. Accessed April 27, 2017.
6. Combs H, Markman J. Anxiety disorders in primary care. *Med Clin.* 2014;98(5):1007-1023.
7. Fernández de la Cruz L, Rydell M, Runeson B, et al. Suicide in obsessive–compulsive disorder: a population-based study of 36,788 Swedish patients. *Mol Psychiatry.* 2016. doi:10.1038/mp.2016.115.
8. Seibell P, Pallanti S, Bernardi S, Hughes-Feltenberger M, Hollander E. *Obsessive-compulsive disorder;* 2017. Retrieved May 28, 2017 from: https://online.epocrates.com/diseases/36243/Obsessive-compulsive-disorder/Emerging-Therapies.
9. Ayers CR, Saxena S, Golshan S, Wetherell JL. Age at onset and clinical features of late life compulsive hoarding. *Int J Geriatr Psychiatry.* 2010;25(2):142-149.
10. Keren M, Ron-Miara A, Feldman R, Tyano S. Some reflections on infancy-onset trichotillomania. *Psychoanal Study Child.* 2006;61:254-272.
11. Simpson H. Pharmacotherapy for obsessive-compulsive disorder in adults. In: UpToDate. 2017. Accessed April 27, 2017.
12. Rosenberg D. Treatment of obsessive-compulsive disorder in children and adolescents. In: UpToDate. 2017. Accessed April 27, 2017.
13. Abramowitz J. Psychotherapy for obsessive-compulsive disorder in adults. In: UpToDate. 2017. Accessed April 27, 2017.
14. Abramowitz J. *Getting over OCD: A 10-Step Workbook for Taking Back Your Life.* New York: The Guilford Press; 2009.
15. Mataix-Cols D, Fernandez de la Cruz L, Alonso P. Treatment of hoarding disorder in adults. In: UpToDate. 2017. Accessed April 27, 2017.
16. Koran L, Hanna G, Hollander E; American Psychiatric Association. Practice guideline for the treatment of patients with obsessive-compulsive disorder. *Am J Psychiatry.* 2007;164:1-56.
17. Koran L, Simpson H. *Guideline Watch (March 2013): Practice Guideline for the Treatment of Patients with Obsessive-Compulsive Disorder;* 2013. Psychiatry Online. Retrieved from http://psychiatryonline.org/pb/assets/raw/sitewide/practice_guidelines/guidelines/ocd-watch.pdf.

7

TRAUMA-RELATED DISORDERS

Maria L. Tiamson-Kassab, MD, DFAPA, FACLP and Jea-Hyoun Kim, MD

A 45-year-old woman with a history of fibromyalgia and chronic back pain complains of headaches and difficulty with sleep. She says she cannot sleep and requests medications to help her. Although initially not forthcoming about the details, she admits to having very vivid nightmares multiple times a week, waking up sweating and her heart racing. She recently started a new job working at a home for abused children, and hearing the children's stories have brought up old memories of her own abuse as a child. She goes on to report that she frequently has intrusive thoughts about the abuse throughout the day. She has also recently felt more depressed and irritable. She has had symptoms like this in the past, but they are more severe now and she has been missing work.

CLINICAL HIGHLIGHTS

- Ask the question: Have you ever experienced a traumatic event in your life?
- Use a screening tool specially designed for primary care settings (PC-PTSD-5).
- Symptoms of posttraumatic stress disorder (PTSD) are divided into four clusters.
- Evaluate patient safety. Is the patient suicidal? Does he or she have access to firearms?
- PTSD has a high rate of comorbidity (depression, substance use disorders).
- Treatment involves trauma-focused, evidence-based psychotherapies and pharmacotherapy using SSRIs, SNRIs, and prazosin. Use benzodiazepines sparingly.

CLINICAL SIGNIFICANCE

Posttraumatic stress disorder (PTSD) is a psychiatric condition that is associated with increased health care utilization, medical comorbidity, and psychiatric comorbidity including depression, substance use disorders, and an increased

risk of suicide. Many studies have shown that patients with psychiatric conditions are more likely to seek treatment of psychiatric disorders from primary care physicians rather than from mental health clinicians.[1] PTSD has often been missed or incorrectly diagnosed in primary care settings, hence the importance of early recognition and treatment.

Patients are exposed to traumatic events of various forms, including war, natural disasters, assault, abuse, or acute medical events. Exposure to trauma can result in sleep disturbances, losing a sense of safety, and social isolation. Although many people may have symptoms acutely following a traumatic event, the majority of people do not subsequently develop any long-term impairment. Each year, the prevalence of PTSD is about 3.6% in men and 9.7% in women.[2] Lifetime, past 12-month, and past 6-month PTSD prevalence using the Same Event definition for *DSM-5* was 8.3%, 4.7%, and 3.8%, respectively.[3] The prevalence of patients meeting criteria for PTSD in the primary care setting ranges widely from 12% to as much as 39%.[4,5]

Exposure to trauma does not necessarily result in PTSD, but patients who are symptomatic often are not treated adequately and this results in significant economic burden due to loss of productivity and disability.[6] In addition, studies showed that patients with PTSD reported more current and lifetime medical conditions than those without PTSD.[1]

Traumatic events can include exposure to war or physical assault, threatened or actual sexual violence, natural or man-made disasters, and severe motor vehicle accidents. Although a life-threatening illness or a debilitating medical condition is not necessarily considered to be traumatic, some sudden, catastrophic medical events (such as massive hemorrhage and AICD [automatic implantable cardiac defibrillator] firing) can qualify. Traumatic events may also have been witnessed or observed to have occurred to close relatives or friends.[7]

DIAGNOSIS
DIAGNOSTIC CONSIDERATIONS

Exposure to traumatic events, such as threatened death, serious injury, or sexual violence, can result in symptoms

TABLE 7-1 Diagnostic Criteria for Trauma and Stressor-Related Disorders

Adjustment disorder	• Alteration in mood with marked distress and decreased functioning • Occurs within 6 months of stressor
Posttraumatic stress disorder (PTSD)	• Experience of a traumatic event • Reexperiencing (intrusive distressing memories, distressing dreaming, or flashbacks) • Avoidance/numbing (avoiding distressing memories or external reminders, lack of reaction/response to emotional triggers) • Negative cognition or mood (a distorted sense of blaming oneself or others, inability to remember events, decreased interest in activities) • Increased arousal and reactivity due to perceived persistent threat (irritability or aggressive behavior, hypervigilance, exaggerated startle, or sleep disturbances) • Symptoms lasting beyond 4 weeks from the traumatic event
Acute stress disorder	• Symptoms of PTSD within first 4 weeks after a traumatic event

of reexperiencing (intrusive distressing memories, distressing dreams, or flashbacks), avoidance/numbing (avoiding distressing memories or external reminders, lack of reaction/response to emotional triggers), negative cognition or mood (a distorted sense of blaming oneself or others, inability to remember events, decreased interest in activities), and increased arousal and reactivity due to perceived persistent threat (irritability or aggressive behavior, hypervigilance, exaggerated startle, or sleep disturbances)[1] (*Box 7-1*). In the first 4 weeks after exposure to a traumatic event, patients with qualifying symptoms in each of these symptom clusters are diagnosed with *acute stress disorder* (ASD). If symptoms persist beyond 4 weeks, a diagnosis of PTSD is made. Symptoms must cause a significant impairment in function. Some patients may not exhibit symptoms in the acute period after a traumatic exposure, which may result in delayed expression, a subtype of PTSD. In addition, some patients may present with dissociative symptoms, which are depersonalization (an "out-of-body experience" and feeling like an individual is watching oneself from outside) or derealization (feeling like "things are not real," associated with decreased emotional intensity) (*Table 7-1*).[8]

BOX 7-1 SYMPTOMS OF POSTTRAUMATIC STRESS DISORDER (PTSD)

Symptoms of PTSD are divided into the following clusters:

• Reexperiencing (e.g., nightmares, flashbacks, intrusive memories)

• Avoidance (e.g., avoidance of trauma-related stimuli)

• Increased arousal (e.g., irritability, exaggerated startle response, hypervigilance, sleep disturbance)

• Negative emotions/moods (e.g., diminished interest, feelings of detachment, persistent inability to experience positive emotions)

A primary care provider may be aware of traumatic events to which a patient has been exposed, but often patients have not disclosed any specific exposure to trauma, particularly

sexual violence or a history of abuse as a child. Patients may present with predominantly somatic symptoms, such as headache, chest pain, fatigue, dizziness, or sleep disturbances. Symptoms can change over time and not present until years after the traumatic event. Symptoms may also recur when patients are exposed to triggers that remind them of the event or when they are facing new life stressors.

The risk of suicide increases following a traumatic injury, and patients may have more frequent contact with a primary care physician than with a mental health provider. Screening for suicidality is important, as up to 83% of people who complete suicide have contact with their primary care provider in the year prior.[9] The risk of suicidality is related to a diagnosis of PTSD, depression, anxiety, or substance use disorder, in addition to level of pain resulting from the traumatic injury and other life stressors.[10]

Often, after exposure to trauma or a stressor, patients will present with negative alterations in mood, including depression and anxiety. Within 3 months of experiencing a stressor, these patients express marked distress and impairment in functioning. When there is a specific stressor that is not necessarily traumatic, an *adjustment disorder* is diagnosed, as long as the symptoms do not persist for more than 6 months after the stressor or its consequences have abated. Patients who present with depressed mood and who are diagnosed with major depressive disorder could have co-occurring PTSD that may be missed without a careful history.[11]

In primary care settings, PTSD may be missed or not recognized because of several factors: lack of clinician awareness of PTSD symptoms, failure to ask patients about traumatic experiences, overlapping psychiatric symptoms with more common disorders such as depression, and time restrictions that interfere with the clinician obtaining a trauma history.[12]

The PTSD Checklist (PCL) has been widely used in the Department of Defense and Veterans Affairs primary care clinics, with both been used successfully across various settings. The PCL was updated to a 20-item questionnaire (PCL-5) following the changes made in DSM-5 to the diagnostic criteria for PTSD. Using this screen in primary care would increase awareness and recognition of PTSD.[13,14] More recently, a five-item screening tool for PTSD for use in the primary care setting was revised and validated and is known as PC-PTSD-5 (https://www.ptsd.va.gov/professional/assessment/screens/pc-ptsd.asp). In all tools, the first step is to assess whether the respondent has had exposure to traumatic events. If none, then the screening is complete and there is no need to proceed further.[15]

DIFFERENTIAL DIAGNOSIS

Differential diagnoses for PTSD include adjustment disorders, ASD, anxiety disorders, OCD, major depression, dissociative disorders, and traumatic brain injury. It is important to remember that patients with PTSD are 80% more likely than those without PTSD to have comorbid psychiatric disorders, especially depression and substance use disorders (*Box 7-2*).[1]

BOX 7-2 DIFFERENTIAL DIAGNOSIS OF POSTTRAUMATIC STRESS DISORDER

Adjustment disorder
Dissociative disorder
Generalized anxiety disorder
Major depressive disorder
Obsessive–compulsive disorder
Traumatic brain injury

BIOPSYCHOSOCIAL TREATMENT

The first thing that needs to be established is the safety of the patient. Patients with PTSD have a high suicide risk and therefore when it is determined that the patient has PTSD, a suicide assessment should follow, specifically asking about access to firearms. Access to firearms dramatically increases risk of suicide, and efforts should be made to remove them from the home (see Chapter 22).

Recommendations for first-line treatment for PTSD include evidence-based psychotherapeutic interventions with or without pharmacologic intervention, and pharmacologic management alone with selective serotonin reuptake inhibitors (SSRIs) or serotonin–norepinephrine reuptake inhibitors (SNRIs).[16]

Adjustment disorder and ASD are treated with various evidence-based psychotherapeutic interventions. Trauma-focused cognitive behavioral therapy (CBT) has consistently been found to be the most effective treatment for PTSD in the short term and the long term.

Trauma-focused psychotherapies, including eye movement desensitization and reprocessing (EMDR), prolonged exposure, cognitive processing therapy (CPT), and imaginal exposure, have been shown to result in significant reduction in symptoms that persist over time.[16] These modalities involve components of exposure and cognitive restructuring. Although the availability of psychotherapy for trauma may be limited in the community, these specific types of psychotherapy have proven efficacy.

TABLE 7-2 Treatment of Trauma and Stressor-Related Disorders

DISORDER	TREATMENT
Adjustment disorder	• Cognitive behavior therapy
Acute stress disorder	• Cognitive behavior therapy
Posttraumatic stress disorder	• SSRI (sertraline or paroxetine) or SNRI (venlafaxine) • Prazosin • Trauma-focused therapies (EMDR, PE, CPT, IE)

CPT, cognitive processing therapy; EMDR, eye movement desensitization and reprocessing; IE, imaginal exposure; PE, prolonged exposure; SNRI, serotonin–norepinephrine reuptake inhibitor; SSRI, selective serotonin reuptake inhibitor.

The pharmacologic treatment of PTSD continues to be challenging. There are two antidepressants that are FDA-approved for PTSD: sertraline (Zoloft) and paroxetine (Paxil).

Studies have shown that other medications, such as venlafaxine (Effexor), also show some benefits in PTSD. Medications may act mostly to blunt the symptoms of PTSD rather than changing any underlying pathophysiologic mechanisms. Adjunctive therapy with prazosin to target hyperarousal and nightmares has also been shown to be effective. However, augmenting with antiepileptics, antipsychotics, or benzodiazepines has not been shown to improve symptoms when compared with placebo.[17]

Those individuals with PTSD whose symptoms are due to prolonged and repeated trauma, such as childhood sexual abuse, domestic violence, and political violence, are thought to have "complex PTSD" (not a DSM-5 diagnosis). These disturbances contribute to distressed lives and disability. The International Society for Traumatic Stress Studies published guidelines for the treatment of complex PTSD. The recommended treatment model is a phase-oriented or sequential treatment guided by a hierarchy of treatment needs assessed before treatment and includes elements of pharmacotherapy, psychoeducation, skills building, meditation, and psychotherapy (*Table 7-2*).[18]

Primary care physicians can initiate pharmacologic treatment for PTSD.

WHEN TO REFER

- When symptoms have not responded to at least one systematic medication trial that is adequate in dose and duration
- In the presence of comorbid substance use or psychiatric disorders that are not improving with treatment, especially psychotic symptoms
- When the patient is experiencing other life stressors and/or has limited social support[19]

CASES AND QUESTIONS

CASE 1:

A 45-year-old woman with a history of fibromyalgia and chronic back pain complains of headaches and difficulty with sleep. She says she cannot sleep and requests medications to help her. Although initially not forthcoming about the details, she admits to having very vivid nightmares multiple times a week, waking up sweating and her heart racing. She recently started a new job working at a home for abused children, and hearing the children's stories have brought up old memories of her own abuse as a child. She goes on to report that she frequently has intrusive thoughts about the abuse throughout the day. She has also recently felt more depressed and irritable. She has had symptoms like this in the past, but they are more severe now and she has been missing work.

1. Which of the following is a likely diagnosis?
   A. Major depressive disorder
   B. Sleep disorder
   C. Depression due to general medical condition (fibromyalgia)
   D. PTSD
   E. Complex PTSD

   Correct answer: E. *Although the patient may also have comorbid major depressive disorder and depression due to a general medical condition should be on the differential, the symptoms described are more specific to PTSD. The patient's nightmares, when combined with her other symptoms, are better attributed to PTSD than to a parasomnia. She meets criteria for a DSM-5 diagnosis of PTSD, but PTSD due to prolonged and repeated exposure to trauma is better described as complex PTSD.*

2. What would be your first choice to help this patient's insomnia and nightmares?
   A. Zolpidem
   B. Hydroxyzine
   C. Paroxetine
   D. Prazosin
   E. Sertraline

   Correct answer: D. *Prazosin has been proven to help insomnia and nightmares due to PTSD. Paroxetine and sertraline help attenuate other symptoms of PTSD but would not be the first choice specifically for insomnia or nightmares. Zolpidem and hydroxyzine have no proven benefit for PTSD or nightmares.*

3. Which of the following is an U.S. FDA–approved treatment for PTSD?
   A. Nefazodone
   B. Sertraline

C. Venlafaxine
D. Olanzapine
E. Duloxetine

Correct answer: B. *The two SSRI antidepressants sertraline and paroxetine are the only FDA-approved medications for PTSD. Antipsychotics, such as olanzapine, have limited efficacy in PTSD and have no FDA indication for treatment of PTSD.*

CASE 2:

A 37-year-old man comes in for follow-up of chronic neck and back pain following a motor vehicle accident 3 months earlier. He has severely limited range of motion of his neck and he is constantly in pain. He was a passenger in a car with his friend when they were rear-ended by a car going full speed on the freeway causing them to hit another car in front of them. The patient was trapped in the car and initially had difficulty getting out and remembers feeling panicked. He currently avoids riding in cars on the freeway because he is constantly looking around him and feels very anxious. He frequently has flashbacks of the accident especially when he tries to turn too quickly and has severe neck pain. He feels frustrated and angry about being physically limited and needing to take time off from work.

1. What are some of the symptom clusters of PTSD did this patient experience?
   A. Avoidance and reexperiencing
   B. Avoidance and numbing
   C. Avoidance and dissociation
   D. Numbing and hyperarousal
   E. Avoidance and delayed expression

   Correct answer: A. *The patient avoids riding in cars and has flashbacks, demonstrating avoidance and reexperiencing. He does not describe numbing or dissociation. His symptom onset is within 6 months and thus is not delayed expression.*

2. What is the first-line treatment for this patient?
   A. Propranolol
   B. Transcranial magnetic stimulation (TMS)
   C. Psychodynamic psychotherapy
   D. Combination of sertraline and trauma-focused CBT
   E. Prazosin

   Correct answer: D. *Trauma-focused psychotherapy has the best evidence for treatment of PTSD and would be preferred over other psychotherapeutic modalities. Of the choices listed, the combination of sertraline, an SSRI that is U.S. FDA–approved for PTSD, and trauma-focused CBT would be best, although either treatment in monotherapy may also* *be appropriate. Propranolol has limited evidence in treating symptoms of PTSD, and this patient is not endorsing nightmares and thus prazosin would not be a first-line treatment. TMS does not have an indication for PTSD.*

3. Which of the following statements is true in the management of this patient?

  A. He should start divalproex for his irritability and anger.
  B. He should be forced to ride in the car along the freeway immediately.
  C. He should be given IV morphine for his pain.
  D. He should be referred to physical therapy (PT).
  E. He should be given haloperidol for his flashbacks.

  Correct answer: D. *Antiepileptics and antipsychotics such as divalproex and haloperidol have no proven benefit in PTSD. Forced exposure, out of context of psychotherapy, is unlikely to produce benefit. A PT referral is appropriate—he has limited range of motion and pain and he can benefit from PT for this. IV morphine would not be appropriate.*

CASE 3:

A 25-year-old woman presents with palpitations that were concerning to her. She appeared very anxious and did not want the male medical assistant to touch her. She has no history of medical problems. She reports that she is a military veteran who was discharged 1 month ago. Since her discharge, she has been staying home most of the time and does not want to be in crowded places such as supermarkets and malls. She tells the female medical assistant that she is afraid of men and when she is around men, she gets palpitations. Eventually, she reports that she was raped 1 month before discharge by a group of men in her battalion, one of which was the supervisor. She never reported this as she was afraid of retaliation. However, since she has been discharged she has been having terrible nightmares that often cause her to wake up suddenly in the middle of the night. As a result, she has not been sleeping. She has been isolating herself and has become increasingly anxious and depressed.

1. What is the diagnosis in this case?

  A. Adjustment disorder
  B. Acute stress reaction
  C. Specific phobia
  D. Panic disorder
  E. PTSD

  Correct answer: E. *The patient is endorsing symptoms consistent with PTSD that have lasted for greater than 1 month, exceeding what would*

be expected from an acute stress reaction. The diagnosis of PTSD precludes a diagnosis of adjustment disorder, panic disorder, or phobia as her fears are rooted in trauma and are not specific or out of proportion to her experiences.

2. What kind of psychotherapy would be best in this situation?

  A. Psychodynamic psychotherapy
  B. Interpersonal therapy
  C. Virtual reality therapy
  D. CPT
  E. Dignity therapy

  Correct answer: D. *Of the therapies listed, CPT is the only trauma-focused, evidence-based type. Virtual reality therapy is being investigated as a way to simulate triggers in a safe environment for individuals who have difficulty visualizing or emotionally engaging with their traumatic memories. However, it is still considered investigational and cognitive processing would be the preferred modality.*

3. If SSRIs do not work, what is the next step?

  A. Propranolol
  B. Venlafaxine
  C. Risperidone
  D. Quetiapine
  E. Amitriptyline

  Correct answer: B. *After sertraline and paroxetine, SNRIs such as venlafaxine have shown benefits to patients with PTSD. Beta-blockers, antipsychotics, and tricyclic antidepressants lack evidence for efficacy.*

PRACTICAL RESOURCES

- www.ptsd.va.gov: **Expert Consensus Guidelines Series: Treatment of Posttraumatic Stress Disorder, V. Primary Care Treatment Guide. J Clin Psych Suppl. 1990;16:32.**
- www.psychiatryonline.org: **Practice Guideline on the Treatment of Acute Stress Disorder and Posttraumatic Stress Disorder. APA. 2010.**

REFERENCES

1. Weisberg RB, Bruce SE, Machan JT, et al. Nonpsychiatric illness among primary care patients with trauma histories and posttraumatic stress disorder. *Psychiatr Serv.* 2002;53(7):848-854.

2. American Psychiatric Association, Diagnostic and Statistical Manual of Mental Disorders (DSM-5); 2013. doi:10.1176/appi.books.9780890425596.

3. Kilpatrick DG, Resnick HS, Milanak ME, et al. National estimates of exposure to traumatic events and PTSD prevalence using DSM-IV and DSM-5 criteria. *J Trauma Stress*. 2013;26(5):537-547.

4. Samson AY, Bensen S, Beck A, et al. Posttraumatic stress disorder in primary care. *J Fam Pract*. 1999;48:222-227.

5. Stein MB, McQuaid JR, Pedrelli P, Lenox R, Mc Cahill ME. Posttraumatic stress disorder in the primary care medical setting. *Gen Hosp Psychiatry*. 2000;22:261-269.

6. World Health Organization (WHO) Post-traumatic Stress Disorder. ICD-11 Beta Draft (Joint Mortality and Morbidity Statistics); 2015.

7. Stein DJ, McLaughlin KA, Koenen KC, et al. DSM-5 and ICD-11 definitions of posttraumatic stress disorder: investigating "narrow" and "broad" approaches. *Depress Anxiety*. 2014;31(6):494-505.

8. Zlotnick C, Johnson J, Kohn R, et al. Epidemiology of trauma, posttraumatic stress disorder (PTSD) and co-morbid disorders in Chile. *Psychol Med*. 2006;36(11):1523-1533.

9. Perkonigg A, Kessler RC, Storz S, et al. Traumatic events and posttraumatic stress disorder in the community: prevalence, risk factors and co-morbidity. *Acta Psychiatr Scand*. 2000;101(10):46-59.

10. Creamer M, Burgess P, McFarlane AC, et al. Posttraumatic stress disorder: findings from the Australian National Survey of mental health and well being. *Psychol Med*. 2001;31(7):1237-1247.

11. Kessler RC, Sonnega A, Bromet E, et al. Posttraumatic stress disorder in the national co-morbidity survey. *Arch Gen Psychiatry*. 1995;52(12):1048-1060.

12. Bruce SE, Weisberg RB, Dolan RT, et al. Trauma and post-traumatic stress disorder in primary care patients. primary care companion. *J Clin Psychiatry*. 2001;3(5):211-217.

13. McCutchen PK, Freed MC, Low EC, et al. Rescaling the posttraumatic stress disorder checklist for use in primary care. *Mil Med*. 2016;181(9):1002-1006.

14. Prins A, Oulmette P, Kimerling R, et al. The primary care PTSD screen (PC-PTSD): development and operating characteristics. *Prim Care Psychiatry*. 2003;6(1):8-14.

15. Prins A, Bovin MJ, Kimerling R, et al. The primary care screen for DSM-5 (PC-PTSD-5): development and evaluation within a veteran primary care sample. *J Gen Intern Med*. 2015;31:1206-1211.

16. Stein DJ, Ipser J, McAnda N. Pharmacotherapy of posttraumatic stress disorder: a review of meta-analyses and treatment guidelines. *CNS Spectr*. 2009;14(1 suppl 1):25-31.

17. Moreau C, Zisook S. Rationale for a posttraumatic stress disorder spectrum. *Psychiatr Clin North Am*. 2002;25(4):775-790.

18. Cloitre M, Courtois CA, Ford JD, et al. The ISTSS Expert Consensus Treatment Guidelines for Complex PTSD in Adults. The ISTSS Expert Consensus Treatment Guidelines for Complex PTSD in Adults; 2012. Retrieved from www.istss.org/.

19. Foa EB, Davidson JRT, Frances A. The expert consensus guideline series: treatment of posttraumatic stress disorder. *J Clin Psychiatry*. 1999;60(suppl 16):3-76.

8

MOOD DISORDERS—DEPRESSION

Jeffrey T. Rado, MD, MPH and Chandan Khandai, MD

A 48-year-old Hispanic woman presents to your office complaining of low energy. She also reports 4 weeks of sleeping more than usual, overeating, and difficulty concentrating at work and at home. She notes less interest in socializing and stopped knitting, which she normally enjoyed. Of note, 1 month ago her son moved away to college, and she was transitioned into a lower-paying, higher-demanding position at work. She denies feeling consistently down—"I don't have time to be depressed"—but admits to crying spells "on occasion." She has never been on medications for mood or sleep and has no family history of mental illness. She adamantly denies any suicidal ideation and denies access to firearms. Physical examination is normal, although the patient seems somewhat tearful and constricted in affect.

CLINICAL HIGHLIGHTS

- Major depressive disorder is characterized by a depressed mood most of the day nearly every day or a significant loss of interest or pleasure in almost all activities (anhedonia) for a period of 2 weeks or more. Various other specific depressive syndromes are characterized by both duration and number of mood symptoms.
- Up to 15% of patients in primary care settings meet the criteria for major depressive disorder.
- Depression is common among postpartum women and patients with a personal or family history of depression, the experience of a recent trauma or loss, ongoing substance abuse, and comorbid systemic medical illnesses such as cancer, diabetes mellitus, HIV, neurologic illness, and cardiovascular disease.
- The U.S. Preventive Services Task Force recommends that primary care practices should screen all adults for depression. Systems should be in place to formally diagnose, treat, and follow patients with depression.

- The Physician Health Questionnaire, or PHQ-9, is a self-administered screening tool for depression that can be easily used in the primary care setting.
- Most patients with depression respond well to psychotherapy, antidepressants, or a combination of both.
- Sixty percent of those with major depressive disorder will have a second episode. Individuals who have had two to three major depressive episodes have an 80% to 90% chance of having yet another episode. Patients with recurrent depression should be educated about the early signs of depression and be on lifelong antidepressant therapy.
- Suicide can occur at any phase of treatment for depression. More than half of all patients who die by suicide have visited their primary care provider within 1 month of their death.
- More than 70% of men and 50% of women who die by suicide used a firearm. Physicians should ask depressed or anxious patients about suicidal ideation and access to firearms at each visit.

CLINICAL SIGNIFICANCE

Depression is a major cause of disability and loss of years of productivity across the globe.[1] Depression is commonly encountered in the primary care setting. Up to 15% of patients seen in primary care settings meet the criteria for major depressive disorder. The prevalence of major depressive disorder is higher—30% to 50%—among patients with chronic medical illnesses such as coronary artery disease (CAD), cerebrovascular disease, diabetes mellitus, obesity, and human immunodeficiency virus (HIV). Depression is the leading cause of disability and premature death in people aged 18 to 44 years and is associated with worsening medical morbidity and mortality.[2] For example, depression in patients with CAD has been consistently demonstrated to be an independent risk factor for increased cardiac mortality.[3] Furthermore, untreated depression may worsen the long-term course of these illnesses.[4]

Up to one-quarter of adults will have a major depressive episode during their lifetime.[3] For the primary care clinician, untreated depression may help explain poor adherence to appointment keeping and prescribed treatments for medical conditions. Women are affected by depression twice as often as men. The lifetime risk of depression increases by two to three times in patients with an affected first-degree relative.[5] Onset of depression is most common among patients aged 12 to 24 years and those over 65 years. The suicide rate is similarly high in both groups.

DIAGNOSIS

Early diagnosis and treatment of depression usually improve a patient's quality of life and health outcomes and may prevent suicide. Most patients with depression initially seek care from their primary care provider before presenting to a mental health provider. Increasingly, primary care physicians are managing depression alone or in consultation with a mental health provider. Major depression is defined by the *Diagnostic and Statistical Manual of Mental Disorders*, Fifth Edition (*DSM-5*), as the presence of five or more depressive symptoms over a 2-week period (depressed mood or lack of interest in pleasurable activities must be present). Symptoms must be present most of the day nearly every day during this period. The collective symptoms cause significant dysfunction and cannot be due to other illnesses such as anxiety, hypothyroidism, or alcohol- or substance-related disorders[6] (*Table 8-1*).

Patients who do not meet the criteria for major depression may have a subsyndromal depression (unspecified depressive disorder in *DSM-5*) or persistent depressive

---

disorder (PDD, formerly called dysthymia). These types of depression are distinguished by the length and number of symptoms in addition to sad mood and anhedonia, the degree of functional impairment, and the severity of symptoms. Unspecified depressive disorder applies to cases when the depressive symptoms cause significant distress or impairment in social or occupational functioning but do not meet full criteria for another depressive disorder. For instance, a patient presenting with two to four depressive symptoms (including depressed mood or anhedonia) or for duration <2 weeks, would fit this criteria. PDD is usually described as a chronic feeling of "being down in the dumps" and is characterized by at least 2 years of three or more depressive symptoms, including depressed mood, for more days than not. Also, to meet *DSM-5* criteria, depressive symptoms will not have been absent for more than 2 months during the 2 or more year-long period of PDD. Depressive symptoms may also present in the context of bereavement or an adjustment disorder. Bereavement presents as sadness and grief, although rarely do patients meet criteria for a full depressive episode. Adjustment disorder is characterized by marked distress in response to an identifiable stressor (e.g., divorce, job loss) that may involve depression and/or anxiety symptoms but does not meet criteria for major depression.

Major depression can be stratified into three levels of severity: mild, moderate, or severe. A diagnosis of mild depression is indicated when no or few additional symptoms beyond the number required for diagnosis of major depression are present in the setting of minor functional impairment. Moderate depression is diagnosed when more than the required number of symptoms for the diagnosis of major depression are present and there is moderate impairment in functioning. Severe depression is suggested by the presence of many more symptoms than required for the diagnosis of major depression and related disabling functional impairment. Psychotic features such as hallucinations or delusions may be present in severe depression. Suicidal ideation may accompany mild, moderate, or severe depression (*Table 8-2*).

IDENTIFYING HIGH-RISK POPULATIONS

Currently there are no diagnostic tests or laboratory makers that reliably estimate risk for the development of depression. Moreover, there is significant debate regarding the actual cause of depression. Although there is strong evidence to support a familial link among first-degree relatives who have depression, there is currently no definitive genetic association with the development of major depressive disorder.

The U.S. Preventive Services Task Force recommends that primary care practices should screen the general adult population for depression, including pregnant and postpartum women. Furthermore, adequate systems should be in place to formally diagnose, effectively treat, and follow patients with depression.[7] The following section provides an overview of risk factors for the development of depression. Patients with risk factors should be screened on the initial primary care visit and at least yearly thereafter.

TABLE 8-1 *DSM-5* Definition of Major Depression

Five or more of the following symptoms have been present during the same 2-week period and represent a change from previous functioning.

- At least one of the symptoms is either *depressed mood* or *loss of interest or pleasure*
- Depressed mood most of the day, nearly every day, as self-reported or observed by others
- Diminished interest or pleasure in all or almost all activities most of the day, nearly every day
- Significant weight loss when not dieting, or weight gain; or decrease or increase in appetite nearly every day
- Insomnia or hypersomnia nearly every day
- Psychomotor agitation or retardation as described by people who know the patient
- Fatigue or loss of energy nearly every day
- Feelings of worthlessness or excessive or inappropriate guilt nearly every day
- Diminished ability to think or concentrate nearly every day
- Recurrent thoughts of death; recurrent suicidal ideation without a specific plan

From Diagnosis and Statistical Manual of Mental Disorders. 5th ed. Washington, DC: American Psychiatric Association; 2013.

TABLE 8-2 ICD-9 and ICD-10 Diagnostic Codes

MAJOR DEPRESSION	ICD-9	ICD-10		
Single episode	296.2x	F32.x		
Recurrent episode	296.3x	F33.x		
	X=	X=		
Unspecified	0	9		
Mild	1	0		
Moderate	2	1		
Severe, without psychosis	3	2		
Severe, with psychosis	4	3		
			Single episode	Recurrent episode
In partial or unspecified remission	5	4	41	
In full remission	6	5	42	
Depressive disorder NOS	311	F32.89		
Dysthymic disorder	300.4	F34.1		
Adjustment disorder with depressed mood	309.0	F43.21		
Mood disorder due to [general medical condition]	293.83	F06.30		

Postpartum Women

Postpartum women may have abrupt hormonal shifts and related short-lived depression commonly referred to as "the blues." Symptoms include weepiness, irritability, and sadness. Most such subsyndromal, postpartum depressive episodes will peek at 2 to 5 days postpartum and subside gradually with supportive care over 1 to 2 weeks after the delivery. A smaller number of women will progress to full-spectrum postpartum depression, but women with a previous mood disorder, poor social support, and delivery following an unplanned or unwanted pregnancy are at particularly high risk for postpartum depression. Continued clinical vigilance for up to 1 year after the delivery is indicated for all postpartum women.

Studies indicate that up to 1 in 10 women in the postpartum period will develop major depression.[8] Risk factors include a personal history of mood and anxiety problems, particularly untreated depression during pregnancy. Clinicians can screen for postpartum depression using the Edinburgh Postnatal Depression Scale at all postpartum office visits. Postpartum women who are depressed should be screened for bipolar disorder and psychosis. Indeed, severe cases of postpartum depression may be complicated by psychotic symptoms, which may lead to poor infant care, infanticide, or suicide. Postpartum psychosis is an emergency and requires hospitalization owing to high risk of harm to the infant. Roughly 20% of women will still be depressed beyond the first year after birth.[8]

Personal or Family History of Depression

A personal history of major depression or bipolar disorder is the most significant risk factor for recurrent depression. Major depressive disorder is up to three times more likely among those with first-degree relatives who have either depression or bipolar disorder.[8] A family history of depression is also associated with longer depressive episodes, greater risk of recurrence, and persistent thoughts of death and suicide.[5]

Advanced Age

Elderly patients with depression can present with apathy, diminished self-care, or severe cognitive deficits. Depression is also common among caregivers of the elderly.[9] Elderly depressed patients often have increased primary care utilization for nonspecific physical complaints and may present with significant weight loss and failure to thrive. Depression is also common in patients with dementia.

Neurologic Disorders

The risk of depression is very high in the first year following a stroke. Nearly one-third of patients develop depression in the 5 years after a stroke.[10] Poststroke depression correlates with failure to regain motor function, more medical complications, and cognitive impairment. Parkinson disease, epilepsy, and migraine are also frequently complicated by depression. The depression in Parkinson disease may have a greater impact on quality of life than impairment from the associated movement disorder. Epilepsy and stroke appear to have a bidirectional relationship with depression.[11] Patients with chronic neurologic disorders such as stroke and Parkinson disease should be watched closely for the emergence of depression or anhedonia.

Comorbid Systemic Physical Illnesses

Patients with diabetes mellitus, cancer, rheumatologic disease, thyroid disease, HIV, myocardial infarction, and obesity have significantly higher rates of depression. At least one-quarter of those with cardiac disease or diabetes will develop major depressive disorder. Depression is frequently missed in patients with comorbid medical disorders, particularly diabetes.[12] Patients may present atypically with nonadherence, multiple unexplained physical symptoms, or chronic pain syndromes.[13-20] When depression and a chronic medical condition are present, the outcomes of both conditions are worsened by the presence of the other.[12] Patients should be regularly screened for depression. Early recognition and treatment of depression can improve morbidity, mortality, and quality of life.

PATIENT ASSESSMENT

The U.S. Preventive Services Task Force encourages routine depression screening for adults in primary care practices, including older adults and pregnant or postpartum women. Furthermore, adequate resources should be available to diagnose, treat, and follow the identified patients.[7] Clinicians should consider repeated screenings of patients with a history of depression or other psychiatric symptoms, comorbid medical illness, multiple unexplained somatic complaints, high rates of clinical utilization, substance abuse, chronic pain, or nonadherence. Patients should also be asked about the use of recent or current medications that have been associated with depressive symptoms or suicidal ideation (e.g., corticosteroids, interferon, montelukast sodium, varenicline, isotretinoin, efavirenz and rilpivirine [non-nucleoside reverse transcriptase inhibitors], and primidone). Of note, depression may initially present with vague complaints of "not feeling myself," fatigue or somatic complaints such as headache, generalized pain, or stomach upset. When there are multiple vague unexplained physical symptoms, it is important to consider depression as a possible explanation.

There are no definitive findings of depression on physical examination, although many patients demonstrate a tearful, blunted, or restricted affect. Depressed patients may also have psychomotor retardation or a quiet and slow speech pattern. The physical examination may be useful in helping to rule out common conditions that are often confused with depression (e.g., hypothyroidism, dementia) and in looking for commonly co-occurring illnesses (e.g., obesity, cancer, CAD). When clinical suspicion is high, laboratory testing might include tests for anemia, hypothyroidism, vitamin B_{12} deficiency, and Cushing disease.

Screening Tools and Rating Scales for Depression

Numerous depression screening tools and rating scales have been developed for primary care practice, both self-report questionnaires and clinician-administered instruments.[20,21] Any positive screen warrants a more in-depth evaluation, taking into account the *DSM-5* criteria for major depression (*Figure 8-1*).

The most widely used screening tool in clinical practice is the Patient Health Questionnaire-9[22], or PHQ-9 (*Figure 8-2*). It is a nine-item self-reported questionnaire that classifies current symptoms on a scale of 0 (not at all) to 3 (nearly every day).[23] Items 1 to 9 are summed to yield a score ranging from 0 to 27. A score of 0 to 4 is considered nondepressed, 5 to 9 mild depression, 10 to 14 moderate depression, 15 to 19 moderately

severe depression, and 20 to 27 severe depression; a score of ≥10 is commonly accepted as a positive screen. The PHQ-9 can also be used both to aid in diagnosis, as well as monitor disease progression and response to treatment: a 50% reduction in score suggests adequate response, 25% to 50% reduction suggests partial response, while <25% reduction suggests minimal to no response to current treatment.[24] Any positive response for suicidality should be followed up with direct questioning about suicidal ideation, intent, and planning (see Chapter 22).

An even simpler screening tool is the Patient Health Questionnaire-2, or PHQ-2,[25] which focuses on the two cardinal symptoms of major depression, again on a scale of 0 (not at all) to 3 (nearly every day):

> "Over the past two weeks how often have you felt down, depressed, or hopeless?"

> "Over the past two weeks how often have you had little interest or pleasure in doing things?"

A score of 2 or higher has a higher sensitivity, though lower specificity, than the PHQ-9 in screening for depression.[26]

Another well-known self-report tool is the Beck Depression Inventory for Primary Care (BDI-PC), a 7-item screening tool designed for primary care and based on the popular Beck Depression Inventory.[27] Other commonly encountered self-report tools include the Center for Epidemiological Studies Depression Scale (CES-D), initially designed to identify depression in the general population and consisting of 20 self-report items focusing on affect, and the Zung Self-Rating Depression Scale (SDS), a 20-item scale with 10 positively scored items and 10 negatively scored items.[28,29]

Other self-report assessments have been developed for particular high-risk populations, such as perinatal women, the elderly, and the medically ill. The Edinburgh Postnatal Depression Scale (EPDS) is a 10-item self-report scale initially developed for detection of postpartum depression and has since been adapted for the antenatal period, as well as across cultures and languages.[30,31] The Geriatric Depression Scale (GDS) is a 15- or 30-item assessment comprising "yes/no" questions, simplifying screening in the elderly population where assessment is often confounded by cognitive impairment and/or medical illness.[32] The Hospital Anxiety and Depression Scale (HADS) is a 14-item self-report scale specifically designed for evaluation of psychiatric symptoms in patients with medical comorbidities, by avoiding reliance on somatic symptoms frequently found in the medically ill such as fatigue and insomnia.[33]

Although self-report tools are frequently used due to ease and brevity, scores can be easily exaggerated or minimized by the person completing them. Thus, some providers prefer clinician-administered rating scales, which have the advantage of incorporating clinician behavioral observations into the overall score. The Hamilton Rating Scale for Depression (HAM-D) is the most widely used clinician-rated instrument and has also been used in many clinical trials. The HAM-D has

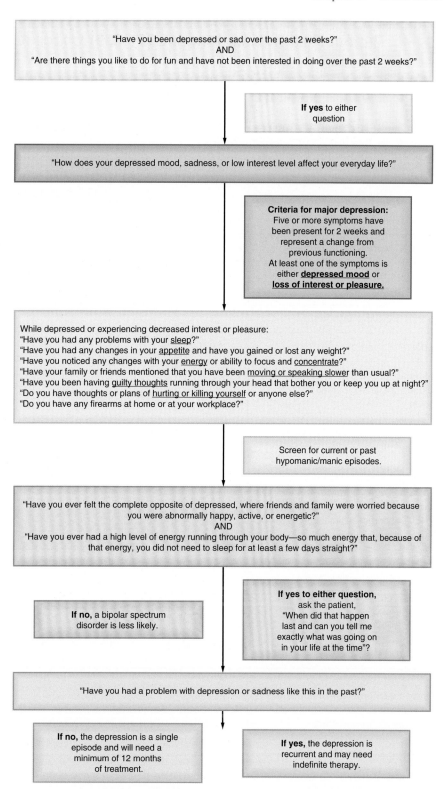

FIGURE 8-1 Diagnosing depression in the primary care setting.

both 17-item and 29-item versions and relies on both patient-reported symptoms and clinical observations of in-session behavior; however, the length of time needed (up to 20 minutes) may make it impractical for some clinicians. The Montgomery-Asberg Depression Rating Scale (MADRS) similarly is clinician administered, consisting of 10 items including both patient-reported and clinician-observed factors, and is thought to be even more sensitive than the HAM-D in detecting changes in depressed clinical state. However, both these scales require training and are primarily utilized in clinical trials of antidepressants.[34]

Patient Health Questionnaire (PHQ-9)
Nine-Symptom Depression Checklist

Name: _____   Date: _____

Over the *last 2 weeks*, how often have you been bothered by any of the following problems? (Please circle your answer.)

	Not at All	Several Days	More than Half the Days	Nearly Every Day
1. Little interest or pleasure in doing things	0	1	2	3
2. Feeling down, depressed, or hopeless	0	1	2	3
3. Trouble falling or staying asleep, or sleeping too much	0	1	2	3
4. Feeling tired or having little energy	0	1	2	3
5. Poor appetite or overeating	0	1	2	3
6. Feeling bad about yourself—or that you are a failure or have let yourself or your family down	0	1	2	3
7. Trouble concentrating on things, such as reading the newspaper or watching television	0	1	2	3
8. Moving or speaking so slowly that other people could have noticed. Or the opposite—being so fidgety or restless that you have been moving around a lot more than usual	0	1	2	3
9. Thoughts that you would be better off dead or of hurting yourself in some way	0	1	2	3

Add Columns, ☐ + ☐ + ☐

Total Score*, ☐   *Score is for healthcare provider

10. If you circled *any* problems, how *difficult* have these problems made it for you to do your work, take care of things at home, or get along with other people? (Please circle your answer.)	Not Difficult at All	Somewhat Difficult	Very Difficult	Extremely Difficult

A score of: 0–4 is considered non-depressed; 5–9 mild depression; 10–14 moderate depression; 15–19 moderately severe depression; and 20–27 severe depression.

FIGURE 8-2 Patient Health Questionnaire (PHQ-9) nine-symptom depression checklist. (Developed by Drs. Robert L. Spitzer, Janet B.W. Williams, Kurt Kroenke and colleagues, with an educational grant from Pfizer Inc. No permission required to reproduce, translate, display, or distribute.)

Suicide Risk Assessment

Clinicians must remain vigilant to the risk of suicide as up to 15% of those with major depressive disorder die by suicide.[6] Suicide is consistently a leading cause of death in the United States; nearly 43,000 individuals die by suicide in the United States each year.[35] Many patients who die by suicide meet criteria for a depressive disorder, and nearly half have seen a primary care physician within a month of their death.[36,37] Older, single white men are at elevated risk. While it is difficult to accurately predict who will commit suicide, clinicians should routinely ask (and document asking) depressed patients if they have had or currently have any thoughts of suicide, of ending their life, or that they would be better off dead. Positive responses should be followed by assessment of the content of suicidal thoughts (including specific plans or actual intent of suicide) and reduction of access to lethal means (especially firearms and medications that may be harmful if taken in large quantities). Asking about suicidal thoughts will not induce such thoughts in patients.[38] Clinicians should consult a psychiatrist if there is any uncertainty regarding suicidal risk or need for hospitalization.

DIFFERENTIAL DIAGNOSIS

Depressive symptoms occur in numerous systemic illnesses, or as an adverse effect of medications, frequently complicating diagnosis. Thus, a comprehensive clinical history and review of systems, physical examination including neurologic examination, and appropriate use of laboratory tests and/or imaging are needed to avoid diagnostic errors.[39] The primary care provider must pay particular attention to relevant medical or family medical history, significant constitutional changes, focal somatic complaints or findings on physical examination, or if depressive symptoms occur suddenly or in the absence of psychiatric history, particularly after the age of 40 years. A focused diagnostic workup is presented in *Table 8-3*.

Depressive symptoms may also be present with psychiatric disorders other than major depression. In bipolar spectrum disorders, patients may initially present with depressive symptoms as part of a depressive or mixed mood episodes. Therefore, it is essential to ask about history of mania or hypomania. Patients with psychotic disorders—schizophrenia, schizoaffective disorder—may at some point present with prominent symptoms of depression. Anxiety and trauma-related disorders, particularly panic disorder and posttraumatic stress disorder (PTSD), may either coexist with depression or feature prominent depressive symptoms. Eating disorders are also highly comorbid with depressive symptoms. Substance-induced mood disorders may also present with depressive symptoms, during periods of either abuse or withdrawal. Dementia is a consideration in older patients who experience cognitive impairment in the context of depressive symptoms. We recommend using the AMPS (Anxiety, Mood, Psychotic, Substance) approach to the psychiatric review of systems when assessing anyone who presents with sadness or anhedonia (see Chapter 1).

NOT TO BE MISSED

- Suicidal thoughts
- Homicidal thoughts
- Opportunities to reduce access to firearms and medications that may be harmful if taken in large quantities (e.g., tricyclic antidepressants)
- Psychotic symptoms
- Illicit drug or alcohol abuse
- Systemic medical causes of depression (e.g., hypothyroidism)
- Bipolar disorder with depressed or mixed episode

BIOPSYCHOSOCIAL TREATMENT
GENERAL PRINCIPLES

The American Psychiatric Association (APA) has recently published updated treatment guidelines for depression.[40] Regardless of treatment modality, the initial goal of treatment is remission of the major depressive episode and full return to the patient's baseline level of functioning. Remission is defined as at least 3 weeks without depressed mood or anhedonia and no more than three remaining symptoms of the major depressive episode. Patients who experience full remission have improved prognosis over patients with only a partial response to therapy.[37,41] Other treatment goals include eliminating suicidal thoughts, minimizing treatment adverse effects, improving quality of life, and preventing relapse.

There are several primary care treatment models for the management of depression. One model is that of a physician or other general medical practitioner (e.g., nurse practitioner, physician assistant) as the sole provider of clinical care. In such models, psychiatric or other mental health care must be obtained on a consultation or referral basis from external mental health systems. There is also the same-site consultation model, where a psychiatrist or other mental health professional maintains an office colocated with the primary care provider. This model facilitates comanagement of depression in a combined model often called "collaborative care." Some collaborative care models use nurses in a disease management model for depression where they follow up with patients, by phone or in person, between clinic visits. Finally, with the use of video teleconferencing equipment, primary care clinicians obtain psychiatric consultation from a distance. This model is referred to as "telepsychiatry," and it is often used in rural or underserved areas. The primary care practitioner is advised to avail himself or herself of consultation (and comanagement, where and when available) within the local clinical care models. Cultural consultations are available in some settings to aid in the diagnosis and treatment of depression in culturally diverse populations.[41]

Initial choice of treatment modality is based on severity of symptoms, as well as patient preference, prior treatment experiences, co-occurring stressors and medical

TABLE 8-3 General Medical Evaluation for Depressive Symptoms	
SCREENING TEST OR PROCEDURE	**MEDICAL CONDITION(S) WITH DEPRESSIVE SYMPTOMS**
Complete blood count (CBC)	Anemia, infection (influenza, pneumonia, mononucleosis), cancer (leukemia, lymphoma)
Basic chemistry panel	Dehydration, hypo/hypernatremia, hypo/hyperkalemia, hypoglycemia, diabetes, adrenal insufficiency, kidney disease
Thyroid stimulating hormone (TSH) and/or free T4	Hypothyroidism, hyperthyroidism
Hepatic panel	Hepatic encephalopathy, hepatitis
Vitamin D level, vitamin B12 level, folate level	Vitamin D deficiency, vitamin B12 deficiency, folate deficiency
Urine pregnancy test	Pregnancy (somatic symptoms of pregnancy may overlap with depression)
Neurologic examination, head imaging	Multiple sclerosis, neoplasms, stroke, Parkinson disease
24-hour urinary cortisol, blood cortisol	Cushing disease
Fluorescent treponemal antibody absorption test	Syphilis
HIV antibody	HIV/AIDS
Antinuclear antibody (ANA)	Systemic lupus erythematosus, rheumatoid arthritis
Medication review	Adverse effect of medications: sedative/hypnotics, steroids, interferon, anticonvulsants, H2-blockers, non steroidal anti-inflammatory drugs (NSAIDs), anti-parkinsonian medications, oral contraceptives, isotretinoin
Cognitive testing—Montreal Cognitive Assessment (MoCA), Mini-Mental Status Examination (MMSE)	Mild cognitive impairment, dementia
Sleep history, review of systems	Obstructive sleep apnea, narcolepsy, restless legs syndrome, primary insomnia
Perimenstrual symptoms	Premenstrual dysphoric disorder (occurs in a week before menses, resolves with menses)
Anxiety review of systems	Anxiety disorders: generalized anxiety disorder, panic disorder, social anxiety disorder, obsessive-compulsive disorder
History of trauma/abuse	Posttraumatic stress disorder, acute stress disorder
Mania/hypomania review of systems	Bipolar disorder, cyclothymia
Psychosis review of systems	Depression with psychotic features (mood-congruent hallucinations/delusions), schizophrenia, schizoaffective disorder
Substance use history, urine drug screen, blood alcohol level	Substance-induced mood disorder: substance use or withdrawal (at least 4 weeks of abstinence necessary when ruling out depression due to substances)
Recent losses, stressors	Adjustment disorder, bereavement (symptoms do not meet full criteria for major depressive episode)

conditions, and concurrent treatments. Patients with mild to moderate depression may do well with either psychotherapy or pharmacotherapy alone.[40] Combination psychotherapy and medication treatment offer no demonstrated short-term advantage in patients with mild to moderate depression. Patient preference and local psychotherapeutic resources should guide the initial choice of depression therapy. For severe, chronic or recurrent depression, however, pharmacotherapy or pharmacotherapy combined with psychotherapy is the treatment of choice.[42] Primary care–based psychotherapy (e.g., interpersonal or cognitive behavioral therapy [CBT]) coupled with medication management may also be effective.[43]

For patients with mild depression who decline medications or psychotherapy, limited evidence exists for exercise, meditation, music therapy, and animal-assisted therapy.[39] Bright light therapy may benefit both seasonal affective disorder (SAD) as well as general depression.

Some evidence supports herbal remedies or supplements for mild depressive symptoms and may be better tolerated. St. John's wort is the most well studied[44]; however, primary care providers must remember that, given its serotonergic mechanism, it must be discontinued before prescription antidepressants to avoid drug–drug interactions and serotonin syndrome and has also been associated with psychotic symptoms. Other complementary alternative medicine option with limited evidence includes saffron, lavender, rhodiola, echium, S-adenosyl methionine (SAMe), and omega-3 fatty acids.[40,45]

PHARMACOTHERAPY

When choosing pharmacotherapy, factors to consider include prior positive response to antidepressants, positive response to a specific antidepressant in a first-degree relative, presence of significant sleep or appetite disturbances or agitation, and anticipation of the need for maintenance therapy.

There are a variety of first-line pharmacologic options for the treatment of depression (*Table 8-4*); these generally enhance serotonin, norepinephrine, and/or dopamine activity in the brain. Regardless of the drug, medication therapy is effective in the majority of cases[43]; within 6 weeks, half of persons receiving antidepressants have at least a 50% reduction in symptoms.[46] The most commonly prescribed antidepressants are classified as selective serotonin reuptake inhibitors (SSRIs), such as fluoxetine (Prozac) and sertraline (Zoloft). Other first-line agents include serotonin norepinephrine reuptake inhibitors (SNRIs), such as venlafaxine (Effexor), desvenlafaxine (Pristiq), and duloxetine (Cymbalta); bupropion (Wellbutrin), a norepinephrine-dopamine reuptake inhibitor (NDRI); and mirtazapine (Remeron), a noradrenergic and specific serotonergic antidepressant (NaSSA). For the purpose of this chapter, we shall focus discussion on these first-line medications. Second-line medications, such as tricyclic antidepressants (TCAs) and

TABLE 8-4 First-Line Antidepressant Medications

CLASS	INITIAL DOSE (mg/day)[a]	THERAPEUTIC DOSE (mg/day)	PRACTICAL POINTERS FOR THE PCP[b]
Selective serotonin reuptake inhibitors (SSRIs)			
Sertraline (Zoloft)	50	50-200	Serotonin and dopamine reuptake inhibition Possible early and temporary diarrhea and dyspepsia Relatively low risk for drug interactions
Paroxetine Paroxetine CR (Paxil, Paxil CR)	20 12.5-20	20-60 25-75	High anticholinergic and antihistamine side effect profile Risk for sedation, weight gain, and dry mouth Short half-life with more risk for discontinuation syndrome High chance for drug interactions Unsafe during pregnancy—class D
Fluoxetine (Prozac)	20	20-60	Long half-life and ideal for intermittently compliant patients Relatively inexpensive High chance for drug interactions
Fluvoxamine (Luvox)	50	50-300	Rarely used owing to high side effect profile
Citalopram (Celexa)	20	20-60	Structurally similar to escitalopram Low risk for drug interactions
Escitalopram (Lexapro)	10	10-20	Structurally similar to citalopram Low risk for drug interactions
Serotonin norepinephrine reuptake inhibitors (SNRIs)			
Venlafaxine XR (Effexor XR)	37.5	75-300	Structurally similar to desvenlafaxine (do not use concurrently) Dual action on serotonin and norepinephrine receptors *Not* consistently "activating" but usually does not cause sedation Sometimes used as an adjunct for chronic pain Not to be used in those with difficult-to-treat hypertension May increase blood pressure and heart rate, especially at higher dosing range (>150 mg/day) Non-XR formulation is rarely used due to side effect profile and twice-per-day dosing Short half-life with more risk for discontinuation syndrome Reduce dose with renal insufficiency

(continued)

TABLE 8-4 First-Line Antidepressant Medications (continued)

CLASS	INITIAL DOSE (mg/day)[a]	THERAPEUTIC DOSE (mg/day)	PRACTICAL POINTERS FOR THE PCP[b]
Desvenlafaxine (Pristiq)	50	50-100	Structurally similar to venlafaxine (do not use concurrently) Dual action on serotonin and norepinephrine receptors *Not* consistently "activating" but usually does not cause sedation Not to be used in those with difficult-to-treat hypertension Short half-life with more risk for discontinuation syndrome Reduce dose with renal insufficiency
Duloxetine (Cymbalta)	30	30-60	Dual action on serotonin and norepinephrine receptors *Not* consistently "activating" but usually does not cause sedation FDA approved for fibromyalgia and diabetic peripheral neuropathic pain Sometimes used for chronic neuropathic pain Short half-life with more risk for discontinuation syndrome Increased risk for drug interactions
Other			
Bupropion	75-150	300-450	
Bupropion SR (Wellbutrin SR)	100	300-400	Given twice per day Likely dual action on dopamine and norepinephrine receptors Contraindicated with seizure and eating disorders
Bupropion XL (Wellbutrin XL)	150	300-450	Increased risk for seizures in those with alcohol withdrawal Not used for anxiety disorders May worsen anxiety associated with depression No serotonin activity and no related sexual side effects XL formulation is supposed to have slower release and lower side effect profile (permits higher dosing and lower seizure risk) Less frequently used owing to side effect profile
Mirtazapine (Remeron)	15	15-45	Increases central serotonin and norepinephrine activity (possibly through presynaptic α_2-adrenergic receptor inhibition) Decreased frequency of sexual side effects Increased sedation and sleepiness at mainly *lower* doses Although not indicated for anxiety disorders, it may be helpful Remeron Soltab is orally dissolving for patients who cannot swallow

[a]*Initial dose should be decreased by half when treating an anxiety disorder or an elderly person.*
[b]*Drug interactions refer to commonly used medications that are principally metabolized by the P450 2D6 pathway.*
FDA, Food and Drug Administration; PCP, primary care physician.

monoamine oxidase inhibitors (MAOIs), will be reviewed in the chapter on treatment-resistant depression.

When choosing a medication, note there are no important clinical differences in response rates among first-line antidepressants. Thus, choosing a medication is largely based on the following: evidence of effectiveness with the patient or first-degree relative; safety, tolerability, and anticipated side effects; co-occurring medical conditions; drug–drug interactions and other pharmacologic properties; and patient preference as well as cost.

Medication Side Effects

Side effects from antidepressant medications are common; more than 60% of people on antidepressants will experience at least one side effect. It is difficult to predict which drug will cause which side effect in any one patient, and even within classes, both response and side effects are not reliably consistent. The most common side effects include nausea, diarrhea, headache, sedation or insomnia, dizziness, and dry mouth and often remit within the first few weeks of treatment. Sexual side effects and weight gain tend to be more persistent. Side effects typically occur during the first two weeks and often remit within a few weeks. Side effects are a significant source of patient nonadherence, as beneficial effects may occur as early as 1 to 2 weeks, but often do not occur until 4 to 8 weeks. Thus, guidelines recommend monitoring patients during the first two weeks and addressing side effects as needed (*Table 8-5*). Primary care providers can lessen side effects by starting at a low dose and titrating upward slowly and as tolerated, lowering the dose if intolerable side effects occur, or switching to another antidepressant.

One particular and controversial side effect is increased suicidal ideation. Severely depressed patients who harbor suicidal ideation may initially lack the

TABLE 8-5 Side Effect Profiles of Antidepressant Classes

	SEXUAL DYSFUNCTION/ DECREASED LIBIDO	WEIGHT GAIN	SEDATION	CARDIAC
SSRIs	+++	+[a]	+/–[a]	0
SNRIs	+++	+/–	+/–	+ (↑ BP)
Mirtazapine	+	+++	++	+/–
Bupropion	0	0	0	+/– (↑ BP)

[a]Paroxetine and fluvoxamine are more likely to cause sedation and weight gain.
BP, blood pressure; SNRIs, serotonin norepinephrine reuptake inhibitors; SSRIs, selective serotonin reuptake inhibitors.

"energy" or initiative to follow through on suicidal thoughts. As their depression is in early response, they may have increased energy to act on their persisting suicidal thoughts. A series of meta-analyses demonstrated that antidepressants were associated with a small but significant increase in suicidal ideation, as well as attempts (though none fatal). As a result, in 2004 the FDA imposed a "black box warning" on package inserts for antidepressants. Of note, subsequent age-stratified analyses showed that this increased risk was significant only among children and adolescents younger than 18 years. There was no evidence of increased risk among adults older than 24 years, and among adults aged 65 years or older, antidepressants had a clear protective effect against the development of suicidal ideation and behavior.[47] However, we still recommend close monitoring of suicidal ideation during the first two weeks and at all encounters as a routine part of depression management.

Psychotropic drug–drug interactions have also been the subject of increasing clinical observation and research.[48] The use of two or more serotonergic medications increases the risk of serotonin syndrome—a potentially dangerous syndrome marked by elevated body temperature, sweating, diarrhea, agitation, tremor, hyperreflexia, and in severe cases seizure and death. Thus, careful attention must be paid to the potential for interactions with other proserotonergic agents that a patient may be taking, including not only other antidepressants such as TCAs and MAOIs but also nondepression medications such as amphetamines, tramadol, dextromethorphan, triptans, metoclopramide, and ondansetron. In addition, individual SSRIs have distinct profiles of P450 inhibition; medications such as fluoxetine, fluvoxamine, and paroxetine have the potential for dangerous interactions, such as increasing serum levels of beta-blockers. Other medications, such as citalopram, escitalopram, and sertraline, show fewer interactions and so may be preferred in the elderly and medically ill, where polypharmacy often occurs.

Continuation, Titration, and Maintenance

After medication initiation, symptoms can improve in as little as 1 week.[49] Clinicians should follow up with patients 1 to 2 weeks after initiating therapy to help curb the high rate of medication discontinuation during this period. If patients are unable to follow up within this time frame, a check-in phone call may be substituted. Clinicians should reinforce adherence, address concerns about adverse effects, and monitor for suicidality and emerging psychosocial stressors. Clinical improvement can be quantified with the PHQ-9. Symptom remission (PHQ-9 score <5) and return to normal functioning are the goals of therapy. After about 4 weeks of therapy with little response, clinicians can (1) increase the dose of the current medication; (2) switch to a different agent from the same or another class (if a therapeutic dose has been reached); (3) start combination therapy by adding a second antidepressant (e.g., adding bupropion or mirtazapine to an SSRI); (4) in consult with a psychiatrist, start augmentation with nonantidepressants; (5) add psychotherapy (CBT as augmentative therapy is just as effective, albeit with a slower response time, when compared with the addition of a second antidepressant agent)[37,41]; or (6) refer to a psychiatrist for medication management. See *Figure 8-3* for guidance in the treatment of depression in the primary care setting.

Before changing medications, it is important to ensure that the antidepressant is dosed high enough (maximum Food and Drug Administration [FDA]-recommended doses with tolerable side effects) and long enough (4 weeks) before a medication trial is considered to have failed. If this doesn't work, switching to another antidepressant within the same class or another class leads to a response in many patients.

Duration of Treatment

In the first episode of depression, patients may require 3 to 6 months of treatment before achieving full remission. Once in remission, medication should continue to be used up to 12 months, generally at the same dose used to achieve remission. During this time, providers should reinforce adherence, continue to address any concerns about adverse effects, and continue to monitor suicidality and emerging psychosocial stressors.

Recurrence of depression is common, occurring in 20% of patients within 6 months following remission. Between 50% and 85% of patients will experience at least one lifetime recurrence; individuals who have had two to

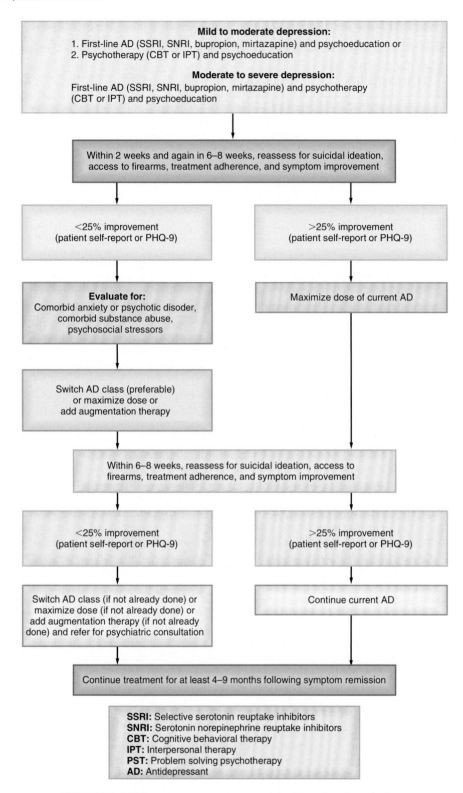

Mild to moderate depression:
1. First-line AD (SSRI, SNRI, bupropion, mirtazapine) and psychoeducation or
2. Psychotherapy (CBT or IPT) and psychoeducation

Moderate to severe depression:
First-line AD (SSRI, SNRI, bupropion, mirtazapine) and psychotherapy
(CBT or IPT) and psychoeducation

Within 2 weeks and again in 6–8 weeks, reassess for suicidal ideation, access to firearms, treatment adherence, and symptom improvement

<25% improvement (patient self-report or PHQ-9)

>25% improvement (patient self-report or PHQ-9)

Evaluate for: Comorbid anxiety or psychotic disoder, comorbid substance abuse, psychosocial stressors

Maximize dose of current AD

Switch AD class (preferable) or maximize dose or add augmentation therapy

Within 6–8 weeks, reassess for suicidal ideation, access to firearms, treatment adherence, and symptom improvement

<25% improvement (patient self-report or PHQ-9)

>25% improvement (patient self-report or PHQ-9)

Switch AD class (if not already done) or maximize dose (if not already done) or add augmentation therapy (if not already done) and refer for psychiatric consultation

Continue current AD

Continue treatment for at least 4–9 months following symptom remission

SSRI: Selective serotonin reuptake inhibitors
SNRI: Serotonin norepinephrine reuptake inhibitors
CBT: Cognitive behavioral therapy
IPT: Interpersonal therapy
PST: Problem solving psychotherapy
AD: Antidepressant

FIGURE 8-3 Primary care treatment algorithm for depression.

three depressive episodes have an 80% to 90% chance of having yet another episode. Risk factors for recurrence include severity of initial and subsequent episodes; history of multiple episodes; earlier age of onset; presence of other psychiatric diagnoses or chronic medical conditions; family history of psychiatric illness, particularly mood disorders; and persistent sleep disturbances or subthreshold depressive symptoms. All patients should be educated about the risk of relapse. Patients with three or more prior depressive episodes, or at otherwise high risk of recurrence, should receive lifelong maintenance treatment.[40]

Discontinuation

At times, a patient may request discontinuation of an antidepressant during remission. How and when to discontinue treatment has not been systematically studied; however, providers should carefully assess risk of recurrence as above, before discontinuing antidepressants. Of note, risk of relapse is highest in the first two months after discontinuation of treatment; thus, patients should be closely monitored during this period. Given the high risk of relapse, patients with history of two or more episodes should be on lifelong antidepressant therapy.

In general, we recommend gradual taper to prevent withdrawal symptoms. Agents with short half-lives, such as paroxetine and venlafaxine, are associated with a discontinuation syndrome, marked by acute headache, dizziness, nausea, insomnia, anxiety, and an electrical "tingling" sensation (often by the ears).[40] If discontinuation syndrome occurs, we recommend returning to dosage before discontinuation, followed by a slower taper over weeks or months as needed. If tapering still results in discontinuation symptoms, an alternate strategy may be switching to fluoxetine, least likely to result in discontinuation owing to its particularly long half-life.[50]

TRANSCRANIAL MAGNETIC STIMULATION AND ELECTROCONVULSIVE THERAPY

Transcranial magnetic stimulation (TMS) and electroconvulsive therapy (ECT) are usually reserved for patients with medication-refractory or unresponsive depression or when urgent treatment response is critical (e.g., in the severely medically compromised or in patients with psychotic depression). TMS is approved for patients who have failed at least one adequate antidepressant trial. ECT is a safe and effective treatment for severe depression.[51] Primary care providers should refer TMS and ECT candidates to an experienced psychiatrist (especially one who performs these treatments ECT regularly) to address the risks, benefits, and side effect issues of these procedures.

PSYCHOSOCIAL TREATMENT

Although several different types of psychotherapy have been shown to treat depression, CBT and interpersonal psychotherapy (IPT) provide the strongest evidence to support their use in patients suffering from depression. Both forms of psychotherapy have an evidence base in primary care and are brief enough for incorporation into the primary care setting. The busy practitioner can easily employ concepts of behavioral activation (BA) to help combat depression in their patients. The following is an overview that is designed to provide an introduction to these three psychotherapies.

Cognitive Behavioral Therapy

The essential construct of CBT is the interrelationship between how one feels, thinks, and acts (see *Figure 8-4*). The goals of are to modify thoughts and behavior to improve mood. The three "R's" can be used to help the patient

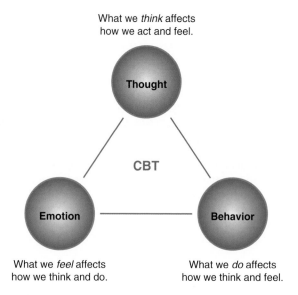

What we *think* affects how we act and feel.

What we *feel* affects how we think and do.

What we *do* affects how we think and feel.

FIGURE 8-4 Cognitive behavioral theory (CBT).

(recognize, reconstruct, repeat) and the provider (read, refer, review) understand and use CBT in the context of treating and recovering from depressive, anxiety disorders.

Three R's for the patient
Recognize

Most patients who are depressed know it. They do not have to contemplate or analyze the "feeling" or "emotion" to understand what they are experiencing. The first step with CBT is to simply identify the unhappy emotion or feeling (e.g., "depression" or "sadness"). Patients should also learn to quantify the degree or severity of the emotion by using a Likert scale (e.g., a scale from 1 to 10 can be used, where 10 indicates the most severe depression and 1 indicates no depression).

The next step is the most critical and often the most difficult to initially conceptualize. After labeling and quantifying the emotion, the patient is then encouraged to *recognize* associated dysfunctional thought patterns. One way to teach the patient to do this is to ask, "When you get really depressed, what thoughts run through your head?" Initially, the patient may confuse emotion with thought and answer, "I'm just very depressed." Another way to help the patient recognize dysfunctional thought patterns is to ask, "You mentioned your depression was really bad last night. What thoughts were running through your head when you felt sad?" Common examples of dysfunctional patterns include "Nobody likes me," "I'm a failure at everything I do," "I will never amount to anything," "I will never feel normal again," and "I have always been depressed." The common denominators with these "dysfunctional thoughts" are twofold. First, these thoughts are negative. Second, persistent thoughts are all or none and absolute and therefore usually inaccurate.

Reconstruct

Once the patient learns how to recognize persistent dysfunctional thoughts, he or she can then begin to critically analyze the thoughts by writing them down and *reconstructing* accurate and less absolute or rigid thoughts onto a dysfunctional thought record (DTR). Completion of a DTR requires the patient to write down a specific unhappy and distressing "emotion" or "feeling" followed by the dysfunctional thought that occurs with it. The dysfunctional thought is then analyzed by the patient for accuracy and reconstructed into a more realistic thought. In this context, patients identify thoughts that are not validated by evidence. The process is usually completed immediately following or at the time a distressful emotion is experienced. The DTR is usually completed outside of the practitioner's office in the form of CBT "homework." Examples of reconstructed thoughts and a DTR are listed in *Tables 8-6* and *8-7*, respectively.

Repeat

CBT is a lifelong tool that can be used by patients to recognize early signs of depression and initiate treatment. A DTR should be used indefinitely by all patients who have a history of major depressive disorder. The patient is encouraged to use the DTR during times of worsening depression or stress, and a prethought reconstruction and postthought reconstruction Likert scale should be used to quantify the improvement in mood, as illustrated in *Table 8-6.*

Three R's for the Practitioner Read

Time constraints and inexperience may prevent primary care practitioners from providing the traditional form of CBT. Abbreviated CBT (ACBT) can be used in the medical setting. This chapter provides only a brief overview of ACBT; interested providers should consult with additional resources to become more proficient with this mode of therapy. The first few sections of

Feeling Good: The New Mood Therapy by Dr. David Burns provides a nice introduction for both the patient and the practitioner.[52]

Refer

Patients who have severe depression or suicidal ideation should be immediately referred to a psychiatrist. Patients who are not benefitting or lack motivation to complete the CBT homework should be referred to a CBT therapist. Many primary care practitioners may elect to refer depressed patients for regularly scheduled CBT sessions and briefly follow up with them in the medical clinic.

TABLE 8-6 Examples of Dysfunctional Thoughts and Reconstruction Strategies

AUTOMATIC DYSFUNCTIONAL THOUGHTS	RECONSTRUCTED THOUGHTS
"*Nobody* likes me."	"That can't be true because my wife and kids love me."
"I'm a failure at *everything* I do."	"Maybe I'm just not good in this one area."
"I will *never* amount to *anything.*"	"I already have a good job and I might get a promotion next year."
"I will *never* feel normal again."	"Depression can get better with medication and therapy."
"I have *always* been depressed."	"Not true—I was very happy when I got married and graduated from college!"

TABLE 8-7 Sample Dysfunctional Thought Record (DTR)

EMOTIONS	AUTOMATIC DYSFUNCTIONAL THOUGHTS	RECONSTRUCTED THOUGHTS	OUTCOME
Specify feeling Rate 1-10 (10 rated as most intense)	**"What is running through your head?" (NOT an emotion or feeling)**	**"Why is the automatic thought inaccurate (be specific)?"**	**Respecify feeling Rerate feeling using 1-10 scale**
"Sad" 9/10	"*No one* will ever really care about me."	"Not true—my parents and wife love me even when I am irritable and unhappy."	"Sad" 3/10
"Depressed" 8/10	"I will never amount to anything."	"I actually have a great job and my kids see me as a great dad.... I think I am just feeling low today."	"Depressed" 2/10
"Really down" 9/10	"I would be much better off dead." "I'm worthless and have no energy."	"Who would take care of my family if I were actually dead?" "The depression makes my energy lower but I can still function." "I feel worthless at this moment but I know my boss relies on me."	"Down" 5/10

Understanding CBT principles will improve communication between primary care providers, CBT providers, and their shared patients.

Review the DTR

Regardless of whether a depressed patient undergoes CBT through self-study or an external therapist, it may be helpful to briefly review the DTR on each visit. Much like the blood glucose log of a diabetic patient, reviewing the DTR can create a "team approach" to the treatment of depression while supplementing the treatment rendered by the psychotherapist.

Interpersonal Psychotherapy

Interpersonal psychotherapy is also effective in treating depression but is not readily provided by primary care practitioners. IPT is a brief therapy (lasting about 3 to 4 months) and focuses on examining relationships. During stressful times in a relationship, many depressed patients will deliberately self-isolate due to dysfunctional thought patterns and a related transient drop in self-esteem. The therapist helps the patient discover healthy coping mechanisms to replace the maladaptive interpersonal conflicts. Depressed patients who have interpersonal isolation or numerous conflicts with relationships should be referred for IPT.

Behavioral Activation

The goal of BA is to increase involvement in enjoyable activities. This approach, based in the principles of CBT, focuses on creating structure, building routine, and planning activities. Instead of letting the mood "take over," the emphasis is on following a focused behavioral plan. As a result, motivation improves and self-efficacy increases.

There are 5 "A's" that are essential to implementing BA in the clinical setting. The first A is to Assess. This has likely already been done, for instance, when the provider has the patient complete a depression assessment such as the PHQ-9. Activities that the patient is no longer engaging in are also identified. The second A is "Advise." Here the provider advises on the cycle of fatigue wherein low energy and motivation leads patients to isolate and avoid participating in activities they normally would enjoy. Sleep hygiene may need to be addressed in this context. "Agree" is the third A: Patients agree to set realistic goals to gradually increase activities. It is best to start with small goals that can build on themselves over time. The more detailed and specific plan works best and should be tracked by the patient at each visit. Examples could be as simple as going for a walk to more complex undertaking such as taking a class. The primary care provider then "Assists" the patient to problem-solve barriers to meeting goals. Simultaneously, patients are encouraged to acknowledge enjoyment of completed activities. Finally, a plan to follow up on goals set at each visit should be "arranged" at the end of the encounter. Addis and martell provide behavioral techniques that clinicians can easily implement in primary care practice.[53]

Reasons for Routine Psychiatric Referrals

- Primary care provider is uncertain of diagnosis or uncomfortable with managing the treatment plan
- Suboptimal response to adequate dose and duration of commonly prescribed antidepressants
- Intolerable and recurrent or persistent adverse effects to medications
- Atypical symptoms (e.g., increased appetite and hypersomnolence)
- Psychotic or manic symptoms
- Comorbid anxiety disorder

Reasons for Urgent Psychiatric Referrals

- Suicidal ideation, intent, or plan
- Homicidal ideation, intent, or plan
- Inability to care for self or dependents due to psychopathology (e.g., unable to provide shelter, food, or clothing)
- Worsening baseline psychotic symptoms
- Need for alcohol or illicit drug detoxification
- Need for ECT

CASES AND QUESTIONS

CASE 1: Screening for Depression

1. A 48-year-old Hispanic woman presents to your office complaining of low energy. She also reports 4 weeks of sleeping more than usual, overeating, and difficulty concentrating at work and at home. She notes less interest in socializing and hobbies such as knitting. Of note, 1 month ago her son moved away to college, and she was transitioned into a lower-paying, higher-demanding position at work. She denies feeling consistently down—"I don't have time to be depressed"—but admits to crying spells "on occasion." She has never been on medications for mood or sleep and has no family history of mental illness. She adamantly denies any suicidal ideation and denies access to firearms. Physical examination is normal, although the patient seems somewhat tearful and constricted in affect. In addition to possible somatic symptoms disorder, what the most likely diagnosis in this patient?

   A. Illness anxiety disorder
   B. Generalized anxiety disorder
   C. Adjustment disorder
   D. Major depressive disorder
   D. Bipolar disorder

   Correct answer: D. *Despite initial somatic complaints, the clinician should broaden the*

continued

initial differential and screen this patient for major depressive disorder, utilizing a screening tool such as the PHQ-9. The patient should also be screened for past or current manic, psychotic, or anxious symptoms. Despite the presence of recent identifiable stressors, which may prompt a diagnosis of adjustment disorder, the patient meets criteria for a major depressive episode.

2. For the treatment of major depressive disorder, which of the following is the best intervention?

   A. Bupropion
   B. SSRI
   C. CBT
   D. Supportive psychotherapy
   E. Any of the above

   Correct answer: E. Once the diagnosis of major depressive disorder has been established and discussed with the patient, she should be asked about her preference for psychotherapy or medications. Should she prefer psychotherapy, the primary care physician should assist with a referral to a local therapist and briefly introduce her to CBT. Should she prefer medication, an SSRI is a reasonable choice to start and the primary care provider should clearly discuss potential side effects. Bupropion is also a reasonable alternative to SSRI in individual concerned about sexual side effects with no history of seizure disorder.

3. If the patient decides to start medication treatment, how long should the treatment course last?

   A. 3 to 4 months
   B. 4 to 6 months
   C. 6 to 9 months
   D. 9 to 12 months
   E. 12 to 36 months

   Correct answer: D. If she tolerates the initial dose well and with minimal side effects, the clinician should repeat her PHQ-9 within 4 to 8 weeks of initiation to test for treatment response. She should be treated for at least 9 to 12 months after symptom remission, and her clinician should continue to assess for recurrent depression and suicidal thoughts during subsequent routine primary care visits.

CASE 2: Decision-Making around Antidepressant Therapy

Mr. H is a 26-year-old man coming to you reporting that his depression is getting worse. He no longer enjoys playing the guitar and his energy is low. His girlfriend has complained to him that he is no longer interested in sex. He responds that getting erections is more difficult. Passive suicidal ideation is present, but there is no plan and he has no access to firearms. His mother has struggled with depression for many years and did well on venlafaxine. The patient has had two previous depressive episodes. He is currently prescribed citalopram 40 mg, which he has taken for the last 2 years until the current symptoms recurred about 8 weeks ago. Headache and dizziness are also among his complaints. He is not suicidal at this time and does not have access to firearms or prescription medications at home. You diagnose him with recurrent major depression and discuss the possibility of either increasing citalopram or changing to a different antidepressant. He attributes erectile dysfunction to the citalopram and admits to intermittently missing doses as a result. BMI is 31.

1. What is this patient's diagnosis?

   A. Bipolar I, most recent episode, depression
   B. Bipolar I, most recent episode, manic
   C. Bipolar II
   D. Major depressive disorder, single episode
   E. Major depressive disorder, recurrent

   Correct answer: E. Despite previous response to citalopram, this patient is now experiencing a recurrence of depression.

2. What is the best treatment approach?

   A. Change citalopram to bupropion
   B. Change citalopram to venlafaxine
   C. Add CBT
   D. Add supportive psychotherapy
   E. Any of the above

   Correct answer: A. Although recurrent or severe depression is best managed in consultation with a psychiatrist, there are approaches that can be employed in primary care settings. This patient is reporting erectile dysfunction related to treatment with SSRI. He is also mildly obese. Given that his depression has recurred, this may be a good time to reevaluate choice of antidepressant. Bupropion may be a good choice given its low propensity to cause weight gain and sexual dysfunction. Although his mother responded to venlafaxine in the past, there's high likelihood the venlafaxine may also cause sexual side effects. Considering this patient's overall situation, bupropion may still be a better choice. Adding psychotherapy will be helpful for this patient because combination medication and psychotherapy tend to be more effective than either alone; the sexual side effects should still be addressed first. Another option would be to add bupropion as combination therapy to citalopram for depression treatment and to reduce sexual side effect. However, the patient must be agreeable to taking two medications rather than one.

3. How long should this patient be on antidepressant treatment?

   A. 3 to 6 months
   B. 6 to 9 months
   C. 9 to 12 months
   D. 12 to 36 months
   E. Lifelong

Correct answer: E. *Given his history of two previous depressive episodes, he should be on lifelong antidepressant therapy. Mr. H should be followed closely and monitored for changes in depressive symptoms, medication side effects, and suicidal ideation.*

PRACTICAL RESOURCES

- Screening for Depression: U.S. Preventive Services Task Force (USPSTF): http://www.ahrq.gov/clinic/3r-duspstf/depression/depressrr.htm
- Geriatric Depression Scale: http://www.stanford.edu/~;yesavage/GDS.html
- Edinburgh Postnatal Depression Scale: http://www.dbpeds.org/media/edinburghscale.pdf
- National Alliance on Mental Illness: http://www.nami.org/
- National Institute for Mental Health: http://www.nimh.nih.gov/
- The MacArthur Foundation on Depression and Primary Care at Dartmouth and Duke: http://www.depression-primarycare.org/
- National Institutes of Health (NIH) Medline Plus: www.nlm.nih.gov/medlineplus/depression.html
- Agency for Healthcare Research and Quality (AHRQ) review of effective depression treatments: http://effectivehealthcare.ahrq.gov/reports/index.cfm
- FDA Drug Safety Guide: http://www.fda.gov/cder/drug/DrugSafety/DrugIndex.htm)
- Patient education: Mayo Clinic overview of Depression: http://www.mayoclinic.org/diseases-conditions/depression/home/ovc-20321449

REFERENCES

1. Global Burden of Disease Study 2013 Collaborators. Global, regional and national incidence, prevalence, and years lived with disability for 301 acute and chronic diseases and injuries in 188 countries, 1990-2013: a systematic analysis for the Global Burden of Disease Study 2013. *Lancet.* 2015:386:743-800.
2. Frasure-Smith N. The montreal heart attack readjustment trial. *J Cardiopulm Rehabil.* 1995;15:103-106.
3. Katon W, Schulberg H. Epidemiology of depression in primary care. *Gen Hosp Psychiatry.* 1992;14:237-247.
4. Arseniou S, Arvaniti A. HIV infection and depression. *Psychiatry Clin Neurosci.* 2014;68:96-108.
5. Wilde A, Chan H-N, Rahman B, et al. A meta-analysis of the risk of affective disorder in relatives of individuals affected by major depressive disorder or bipolar disorder. *J Affect Disord.* 2014;158:37-47.
6. *Diagnostic and Statistical Manual of Mental Disorder.* 5th ed. Arlington, VA: American Psychiatric Association; 2013.
7. Siu AL; and the US Preventive Services Task Force (USPSTF). Screening for depression in adults: US preventive services task force recommendation statement. *JAMA.* 2016;315(4):380-387.
8. Stewart DE, Vigood S. Postpartum depression. *N Engl J Med.* 2016;375(22):2177-2186.
9. Bergman-Evans B. A health profile of spousal Alzheimer's caregivers. Depression and physical health characteristics. *J Psychosoc Nurs Ment Health Serv.* 1994;32:25-30.
10. Robinson RG, Jorge RE. Post-stroke depression: a review. *Am J Psychiatry.* 2016;173:221-231.
11. Hersdorffer DC. Comorbidity between neurological illness and psychiatric disorders. *CNS Drugs.* 2016;21(3):230-238.
12. Holt RIG, De Groot M, Golden SH. Diabetes and depression. *Curr Diab Reports.* 2014:14:491-510.
13. Popkin MK, Callies AL, Lentz RD, et al. Prevalence of major depression, simple phobia, and other psychiatric disorders in patients with long-standing type I diabetes mellitus. *Arch Gen Psychiatry.* 1988;45:64-68.
14. Anderson RJ, Freedland KE, Clouse RE, et al. The prevalence of comorbid depression in adults with diabetes: a meta-analysis. *Diabetes Care.* 2001;24:1069-1078.
15. House A, Dennis M, Mogridge L, et al. Mood disorders in the year after first stroke. *Br J Psychiatry.* 1991;158:83-92.
16. Schleifer SJ, Macari-Hinson MM, Coyle DA, et al. The nature and course of depression following myocardial infarction. *Arch Intern Med.* 1989;149:1785-1789.
17. de Maat MM, Hoetelmans RM, Math t RA, et al. Drug interaction between St John's wort and nevirapine. *AIDS.* 2001;15:420-421.
18. Stunkard AJ, Faith MS, Allison KC. Depression and obesity. *Biol Psychiatry.* 2003;54:330-337.
19. Onyike CU, Crum RM, Lee HB, et al. Is obesity associated with major depression? Results from the third national health and nutrition examination survey. *Am J Epidemiol.* 2003;158:1139-1147.
20. Screening for depression: recommendations and rationale. *Ann Intern Med.* 2002;136:760-764.
21. Beck CT. Predictors of postpartum depression: an update. *Nurs Res.* 2001;50:275-285.
22. Mulrow CD, Williams JW Jr, Gerety MB, et al. Case-finding instruments for depression in primary care settings. *Ann Intern Med.* 1995;122:913-921.
23. Spitzer RL, Kroenke K, Williams JB. Validation and utility of a self-report version of PRIME-MD: the PHQ primary care study. Primary care evaluation of mental disorders. Patient health questionnaire. *JAMA.* 1999;282:1737-1744.
24. Lowe B, Unutzer J, Callahan CM, et al. Monitoring depression treatment outcomes with the patient health Questionnaire-9. *Med Care.* 2004;42:1194-1201.
25. Whooley MA, Avins AL, Miranda J, et al. Case-finding instruments for depression: two questions are as good as many. *J Gen Intern Med.* 1997;12:439-445.
26. Arroll B, Goodyear-Smith F, Crengle S, et al. Validation of PHQ-2 and PHQ-9 to screen for major depression in the primary care population. *Ann Fam Med.* 2010;8(4):348-353.
27. Deneke DE, Schultz HE, Fluent TE. Screening for depression in the primary care population. *Psychiatr Clin North Am.* 2015;38(1):23-43.
28. Shafer AB. Meta-analysis of the factor structures of four depression questionnaires: Beck, CES-D, Hamilton, and Zung. *J Clin Psychol.* 2006;62(1):123-146.
29. Zung WW. A self-rating depression scale. *Arch Gen Psychiatry.* 1965;12:63-70.

30. Cox JL, Holden JM, Sagovsky R. Detection of postnatal depression. Development of the 10-item Edinburgh post-natal depression scale. *Br J Psychiatry*. 1987;150:782-786.

31. Chorwe-Sungani G, Chipps J. A systematic review of screening instruments for depression for use in antenatal services in low resource settings. *BMC Psychiatry*. 2017;17(1):112.

32. Dennis M, Kadri A, Coffey J. Depression in older people in the general hospital: a systematic review of screening instruments. *Age Ageing*. 2012;41(2):148-154.

33. Bjelland I, Dahl AA, Haug TT, Neckelmann D. The validity of the hospital anxiety and depression scale. An updated literature review. *J Psychosom Res*. 2002;52(2):69-77.

34. Hirschfeld RM. Differential diagnosis of bipolar disorder and major depressive disorder. *J Affect Disord*. 2014;169(suppl 1):S12-S16.

35. *Centers for Disease Control FASTSTATS Suicide and Self-injury*; https://www.cdc.gov/nchs/fastats/suicide.htm. Accessed May 25, 2017.

36. Luoma JB, Martin CE, Pearson JL. Contact with mental health and primary care providers before suicide: a review of the evidence. *Am J Psychiatry*. 2002;159:909-916.

37. Rush AJ, Trivedi MH, Wisniewski SR, et al. Acute and longer-term outcomes in depressed outpatients requiring one or several treatment steps: a STAR*D report. *Am J Psychiatry*. 2006;163:1905-1917.

38. Dazzi T, Gribble R, Wessely S, et al. Does asking about suicide and related behaviours induce suicidal ideation? What is the evidence? *Psychol Med*. 2014;44:3361-3363.

39. Bentley SM, Pagalilauan GL, Simpson SA. Major depression. *Med Clin North Am*. 2014;98(5):9815-1005.

40. American Psychiatric Association (APA). *Practice Guideline for the Treatment of Patients with Major Depressive Disorder*. 3rd ed. 2010. Retrieved from http://psychiatryonline.org/pb/assets/raw/sitewide/practice_guidelines/guidelines/mdd.pdf. Accessed May 30, 2017.

41. Thase ME, Friedman ES, Biggs MM, et al. Cognitive therapy versus medication in augmentation and switch strategies as second-step treatments: a STAR*D report. *Am J Psychiatry*. 2007;164:739-752.

42. Thase ME, Greenhouse JB, Frank E, et al. Treatment of major depression with psychotherapy or psychotherapy–pharmacotherapy combinations. *Arch Gen Psychiatry*. 1997;54:1009-1015.

43. Schulberg HC, Katon W, Simon GE, et al. Treating major depression in primary care practice: an update of the Agency for Health Care policy and Research Practice Guidelines. *Arch Gen Psychiatry*. 1998;55:1121-1127.

44. Apaydin EA, Maher AR, Shanman R, et al. A systematic review of St. John's wort for major depressive disorder. *Syst Rev*. 2016;5(1):148.

45. Dwyer AV, Whitten DL, Hawrelak JA. Herbal medicines, other than St. John's Wort, in the treatment of depression: a systematic review. *Altern Med Rev*. 2011;16(1):40-49.

46. Trivedi MH, Fava M, Wisniewski SR, et al. Medication augmentation after the failure of SSRIs for depression. *N Engl J Med*. 2006;354:1243-1252.

47. Friedman RA. Antidepressants' black-box warning–10 years later. *N Engl J Med*. 2014;371(18):1666-1668.

48. Sandson NB, Armstrong SC, Cozza KL. An overview of psychotropic drug-drug interactions. *Psychosomatics*. 2005;46:464-494.

49. Taylor MJ, Freemantle N, Geddes JR, et al. Early onset of selective serotonin reuptake inhibitor antidepressant action: systematic review and meta-analysis. *Arch Gen Psychiatry*. 2006;63:1217-1223.

50. Haddad PM. Antidepressant discontinuation syndromes. *Drug Saf*. 2001;24(3):183-197.

51. Fink M, Taylor MA. Electroconvulsive therapy: evidence and challenges. *JAMA*. 2007;298:330-332.

52. Burns DD. *Feeling Good: The New Mood Therapy*. New York: Avon Books; 1999.

53. Addis ME, Martell CR. *Overcoming Depression One Step at a Time*. Oakland, CA: New Harbinger Publications; 2004.

9

TREATMENT-RESISTANT DEPRESSION

Jeffrey T. Rado, MD, MPH and Molly Lubin, MD

Mr. L is a 34-year-old man with a history of poor response to antidepressant treatment. He has comorbid diabetes and often forgets to take his insulin. His PCP has tried sertraline, bupropion, and venlafaxine. None of these medications have been helpful. He thought sertraline worked a bit initially but then seemed to lose its effect.

CLINICAL HIGHLIGHTS

- 10% to 30% of patients with major depression develop a chronic, frequently relapsing, difficult-to-treat depression.
- The antidepressant dose should be increased at least above starting dose before considering it a treatment failure.
- TRD is associated with significant clinical burden, increased health care costs and reduced quality of life.
- Although many treatment options exist, none are consistently effective.
- A majority of patients do not remit after an initial antidepressant trial, although most eventually remit after trying multiple agents.
- There is a broad array of pharmacologic strategies available for the treatment of depression including augmenting, switching, and combining antidepressants.
- Providers should be proactive at initiating trials of alternative medications or neuromodulatory approaches to get patients into remission.

INTRODUCTION

Depression is a major cause of disability worldwide. Roughly 50% of patients with depression respond to antidepressants.[1] Among those suffering from depression, approximately 10% to 30% of individuals experience a more severe, difficult-to-treat form of the illness.[2]

These patients undergo switching and augmenting pharmacologic trials as well as electroconvulsive therapy (ECT) and transcranial magnetic stimulation (TMS), often while continuing to receive psychotherapy and having significant symptoms. There is no agreement on the exact definition of treatment-resistant depression (TRD), although the term most frequently refers to a patient who has failed to respond to two adequate trials of an antidepressant.[3] Therefore, when assessing TRD, it is essential to assess whether the patient truly underwent an antidepressant trial of adequate dose (usually at least a middle or high dose) and duration (typically at least 4 weeks), as well as attention to evidence-based psychotherapy. Adherence to medication also needs to be verified, as nonadherence to antidepressant medication is a common cause of "pseudoresistance." Treatment strategies include pharmacologic augmentation or switching, combinations of agents, the addition of psychotherapy, and neuromodulation.

CLINICAL SIGNIFICANCE
PREVALENCE AND COSTS

The STAR*D study, which utilized a treatment algorithm in both primary care and specialty psychiatric practices, highlighted the relatively common problem of treatment resistance.[4] In that study, 37% of patients responded to initial treatment with the SSRI citalopram. Of those who received a second line of treatment (switch to another SSRI [selective serotonin reuptake inhibitor] or an SNRI [serotonin–norepinephrine reuptake inhibitor]), only 31% reached remission (or 19% of the original sample). This means that only 56% of patients remitted after two adequate antidepressant trials and the remaining 44% had TRD. Eighteen of the clinical sites for the STAR*D were primary clinic office indicating a high prevalence of TRD in primary care. Furthermore, study of more than 1,200 primary care patients with major depression found an overall TRD prevalence of 21.7%.[5] In this study, TRD patients had longer episode duration, were more likely to receive polypharmacy, and reported more adverse events from antidepressants.

The societal impact of TRD includes higher health care costs and lost productivity.[6] One review found that TRD added $29 to 48 billion to the financial costs of depression to society.[6] This same study found worse quality of life in patients with TRD versus other depressed patients. Seventeen percent of TRD patients had attempted suicide. Another study found that major depression cost the United States $80 to $130 billion annually, of which 40% could be attributed to TRD.[7]

CLINICAL BURDEN, SUICIDE, MEDICAL COMORBIDITIES

TRD is associated with worse psychiatric and medical outcomes. Scherrer et al. (2012) found that increased mortality following a myocardial infarction was associated with treatment resistance.[8] TRD patients are more likely to be hospitalized for psychiatric and medical reasons, have more outpatient visits, and take more psychotropic medications.[9] Reduced work productivity, decreased involvement in activities, and impaired sexual enjoyment have also been noted.[10] A systematic review of nine TRD studies found that less than 20% of TRD patients remitted at 1 year and relapse was frequent.[11] This was associated with poor quality of life and higher mortality.

DIAGNOSIS
STAGING MODELS

Several models have been developed to stage TRD as an aid to clinicians in their care of these patients.[3,11] The Thase and Rush Staging Model proposes five successive stages of increasing resistance. It separates antidepressants into a hierarchy of effectiveness, which may not reflect real-world experience. It also does not account for resistance to psychotherapy. The Massachusetts General Hospital staging approach assesses resistance based on the number of failed antidepressants. This model assesses for adequacy and duration of each antidepressant trial and also considers augmentation and combined treatments. Finally, the Maudsley Staging Model uses a multidimensional approach that monitors the number of failed antidepressant trials but does not differentiate between classes.

RISK FACTORS FOR TREATMENT-RESISTANT DEPRESSION

Patients who do not reach remission in their first depressive episode and therefore continue to have residual symptoms are more likely to develop a more severe and chronic depression that is more difficult to treat.[12] This is one reason that guidelines recommend treating patients to complete, rather than partial remission. Risk factors for TRD include the presence of psychiatric comorbidity such as panic disorder, social phobia, substance use disorders, and personality disorder. Patients with comorbid anxiety disorders may have the strongest risk to develop hard-to-treat depression.[13] Other risk factors associated

with TRD include early age of onset, current suicidal risk, melancholic features, nonresponse to first antidepressant ever tried, experiencing more adverse events from medications, and more frequent disease recurrences.[13] Low social support, negative social interactions, and weak social integration are also linked to chronic, poorly controlled depression. Balestri and colleagues found that TRD was predicted by longer duration and greater severity of depressive episode, presence of antidepressant side effects, higher suicidal risk, and presence of first- and second-degree relatives with psychiatric illness.[14]

DIFFERENTIAL DIAGNOSIS

Patients who do not respond to initial antidepressant therapy should be evaluated for comorbid psychiatric and medical conditions that may be contributing to their lack of response. Especially important considerations are bipolar depression, i.e., depression in someone with previous hypomania or mania, which would require a different treatment approach (see Chapter 10), and mixed states, which refer to the presence of significant irritability, mood lability, mental overactivity, and psychomotor overactivity and often do not respond well to conventional antidepressant treatment.[15,16] For instance, agitation occurring in the context of bipolar depressed or mixed states may respond better to antipsychotics. Additional considerations include undiagnosed psychosis, eating disorders, substance use disorders, obsessive–compulsive disorder, posttraumatic stress disorder, or neurocognitive disorders, especially in older individuals in whom dementia can resemble depression. The presence of these untreated psychiatric comorbidities may hinder improvement in the depression (*Figure 9-1*). Other psychiatric concerns to evaluate for include a history of significant trauma that is impeding recovery, as well as personality disorders and long-standing psychological issues that are more amenable to long-term psychodynamic psychotherapy.

Depression that has not responded to initial treatment, including when there are atypical symptoms such as lack of cognitive symptoms commonly found in depression (e.g., hopelessness), should prompt consideration and evaluation for other medical causes of TRD presentations. Medical conditions that can masquerade as TRD include hypothyroidism, anemia, sleep apnea, vitamin deficiencies, and less commonly, malignancy and autoimmune disorders. Any patient failing to respond to an optimized trial of at least one antidepressant should receive further medical evaluation that includes a focused physical examination, vitamin D levels, thyroid function tests, complete blood count (CBC), liver and renal function, cortisol level, and workup for anemia or chronic inflammatory conditions.[17] Furthermore, the patient's existing medications should be reviewed for any agents that may be contributing to the depression.

Lastly, patients should always be evaluated for nonadherence to antidepressant treatment, as failure to take antidepressants consistently and at prescribed doses will limit their effectiveness. A number of factors may affect patient adherence with medications and dosing. These include personal ambivalence about their diagnosis and treatment as well as social stigma, negative family or peer attitudes toward the illness, cognitive issues leading to misunderstanding about the purpose of the medication or how it should be taken, the cost, and the side effects of the medication.

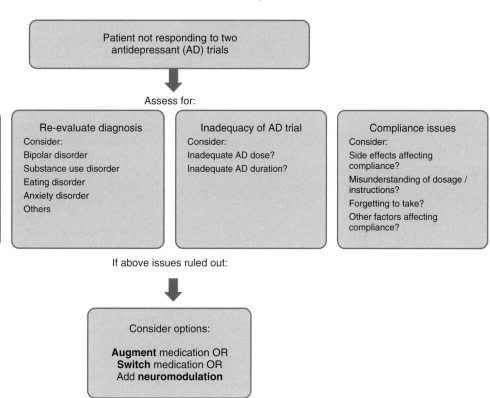

FIGURE 9-1 Options in treatment-resistant depression.

BIOPSYCHOSOCIAL TREATMENT

PHARMACOTHERAPY

It is important to know that no medications are FDA approved for "treatment-resistant depression." When a patient has not responded to a first trial of an antidepressant, it is useful to reassure the patient that this is not unusual, given that only about one-third of patients remit with the initial antidepressant trial. In terms of next steps, there are four general psychopharmacologic strategies to consider:

• optimization of the initial medication;
• augmentation, which refers to the addition of a nonantidepressant medication shown to have depression-relieving properties;
• combination, which refers to the addition of a second antidepressant; and
• switch to a different medication.

Much of our knowledge of these strategies comes from the STAR*D study, which is the largest prospective clinical trial of major depression ever conducted in primary care settings, and which specifically compared different next-step options for patients who did not remit after a trial of citalopram prescribed at its maximum tolerable dose.[18] After failure of citalopram, patients were offered a choice of adding another agent, or switching medications altogether, with patients then being randomized to different augmentation or switch strategies. Those whose depression did not remit after this second step were then augmented or switched again at their choice, and those whose depression still did not remit after this third step were switched again,

with about two-thirds of patients achieving remission by the last level of the study.

The STAR*D used an aggressive dosing strategy, that is, medications were prescribed at their maximum approved or tolerable doses. Accordingly, medications should be similarly optimized in the real world, before being declared ineffective. That is, they should generally be increased to their highest tolerable doses, their maximum approved doses, or at a minimum to an above starting dose.[19] The medication should be maintained at that dose for 6 to 12 weeks to assess for efficacy. In cases where there is absolutely no improvement at moderate (at least above starting dose) doses, switching to a different agent or augmentation may be considered.

AUGMENTATION

When a patient has had partial but incomplete response to the first agent, an appropriate next step is augmentation of that agent (*Table 9-1*). Although the organization of the STAR*D trial did not permit direct comparison of medication augmentation versus switch as a best next step for patients with resistance to a first agent, there is some evidence from STAR*D that patients with partial response to the initial SSRI benefit more from augmentation than from switch.[20] An obvious advantage of adding a second medication over switching medications is that the partial benefit from the first medication will not be lost in the process of discontinuing the first and starting the second.

Although many augmentation agents have been studied, three have the most evidence demonstrating their benefit in unipolar depression: atypical antipsychotics, lithium, and thyroid hormone. Of these, atypical

TABLE 9-1 Augmentation Options for Treatment-Resistant Depression

MEDICATION	THERAPEUTIC DOSE RANGE	SIDE EFFECTS
Atypical antipsychotics		
Aripiprazole	2-15 mg	Sedation, abnormal metabolic labs, weight gain, akathisia, increased prolactin, QTc prolongation
Quetiapine	150-300 mg	
Olanzapine (adjunctive to fluoxetine)	6-18 mg	
Risperidone	1-3 mg	
Ziprasidone	40-160 mg	
Brexpiprazole	2-3 mg	
Others		
Lithium	600-900 mg/0.6-0.9 mmol/L blood level	Ataxia, tremor, nausea, diarrhea, polyuria, renal dysfunction, hypothyroidism
T3	25-50 μg	
Modafinil	100-400 mg	Rare cutaneous reactions (TEN, SJS), cytochrome p450 interactions
SAM-e	800-1,600 mg	
Methylfolate	15-30 mg	
Omega-3 (EPA)	1-2 g	
Bupropion	150-450 mg	HTN, seizures (do not give in patients with epilepsy or other risk factors predisposing to seizure)
Mirtazapine	15-45 mg	Sedation, increase in cholesterol, weight gain
Lamotrigine	25-100 mg	Cutaneous reactions (TEN, SJS)
Pramipexole	1-5 mg	Sedation, nausea, dizziness, tremor, compulsive behavior
Lisdexamfetamine	20-70 mg	Dry mouth, anxiety, appetite suppression, increase in BP

TEN, toxic epidermal necrolysis; SJS, Stevens–Johnson syndrome; HTN, hypertension; BP, blood pressure.

antipsychotics are the best-studied, with multiple studies demonstrating their superior efficacy compared with placebo. Efficacy of these agents for treating depression is likely due to their effects on serotonin, norepinephrine, and dopamine receptors. Moreover, they have demonstrated utility in the treatment of mixed depression likely because of their reduction in agitation and, although not FDA-approved for it, are recommended by expert consensus as first-line treatment for mixed depression.[16]

Aripiprazole has the most evidence supporting its use in depression. For instance, a recent post hoc analysis pooled data from three randomized placebo-controlled trials in patients with minimal or no response to 8 weeks of SSRI or SNRI monotherapy. Compared with placebo, adjunctive aripiprazole 5 to 20 mg daily was associated with significantly greater rates of response, defined as ≥50% reduction in MADRS score, and remission, defined as MADRS score <10.[21]

There is also an evidence base for the use of quetiapine, risperidone, and the combination of the antipsychotic olanzapine and the SSRI fluoxetine (OFC) as adjunctive treatment for depression. A meta-analysis of multiple randomized placebo-controlled studies of patients with major depression who had had inadequate response to at least one prior antidepressant trial and then were randomized to an adjunctive antipsychotic or placebo compared the odds of achieving remission with the various antipsychotics versus placebo.[22] The authors found statistically significant improved odds of remission with aripiprazole (number needed to treat (NNT) = 9), OFC (NNT = 19), quetiapine (NNT = 9), and risperidone (NNT = 9) as compared with placebo. Aripiprazole was associated with akathisia, sedation, and weight gain; OFC was associated with weight gain, sedation, abnormal blood glucose and lipids, and elevated prolactin; quetiapine was associated with sedation and abnormal glucose and lipids levels, while risperidone was not significantly associated with any adverse events.

There is promising evidence for the use of the atypical antipsychotics ziprasidone and brexpiprazole for augmentation of depression treatment. There is one randomized trial of 8 weeks of add-on ziprasidone versus placebo in patients who had been on escitalopram for 8 weeks and still met criteria for major depressive disorder (MDD) based on the DSM-IV or had a QIDS-SR score ≥10.[23] The ziprasidone group showed significantly greater rates of clinical response on the HAM-D at doses of 40 to 160 mg daily (mean dose = 98 mg) than those randomized to placebo, although with significantly greater rates of fatigue, irritability, anxiety/agitation, and muscle twitching than the placebo group. Adjunctive brexpiprazole, a newer atypical antipsychotic, was studied in two recent phase III clinical trials of patients with less than 50% symptom improvement after 8 weeks of antidepressant treatment. Brexpiprazole 2 or 3 mg daily dose was associated with significantly greater reduction in MADRS score versus placebo.[24] The most frequent reported adverse events in the brexpiprazole group were weight gain and akathisia.

Significant evidence supports the use of adjunctive lithium and thyroid hormone in TRD. Their use has been more studied as adjuncts to the older, tricyclic antidepressants (TCAs) and comparatively less when combined with newer antidepressants. Nonetheless, the literature regarding their use as adjuncts to SSRIs and SNRIs is promising. Lithium was used as a level 3 augmenting agent in STAR*D: after failure of citalopram and failure of a second step (either augmentation or switch), and led remission rates of about 15%.[18] A 2014 meta-analysis of three randomized placebo-controlled trials of lithium augmentation for SSRI and SNRIs in MDD found that the odds ratio for response with lithium augmentation (600 to 900 mg daily) after at least 4 weeks of antidepressant treatment was 3.06 compared with placebo, with response defined as >50% symptom improvement in whatever scale the primary authors were using.[25] The STAR*D trial helped establish the efficacy of T3, as well as lithium, as an augmenting agent for antidepressants, in fact showing slightly improved efficacy and tolerability of T3 over lithium.[18] Three augmentation studies of T3 in doses of 25 to 50 µg daily in SSRI nonresponders showed that the majority of subjects experienced response or remission, with definition of response varying per study but remission defined in all as a HAM-D score <7.[26]

Other psychopharmacologic agents demonstrate a less robust, but still promising, evidence base. These include SAM-e, L-methylfolate, Omega-3, modafinil, and celecoxib. A 2016 review and meta-analysis of adjunctive nutraceuticals for the treatment of depression found benefit from the use of folate metabolites and Omega-3.[27] Of 15 trials of adjunctive folate in subjects with treatment resistance (failure to respond to a trial of a newer antidepressant, most commonly fluoxetine), 10 showed that these agents improved depression symptoms as measured by the HAM-D or BDI. The effective doses were 15 to 30 mg daily L-methylfolate monotherapy or 800 to 1600 mg of SAM-e daily monotherapy. Eight randomized placebo-controlled trials examined Omega-3 as adjunct to antidepressants, although not specifically in the setting of treatment resistance. Meta-analysis of the data showed a benefit of Omega-3 over placebo on HAM-D score, with the EPA or ethyl-EPA formulation having an additional advantage over the DHA formulation, in doses ranging from 930 mg to 4.4 g daily and most common doses being 1 to 2 g daily. A 2013 meta-analysis included four randomized controlled trials of adjunctive modafinil versus placebo for unipolar depression. Two of these were composed of patients demonstrating treatment resistance to ≥4 weeks of SSRIs, suggesting a positive effect of modafinil on depression scores measured by HAM-D or IDS (Inventory of Depressive Symptomatology), which approached significance.[28] Doses range was 100 to 400 mg daily.

Similarly, evidence is accumulating for the use of the anti-inflammatory celecoxib. A 2014 meta-analysis of four randomized placebo-controlled trials of celecoxib versus placebo augmentation found significantly greater odds of response and remission, measured by the HAM-D, in the celecoxib groups, at doses of 200 to 400 mg daily.[29] Three of the trials used SSRIs as the antidepressant that was being augmented, and one used the norepinephrine reuptake inhibitor reboxetine (only available in Europe). Moreover it has been shown that elevated inflammatory markers such as C-reactive protein (CRP) are associated with treatment resistance, and although not routinely carried out at this time, measurement of CRP levels may increase ability to detect TRD and thus inform treatment.[30]

Benzodiazepines reduce symptoms of depression when used as augmenting agents, and reduce baseline anxiety and improve adherence to antidepressants.[19] However, benzodiazepines should be used with caution because of their potential for adverse effects such as sedation, falls, cognitive slowing, addiction, tolerance, and withdrawal.

There are a number of augmentation strategies that are commonly used and theoretically promising, yet have a more mixed evidence base regarding their use. These include lamotrigine, buspirone, pramipexole, pindolol, and stimulants. Buspirone was used as a second-step augmenting agent in STAR*D, that is, after failure of a trial of citalopram, at a mean dose of 40.9 mg daily. About 30% of those initial nonresponders randomized to buspirone experienced remission, which was a similar rate to those randomized to bupropion (discussed below as a combination strategy option), although there was slightly better reduction in depression scores as measured by QIDS-SR (Quick Inventory of Depressive Symptoms—Self Report) and improved tolerability in the bupropion group.[18]

The anticonvulsant lamotrigine is commonly used as an augmentation agent in the treatment of unipolar depression, with retrospective chart reviews and open label studies suggesting significant benefit. However, a large, multicenter, randomized controlled trial of 10 weeks of add-on lamotrigine up to 400 mg daily versus placebo in unipolar patients who had failed one antidepressant trial and then had insufficient response to 8 weeks of paroxetine, did not show a difference between the two groups on depressive symptoms as measured by MADRS scores.[31] The authors noted, however, that lamotrigine did have a superior benefit to placebo in the patients who were more severely depressed and treatment resistant, so it may be that lamotrigine's efficacy is enhanced in this population and that future studies of lamotrigine should focus on a more refractory group.

Pindolol, a β-adrenergic agent, has been shown in some studies to accelerate the response to antidepressant treatment. A meta-analysis was conducted of four randomized controlled trials of adjunctive pindolol versus placebo and one randomized trial of pindolol versus SSRI alone in patients with treatment-resistant unipolar depression. The authors found that pindolol added to SSRIs did not have a significant effect on response rates.[32] Most trials administered pindolol 2.5 mg three times daily, while one dosed it at 7.5 mg once daily and found significant benefit in highly treatment-resistant patients.

Pramipexole, a dopamine receptor agonist, utilized to improve mood in Parkinson disease patients, is also used in major depression. The two randomized controlled trials of pramipexole augmentation for depression demonstrated conflicting results, one showing no added benefit of pramipexole added to escitalopram, while the other showed that pramipexole added to various antidepressant agents versus placebo add-on in treatment-resistant patients was well tolerated and led to greater response rates.[33,34] Further studies of pramipexole in TRD are needed.

Methylphenidate and amphetamines have been studied as adjuncts for TRD, but the evidence for their use is less robust compared with modafinil. One double-blind randomized placebo-controlled study found greater improvement in depressive symptoms with the addition of lisdexamfetamine compared with placebo among participants with partial response to escitalopram. However, this has not been replicated and the two prior randomized placebo-controlled studies of dopaminergic stimulants in TRD were negative.[35]

COMBINATIONS

The combination of two antidepressants has also been studied. Antidepressants of the same class should not be combined. Combination should be reserved for antidepressants of different classes so as to target different mechanisms of action.[19] When using multiple antidepressants, it is important to check for potential drug–drug interactions and be wary of potential complications including serotonin syndrome. Although combinations are commonly used to treat depression, there is not a large evidence base to support this strategy. The one exception is bupropion, a norepinephrine-dopamine reuptake inhibitor. It is commonly used in combination with SSRIs, with the additional advantage of its tendency to reduce SSRI-associated side effects such as sedation, sexual dysfunction, and weight gain. It was evaluated as a combination agent in STAR*D after citalopram monotherapy, with about 30% of those randomized to combination bupropion achieving remission. It also showed slightly improved tolerability and greater total reduction in QIDS-SR scores compared with buspirone.[18] Despite this, there are no placebo-controlled data to support its use in TRD. However, a recent randomized placebo-controlled trial of 6 weeks add-on bupropion (150 to 300 mg daily) versus aripiprazole was conducted in patients with depression unresponsive to 4 weeks of SSRI monotherapy. Although both agents significantly reduced depressive symptoms, bupropion demonstrated a trend toward greater reduction in MADRS score compared with aripiprazole.[36]

SWITCHING AGENTS

An alternative to augmentation or combination of agents is to switch agents. Although response rates to switching versus augmenting after initial antidepressant failure appear to be similar, switching agents is a reasonable strategy when the patient has had no response to the first agent[19] (*Table 9-2*). Although the STAR*D trial did show comparable gains from augmenting and switching, further analysis of STAR*D data suggested that switch may be a better option in those who have had complete non-response to the first antidepressant.[20] STAR*D showed that among patients switched to a second SSRI versus a non-SSRI antidepressant (venlafaxine or bupropion), remission rates were similar across all three groups.[24] However, a meta-analysis examining the effectiveness of within-class versus between-class antidepressant switches found a slight advantage of switching from an SSRI to a non-SSRI (venlafaxine, mirtazapine, or bupropion), in terms of the likelihood of achieving remission.[37]

Venlafaxine, a SNRI, was used as a second-level switch agent in STAR*D. That is, after failure of citalopram,

TABLE 9-2 Switch Options After SSRI Failure		
MEDICATION	**THERAPEUTIC DOSE RANGE**	**SIDE EFFECTS**
Serotonin–norepinephrine reuptake inhibitors		
Venlafaxine	75-375 mg	HTN, sexual dysfunction, weight gain
Desvenlafaxine	60 mg	
Duloxetine	60-120 mg	
Atypical antidepressants		
Bupropion	300-450 mg	HTN, seizures (do not give in patients with epilepsy or other risk factors predisposing to seizure)
Mirtazapine	15-45 mg	Sedation, increase in cholesterol, weight gain
Tricyclic antidepressants		
Nortriptyline	50-200 mg	Anticholinergic side effects, cardiac arrhythmia (avoid in patients with cardiac instability or ischemia), sedation, sexual dysfunction
Imipramine	100-300 mg	
Desipramine	100-300 mg	
Monoamine oxidase inhibitors		
Tranylcypromine	30-60 mg	Hypertensive crisis, severe serotonin syndrome, weight gain, sexual dysfunction
Phenelzine	45-90 mg	

HTN, hypertension.

subjects were randomized to venlafaxine, bupropion or sertraline. Rates of remission were similar across all three groups, with about one-quarter in each achieving remission. A separate pooled analysis was conducted of three trials involving patients unresponsive to an initial SSRI who were randomized to either switch to venlafaxine (75 to 300 mg daily) or to another SSRI. The authors found that the venlafaxine group was more likely to achieve remission, with no difference in the rates of discontinuation.[37] Thus, switching to venlafaxine or another SNRI is a reasonable next strategy after initial failure of an SSRI.

An option to try after SSRI or SNRI failure is an atypical antidepressant such as mirtazapine or bupropion. Bupropion generated comparable remission rates to venlafaxine when studied as a first-line switch agent in STAR*D.[24] Although there are fewer studies of bupropion as a switch agent compared with venlafaxine, bupropion may be especially useful for patients not tolerating SSRIs because of sexual dysfunction. Mirtazapine, a noradrenergic and serotonergic atypical antidepressant, was a third-step switch option in STAR*D (after failure of citalopram and a second-step treatment), with 12% achieving remission on mirtazapine at a mean daily dose of 42.1 mg.[18] At this level of the trial, treatment with mirtazapine did not show a significant difference in efficacy or tolerability as compared with nortriptyline, which was also offered as a third-step switch option.

Although no longer considered first-line treatments for depression given greater tolerability of SSRIs, TCAs still have a role in the management of TRD. Nortriptyline was offered at doses up to 200 mg daily as a third-line switch option in STAR*D, resulting in an additional 20% of subjects achieving remission.[18] This was not significantly different from the remission rates seen with its comparator, mirtazapine. Although nortriptyline was well-tolerated in the STAR*D trial, TCAs can cause side effects related to their antimuscarinic properties. Similarly, monoamine oxidase inhibitors (MAOIs) are no longer routinely used in the treatment of depression, because of tolerability and safety concerns, but may be efficacious in TRD. When prescribing MAOIs, providers must be sure to first discontinue and allow for minimum 2 week washout of other serotonergic agents given the risk of serotonin syndrome when MAOIs are combined with other serotonergic agents. Patients must also be counseled to avoid tyramine-rich foods because of their risk of provoking hypertensive crisis. The MAOI tranylcypromine at a mean dose of 36.9 mg daily was used as a fourth-step switch option in STAR*D. Although it achieved a 7% remission rate, efficacy and tolerability were lower than its fourth-step comparator, a mirtazapine–venlafaxine combination.[18] MAOIs may also be especially useful for patients with features of atypical depression, which has been found to be more responsive to MAOIs than to TCAs. Atypical depression is characterized by increased appetite, weight gain, hypersomnia, heavy sensation in the limbs, rejection sensitivity, and brief mood improvement in response to positive events.

BRIGHT LIGHT THERAPY

Bright light therapy has not been specifically studied for TRD. However, it is not considered a first-line approach for depression and, as a result, is more often utilized in patients who have not responded to first-line antidepressant medications. The efficacy is supported by a meta-analysis of 20 RCTs using bright light therapy for nonseasonal depression.[38] It is effective both as monotherapy and in combination with antidepressants. Given its minimal side effects, light therapy should be considered in those who are unable to tolerate antidepressants. Alternatively, it may augment antidepressants in individuals hesitant to take additional medications. Treatment involves a 10,000 lux lamp positioned 12 inches from the face for 30 minutes every morning. The cost of the lamp is not typically covered by insurance but is widely available from internet vendors. The treatment is generally well tolerated although it can induce hypomania in susceptible individuals.

ADJUNCTIVE PSYCHOTHERAPIES

Medications have traditionally been recommended as the primary treatment of TRD. However, failure to respond to antidepressants does *not* predict lack of response to psychotherapy. Although there is an established evidence base for cognitive behavioral therapy (CBT) and other psychotherapies in the treatment of depression, the overall evidence base supporting psychosocial therapies for TRD is small, although an emerging literature supports the use of various psychotherapeutic modalities. In STAR*D, subjects were offered CBT after they failed an antidepressant trial. Introduction of CBT led to remission rates comparable to antidepressants in that trial[11] The addition of CBT or dialectical behavior therapy has also demonstrated benefit in small studies.[11] Primary care–based CBT was shown to be effective as an adjunct treatment to antidepressants in 469 patients with TRD. A significant greater number of patients achieved clinical response with CBT versus medications alone.[39] In contrast, the addition of interpersonal psychotherapy to pharmacotherapy did not lead to improvement in a small sample of 40 patients with TRD.[40] Themes such as hopelessness, low self-esteem, and emotional reactivity often prevail in patients with TRD.[41] Psychotherapy should be considered in patients with these traits and who are motivated to engage in psychotherapy. In some cases, emphasizing learning to live with symptoms may be more helpful than attempting complete eradication. This approach focuses on well-being despite presence of illness and the importance of setting realistic expectations. In this context, it is argued that TRD may be best managed as a chronic condition similar to diabetes and heart disease. A small trial that focused on a chronic disease management intervention resulted in improved social functioning and quality of life despite persistence of depression symptoms.[42] Primary care providers (PCPs) can be actively involved, utilizing this approach in their

TABLE 9-3 Neuromodulatory Approaches to Treatment-Resistant Depression

TREATMENT	INDICATION	ADVANTAGES	DISADVANTAGES
Electroconvulsive therapy	Severe refractory depression; malnutrient, psychotic depression; severe suicide risk	Proven approach; high remission rates; widely available; covered by insurance	Antegrade and retrograde amnesia; high relapse rate without maintenance therapy
Transcranial magnetic stimulation	Failure to respond any number of adequate antidepressant trials	Well tolerated; no cognitive impairment	Limited availability or insurance coverage
Vagal nerve stimulation	Failure to respond to four adequate antidepressant trials	Well tolerated	Weak evidence to support efficacy

patients with TRD.[11] Educating patient and family members about depression is essential. Teaching self-management skills gives patients a sense of self-control.

NEUROMODULATORY APPROACHES

Neuromodulation utilizes different techniques to directly stimulate the areas of the brain thought to be responsible for depression. These approaches are generally employed only after multiple failed trials of antidepressants (*Table 9-3*).

Electroconvulsive Therapy

ECT utilizes electrical current applied to the brain to induce a seizure. A well-established and safe procedure, it is a widely available treatment option for those with inadequate response or poor tolerability to medications. ECT is administered in a hospital setting and requires anesthesia. Remission rates are between 50% and 80%,[43] making it the most effective antidepressant treatment. Relapse rates are high in the 6 months after a successful treatment course; therefore maintenance treatment is often employed. Although ECT is extremely effective, its use is hampered by concern over perceived cognitive side effects, most notably short-term memory loss, although this may be reduced by unilateral electrode placement. It is particularly useful in urgent situations when rapid improvement is needed, such as malnutrition, agitated psychosis, or severe suicide risk.[44] Treatment is three times weekly for 6 to 12 treatments and can be performed on inpatient or outpatient basis. Continuous and maintenance treatment should be offered to those with severe, highly recurrent disease. ECT treatment is considered underutilized for depression in the United States.

Transcranial Magnetic Stimulation

Repetitive transcranial magnetic stimulation (rTMS) is approved as monotherapy for patients who have failed any number of adequate antidepressant medication trials.[45] At the current time, it is most often used adjunctively with antidepressant medications. Its noninvasive approach involves the application of pulsed magnetic fields to the left dorsolateral prefrontal cortex via application of a magnetic coil to the scalp. In contrast to ECT, it does not involve seizure induction. Its mechanism of action is unknown but is thought to involve activation of cortical neurons with secondary activation of deeper brain structures. Currently, treatment is most often delivered on a daily basis for approximately 6 weeks (5 days per week) plus a taper period. Treatments last 38 minutes, are administered by a nurse or technician, and can be delivered in the outpatient setting while the patient is awake reclining in a chair. Side effects are mild and include transient headache and scalp pain, with no long-term cardiovascular or neurologic sequelae. Seizures are a rare side effect and nearly nonexistent when standardized treatment parameters are employed. Cognition and memory are not affected by the treatment, making it significantly better tolerated compared with ECT. Deep rTMS is a modified approach that reaches deeper into the brain. More recently, handheld TMS devices have been approved by the FDA for treatment of MDD.

Vagal Nerve Stimulation

Vagal nerve stimulation (VNS) involves implantation of a programmable neurostimulator under the skin in the anterior chest wall.[43] Intermittent low frequency electrical impulses are sent to the vagus nerve every 5 minutes, making this a chronic treatment. This procedure is approved for failure of at least four antidepressant treatments. Possible side effects include infection at the site of implantation, cough, hoarse voice and dysphagia. The efficacy of VNS has been questioned, and as a result, this is not a commonly utilized treatment for depression.

EXPERIMENTAL THERAPIES

This section briefly reviews experimental treatments that currently lack FDA approval.

Deep Brain Stimulation

Deep brain stimulation (DBS) is the most invasive neuromodulatory approach. It involves the implantation of stimulating electrode wires directly into the brain regions responsible for depression.[46] These wires are connected to a programmable neurostimulator implanted in the anterior chest wall. Based on several small open label trials, greater than 50% response rates are achievable in the most extremely resistant cases and benefits may last for years. Larger controlled trials have not replicated these findings. In a 16 weeks placebo-controlled industry-sponsored trial in 30 patients, DBS did not lead to greater clinical benefit compared with placebo.[47] A second placebo-controlled trial in 75 patients was terminated early because of lack of clinical benefit.[48] Issues in study design may have contributed to lack of positive findings. Side effects include infection, headache, seizure, and infection. Cognitive function does not seem to be negatively impacted. As this is not an FDA-approved therapy, it is only conducted at highly specialized academic centers.

Magnetic Seizure Therapy

Magnetic seizure therapy employs magnetic waves to induce seizures. It resembles ECT with the goal of inducing more focal seizures while reducing cognitive side effects. Several open label trials indicate good efficacy although longer-term placebo-controlled randomized trials are needed. This treatment remains in the research realm and is not currently FDA approved.

Ketamine

Ketamine is a glutamatergic *N*-methyl-D-aspartate receptor antagonist that is used as an anesthetic in the United States. Several small studies support its use as a treatment option for refractory depression. Interest in ketamine is partly due to its potential rapid antidepressant effect—within hours versus weeks with standard antidepressants. Research indicates that infusion of subanesthetic doses over 40 minutes may lead to a rapid antidepressant effect. The exact antidepressant mechanism is unknown but may involve brain derived neurotrophic factor. In light of its growing off-label use in major depression, the American Psychiatric Association (APA) Council of Research Task Force on Novel Biomarkers and Treatment issued a consensus statement on the use of ketamine in mood disorders. Given the low numbers of subjects in clinical trials and a lack of long-term safety and efficacy data, the authors caution that before expanding clinical access, guidelines are needed regarding treatment setting, standard operating procedures, medication delivery, safety monitoring, and follow-up assessment.[49]

Finally, the naturally occurring plant alkaloid psilocybin has recently been evaluated for depression in several small studies. For instance, Carhart-Harris and colleagues found a significant improvement in 20 patients with treatment-refractory depression after 5 weeks of open label psilocybin treatment, with sustained improvements at 3 and 6 months.[50] Larger controlled trials are needed to further evaluate this molecule's efficacy.

WHEN TO REFER

It is reasonable to refer to a psychiatrist any patient who fails to respond to two or more adequate trials of a standard first-line antidepressant at a therapeutic dose. Any candidate for a neuromodulatory treatment, such as ECT or TMS, should be referred to a treatment center with experience in these procedures.

CONCLUSION

All too often depression lingers because patients are on a pharmacologic regimen that is ineffective or only partly effective. As medicine becomes more personalized, we will have a better ability to predict which patient will respond to which antidepressant, but at this point it is still often necessary to try multiple antidepressants and augmenting agents in patients who do not respond to initial antidepressants. Although it is appropriate to start with agents that have a greater evidence base for the treatment of resistant depression, some patients will respond to a medication that is less often used or less widely studied. Thus, it is crucial to keep trying different strategies and to keep persisting in efforts to treat the condition, remembering that no patient with depression should be deemed untreatable.

CASES AND QUESTIONS

CASE 1:

Mr. L is a 34-year-old man with a history of poor response to antidepressant treatment. He has comorbid diabetes and often forgets to take his insulin. His PCP has tried sertraline, bupropion, and venlafaxine. None of these medications have been helpful. He thought sertraline worked a bit initially but then seemed to lose its effect.

1. What is the percentage of patients who respond to an initial trail of antidepressant medication?

   A. Less than 2%
   B. 30% to 40%
   C. About 50%
   D. Two-thirds

   Correct answer: B. *The overall goal of the STAR*D trial was to assess the effectiveness of depression treatments in patients diagnosed with MDD, in both primary and specialty care settings. It is the largest and longest study ever conducted to evaluate depression treatment. The STAR*D study showed 37% of patients responded to initial treatment with the SSRI citalopram.*

2. What needs to be done before confirming this case as "treatment resistant"?

   A. Initiate a trial of mirtazapine to confirm treatment resistance.
   B. Refer patient for psychotherapy.
   C. Confirm that each trial was of adequate duration at a therapeutic antidepressant dose.
   D. Refer to psychiatry for further evaluation.

   Correct answer: D. *The definition of TRD varies from provider; however, the term most frequently refers to a patient who has failed to respond to two adequate trials of an antidepressant. Therefore, it would be beneficial to have a psychiatrist assess whether the patient truly had trials of adequate dose and duration.*

continued

3. Clinical predictors of TRD include all of the following except:
   A. Having first degree relative with psychiatric illness
   B. Presence of comorbid anxiety disorder
   C. Low social support
   D. Low birth weight

   Correct answer: D. *Risks for development of TRD include psychiatric comorbidity (anxiety disorders, panic disorder, substance use disorder), early age of onset of depression, low social support, negative social interaction, and weak social integration.*

CASE 2:

Mrs. H is a 62-year-old African-American woman with history of osteoarthritis, hypertension, and major depression. Her symptoms include anhedonia, hopelessness, and anxiety. She has undergone trials of fluoxetine 60 mg daily for 3 months, mirtazapine 30 mg daily for 2 months, duloxetine 60 mg daily for 1 year, and nortriptyline 150 mg, which has been taken for the last 9 months. She has been hospitalized multiple times in the past for suicidal ideation including two suicide attempts when she overdosed on her medications and spent a week in the intensive care unit. She is currently feeling suicidal again with some transient thoughts of overdosing on her pills.

1. Does this patient have TRD?
   A. No, because she has not tried a combination of antidepressants.
   B. Yes, because she has failed to get better with nortriptyline.
   C. No, because she has not failed augmentation with an antipsychotic.
   D. Yes, because she has failed to respond to two adequate antidepressant trials.

   Correct answer: D. *The definition of TRD refers to a patient who has failed to respond to two adequate trials of an antidepressant. However, providers should assess whether the patient truly had trials of adequate dose and duration before determining the medications are ineffective. Medication should be prescribed at their maximum approved or tolerable doses before being declared ineffective. For instance, they should generally be increased to their highest **tolerable** doses, their maximum approved doses, or at a minimum to an above starting dose, and that medication should be maintained at that dose for 6 to 12 weeks to assess for efficacy.*

2. Regarding neuromodulatory approaches, all of the following are true except:
   A. TMS requires anesthesia.
   B. ECT leads to remission rates as high as 90%.
   C. DBS is not FDA approved for major depression.
   D. VNS is approved for failure to respond to four antidepressant medication trial.

Correct answer: A. *Neuromodulation approaches utilize different techniques to directly stimulate the areas of the brain thought to be responsible for depression. TMS is a noninvasive approach and involves utilizing pulsed magnetic fields to the left dorsolateral prefrontal cortex via application of a magnetic coil to the scalp. Treatment can be administered in the outpatient setting while the patient is awake **without the need for anesthesia**. ECT utilizes electrical current applied to the brain to induce a seizure. ECT is administered in a hospital setting and **requires anesthesia**. DBS is the most invasive neuromodulatory approach. It involves the implantation of stimulating electrode wires directly into the brain regions responsible for depression. DBS is not FDA approved. VNS involves implantation of a programmable neurostimulator under the skin in the anterior chest wall. This procedure is approved for failure of at least four antidepressant treatments.*

3. Which of the following factors in this case might make ECT a particularly appropriate next treatment?
   A. Severe suicidality
   B. Comorbid psychosis
   C. Comorbid anxiety
   D. Failure to respond to an SSRI

   Correct answer: A. *ECT is indicated in urgent situations when rapid improvement is needed, such as malnutrition due to catatonia, agitated psychosis, or severe suicide risk.*

CASE 3:

Jane is a 38-year-old single accountant with hypothyroidism, who after being laid off from her job begins to feel like she is a failure and to avoid her friends as she no longer finds social outings enjoyable. She has trouble concentrating on job applications because of negative ruminations about the state of her life; she has minimal appetite, stays in bed most of the day, and feels as if her situation will never improve. You diagnose her with major depression and start her on sertraline at 50 mg daily, increasing it over the next 4 weeks to a dose of 200 mg daily, and maintain her on this dose for 6 weeks. At this point she is able to get out of bed more and does socialize occasionally, but still has trouble completing job applications, continues to feel ashamed and worthless, and her appetite and energy level, while a bit improved, are still lower than before.

1. At this point you should:
   A. Check her TSH.
   B. Screen for bipolar disorder, eating disorder, and substance use disorders.
   C. Assess for medication adherence.
   D. All of the above.

   Correct answer: D. *Patients who do not respond to initial antidepressant therapy should be evaluated for comorbid psychiatric and medication conditions,* *as they can hinder the treatment of depression. One should consider undiagnosed psychosis, eating disorders, substance use disorders, obsessive–compulsive disorder, posttraumatic stress disorder, or neurocognitive disorders (such as dementia), which can resemble depression. Additionally, medical conditions that can mimic depression include hypothyroidism, anemia, sleep apnea, vitamin deficiencies, certain malignancy (pancreatic cancer), and autoimmune disorders. For patients not responding to an optimized dose of antidepressant, it would be beneficial to conduct thorough medical evaluation and obtain basic laboratory workup, which include a focused physical examination, vitamin D levels, thyroid function tests, CBC, liver and renal function, cortisol level, and workup for anemia or chronic inflammatory conditions.*

2. After further assessment and workup, you find no evidence of other psychiatric or medical pathology, and no adherence issues. What should you tell Jane?

   A. It is very unusual to not respond to a trial of SSRI at a therapeutic dose.
   B. This is not unusual; about one-third of patients do not respond to their first antidepressant trial.
   C. This is not unusual; about two-thirds of patients do not respond to their first antidepressant trial.
   D. Because sertraline hasn't been effective, she will likely need ECT.

   Correct answer: B. *When a patient has not responded to a first trial of an antidepressant, it is useful to inform him or her that only about one-third of patients remit with the initial antidepressant trial. The STAR*D study showed 37% of patients responded to initial treatment with the SSRI. Furthermore, of those who received a **second line** of treatment (switch to another SSRI or an SNRI), only 31% reached remission (or 19% of the original sample). This means that only 56% of patients remitted after two adequate antidepressant trials.*

3. What should you do at this point, in terms of medications?

   A. Switch from sertraline to a different SSRI.
   B. Switch from sertraline to a different class of antidepressant.
   C. Add an augmenting agent.
   D. Add a second antidepressant.

   Correct answer: A. *Several strategies are available for patients who do not respond to the first trial of antidepressant pharmacotherapy. Switching from one SSRI to another can be effective given that significant chemical and pharmacologic differences between SSRIs. The STAR*D study showed that among patients switched to a second SSRI versus a non-SSRI antidepressant (venlafaxine or bupropion), remission rates were similar across all three groups. However, a meta-analysis examining the effectiveness of within-class versus between-class antidepressant switches found a slight advantage of switching from an SSRI to a non-SSRI in terms of the likelihood of achieving remission.*

REFERENCES

1. Underagga J, Baldessarini RJ. Randomized, placebo-controlled trials of antidepressants for acute major depression: thirty-year meta-analytic review. *Neuropsychopharmacology.* 2011;37:851-862.
2. Blanco C, Okuda M, Markowitz JC, et al. The epidemiology of chronic major depressive disorder and dysthymic disorder: results from the National Epidemiologic Survey on alcohol and related conditions. *J Clin Psychiatry.* 2010;71(12):1645-1656.
3. Gaynes B. Assessing the risk factors for difficult-to-treat depression and treatment-resistant depression. *J Clin Psychiatry.* 2016;77(suppl 1):4-8.
4. Rush AJ, Trivedi MH, Wisniewski SR, et al. Bupropion-SR, sertraline, or venlafaxine-XR after failure of SSRIs for depression. *N Engl J Med.* 2006;354(12):1231-1242.
5. Rizvi SJ, Grima E, Tan M, et al. Treatment resistant depression in primary care across Canada. *Can J Psychiatry.* 2014;59(7):349-361.
6. Mrazek DA, Hornberger JC, Altar CA, Degtiar I. A review of the clinical, economic, and societal burden of treatment-resistant depression: 1996-2013. *Psychiatr Serv.* 2014;65(8):977-987.
7. Gaynes BN. Identifying difficult-to-treat depression: differential diagnosis, subtypes and comorbidities. *J Clin Psychiatry.* 2009;70(suppl 6):10-15.
8. Scherrer JF, Chrusciel T, Garfield L, et al. Treatment-resistant and insufficiently treated depression and all-cause mortality following myocardial infarction. *Br J Psychiatr.* 2012;200:137-142.
9. Lepine BA, Moreno BA, Compos RN, et al. Treatment-resistant depression increases health costs and resource utilization. *Rev Bras Psiquatr.* 2012;34(4):379-388.
10. Peterson T, Papkostas GI, Hahal Y, et al. Psychosocial functioning in patients with treatment resistant depression. *Eur Psychiatry.* 2004;19(4):196-201.
11. Keitner GI, Mansfield AK. Management of treatment-resistant depression. *Psychiatr Clin N Am.* 2012;35:249-265.
12. Bennabi D, Aouizerate B, El-Hage W, et al. Risk factors for treatment resistance in unipolar depression. *J Affect Disord.* 2015;171:137-141.
13. Souery D, Oswald P, Massat I, et al. Clinical factors associated with treatment resistance in major depressive disorder: results from a European multicenter study. *J Clin Psychiatry.* 2007;68(7):1062-1070.
14. Balestri M, Calati R, Souery D, et al. Socio-demographic and clinical predictors of treatment resistant depression: a prospective European Multicenter study. *J Affect Disord.* 2016;189:224-232.
15. Perugi G, Quaranta G, Dell'Osso L. The significance of mixed states in depression and mania. *Curr Psychiatr Rep.* 2014;16:486.
16. Stahl S, Morrissette DA, Faedda G, Fava M. Guidelines for the recognition and management of mixed depression. *CNS Spectr.* 2017;22:203-219.
17. Epstein I, Szpindel I, Katzman MA. Pharmalogical approaches to manage persistent symptoms of major depressive disorder: rationale and therapeutic strategies. *Psychiatr Res.* 2014: S15-S33.
18. Gaynes BN, Warden D, Madhukar T, Wisniewski S, Fava M, Rush A. What did STAR*D teach us? Results from a large-scale, practical, clinical trial for patients with depression. *Psychiatr Serv.* 2009;60(11):1439-1445.

19. Ionescu DF, Rosewbaum JF, Alpert JE. Pharmacological approaches to the challenges of treatment resistant depression. *Dialogues Clin Neurosci.* 2015;17(2):111-126.

20. Gaynes BN, Dusetzina SB, Ellis AR, et al. Treating depression after initial treatment failure: directly comparing switch and augmenting strategies in STAR*D. *J Clin Psychopharmacol.* 2012;32:114-119.

21. Casey DE, Laubmeier KK, Eudicone JM, et al. Response and remission rates with adjunctive aripiprazole in patients with major depressive disorder who exhibit minimal or no improvement on antidepressant monotherapy. *Int J Clin Pract.* 2014;68(11):1301-1308.

22. Spielmans GI, Berman MI, Linardatos E, Roselicht NZ, Perry A, Tsai AC. Adjunctive atypical antipsychotic treatment for major depressive disorder: a meta-analysis of depression, quality of life, and safety outcomes. *PLoS Med.* 2013;10(3):e1001403.

23. Papkostas G, Fava M, Baer L, et al. Ziprasidone augmentation of escitalopram for major depressive disorder: efficacy results from a randomized, double-blind placebo-controlled study. *Am J Psychiatry.* 2015;172(12):1251-1258.

24. Thase ME, Youakim JM, Skuban A, et al. Efficacy and safety of adjunctive brexpiprazole 2 mg in major depressive disorder: a phase 3, randomized, placebo-controlled study in patients with inadequate response to antidepressants. *J Clin Psychiatry.* 2015;76(9):1224-1232.

25. Nelson JC, Baumann P, Delucchi K, Joffe R, Katbna C. A systematic review and meta-analysis of lithium augmentation of tricyclic and second-generation antidepressants in major depression. *J Affect Disord.* 2014;168:269-275.

26. Touma K. Liothyronine for depression: a review and guidance for safety monitoring. *Innov Clin Neurosci.* 2017;14 (3-4):24-29.

27. Sarris J, Murphy J, Mischoulon D, et al. Adjunctive nutraceuticals for depression: a systematic review and meta-analyses. *Am J Psychiatry.* 2016;173:575-587.

28. Goss A, Kaser M, Costafreda SG, Sahakiaw BJ, Fu CHY. Modafinil augmentation therapy in unipolar and bipolar depression. *J Clin Psychiatry.* 2013;74(11):1101-1107.

29. Faridhosseini F, Sadeghi R, Faeid L, Pourgholami M. Celecoxib: a new augmentation strategy for depressive mood episodes. A systematic review and meta-analysis of randomized placebo-controlled trials. *Hum Psychopharmacol Clin Exp.* 2014;29:216-223.

30. Strawbridge R, Anone D, Danese A, Papadopoulos A, Herane Vives A, Cleare AJ. Inflammation and clinical response to treatment in depression: a meta-anaysis. *Eur Neuropsychopharmacol.* 2015;25(10):1532-1543.

31. Barbee JG, Thompson TR, Jamhour NJ, et al. A double blind placebo-controlled trial of lamotrigine as an antidepressant augmentation agent in treatment-refractory unipolar depression. *J Clin Psychiatry.* 2011;72(10):1405-1412.

32. Liu Y, Zhou X, Zhu D, et al. Is pindolol augmentation effective in depressed patients resistant to selective serotonin reuptake inhibitors? A systematic review and meta-analysis. *Hum Psychopharmacol Clin Exp.* 2015;30:132-142.

33. Kleeblatt J, Betzler F, Kilarski LL, Bschor T, Kohler S. Efficacy of off-label augmentation in unipolar depression: a systematic review of the evidence. *Eur Psychopharmacol.* 2017;27(5):423-441.

34. Cusin C, Iovieno N, Iosifescu DV, et al. A randomized, double-blind, placebo-controlled trial of pramipexole augmentation in treatment-resistant major depressive disorder. *J Clin Psychiatry.* 2013;74(7):e636-e641.

35. Corp SA, Gitlin MJ, Altshuler LI. A review of the use of stimulants and stimulant alternatives in treating bipolar depression and major depressive disorder. *J Clin Psychiatry.* 2014;75(9):1010-1018.

36. Cheon EJ, Lee JB, Park YW, et al. Comparison of the efficacy and safety of aripiprazole versus bupropion augmentation in patients with major depressive disorder unresponsive to selective serotonin reuptake inhibitors: a randomized, prospective, open-label study. *J Clin Psychopharmacol.* 2017;37(2):193-199.

37. Papakostas GI, Fava M, Thase ME. Treatment of SSRI-resistant depression: a meta-analysis comparing within-versus across-class switches. *Bioi Psychiatry.* 2008;63(7):699-704.

38. Perera S, Eisen R, Bhatt M, et al. Light therapy for non-seasonal systematic review and meta-analysis. *BJPsych Open.* 2016;2:116-126.

39. Wiles N, Thomas L, Abel A, et al. Cognitive behavioural therapy as an adjunct to pharmacotherapy for primary care based patients with treatment resistant depression: results of the CoBalT randomized controlled trial. *Lancet.* 2013;381:375-384.

40. Souza LH, Salum GA, Mosquiro BP, et al. Interpersonal psychotherapy as add-on for treatment-resistant depression: a pragmatic randomized controlled trial. *J Affect Disord.* 2016;193:373-380.

41. Casey M, Perera DN, Clarke DM. Psychosocial treatment approaches to difficult-to-treat depression. *MJA Open.* 2012;1(suppl 4):52-55.

42. Ryan CE, Keitner GI, Bishop S. An adjunctive management of depression program for difficult-to-treat depressed patients and their families. *Depress Anxiety.* 2009;27(1):27-34.

43. Berewick B, Schlaepfer TE. Update on neuromodulation for treatment-resistant depression. *F1000 Res.* 2015:1-10.

44. Kellner CH, Greenberg RM, Murrough JW, et al. ECT in treatment-resistant depression. *Am J Psychiatry.* 2012;169:1238-1244.

45. Brunoni AR, Chaimani A, Moffa AH, et al. Repetitive transcranial magnetic stimulation for the acute treatment of major depressive episodes: a systematic review of network meta-analysis. *JAMA Psychiatry.* 2016;74(2):143-153.

46. Haddad PM, Talbot PS, Anderson IM, et al. Managing inadequate antidepressant response in depressive illness. *Br Med Bull.* 2015;115:183-201.

47. Dougherty DD, Rezai AR, Carpenter LL, et al. A randomized sham controlled trial of deep brain stimulation of the ventral capsule/ventral striatum for chronic treatment-resistant depression. *Biol Psychiatry.* 2015 78(4):240-248.

48. .Morishita T, Fayad SM, Higuchi MA, et al. Deep brain stimulation for treatment-resistant depression: systematic review of clinical outcomes. *Neurotherapeutics.* 2014;11:475-484.

49. Sanacora G, Frye MA, McDonald WM, et al. A consensus statement on the use of ketamine in the treatment of mood disorders. *JAMA Psychiatry.* 2017;74(4):399-405.

50. Carhart-Harris RL, Bolstridge M, Day MJ, et al. Psilocybin with psychological support for treatment-resistant depression: six month follow up. *Psychopharmacology.* 2017. doi:10.1007/s00213-017-4771-x.

10

PSYCHIATRIC DISORDERS: BIPOLAR AND RELATED DISORDERS

Y. Pritham Raj, MD, Jeremy A. Parker, MD, David Safani, MD, MBA, and Keeban C. Nam, MD

CLINICAL HIGHLIGHTS

- In the primary care setting, patients with bipolar disorder are often misdiagnosed as having unipolar major depression because they seek help only when they are experiencing symptoms of depression rather than mania/hypomania.
- Bipolar patients have the second highest suicide attempt rate (28.5%)—behind only schizophrenia.
- The main feature of bipolar II disorder is the frequency and prominence of the depressive episodes. The ratio of depression to hypomania is an astonishing 39:1 in patients with bipolar II disorder when symptomatic.
- Bipolar disorder is associated with a high rate of suicide completion: typically one suicide for every three attempts.
- Lithium is not just one of the most efficacious mood stabilizers, it is the only pharmacotherapy that has been shown to reduce mortality from suicide (number needed to treat: 23).
- The use of antidepressants in bipolar disorder can contribute to worsening outcomes and may induce mania or rapid cycling (although the risk is typically low). The Systematic Treatment Enhancement Program for Bipolar Disorder (STEP-BD) found no advantage of adding antidepressants to mood stabilizers in the treatment of bipolar depression.[1]
- Postpartum psychosis, which can present days to weeks after delivery, is typically part of the bipolar spectrum.
- When treating women of child-bearing age with mood stabilizers, it is advisable to ensure that some form of birth control is also prescribed/recommended.
- Patients with bipolar disorder are not only at higher risk of substance-use disorders, but so are their relatives without bipolar disorder.[2]

CLINICAL SIGNIFICANCE

Bipolar and related disorders are arguably among the most difficult disorders in all of medicine to diagnose largely because they are spectrum disorders with complex features[3] that tend to overlap with unipolar depression. According to the United States Preventive Services Task Force (USPSTF), nearly 74% of patients with depression are treated by their primary care provider (PCP), thus making screening adults for depression a Grade B recommendation.[4] Unfortunately, there are no formal screening recommendations for bipolar disorder in primary care. However, screening for depression in a primary care setting without assessing for mania or hypomania can lead to incorrect diagnosis and treatment of bipolar disorder.[5] A general rule is that if a PCP is preparing to treat a patient with symptoms of depression, doing so without screening for bipolar disorder would be ill-advised.

Sixty percent of people with bipolar disorder are in the depressed phase when they go to their PCP for help, and up to 30% of patients treated for depression and/or anxiety actually have bipolar disorder. According to the National Depressive and Manic-Depressive Association (NDMDA) 2000 survey of individuals with bipolar disorder, 69% of patients with bipolar disorder reported being misdiagnosed during evaluation, with major depressive disorder (MDD) the most common misdiagnosis.[6] The same study reported that 70% of these patients were misdiagnosed up to three times and 68% of those patients saw up to four physicians (most in primary care or emergency settings) before receiving the proper diagnosis of bipolar disorder. Misdiagnosed patients are the ones who typically do not respond adequately to treatment with antidepressants alone, which may aggravate or trigger a manic or hypomanic episode.[7] or Patients with bipolar disorder are at increased risk of suicide.

The prevalence rate of bipolar I disorder ranges from 0.5% to 1.0% of the population[8,9] with similar rates seen between female and male patients. The prevalence of bipolar II disorder is 0.5% to 1.1%, with a female predominance. The overall estimated lifetime prevalence for all bipolar disorders ranges from 3.0% to 8.3% depending on study methodology.[10,11] Subthreshold bipolarity as described in a multinational, transcultural study is found in 3.3% of the general population, and as much as 47% of all patients with depression.[12] In 2004, the World Health Organization ranked bipolar disorders collectively as the 12th most common moderately to severely disabling condition in the world for any age group.[13]

Although they can occur at any age, bipolar disorders are most common in persons younger than 25 years—one of the key differentiating features of bipolar disorder compared with other mood disorders. The mean age at symptom onset is 18 years in bipolar I disorder and 22 years in bipolar II disorder.[9] This is quite different from MDD, which tends to present in the fourth decade of life. In primary care settings, whenever mood or even physical symptoms are reported as being present "for as long as they can remember," bipolar disorder must enter the differential diagnosis of even the busiest PCP as symptoms often appear early in life.

DIAGNOSIS

DIAGNOSTIC CONSIDERATIONS

Many changes to the mood disorders (DSM IV-TR classification) were proposed during the development of the DSM-5. However, by the time the DSM-5 was published in 2013 and bipolar and related disorders became its own classification,[14] most of the other revisions were minor and the definitions kept mostly intact (*Table 10-1*). The cardinal feature of bipolar I disorder is a history of at least one manic episode (*Box 10-1*) at any point in one's life. A manic episode is a period of abnormally and persistently elevated, expansive, or irritable mood and abnormally and persistently increased goal-directed activity or energy, lasting at least 1 week or any duration if hospitalization is necessary (DSM-5 A Criteria). Although the hallmark of the bipolar I diagnosis is the manic episode, clinicians must remember that patients with bipolar I disorder still spend significantly more time in the depressed phase when symptomatic compared with mania/hypomania at a ratio of 3:1.[15,16] It is important to highlight that *irritability* is part of the criteria for bipolar mania as clinician often associated euphoria with bipolar mania.

BOX 10-1   DIGFAST MNEMONIC FOR MANIA: THREE OR MORE OF THE SEVEN CRITERIA MUST BE MET[17]

Distractibility—poor focus
Insomnia—decreased need for sleep
Grandiosity—inflated self-esteem
Flight of Ideas—racing thoughts
Activity—increased goal-directed activity
Speech—pressured or more talkative
Thoughtlessness—"risk-taking" behavior

TABLE 10-1 Definitions of Bipolar Disorders as Described in the DSM-5[14]

Bipolar I disorder	Manic (at least one lifetime episode) or mixed episode with or without psychosis and/or major depressive episode or hypomanic episode (ratio of 3:1 depressed vs. manic/hypomanic)[15,16]
Bipolar II disorder	Hypomanic episode and/or major depressive episode; no history of manic or mixed episode (ratio of 39:1 depressed vs. hypomanic)[15,16]
Cyclothymic disorder	Hypomanic and/or depressive symptoms over 2 years that do not meet criteria for bipolar I or II disorder; no major depressive episode
Substance/ medication-induced bipolar and related disorder	Elevated, expansive, or irritable mood, with or without depressed mood that is substance/medication related with onset during intoxication or withdrawal
Bipolar and related disorder due to another medical condition	Bipolar symptom disturbance that is the direct pathophysiologic consequence of another medical condition (e.g., hyperthyroidism)
Unspecified bipolar and related disorder	Does not meet criteria or there is insufficient information to make a more specific diagnosis of the other types of bipolar disorder (e.g., less than 1 week of manic symptoms without psychosis or hospitalization or in emergency room settings)

Bipolar II disorder is among the most challenging disorders to diagnose because of the tremendous overlap with MDD. A hallmark of bipolar II disorder is the hypomanic episode that, although similar to manic episodes, is not as severe and typically does not last as long, with a 4-day threshold to meet criteria. Hypomania is not severe enough to cause marked impairment in social or occupational functioning, or to necessitate hospitalization. In fact, hypomania is often associated with increased creativity and energy, which patients actually like, and thus, do not seek medical attention. The main feature of bipolar II disorder is the frequency and prominence of the depressive episodes. The ratio of depression to hypomania is an astonishing 39:1 in patients with bipolar II disorder when symptomatic.[15,16]

Diagnosing bipolar disorder is not just a challenge for the busy PCP but can be difficult for even the most seasoned psychiatrist. A recent poll demonstrated the lack of uniformity in diagnostic approach that providers take when assessing for bipolar disorder (*Figure 10-1*).[18] What a challenge it would be to have four different approaches when evaluating chest pain or screening for diabetes. We find that the best approach to diagnosing bipolar

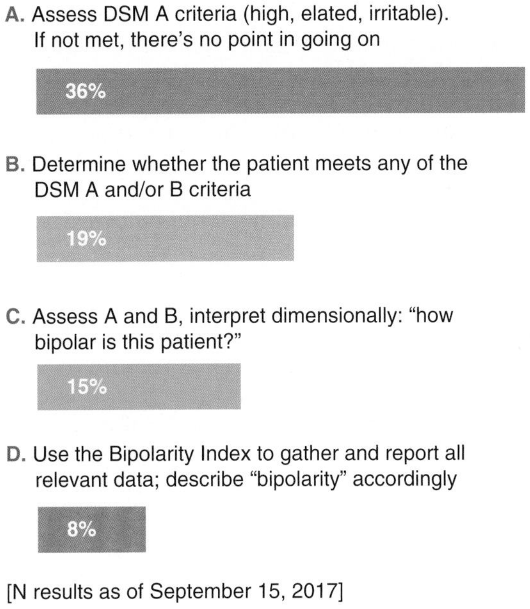

A. Assess DSM A criteria (high, elated, irritable). If not met, there's no point in going on

36%

B. Determine whether the patient meets any of the DSM A and/or B criteria

19%

C. Assess A and B, interpret dimensionally: "how bipolar is this patient?"

15%

D. Use the Bipolarity Index to gather and report all relevant data; describe "bipolarity" accordingly

8%

[N results as of September 15, 2017]

FIGURE 10-1 Practitioners' approaches to bipolar diagnosis (*N* = 312).[18]

disorder is having familiarity with the diagnostic criteria and then marrying the clinical impression with a validated screening instrument.

One of the most widely used screens for bipolar disorder is the Mood Disorders Questionnaire (MDQ), which is simple to complete and has been validated in adults and adolescents and in a variety of languages.[19] It is easy to utilize in primary care settings as it is self-rated and has both good sensitivity and very good specificity, correctly identifying 7 of 10 patients with bipolar disorder, while 9 of 10 patients without bipolar disorder would be correctly screened out. The MDQ includes 13 questions plus items assessing clustering of symptoms and functional impairment. Another helpful screening tool is the Bipolar Spectrum Diagnostic Scale (BSDS),[20] which takes the form of a narrative paragraph that is easy to read—and one that bipolar patients typically identify with rather strongly. Ultimately, it is less important *how* one screens than *that* one screens systematically for bipolar disorder especially for the patient with symptoms of depression.

DIFFERENTIAL DIAGNOSIS

The differential diagnosis for depression is rather broad and covered elsewhere in this book. This chapter will focus on the plethora of conditions that can be causally related or mimic the other "pole" of bipolar disorders—namely, mania (*Box 10-2*). Treating the underlying condition is often enough to result in remission of the symptoms of mania. For ease, we have divided the differential diagnosis into seven categories: metabolic, autoimmune, neurocognitive/neurologic, infectious, cancerous, psychiatric, and toxic. A mnemonic that incorporates the first letter of each of these seven categories (see *Box 10-3*) is **MANIC PT** ("**manic patient**").

BOX 10-2   SCREENING QUESTIONS FOR MANIC AND HYPOMANIC EPISODES

1. "Have you ever felt the complete opposite of depressed, where friends and family were worried about you because you were too happy?"
2. "Have you ever had excessive amounts of energy running through your body, to the point where you did not need to sleep for days?"
   - "How long did these symptoms last?"
   - "During these periods, did you feel like your thoughts were going really fast and it was hard to focus?"
   - "During these periods, did people comment that you were talking really fast?"
   - "During these periods, did you ever make impulsive decisions that you regretted later (e.g., spending too much money or being sexually promiscuous)?"
   - "During any of these periods, did your behaviors get you into trouble at work, at home, or with the law, or cause you to end up in the hospital?"
   - "During these periods, were you using any alcohol or substances?"

BOX 10-3   DIFFERENTIAL DIAGNOSIS MNEMONIC FOR MANIA

Metabolic
Autoimmune
Neurocognitive/neurologic
Infectious
Cancerous
Psychiatric
Toxic

Metabolic

This category includes endocrine disorders and electrolyte imbalances. See *Table 10-2* for a list of more specific examples. We recommend checking a comprehensive metabolic panel and complete blood count (CBC) for anyone presenting with manic symptoms, as electrolyte derangements can lead to mood dysregulation that can appear manic. A serum thyroid-stimulating hormone (TSH) level is also a good lab to check as part of your routine workup for most mood disorders.[21]

Autoimmune

This category includes the ever-challenging systemic lupus erythematosus (SLE). Patients with SLE may develop an agitated psychosis that can resemble mania. Studies have found that these symptoms occur in roughly

5% of patients with SLE, are most likely to occur in the first year after diagnosis, may be more severe at night, and may be either catalyzed by or independent of treatment with steroids.[22,23] Hallucinations primarily related to SLE itself (rather than steroids) are more often visual and tactile rather than auditory. Other autoimmune disorders, particularly encephalitides, should also be included in the differential for mania.[24,25]

Neurocognitive/Neurologic

Strokes, traumatic brain injury, multiple sclerosis, and major neurocognitive disorders (dementias) all fall in this category.[26] The most common neurocognitive disorder that masquerades as mania is hyperactive delirium. Shared symptoms include sleep–wake cycle derangement, psychomotor agitation, inattention, affective changes, impulsivity, and sometimes psychosis.[27] Differentiating delirium from mania is a task of great importance, and treatment approaches can differ drastically depending on the underlying cause. Some distinguishing features include the waxing and waning course of symptoms in delirium, as well as thet fact that delirium is more common in older patients, while the mean age of onset for bipolar mania is in the late teens. As for etiology, delirium deserves an entire differential of its own, which is covered elsewhere in this book.

Infectious

Disseminated infections with central nervous system involvement, such as syphilis, can cause manic episodes.[28] Manic symptoms also occur in acute systemic infections, as with human immunodeficiency virus (HIV). AIDS mania is a known clinical entity and less common since the advent of effective antiretroviral therapies, but mania may also occur earlier on in the course of the illness.[29] If a patient presents in a febrile state, in addition to routine lab testing, we would recommend blood cultures along with any other targeted testing (e.g., urinalysis for suspected urinary tract infection, would cultures).

Cancerous

Cerebral neoplasms and paraneoplastic disorders can also present with new-onset mania.[26] As with many of the neurologic etiologies listed in *Table 10-2*, it is common to also observe neurologic deficits, focal and otherwise, associated with the psychiatric symptoms in these cases. These accompanying features can help point one in the direction of where the underlying illness may be found.

Psychiatric

Even if an underlying medical cause for mania has been ruled out and all signs point to a psychiatric illness, it may still be premature to diagnose bipolar disorder. If the symptom complex is present for only a few days and does not cause major functional impairment, the diagnosis may be hypomania instead of mania. Hypomania is not always treated in the same way as mania. Behaviors concerning mania in one person may also be within the range of normal experience for individuals with certain personality disorders (PDs), such as borderline and narcissistic PD. Hyperactivity, impulsivity, and inattention

---

TABLE 10-2 Selection of Conditions That May Cause or Mimic Mania

ETIOLOGIC CATEGORY	EXAMPLES
Metabolic	Adrenal insufficiency (Addison disease), adrenergic storm, hemochromatosis, hypercalcemia, hypercortisolism (Cushing syndrome), hypernatremia, hyperthyroidism, hypocalcemia, hypopituitarism, obstructive sleep apnea (OSA), porphyria, vitamin B12 deficiency, Wernicke encephalopathy, Wilson disease
Autoimmune	Collagen vascular disorders, systemic lupus erythematosus (SLE)
Neurocognitive (or neurologic)	Alzheimer disease, basal ganglia calcification, frontotemporal dementia (FTD), hemorrhagic stroke, Huntington disease, hyperactive delirium, ischemic stroke, multiple sclerosis (MS), normal pressure hydrocephalus (NPH), Parkinson disease, traumatic brain injury (TBI)
Infectious	Central nervous system tuberculosis (CNS TB), systemic human immunodeficiency virus (HIV), tertiary syphilis
Cancerous	Carcinomatosis, cerebral tumors, paraneoplastic cerebellar degeneration, paraneoplastic limbic encephalitis
Psychiatric	Attention deficit hyperactivity disorder (ADHD), bipolar I disorder, bipolar II disorder, borderline personality disorder, cyclothymia, narcissistic personality disorder, schizophrenia-spectrum disorders
Toxic	Alcohol withdrawal, amphetamine intoxications, antidepressants, barbiturate withdrawal, benzodiazepine withdrawal, carbon monoxide poisoning, cocaine intoxication, chemotherapy agents, corticosteroids, cholinesterase inhibitors, cimetidine, hallucinogen intoxication, heavy metal poisoning, inhalant intoxication, interferons, neuroleptic malignant syndrome, opiate withdrawal, serotonin syndrome

may be seen in mania, but they are also the core features of attention deficit hyperactivity disorder (ADHD). Although some patients develop psychosis only when they're manic, those with schizoaffective disorder experience psychosis even when in a euthymic mood state, and they too may require a different treatment strategy.

Toxic

Poisoning from heavy metals such as mercury, intoxication on stimulants, withdrawal from alcohol, and toxicity from prescribed medications (including interferons, corticosteroids, and many others) can all cause symptoms of mania. A thorough clinical history may provide useful clues regarding possible exposures. Careful review of a patient's medication list, as well as collection of a urine drug screen, is recommended in any case of symptoms concerning mania. Respiratory and gastrointestinal symptoms, as well as irritation/inflammation of the mucous membranes, may suggest that a toxic inhalation or ingestion has more likely occurred as the cause of the symptoms.[30]

BIOPSYCHOSOCIAL TREATMENT

Patients who are acutely manic, and consequently impulsive and erratic, and particularly those who are experiencing psychosis as a result of affective disturbance, require emergency evaluation and hospitalization. A patient is expected to resume care in the outpatient setting with a PCP, once a level of stability has been achieved and sustained. As such, most patients who present in the office of a PCP are in maintenance phase.

The focus in treating a chronic episodic illness such as bipolar disorder is functional restoration and preservation. A thorough approach to treatment utilizes a biopsychosocial approach. Medications receive much attention as the mainstay of biological approach to treatment. Psychological intervention begins with a referral to psychotherapy as well as very short educative and motivational interventions that can be offered during even the busiest of primary care clinics. Social interventions consist mostly of referrals to community resources and support groups. A key feature of psychotherapy for patients with bipolar disorder is accepting that they have an illness that requires ongoing treatment for life.

BIOLOGICAL APPROACHES

The following discussion on medications focuses on treatment of all manners of presentation. Management during the maintenance period and depressive states merits particular attention. A simple rule of thumb is to adjust the dose of the medication higher if the patient is experiencing breakthrough mania while on a maintenance regimen. If a patient is already on the highest recommended dose, it is not unusual to prescribe a combination. The classes of medications most commonly used in addressing bipolar disorder are mood stabilizers and antipsychotics; combining one of each is a common practice in psychiatry (see

Tables 10-3, 10-4, and 10-5). If a patient is experiencing depressive symptoms, it is better to avoid antidepressants and focus on alternatives; more will be said on this later.

Mood Stabilizers

Lithium

Lithium is one of the best known and most commonly used mood stabilizers. It has the strongest level of evidence in support of its efficacy as monotherapy treatment for acute mania.[31] The drawback to its therapeutic value is the delay in the expected time to response, which is about 7 days from start of treatment. For this reason, lithium is often paired with another medication, usually an antipsychotic, when targeting acute mania. Lithium has also shown the strongest level of evidence in the prophylaxis of an acute mood episode, or during the maintenance period of bipolar disorder. It has been shown to be more effective in preventing mania than depression, though useful for both ends of the spectrum, and to reduce the frequency and severity of relapse events. It is protective against suicide in patients with bipolar disorder, and some sources suggest value in addressing antidepressant-induced hypomania as well.[32]

Lithium has a narrow therapeutic index, and plasma levels need to be checked regularly to avoid toxicity. Optimal plasma levels against acute manic symptoms range from 0.6 to 1.2 mmol/L, with levels above 0.8 mmol/L ensuring stronger protection. Levels of at least 0.4 mmol/L have been suggested as effective for acute depression and for prophylaxis—during maintenance—against mania.[33] Blood samples should be obtained approximately 5 days after a dosage adjustment, roughly 12 hours post dose. The recommended dosage range as monotherapy treatment for acute mania is 600 to 1,200 mg/day (which is roughly equivalent to serum level 0.8 to 1.3 mmol/L); initial therapy is typically divided in BID dosing for better tolerance. Kidney function and thyroid function tests should be part of the pretreatment workup and periodic monitoring every 6 months. Lithium level is recommended as part of the 6-month monitoring labs.[34]

Side effects are dose dependent, and the most common ones are gastrointestinal discomfort, tremor, and weight gain. Less common but noteworthy ones are renal toxicity, hypothyroidism, hyperparathyroidism, and nephrogenic diabetes insipidus, leading to polyuria and polydipsia.[35] Symptoms of toxicity include nausea, diarrhea, ataxia, seizures, and coma. Risk factors for toxicity involve changes in sodium levels. As such, the use of ACE Inhibitors, thiazide diuretics, carbamazepine, and NSAIDs can lead to unpredictable lithium levels and possible adverse events. Given NSAIDs are easily found over the counter and are self-administered, it is important to recommend regular use, as opposed to PRN, with instructions to check levels more frequently.

Valproic Acid

Valproate has the same level of evidence as lithium in support of its use in addressing acute mania.[31] Therapeutic response is anywhere between 5 and 15 days, prompting a paired agent for acute mania, typically an antipsychotic.

TABLE 10-3 Common Medications Used in the Treatment of Bipolar Mania

TREATMENT OF ACUTE MANIA

MEDICATION	STARTING DOSE	TARGET DOSE	COMMON SIDE EFFECTS	RARE SIDE EFFECTS	PREGNANCY CATEGORY
Lithium	300 mg BID	600-1,200 mg (target level 0.6-1.2 mmol/L)	GI discomfort, tremor, weight gain	Renal toxicity, hypothyroidism, diabetes insipidus	D
Valproate	500-750 mg BID	1,200-3,000 mg (target level 50-100 mg/L)	GI discomfort, sedation, weight gain, tremor	Hepatic failure, pancytopenia, thrombocytopenia	D
Olanzapine	10 mg QHS	20 mg	Sedation, weight gain	Metabolic symptoms, NMS	C
Quetiapine	IR—300 mg QHS; increase by 100 mg Q1-2 days	600-800 mg	Sedation, weight gain, orthostasis	Metabolic symptoms, NMS	C
	XR—300 mg QHS; can double dose within 1-2 days	600 mg	Weight gain		
Aripiprazole	15 mg QHS	30 mg	Akathisia, restlessness		C
Risperidone	1 mg QHS or BID	6 mg	Weight gain, EPS, constipation	Prolactinemia, NMS	C
Asenapine	10 mg QHS	20 mg	Sedation, weight gain, dizziness, EPS	Metabolic symptoms, NMS	C
Haloperidol	5-10 mg QHS or BID	20 mg	Sedation, EPS, constipation	NMS, Parkinsonism	C

BID, dosed twice a day; EPS, extrapyramidal symptom; GI, gastrointestinal; IR, immediate release; NMS, neuroleptic malignant syndrome; QHS, dosed nightly; XR, extended release. Medications indicated for acute mania are typically sedating and, as such, dosed at nighttime to optimize sleep function.

TABLE 10-4 Common Medications Used in the Treatment of Bipolar Depression

TREATMENT OF ACUTE DEPRESSION

MEDICATION	STARTING DOSE	TARGET DOSE	COMMON SIDE EFFECTS	RARE SIDE EFFECTS	PREGNANCY CATEGORY
Lithium	300 mg BID	600-1,200 mg (target level 0.4-1.2 mmol/L)	GI discomfort, tremor, weight gain	Renal toxicity, hypothyroidism, diabetes insipidus	D
Lamotrigine	25 mg/day × 2 weeks, then double every 2 weeks	200 mg		Rash/SJS associated with rapid titration	C
Olanzapine/ fluoxetine	5/20 mg/day or 10/40 mg/day	10/40 mg	Weight gain, sedation (from olanzapine)		C/C
Quetiapine	200-300 mg/night	300-600 mg	Sedation, weight gain, orthostasis	Metabolic symptoms	C
Lurasidone	20-40 mg/day	120 mg	Akathisia		B

BID, dosed twice a day; GI, gastrointestinal; SJS, Stevens–Johnson syndrome.

TABLE 10-5 A Comparison of Medications, Indications, and Advantages/Disadvantages

	INDICATIONS—EVIDENCE	ADVANTAGES	DISADVANTAGES
Lithium	**Acute mania—strong** Acute depression—moderate Acute mixed—weak **Prev mania—strong** Prev depression—moderate **Prev rapid cycling—strong**	• Benefits over suicide risk • Neuroprotective effects • Allows monitoring treatment adherence through plasma levels • Benefits for psychotic symptoms	• Delayed time to response • Requires periodic monitoring • Narrow therapeutic index poses concern for risk of overdose • Possible congenital malformations in fetus • Interactions with diuretics and NSAIDs
Valproate	**Acute mania—strong** Acute depression—moderate Acute mixed—moderate Prev mania—moderate Prev depression—moderate	• Benefits in comorbid anxiety • Better tolerated compared with lithium • Allows monitoring treatment adherence through plasma levels	• Delayed time to response • Requires periodic monitoring • Caution in women of child-bearing age • Unknown effects on psychotic symptoms • Weight gain
Lamotrigine	Acute depression—moderate Prev mania—moderate **Prev depression—strong**	• Well tolerated if following slow titration	• Not ideal for acute situations given prolonged titration schedule • Risk of severe rash/SJS
Haloperidol	**Acute mania—strong** Acute mixed—weak	• Faster time to response • Benefits for agitated behavior • Most efficacious out of antipsychotics against severe mania	• Switch risk to depression • EPS, Parkinsonism, Tardive dyskinesia • Rare risk of NMS • Least tolerable out of antipsychotics
Olanzapine	**Acute mania—strong** **Acute depression—strong** Acute mixed—moderate Acute rapid cycling—moderate **Prev mania—strong** **Prev depression—strong** **Prev mixed—strong**	• Faster time to response • Oral dissolvable formulation available for improved adherence	• Weight gain • Sedation • Not ideal for patients with hyperlipidemia and diabetes • Less tolerable compared with lithium
Quetiapine	**Acute mania—strong** **Acute depression—strong** Acute mixed—weak Acute rapid cycling—moderate **Prev mania—strong** **Prev depression—strong** **Prev rapid cycling—strong**	• Combining with lithium/valproate has strong evidence of benefits for preventing rapid cycling[a] • Benefits in comorbid anxiety • Faster time to response • More efficacious than olanzapine against depression	• Weight gain (not as much as olanzapine) • Sedation • Not ideal for patients with hyperlipidemia and diabetes • Less tolerable compared with lithium
Aripiprazole	**Acute mania—strong** Acute depression—weak Acute mixed—moderate Acute rapid cycling—moderate **Prev mania—strong** Prev depression—weak Prev rapid cycling—moderate	• Faster time to response • Better tolerated compared with lithium	• EPS, Akathisia
Risperidone	**Acute mania—strong** Acute mixed—moderate **Prev mania—strong**[b] Prev depression—weak **Prev rapid cycling—strong**	• Faster time to response • Long-acting injectable form available for improved adherence[b]	• EPS, Parkinsonism • Hyperprolactinemia • Weight gain • Not ideal for patients with hyperlipidemia and diabetes
Lurasidone	**Acute depression—strong**	• Benefits in comorbid anxiety • More efficacious than olanzapine against depression • Category B in pregnancy	• Akathisia

(continued)

TABLE 10-5 A Comparison of Medications, Indications, and Advantages/Disadvantages   (continued)

	INDICATIONS—EVIDENCE	ADVANTAGES	DISADVANTAGES
Asenapine	**Acute mania—strong** Acute mixed—moderate Prev mania—moderate Prev depression—moderate	• Faster time to response • Sublingual formulation	• Weight gain • Sedation, dizziness

[a]Quetiapine as either monotherapy or combined with lithium/valproate has strong level of evidence in prevention against rapid cycling.
[b]Information pertains to long-acting injectable form.
EPS, extrapyramidal side effects; NMS, neuroleptic malignant syndrome; Prev, "prevention of"; SJS, Stevens–Johnson syndrome.

It may be effective as an alternative to and an adjunct to lithium. Some sources support the efficacy of valproate in the treatment of bipolar depression, and some suggest its use in addressing comorbid anxiety as well. Use of valproate during maintenance is not solidly supported but remains a common approach.

Target plasma levels for acute mania range from 50 to 100 mg/L. Recommended doses for monotherapy in acute mania range from 1,200 to 3,000 mg/day, divided in two doses. Loading doses to rapidly achieve therapeutic levels are generally well tolerated, and these correspond to 20 to 30 mg/kg per day (which can be given in divided doses)—for an average weight of 50 kg, this translates to 500 to 750 mg BID. In this way, goal concentrations can be reached in about 3 days. Levels should be checked immediately before the next dose. Pretreatment and periodic workup should include a CBC, liver function, and weight; these, along with valproate level, should be checked every 6 months.

The most commonly reported side effects are gastrointestinal discomfort, nausea, sedation, weight gain, and a dose-dependent tremor. Periodic blood counts and liver functions tests are recommended because of less common but more concerning risks of hepatic failure, hyperammonemia, pancytopenia, and thrombocytopenia. Polycystic ovarian syndrome is an associated risk in females. Women of child-rearing age should not be prescribed valproate given the risk of teratogenicity—neural tube defects.[34] If alternatives are limited and valproate cannot be avoided, preemptive measures ought to be taken through contraceptive means and/or prophylactic folate. Drugs that inhibit CYP enzymes, such as fluoxetine, erythromycin, and cimetidine, can increase levels of valproate. Valproate can in turn inhibit metabolism and increase levels of other drugs, such as lamotrigine, warfarin, quetiapine, and phenobarbital.

Lamotrigine

The strong suit of lamotrigine is in its benefits toward symptoms of bipolar depression. The data are controversial in establishing a solid argument in treating an acute depressive episode, with some evidence suggesting improvements in secondary outcomes only. It has been declared efficacious during the maintenance period, in prophylaxis against depression.[31] It has not demonstrated positive results in

addressing acute manic symptoms or in prophylaxis against mania. The downside of using lamotrigine lies in its lengthy titration process, required to avoid severe rashes and Steven-Johnson Syndrome. Guidelines recommend starting at 25 mg/day over the course of 2 weeks, then 50 mg/day over the course of the next 2 weeks, and then increasing by 50 mg/day every 1 to 2 weeks for a target of 200 mg/day. Doses higher than 200 mg/day have not shown to be more effective. Concomitant use of valproate can increase serum levels of lamotrigine and, as a result, prompts starting at half its original schedule: 12.5 mg/day over 2 weeks, then 25 mg/day over 2 weeks, then increasing by 25 to 50 mg/day every 1 to 2 weeks, for a target of 100 mg/day. On the contrary, concomitant use of carbamazepine, phenytoin, or phenobarbital can decrease levels of lamotrigine and prompts doubling the starting dose, the adjusting increments, and the final target dose.

Antipsychotics

It is inaccurate to consider the use of these medications designed solely for psychosis. The versatility of antipsychotics, particularly the second-generation class, has allowed them to be part of a regimen in addressing many different psychiatric presentations, including various aspects of bipolar disorder. They are markedly effective in addressing psychotic features of acute manifestations.[31]

Haloperidol is one of the oldest and most familiar antipsychotics, in the first-generation class. Studies testing its validity against acute mania have shown positive results. Long-term use has been associated with depression,[31] leading to haloperidol falling out of favor in comparison with the second-generation counterparts. Most commonly noted side effects are extrapyramidal symptoms (EPSs), sedation, and constipation. Typical starting doses range from 5 to 20 mg/day, usually in divided doses to avoid severe EPSs.

Olanzapine had positive results in the treatment of acute mania, with therapeutic response within 2 to 7 days. It has shown to be as effective as lithium and valproate individually, and most effective when combined with these mood stabilizers. It is also accepted for long-term use in maintenance and prophylaxis against mania, depression, and mixed features.[31] Olanzapine alone has been suggested in the treatment of depressive symptoms as well, and the combined use of olanzapine/fluoxetine, with the trade name Symbyax, has been recommended as first-line treatment for acute bipolar depression.[34] Dose range recommendations are 10 to 20 mg/day usually at nighttime, to address acute mania. Commonly noted adverse effects include sedation, dizziness, and weight gain, with considerable long-term metabolic effects.

Quetiapine has demonstrated efficacy against acute mania and acute depression, and in prevention against mania and depression. Studies suggested improvements in co-occurring anxiety and benefits over prophylaxis of rapid cycling moods especially in combination with lithium or valproate. It is similarly efficacious for depression in the setting of bipolar disorder I and bipolar disorder II.[31] Dose range for treatment of bipolar depression is 300 to 600 mg/day, typically given at nighttime. Doses for treatment of acute mania can go as high as 800 mg/day. Most common adverse effects are related to sedation, dizziness, orthostatic hypotension, and weight gain.

Aripiprazole had mostly positive results in the treatment of acute mania. Studies testing its efficacy against bipolar depression were negative, and the evidence for its use in maintenance was in support of prophylaxis against mania but not against bipolar depression.[31] Doses for treatment of mania range from 15 to 30 mg/day. Although the rates of EPS and metabolic symptoms are not as frequent, aripiprazole has commonly been associated with akathisia and anxiety/restlessness.

Risperidone has shown positive results in support of treatment against acute mania, with therapeutic effect within 3 days.[31] Doses range from 1 to 6 mg/day, typically divided BID, and commonly noted side effects are somnolence, constipation, EPS, prolactinemia, and gynecomastia in the long term.

Lurasidone has been approved in the treatment of bipolar depression in response to two studies showing positive results in lurasidone alone or in combination with a mood stabilizer.[31] Doses range from 20 to 120 mg/day. Lurasidone needs to be taken with food (at least 350 calories) to be fully absorbed. Commonly reported side effects include sedation and akathisia.

Asenapine has been shown to be effective in the treatment of bipolar mania and mixed episodes, with effects noted within 2 days[31] It has also been reliably more effective than placebo in preventing recurrence of any mood episodes,[36] though not particularly helpful for bipolar depression. Asenapine is a medication that is dosed sublingually and can be used advantageously with patients who have aversion toward or avoid swallowing tablets. Doses range from 10 to 20 mg/day. Most common adverse effects are dizziness, sedation, weight gain, EPS, dry mouth, and oral hyperesthesia.

In general, the most efficacious the antipsychotic is against mania, the least tolerable it is also. Haloperidol, while frequently used in emergency situations, is not commonly utilized during maintenance phase, because of intolerable EPS and Parkinsonian side effects. On the other hand, the second-generation antipsychotics, which are used commonly for either acute or maintenance phases, are well known to cause metabolic side effects. Weight, fasting lipids, and plasma glucose or hemoglobin A1c should be monitored routinely, every 3 to 6 months,

because of risk of developing hyperlipidemia and diabetes mellitus. The addition of metformin has been implicated in combating weight gain or amenorrhea, when these arise as side effects to antipsychotics.

Antidepressants

The use of classic antidepressants such as selective serotonin reuptake inhibitors (SSRIs) and serotonin norepinephrine reuptake inhibitors (SNRIs) for the treatment of bipolar depression have fallen out of favor, largely because of the potential to induce mania and rapid cycling between affective states.[31] Although the recommendations do not take a hard stance on whether they should or should not be used in the treatment of bipolar depression, monotherapy with an antidepressant is discouraged. As in the case of Symbyax, an SSRI such as fluoxetine is typically paired with either an antipsychotic or a mood stabilizer, and often not initiated without the mood-stabilizing medication (including antipsychotic) having achieved a maintenance dose to protect against mania. Of note, venlafaxine, an SNRI, has been associated with higher risk of switch rates. Bupropion (a norepinephrine dopamine reuptake inhibitor) has been associated with lower risk of switching to mania. In clinical settings, antidepressant use is often associated with worsening insomnia and irritability. Tapering off the antidepressant has been associated with improvement with insomnia and irritability. In general, the use of antidepressants ought to be approached cautiously, consulting a psychiatrist first. Alternative options such as lamotrigine, quetiapine, lurasidone, and lithium are more strongly recommended for the treatment of bipolar depression. Antidepressant may nevertheless be employed cautiously after the aforementioned options have been employed and depression continues to be the predominant symptom.

COMPLEMENTARY REMEDIES

It is not uncommon to encounter patients who seek complementary remedies in the treatment of bipolar disorder. It is important to educate the patient that although such alternatives to treatment-as-usual may be considered helpful, there is insufficient evidence to suggest a substitute function. Omega-3 fatty acids have been implicated in promoting mood stability.[37] Dosages of EPA (eicosapentaenoic acid) and DHA (docosahexaenoic acid) together exceeding 1,000 mg have been observed to benefit emotional health. Bright light therapy has also shown some benefits, primarily for depressive symptoms.[38]

PSYCHOLOGICAL APPROACHES

Because depression and anxiety are not unique to bipolar disorder and have been subjects of focus in other sources of psychological treatments, the psychological approaches in this section will focus primarily on addressing mania and prevention of mania. In most cases, individuals with bipolar disorder will require a maintenance medication throughout their lifetime. This is particularly difficult to accept for many as the episodic nature of the illness prompts the patient to believe that once they are "in the clear," they can consider the option of titrating off medications. Furthermore, individuals with bipolar disorder may enjoy the mania, despite the consequential destructive patterns it brings. It is important to confirm that the patient understand the risks associated with each manic episode including fractured relationships and employment, lost productivity, and self-injury. A helpful tip to offer early on is to inform the patient of the "kindling effect": the threshold for a relapse event is lowered with each subsequent destabilization. In other words, the more frequent relapses a patient has, the more likely he or she is going to experience another relapse. It is imperative therefore that the patient and clinician are fully invested in preventive medicine. Motivational interviewing interventions can be valuable in gauging the degree to which the patient is willing to take ownership of the treatment. Asking questions such as "What do you recall about your state of mind when you were in a manic state/feeling elated/getting into so many frequent arguments?" "How comfortable are you with continuing the medication?" and "How do you see the medication helping you?" can help prompt further discussion and guide intervention.

It is important to note that patients who have demonstrated insight into their past maladaptive and disorganized presentations can still lose sight of reality when symptoms of mania return. As such, it is valuable to discuss with patients the nature of their early warning signs, to teach them to develop strategies in prevention, and to gauge insight and motivation into treatment on each encounter. Early warning signs are harbingers of a much more entrenched and disturbed mood episode, and being aware of them can signal the patient to make minor adjustments and changes in habit. Examples of early warning signs include changes in sleep habit or day-to-day activities, increased energy, irritability, mood swings, trouble with concentration, racing or clouded thoughts, and neglecting responsibilities. These can be addressed through regular mood monitoring, managing social rhythm and sleep hygiene, and education by the provider on needed adjustments on the regimen or maintenance of adherence.[31,39] Spending time in the initial evaluation determining what the patient's early warning signs are will allow you to ask about these signs specifically in later sessions.

Bipolar disorder also presents with functional impairments in cognitive abilities, particularly in the domains of attention, memory, and executive function,[40] even during euthymic states. Training in organizational skills, communication and social skills, and financial management skills have shown to sustain detriments in quality of life.[41,42] Providers can help in these areas by encouraging patients to keep a balance between under- and overactivity in social engagements, maintain stability in sleep–wake rhythms, and placing controls on impulsive activities, such as creating spending limits on credit cards. Encouraging family involvement in supportive family settings can make a big difference in the prognosis of the illness.

SOCIAL APPROACHES

Improving social and occupational functioning has consistently demonstrated positive effects on overall quality of life and illness outcomes.[43] The burden of a chronic illness such as bipolar disorder is significant particularly on families and the surrounding communities. It is helpful to refer both patient and relatives to local chapters of community organizations such as the National Alliance on Mental Illness (NAMI). These organizations not only provide resources for patient education and respite for families, but also function in representing the mentally ill at the legislative level. Patients with a history of suicidal ideation or attempt can benefit from having access to suicide hotlines while those who thrive or seek comfort in communal circles can find strength in support groups. Either of these can easily be found on online search engines. Those who struggle with keeping a job or with financial duress as a result of the burden of their illness can be referred to the local Social Services Agency, to apply for disability. Alternatively, those who hold jobs with irregular shifts (nurses, security guards, etc.) may need letters to the employer informing them it is medically ill-advised to have work shifts that can disrupt their sleep patterns. Similarly, for students who struggle in their academic functions, the provider can write letters to advocate for educational accommodations.

CASES AND QUESTIONS

CASE 1:

Mr. A is a 32-year-old recently divorced, professional writer with metabolic syndrome and periods of "low mood" who presents to establish care in the primary care clinic. He has completed his previsit paperwork including the Patient Health Questionnaire-9 (PHQ-9) screening instrument for depression, scoring in the moderate range (14 out of 27). He reports that he has been prescribed two or three different antidepressants in the past, including fluoxetine, which left him "irritable," another medication that begins with the letter "C" that didn't really do anything for him, and he perhaps one other medication back in college when he felt low after a breakup with a girlfriend. During a review of systems, he discloses that he has trouble falling asleep. He wonders if there is anything that could help him with his mood and initial insomnia.

1. What is a good screening question if you, the busy PCP, is short on time but need to screen for mania?
   A. Have you had severe insomnia recently?
   B. Do you have a family history of bipolar disorder?
   C. Have you had friends tell you that you are going too fast or talking too fast?
   D. Have you been spending too much money?
   E. Do you use any substances like alcohol or marijuana?

   Correct answer: C. *Although all of these questions can be helpful, the following screening question is of greatest value: "Have you had periods of feeling so happy or energetic that your friends told you were talking too fast or that you were too 'hyper'?"*

If this initial screen is positive, the "DIGFAST" mnemonic (Box 10-1) can be used to recall the cardinal symptoms of mania to assess more fully.

2. What feature of the case is most consistent with active mania/hypomania or at least mixed features?

   A. Irritability
   B. Failure of multiple medications
   C. We still need to ask about elevated mood
   D. The fact that he is a writer (artistic)
   E. Active depression

   Correct answer: A. *Irritability. Although elevated mood is a hallmark of bipolar disorder, when a patient describes "irritable mood," that can be considered a manic-equivalent symptom. In fact, irritability has a much higher correlation with bipolar disorder than major depressive episodes (MDE) with 77% of patients with bipolar disorder reporting irritable mood compared with only 46% of patients with MDE.[12]*

3. What percentage of patients with bipolar disorder typically complain of decreased sleep?

   A. 50%
   B. 60%
   C. 70%
   D. 80%
   E. 90%

   Correct answer: E. *Compared to patients with MDE (47%), decreased sleep was seen in 90% of patients with bipolar disorder.[12] Thus, although nonspecific, the association between insomnia and bipolar disorder is very high.*

CASE 2:

Ms. B is a 36-year-old thin, married woman who has been on sertraline in the past. She reports that her mood has been low recently and presents to your primary care office requesting to restart sertraline. She is a rock musician who has purple hair and a rather flamboyant style. You restart the sertraline, but she calls you after a few days stating she has not been sleeping, is feeling "revved," and is contemplating having an affair with a casual acquaintance. You recognize the signs of mania and have her stop the sertraline. Having read this chapter, you are inclined to call in a prescription for lithium but need a little encouragement because you have not prescribed it before.

1. Which of the following statements about lithium therapy is true?

   A. Lithium monotherapy is equally effective compared with the combination of lithium + valproate.
   B. Lithium monotherapy is equally effective compared with valproate.
   C. Lithium monotherapy is less effective compared with the combination of lithium + valproate.
   D. Lithium monotherapy is less effective than valproate.
   E. Lithium monotherapy is less effective than lamotrigine.

   Correct answer: A. *In the United States, prescription of lithium for outpatients nearly halved between 1992 and 1996, and 1996 and 1999, whereas the rate of prescription of valproate almost tripled.[44] Yet according to the BALANCE trial, lithium monotherapy was more effective in relapse prevention of bipolar I disorder than valproate and equally effective to the combination of lithium and valproate.[45] Lithium offers an average 83% probability against an affective relapse after 1 year, 52% after 3 years, and 37% after 5 years.*

2. What are the main concerns in prescribing lithium in this case?

   A. Lithium would not help because this is likely sertraline-induced mania
   B. Lithium is a perfect choice for this patient with no major concerns
   C. Potential to worsen insomnia
   D. Potential for weight gain and patient's age
   E. Child-bearing age and lab-monitoring requirements

   Correct answer: E. *Child-bearing age and labs. The potential for weight gain is a concern. But in this case, this woman is of child-bearing age and thus, any pharmacotherapy recommendation must be made with great care. It is highly recommended that pregnancy be a planned event. Lithium also requires periodic laboratory monitoring including serum lithium level, renal function, and annual TSH as it can lead to renal impairment, hypothyroidism, and even nephrogenic diabetes insipidus if prescribed long term.*

3. What dose of lithium should be prescribed?

   A. 300 mg three times daily is the standard acute mania dose
   B. 300 mg twice daily is better tolerated in acute mania
   C. 15 mg/kg per day
   D. 25 mg/kg per day
   E. 450 mg at bedtime

   Correct answer: E. *450 mg qhs. The starting dose of lithium is typically 15 mg/kg per day, but we would recommend starting more conservatively. It can be divided into twice-daily dosing at the start, but we advocate quickly moving to once-daily dosing of the long-acting formulation in the evening to minimize adverse effects and improve adherence. Of note, 25 mg/kg per day is typically the dose calculation for valproate.*

CASE 3:

Mr. C is a 29-year-old man with a long history of substance-related disorders (intravenous heroin, methamphetamine, and marijuana) who presents to the outpatient clinic following a recent emergency room visit for chest pain. He has a long history of emotional and physical trauma as a child, has been in and out of jail, and although he is concerned about the recent episode of chest pain, he is frustrated by his up and down mood and even a detached feeling that causes him to self-medicate with drugs and even cut himself at times to "feel real." He has felt like this "as long as I can remember." On physical examination he has many piercings, tattoos, a leopard-print suit, and long hair shaved on one side.

1. Which of the following psychiatric diagnoses is NOT high the differential diagnosis?
   A. Borderline PD
   B. Narcissistic PD
   C. Bipolar disorder
   D. ADHD
   E. Generalized anxiety disorder

   Correct answer: B. *Besides the stated substance-related disorder, one must remember that a patient with bipolar disorder (or other mood disorders) often self-medicates to target the symptoms. In this case, the history of trauma and self-injury puts borderline PD firmly in the differential as well. Many experts consider borderline PD part of the bipolar spectrum. ADHD must also be considered and questions about childhood and development will help in the evaluation. Additionally, anxiety disorders and somatic symptom disorders enter the differential of most presentations like this; however, there was nothing in the case that suggested narcissistic PD.*

2. What does the patient's age suggest about the possibility of bipolar disorder?
   A. Bipolar disorder is mostly diagnosed in the fifth decade of life.
   B. Bipolar disorder is mostly diagnosed in the fourth decade of life.
   C. Bipolar disorder is mostly diagnosed in the third decade of life.
   D. Bipolar disorder is mostly diagnosed in the second decade of life.
   E. Bipolar disorder is mostly diagnosed in the first decade of life.

   Correct answer: C. *Whenever patients in their third decade of life talk about how they have had symptoms for "as long as they can remember," bipolar disorder must be firmly in the differential diagnosis because symptoms typically appear earlier than age 25.*

3. What aspect of the physical examination in this case best supports a diagnosis of bipolar disorder?
   A. Piercings
   B. Tattoos
   C. Leopard-print suit
   D. Hairstyle
   E. All of the above

   Correct answer: C. *All of the answers might be considered because many physical appearance and style characteristics have been studied and found to have some associations with bipolar disorder. However, of these, extravagant dressing style was one of the behavioral markers found to be significantly different in a bipolar cohort compared with a group with depression.[46]*

PRACTICAL RESOURCES

- The Mood Disorder Questionnaire, www.psycheducation.org/depression/MDQ
- The Depressive and Bipolar Support Alliance, www.dbsalliance.org
- The National Alliance for the Mentally Illness, www.nami.org
- The National Institute of Mental Health, www.nimh.nih.gov

REFERENCES

1. Sachs GS, Nierenberg AA, Calabrese JR, et al. Effectiveness of adjunctive antidepressant treatment for bipolar depression. *N Engl J Med.* 2007;356:1711-1722.

2. Hulvershorn LA, King J, Monahan PO, et al. Substance use disorders in adolescent and young adult relatives of probands with bipolar disorder: what drives the increased risk? *Compr Psychiatry.* 2017;78:130-139.

3. Fountoulakis K. The contemporary face of bipolar illness: complex diagnostic and therapeutic challenges. *CNS Spectr.* 2008;13:763-779.

4. Final Recommendation Statement: Depression in Adults: Screening. U.S. Preventive Services Task Force. November 2016. Available at https://www.uspreventiveservicestaskforce.org/Page/Document/RecommendationStatementFinal/depression-in-adults-screening1. Accessed September 11, 2017.

5. Das AK, Olfson M, Gameroff MJ. Screening for bipolar disorder in a primary care practice. *JAMA.* 2005;293(8):956-963.

6. Hirschfeld M, Lewis L, Vornik L, et al. Perceptions and impact of bipolar disorder: how far have we really come? Results of the national depressive and manic-depressive association 2000 survey of individuals with bipolar disorder. *J Clin Psychiatry.* 2003;64:161-174.

7. Tohen M, Chengappa KN, Suppes T, et al. Relapse prevention in bipolar 1 disorder: 18-month comparison o folanzapine plus mood stabilizer v. mood stabilizer alone. *Br J Psychiatry.* 2004;184:337-345.

8. Weissman MM, et al. Affective disorders. In: Robins LN, Resler DA, eds. *Psychiatric Disorders in America*; 1991:53-80.

9. Merikangas KR, Akiskal HS, Angst J, et al. Lifetime and 12-month prevalence of bipolar spectrum disorder in the National Comorbidity Survey replication [published correction appears in *Arch Gen Psychiatry.* 2007;64(9):1039]. *Arch Gen Psychiatry.* 2007;64(5):543-552.

10. Angst J. Bipolar disorder: a seriously underestimated health burden. *Eur Arch Psychiatry Clin Neuorsci.* 2004;254:59-60.

11. Weissman MM, Bland RC, Canino GJ, et al. Cross-national epidemiology of major depression and bipolar disorder. *JAMA.* 1996;276:293-299.

12. Angst J, Azorin JM, Bowden CL, et al; BRIDGE Study Group. Prevalence and characteristics of undiagnosed bipolar disorders in patients with a major depressive episode: the BRIDGE study. *Arch Gen Psychiatry.* 2011; 68:791-798.

13. World Health Organization. The global burden of disease: 2004 update. Part 3: disease incidence, prevalence and disability. Available at http://www.who.int/health-info/global_burden_disease/2004_report_update/en/. Accessed September 17, 2017.

14. American Psychiatric Association. *Diagnostic and Statistical Manual of Mental Disorders, Fifth Edition (DSM-5).* Arlington, VA: American Psychiatric Association; 2013.

15. Judd LL, Akiskal HS, Schettler PJ, et al. The long-term natural history of the weekly symptomatic status of bipolar I disorder. *Arch Gen Psychiatry.* 2002;59:530-537.

16. Judd LL, Akiskal HS, Schettler PJ, et al. A prospective investigation of the natural history of the long-term weekly symptomatic status of bipolar II disorder. *Arch Gen Psychiatry.* 2003;60:261-269.

17. Ghaemi SN. Bipolar disorder and antidepressants: an ongoing controversy. *Primary Psychiatry.* 2001;8:28-34.

18. Phelps J. Clinical Conundrum: Approaching Bipolar Diagnosis Four Ways. Psychiatric Times. Available at http://www.psychiatrictimes.com/bipolar-disorder/clinical-conundrum-approaching-bipolar-diagnosis-four-ways. Accessed September 18, 2017.

19. Hirschfeld RMA, Williams JBW, Spitzer RL, et al. Development and validation of a screening instrument for bipolar spectrum disorder: the mood disorder questionnaire. *Am J Psychiatry.* 2000;157:1873-1875.

20. Ghaemi NS, Miller CJ, Berv DA, et al. Sensitivity and specificity of a new bipolar spectrum diagnostic scale. *J Affect Disord.* 2005;84(2-3):273-277.

21. Sajatovic M, Strejilevich SA, Gildengers AG, et al. A report on older-age bipolar disorder from the International Society for Bipolar Disorders Task Force. *Bipolar Disord.* 2015;17:689.

22. Ward MM, Studenski S. The time course of acute psychiatric episodes in systemic lupus erythematosus. *J Rheumatol.* 1991;18:535.

23. Bhangle SD, Kramer N, Rosenstein ED. Corticosteroid-induced neuropsychiatric disorders: review and contrast with neuropsychiatric lupus. *Rheumatol Int.* 2013; 33:1923.

24. Höftberger R, van Sonderen A, Leypoldt F, et al. Encephalitis and AMPA receptor antibodies: novel findings in a case series of 22 patients. *Neurology.* 2015;84:2403.

25. Kayser MS, Titulaer MJ, Gresa-Arribas N, Dalmau J. Frequency and characteristics of isolated psychiatric episodes in anti–N-methyl-D-aspartate receptor encephalitis. *JAMA Neurol.* 2013;70:1133.

26. Satzer D, Bond DJ. Mania secondary to focal brain lesions: implications for understanding the functional neuroanatomy of bipolar disorder. *Bipolar Disord.* 2016;18:205.

27. Francis J. Delirium in older patients. *J Am Geriatr Soc.* 1992;40:829.

28. Zheng D, Zhou D, Zhao Z, et al. The clinical presentation and imaging manifestation of psychosis and dementia in general paresis: a retrospective study of 116 cases. *J Neuropsychiatry Clin Neurosci.* 2011;23:300.

29. Lyketsos CG, Schwartz J, Fishman M, Treisman G. AIDS mania. *J Neuropsychiatry Clin Neurosci.* 1997;9:277.

30. Kanluen S, Gottlieb CA. A clinical pathologic study of four adult cases of acute mercury inhalation toxicity. *Arch Pathol Lab Med.* 1991;115:56.

31. Fountoulakis KN, Yatham L, Grunze H, et al. The international college of neuro-psychopharmacology treatment guidelines for bipolar disorder in adults, part 2: review, grading of the evidence, and a practice algorithm. *Int J Neuropsychopharmacol.* 2017;20(2):121-179.

32. Geddes JR, Burgess S, Hawton K, et al. Long-term lithium therapy for bipolar disorder: systematic review and meta-analysis of randomized controlled trials. *Am J Psychiatry.* 2004;161:217-222.

33. Severus WE, Kleindienst N, Seemuller F, et al. What is the optimal serum lithium level in the long-term treatment of bipolar disorder?—a review. *Bipolar Disorder.* 2008;10:231-237.

34. National Institute for Health and Care Excellence. Bipolar Disorder: The Assessment and Management of Bipolar Disorder in Adults, Children and Young People in Primary and Secondary Care. Draft for Consultation, April 2014. http://www.nice.org.uk/.

35. Gitlin M. Lithium side effects and toxicity: prevalence and management strategies. *Int J Bipolar Disord.* 2016;4:27.

36. Szegedi A, Durgam S, Mackle M, et al. Randomized, double-blind, placebo-controlled trial of asenapine maintenance therapy in adults with an acute manic or mixed episode associated with bipolar I disorder. *Am J Psychiatry.* 2017. doi:10.1176/appi.ajp.2017.16040419.

37. Perica MM, Delas I. Essential fatty acids and psychiatric disorders. *Nutr Clin Pract.* 2011;26(4):409-425.

38. Penders TM, Stanciu CN, Schoemann AM, et al. Bright light therapy as augmentation of pharmacotherapy for treatment of depression: a systematic review and meta-analysis. *Prim Care Companion CNS Disord.* 2016;18(5).

39. Haynes PL, Gengler D, Kelly M. Social rhythm therapies for mood disorders: an update. *Curr Psychiatr Rep.* 2016;18(8):75.

40. Cipriani G, Danti S, Carlesi C, et al. Bipolar disorder and cognitive dysfunction: a complex link. *J Nerv Ment Dis.* 2017;205(10):743-756.

41. O'Donnell LA, Axelson DA, Kowatch RA, et al. Enhancing quality of life among adolescents with bipolar disorder: a randomized trial of two psychosocial interventions. *J Affect Disord.* 2017;219:201-208.

42. Cheema MK, MacQueen GM, Hassel S. Assessing personal financial management in patients with bipolar disorder and its relation to impulsivity and response inhibition. *Cognit Neuropsychiatry.* 2015;20(5):424-437.

43. Miziou S, Tsitsipa E, Moysidou S, et al. Psychosocial treatment and interventions for bipolar disorder: a systematic review. *Ann Gen Psychiatr.* 2015;14:19.

44. Blanco C, Laje G, Olfson M, Marcus SC, Pincus HA. Trends in the treatment of bipolar disorder by outpatient psychiatrists. *Am J Psychiatry.* 2002;159:1005-1010.

45. Geddes JR, Goodwin GM, Rendell J, et al. Lithium plus valproate combination therapy versus monotherapy for relapse prevention in bipolar 1 disorder (BALANCE): a randomised open-label trial. *Lancet.* 2010;375:385-395.

46. Lara DR, Bisol LW, Ottoni GL, et al. Validation of the "rule of three," the "red sign" and temperament as behavioral markers of bipolar spectrum disorders in a large sample. *J Affect Disord.* 2015;183:195-204.

11

PSYCHOTIC DISORDERS

Poh Choo How, MD, PhD, Anne B. McBride, MD, and Glen L. Xiong, MD

David is a 21-year-old man who presents with his friend for worsening depression, anxiety, and insomnia. During the examination, he is nervous and staring intently at the walls. He states that he is afraid of demons, as they have been asking him to do "weird things." His friend reports that David has not been eating or bathing regularly and he has been feeling depressed since failing his midterm exams recently.

CLINICAL HIGHLIGHTS

- Psychosis is a state of disordered thoughts or impairment in reality testing, as manifested by perceptual disturbances (e.g., hallucinations, delusions), disorganized speech, and disorganized behavior.

- Psychotic symptoms can occur owing to primary psychiatric disorders (e.g., schizophrenia, bipolar disorder, depression with psychotic features) or can be caused by general medical conditions (e.g., neurocognitive disorder or delirium), side effects from prescribed medications (e.g., prednisone or opioid analgesics), and/or illicit substance use.

- Positive psychotic symptoms are outward manifestations of thought disorder: hallucinations, delusions, and disorganized behaviors or speech. Negative psychotic symptoms include affective flattening (decreased expressed emotions), alogia (poverty of thoughts), attention deficits, anhedonia, amotivation, and social withdrawal.

- Indefinite antipsychotic medication treatment for recurrent psychosis in patients with primary psychotic disorders is generally recommended, if two or more episodes occur within 5 years.

- Treatment of chronic psychotic disorders, such as schizophrenia, begins with the selection of an appropriate second-generation antipsychotic (SGA) medication and referral for psychosocial services.

- Patients who are treated with any SGA are at an increased risk for developing metabolic syndromes, which include hypertension, hyperglycemia, weight gain, and hyperlipidemia. Patients should be monitored regularly for the development of metabolic syndrome and other side effects of SGAs.

CLINICAL SIGNIFICANCE

The lifetime prevalence of psychotic disorders in the general population is approximately 3%[1,2] with about 0.2% prevalence of psychotic disorders due to a general medical condition.[2] Patients who experienced psychotic symptoms are also more likely to have comorbid depression, anxiety, suicidal thinking, and alcohol abuse.[1] In addition, a retrospective analysis found that 60% of individuals eventually diagnosed with a first episode of a primary psychotic disorder were previously in contact with primary care for a mental health concern.[3]

Management of psychotic disorders and their comorbidities has become a mainstay of primary care practice for a number of reasons. Patients with primary psychotic disorders have a higher risk of morbidity and mortality partly because psychotic symptoms may interfere with their ability to manage comorbid medical conditions. In addition, medications used to treat psychosis have significant metabolic side effects, placing patients at increased risk for developing hyperlipidemia, diabetes mellitus, and cardiovascular disease.[4] Furthermore, secondary psychotic symptoms due to neurocognitive disorder and delirium have contributed to the increased use of antipsychotics in the last decade of life.[5]

DIAGNOSIS
DIAGNOSTIC CONSIDERATIONS

Psychosis is experienced as a constellation of symptoms rooted in the impairment of thought process and reality testing. Psychotic symptoms can be experienced as part of a primary psychiatric disorder (e.g., schizophrenia, bipolar disorder, depression with psychotic features) or can be caused by medical conditions (e.g., neurocognitive disorder with Lewy bodies, epilepsy, traumatic brain injury), substance use, or medication side effects (e.g., steroids, opioids).

Accurate diagnosis of the etiology of psychotic symptoms is important so that the root cause of the psychotic disorder can be appropriately treated. In some patients, psychosis may be limited in the number of symptoms experienced and in the degree and duration of symptom expression. Up to 25% of the general population report psychotic-like experiences and are considered at increased risk of developing clinical psychosis, although only a small proportion of the population go on to develop a psychotic disorder.[6] It is important to distinguish between this high-risk population in which treatment with an antipsychotic is not typically recommended and those individuals who experience full psychotic symptoms and may require treatment with an antipsychotic.

The *Diagnostic and Statistical Manual of Mental Disorders*, Fifth edition (*DSM-5*),[7] characterizes a number of schizophrenia spectrum disorders (*Table 11-1*). Schizophrenia is a primary psychotic disorder characterized by hallucinations, delusions, disorganized speech or thought, disorganized behavior, and/or negative symptoms that cause functional impairment and behavioral changes (*Tables 11-2 and 11-3*). In schizophrenia, symptoms persist for more than 6 months, whereas in schizophreniform disorder, symptoms resolve before 6 months. In schizoaffective disorder, individuals meet *DSM-5* criteria for schizophrenia and additionally meet *DSM-5* criteria for a major mood episode (e.g., mania or depression) for the majority of the illness. This is in contrast to mood disorders with psychotic features where the psychosis occurs only in the context of a primary mood disorder (major depression or bipolar disorder) (see Chapters 8 and 10 for further details). The *DSM-5* no longer makes a distinction among the different subtypes of schizophrenia such as paranoid, undifferentiated, or residual subtypes.

Although not included in the diagnostic criteria, the age of onset of psychotic symptoms is an important consideration, since schizophrenia typically presents in late adolescence and early adulthood (late teens to early 20s) and sometimes later in women (25 to 35 years old at initial onset). It is important to consider other causes of psychosis if a patient presents with new-onset psychotic symptoms at an older age. Childhood-onset schizophrenia (12 years and younger) is significantly less common, with a prevalence of 0.2 to 0.4 per 10,000.[8]

To diagnose a primary psychotic disorder, secondary causes of psychosis need to be ruled out (*Figure 11-1*). In substance- or medication-induced psychotic disorders, the onset of psychotic symptoms can be temporally linked with the use of the substance or medication and symptoms typically resolve when the substance or medication is discontinued. Similarly, psychotic symptoms can occur as a result of a broad array of medical conditions (see *Table 11-4* for common general medical causes of psychosis) and should resolve or improve with the treatment of the medical condition.

Even though symptoms may cause significant distress, the primary etiology of psychosis may not be clear or may

TABLE 11-1 Psychotic Disorders[7]

DIAGNOSIS	CHARACTERISTICS
Schizotypal personality disorder	Persistent pattern of social and interpersonal insufficiencies, with reduced capacity for personal relationships, along with distorted thoughts and perceptions, odd behavior, and thoughts and beliefs that are out of the ordinary realm that is below the threshold for the diagnosis of a psychotic disorder
Delusional disorder	One month of delusions without other psychotic symptoms
Brief psychotic disorder	Psychotic symptoms that last more than 1 day and resolves by 1 month
Schizophreniform disorder	Symptoms equivalent to schizophrenia except for its duration (less than 6 months), decline in functioning not necessary to meet diagnostic criteria
Schizophrenia	Lasts for at least 6 months and includes at least 1 month of active-phase symptoms. Decline in function noted over chronic course
Schizoaffective disorder	Major mood episode (e.g., mania or depressive episode) concurrent with schizophrenia for majority of illness, plus psychotic symptoms that occur in the absence of mood symptoms for a 2-week period
Substance-/medication-induced psychotic disorder	Psychotic symptoms due to the physiological effect of a drug of abuse, a medication, or toxin exposure and cease after removal of the agent
Psychotic disorder due to another medical condition	Psychotic symptoms due to the physiological effect of another medical condition
Other specified and unspecified schizophrenia spectrum and other psychotic disorder	Classifies psychotic presentations that do not meet the criteria for any of the specific psychotic disorders or psychotic symptomatology about which there is inadequate or contradictory information

TABLE 11-2 Description and Examples of Psychotic Symptoms

TYPE OF SYMPTOM	SYMPTOM	EXAMPLE
Positive symptoms	**Delusions** Fixed beliefs that are at odds with reality and held tightly by the patient despite being challenged by evidence otherwise.	A patient believes that their parents have been replaced by other people and does not believe that they are his parents despite being shown documentation.
	Hallucinations Experience of a sensory modality (visual, auditory, olfactory, or tactile) without the presence of an external stimulus.	A patient is verbally responding to hearing voices talking to him; it does not appear that he is communicating with a physical person. (Note: Auditory hallucinations are more common in primary psychotic disorders, whereas visual hallucinations occur more frequently in secondary psychotic disorders.)
	Disorganized thinking or speech Inability to think or communicate in a linear, logical, understandable fashion.	When asked what he would like to eat, a patient states, "The washer and the fluonty are flying, floating."
	Grossly disorganized behavior Inability to behave in a socially appropriate, goal-directed manner, leading to difficulties performing activities of daily living.	Can range from childlike (thumb-sucking), "silly," bizarre (drinking water from the toilet), odd (mismatched attire, smeared makeup) to agitation.
Negative symptoms	**Flat affect (diminished emotional expression)** Reduction in expression of emotion in the face, eye contact, intonation of speech (prosody), and bodily movements that normally provide emotional emphasis to speech.	A patient sits and stares straight ahead despite efforts to engage him in conversation. The patient may speak in an expressionless way.
	Avolition/amotivation Decrease in motivation, purposeful, and self-initiated activities.	A patient may sit for long periods, showing little interest in participating in activities.
	Alogia Diminished speech output.	Patient speaks nonspontaneously (only when spoken to), minimally, with few words, increased latency of response (is quiet for a long time before answering a question).
	Anhedonia Decreased ability to experience pleasure, minimizes previous pleasurable experiences.	A patient who used to enjoy listening to music no longer finds pleasure in this activity.
	Asociality Decreased interest in social interactions.	A patient may decline multiple opportunities and invitations to socialize or relate with others.

be confounded by other factors such as concurrent substance use or another medical condition. In these cases, a diagnosis of *unspecified schizophrenia spectrum and other psychotic disorder* can be used to capture the multifactorial etiology that may give rise to psychosis and to specify the symptoms of concern. This serves as a working diagnosis that may be used while investigating the cause of psychotic symptoms. Examples of clinically significant psychotic symptoms that may not fit into a specific diagnosis include transient stress-induced psychosis and postpartum psychosis in the absence of a mood disorder.

ASSESSMENT AND DIFFERENTIAL DIAGNOSIS

Given the broad differential diagnosis for psychosis, a thorough assessment is required to facilitate the diagnostic process. In the primary care setting, patients may present in a variety of ways such as by themselves, due to concern about specific symptoms, or, more frequently, being brought in by family members who notice a change in behavior (e.g., becoming more isolative or paranoid) or decline in function (e.g.,

TABLE 11-3 Diagnosing Schizophrenia[7]

1. Elicit symptoms
   a. Presence of at least two positive or negative symptoms (see Table 11-2) for at least 1 month. Either delusions, hallucinations, or disorganized speech must be present (see Table 11-1 for definition of symptoms).
   b. Presence of a decline in social, vocational, and personal self-care functioning
   c. Obtain collateral information from caregivers, family, or friends who know the patient well
2. Determine time course
   a. Presence of symptoms for at least 6 months with at least 1 month of symptoms described in (1a).
3. Rule out mood episodes
   a. If mood episodes are present during the time course described in (2), determine the temporal relationship with psychotic symptoms to rule out other diagnoses.
   b. If mood symptoms occur only when psychotic symptoms are present, the patient may have schizoaffective disorder.
   c. If mood episodes occur both independently and/or concurrently with psychotic symptoms, the patient may have a mood disorder with psychotic features.
4. Rule out contribution of substance abuse, medication use, and medical conditions that may contribute to psychosis. Determine temporal relationship between the use of substances, medications, or diagnoses of medical conditions, with onset of psychotic symptoms (see *Tables 11-4, 11-6, and 11-7*).

lack of concern for grooming and hygiene and lack of interest in activities of daily living [ADLs]). Given that psychosis involves impairment in reality testing, it is important to get both the patient's perspective and collateral information from family or friends who know the patient well. Prior medical records may provide additional information to clarify the diagnosis. Ideally, the patient and family member should be interviewed independently. An interpreter should be used if there is a language barrier. In general, consider the stepwise approach discussed below (*Figure 11-2*) in an assessment of new-onset psychosis.

Elicit the Symptoms

Eliciting the symptoms and history from a patient with psychosis can be challenging. Patients may vary in the degree of symptom severity and level of insight into their symptoms. Some patients may have minimal insight into their symptoms and basis in reality. It is important to maintain a neutral and caring stance, neither supporting nor confirming their symptoms, but connecting with their level of distress by making empathic statements (see *Table 11-5*). Patients may present with vague symptoms such as feeling "stressed," which can be viewed as an idiom of distress. In this case, the practitioner may use the patient's idiom of distress to elicit further symptoms. It is also important to consider the patients' symptoms in the context of their own cultural or spiritual beliefs.

Positive psychotic symptoms such as hallucinations, delusions, or bizarre or disorganized behaviors or speech are outward manifestations of psychosis that can be evident to any observer. Negative symptoms such as flat affect, avolition, anhedonia, and asociality (*Table 11-3*) may be subtler and are generally more difficult to treat. Practitioners should elicit the time course and fluctuation of symptoms as well as the impact they have on the patient's behaviors and functioning. In some cases, patients may deny or minimize

their symptoms or level of distress, in which case it is important to not only consider the patient's subjective report, but your own observation by performing a complete mental status examination and obtaining collateral information from family or friends about the patient's behavior and functioning in the community. Finally, it is important to perform a safety assessment by asking patients whether they are experiencing suicidal or homicidal thoughts, which may arise out of the significant distress they are experiencing due to their symptoms.

Evaluate for Secondary Causes of Psychosis

As previously discussed, psychosis may be caused by a variety of medical conditions, medications, and substances. *Table 11-4* provides a review of general medical conditions associated with psychosis and their corresponding workup. Routine initial primary care workup for new-onset psychosis should include a comprehensive chemistry panel, complete blood count, thyroid-stimulating hormone levels, and a urine drug screen. To avoid unnecessary cost, inconvenience, and false positives, further testing should be performed based on clinical suspicion and not as a routine practice. The American Association of Family Physicians recommends that brain imaging for the evaluation of psychosis should only be performed in patients with new, severe, unremitting headache, focal neurologic deficits, or a history of recent significant head trauma.[9]

Delirium is a frequent cause of acute psychosis in the medical setting. It can be differentiated from other causes of psychosis by the presence of fluctuating consciousness, disorientation, and impaired ability to sustain attention. Patients may have difficulty with questions involving orientation, calculation, or spelling (that measure attention) on cognitive screening. Neurocognitive disorder (formerly known as "dementia" in the *DSM-IV*) should also be considered as a causative factor for psychotic symptoms with about 30% of patients with

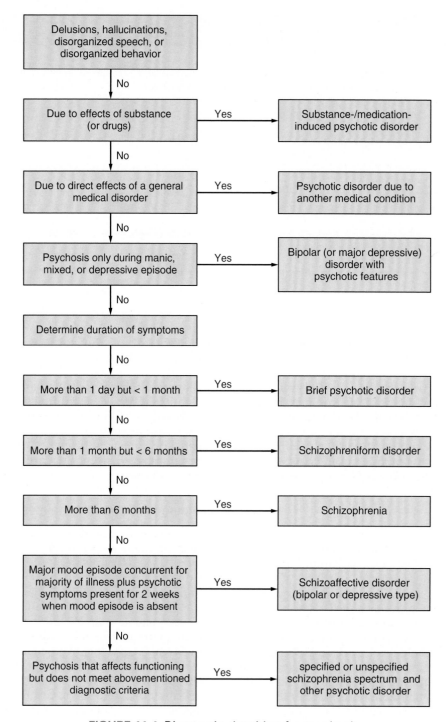

FIGURE 11-1 Diagnostic algorithm for psychosis.

dementia experiencing comorbid psychosis. *Table 11-6* helps to distinguish between delirium, neurocognitive disorder, and primary psychosis.

A variety of medications can cause psychosis (*Table 11-7*). In this case, there should be a temporal link between initiation of the medication and onset of psychotic symptoms. A discontinuation or reduction of the medication will also usually be associated with cessation or reduction of psychotic symptoms. The elderly population is more susceptible to medication-induced psychosis owing to decline in liver or renal function, polypharmacy, and drug–drug interaction. A review of medications should include over-the-counter medications and herbal supplements as well as prescribed medications. Common causes of medication-induced psychosis include anticholinergics, sedative-hypnotics, opioid analgesics, anticonvulsants, antimalarials, theophylline, and digoxin.

TABLE 11-4 General Medical Causes of Psychosis

CONDITIONS	PRESENTATION	ASSESSMENT	COMMENTS
Chronic neurologic disorders (seizure disorder, Parkinson disease, multiple sclerosis, stroke, Huntington disease, dementia with Lewy body, traumatic brain injury, brain tumor)	• Acute or progressive development of delusions, hallucinations, disorganized behavior, agitation, disinhibition, and cognitive deficit • Temporal relationship between the neurologic disorder and the psychotic symptoms • Psychiatric finding may be the only presentation in cases of isolated neurologic lesions (e.g., stroke or occult multiple sclerosis)	• Neurologic examination • Brain imaging to detect underlying neurologic condition • Lumbar puncture for multiple sclerosis • EEG	• Patients with a primary neurologic condition and psychosis should be given a diagnosis of "psychosis due to another medical condition," rather than be diagnosed with schizophrenia • Pharmacotherapy may be similar to schizophrenia but antipsychotic-associated EPS may be more likely in this patient population
Acute neurologic disorders (central nervous system infection or inflammation, e.g., syphilis, herpes encephalitis, HIV, lupus, vasculitides, brain tumor, autoimmune encephalitides	• Acute to subacute onset of hallucinations, delusions, agitation, mania, depression, disorganized behavior, delirium, and cognitive deficits • Often presents with fever and headache may have focal neurologic signs or seizures • Minimal systemic findings may be present in the beginning	• RPR/VDRL • HIV • ANA • ESR/CRP • CBC • Lumbar puncture • Brain imaging	• RPR/VDRL and an HIV test should be considered as part of the workup of psychosis in those who have risk factors (e.g., use of intravenous drugs, unprotected sex with multiple partners, or history of risky sexual behavior) • Inflammatory markers, ANAs, and more specific antibody tests may also be considered, as clinically indicated
Electrolyte disturbance (hypercalcemia, hyponatremia, or uremia)	• Acute to progressive course of lethargy, agitation, disorganization, delirium, hallucinations, and cognitive deficits	• Basic chemistry panel with calcium and magnesium	• Systemic symptoms are often present • In this case, psychosis is probably a component of delirium
Endocrinopathies (hormone-producing tumors, diabetes, parathyroid, and thyroid disease)	• Acute to subacute onset of hallucinations, delusions, agitation, mania, depression, and disorganized behavior • Symptoms related to endocrine dysfunction (e.g., tachycardia, weight loss, proptosis in hyperthyroidism)	• Basic chemistry panel with calcium • TSH/free T4 • HgbA1c	• Psychosis is a component of delirium
Nutritional deficiencies (vitamin B12, thiamine, niacin)	• Progressive onset of hallucinations, delusions, agitation, mania, depression, and disorganized behavior • Accompanied by cognitive deficits and other symptoms of vitamin deficiency (e.g., nystagmus, ataxia with thiamine deficiency)	• Serum folate, thiamine, vitamin B12 levels • CBC	• Psychosis can be corrected with repletion of vitamins

ANA, antinuclear antibody; CBC, complete blood count; CRP, C-reactive protein; EPS, extrapyramidal symptoms; ESR, erythrocyte sedimentation rate; HIV, human immunodeficiency virus; RPR, rapid plasma reagin; VDRL, Venereal Disease Research Laboratories.

Similarly, psychotic symptoms can occur owing to substance use, intoxication, and withdrawal. Psychoactive substances range from stimulants (e.g., phencyclidine [PCP], cocaine, methamphetamines, methylenedioxymethamphetamine [MDMA]), depressants or sedative-hypnotics (e.g., opioids, ketamine, benzodiazepines), psychedelics (e.g., lysergic acid diethylamide [LSD], psilocybin mushrooms), alcohol, and marijuana. Patients with a history of alcoholism or various malnutrition states may have thiamine deficiency and develop Wernicke encephalopathy characterized by delirium, ocular motor deficits, and ataxia or Korsakoff psychosis with resultant confabulation, deficits in memory, and diminished ability to perform ADLs. Patients may also develop transient psychotic symptoms in the setting of alcohol withdrawal or delirium tremens. Cocaine and methamphetamine intoxication–related psychosis is often characterized by paranoia.

Most substance-induced psychosis resolves over a brief period (usually 3 hours to 3 days of detoxification) and therefore does not require prolonged treatment other than counseling about cessation from the offending substance. However, some substances such as methamphetamine, ecstasy, or MDMA and some psychedelics may cause persistent psychotic symptom. Although timing may be difficult to determine, the *DSM-5* suggests that substance-induced psychosis typically resolves within

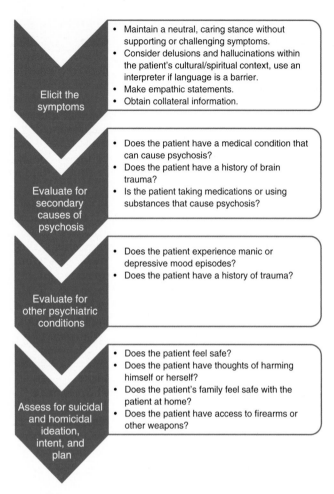

FIGURE 11-2 Algorithm for the assessment of psychosis.

1 month. The causal association may be difficult to establish and usually requires at least a three- to four-week period of sobriety to solidify a diagnosis and treatment plan. Given that primary psychotic disorders are often frequently comorbid with substance use disorders, the two can be hard to disentangle at times.

The use of cannabis is particularly common in young adults with early psychotic symptoms. The evidence is growing that cannabis may cause acute psychosis, increase the risk of schizophrenia, and worsen the course of psychotic disorders. Psychotic symptoms may occur in up to 15% of marijuana users.[10] Use of cannabis increases the risk of later-life psychosis. Also the relationship between cannabis and psychosis is dose dependent, in that increased use is associated with higher risks of psychosis. Genetic polymorphisms, family history of psychosis, and childhood trauma are risk factors associated with cannabis-induced psychosis.[11]

Evaluate for Other Psychiatric Conditions

Psychosis may occur as part of a depressive or manic episode in major depressive disorder and bipolar disorder. When expressed as part of a mood episode, the psychotic thought content is sometimes congruent with

TABLE 11-5 Suggestions for Communicating with Patients Who Have Psychosis

GOAL	WHAT YOU MIGHT SAY
Normalize	• "In my practice, many patients have experienced (symptom); have you experienced this as well?" • "Having schizophrenia is very common. In fact, 1% of people in the United States have schizophrenia at some point in their lives."
Empathize, don't collude	• "If it's all right, I would like to learn more about how the voices affect your life."
Ask, don't tell	• "How do you feel when this happens?" *or* "How do you cope when this happens?" is usually better than "I'd be scared if that happened to me," or "This sounds frightening," unless the patient is indicating a particular emotional state.
Validate, without confirming reality of the patient's symptoms	• *Patient*: "You believe me, don't you, doctor? Can't you see them too?" • *Doctor*: "I believe that these symptoms are very real and troubling to you, and I do not think you are making things up."
Bring up psychotic symptoms in context of more normal experiences	• "The brain is very powerful, and we all have a strong mind–body connection. Have you ever cried or laughed when you watched a movie? Nothing was happening to you when you cried, but you were sad. Your mind lets you experience that sadness, and told you that you were sad. Similarly, your mind has you experiencing voices and visions that others aren't experiencing. Does that make sense?"
Discussing diagnosis: inquiry and biases	• "Have you heard of the term *hallucination* or *delusion*? What does that mean to you? What do you know about people who experience this? What happens to them?"
Preparation of key messages	• For any discussion of diagnosis or prognosis, prepare your key statements in advance. What are the three concise things that you want your patient and their family members to remember? For instance: • "You have a disease called schizophrenia." • "It is common and has many treatments. Together, we'll find the best treatment for you." • "With the right treatment, many people enjoy a good quality of life."

the patient's mood. For example, patients with severe depression may experience nonbizarre delusions associated with guilt, poverty, somatic concerns, or contamination. Such patients may also have auditory hallucinations telling them that they are worthless or commanding

TABLE 11-6 Differentiating between Delirium, Neurocognitive Disorder, and Primary Psychosis

	DELIRIUM	NEUROCOGNITIVE DISORDER	PRIMARY PSYCHOSIS
Description	• Fluctuating mental status, with reduced attention, focus, and cognition • Usually reversible	• Progressive, chronic cognitive and functional decline • Rarely reversible	• Impaired understanding of reality and often accompanied by delusions, hallucinations, mood disturbances, bizarre speech and behaviors, poor insight • Amotivation with affective flattening
Etiology	• Global CNS dysfunction often from a medical illness or drug side effect • Common in older patients, patients with dementia, or those with serious medical problems	• Various areas of dysfunction and/or brain atrophy, depending on the type of neurocognitive disorder	• Although the cause of schizophrenia is not known for certain, positive symptoms appear to be related to dopamine excess in the mesolimbic system of the brain and decreased functioning of frontostriatal pathways
Prototypic diseases	• Infections (e.g., urinary tract infections, pneumonia) • CNS disorders (e.g., stroke, dementia) • Illicit drugs (e.g., cocaine, methamphetamines, alcohol) • Metabolic abnormalities (e.g., end-stage liver disease, untreated renal failure)	• Cortical (Alzheimer disease, frontotemporal disease, Lewy body disease) • Subcortical (Parkinson disease, Huntington disease, Wilson disease) • Infectious (sometimes reversible) (HIV-associated dementia, neurosyphilis) • Other (Korsakoff dementia from thiamine deficiency) • Vascular dementia	• Schizophrenia • Schizoaffective disorder
Differentiating factors	• Fluctuations in attention, distractibility, confusion, disorientation • Symptoms fluctuate and are often worse at night • Condition resolves when offending agent is removed or underlying illness resolves • New-onset psychosis, particularly with visual hallucinations, in older age	• Patients typically present with chronic, progressive decline in cognitive function and memory • In the earlier stages, reality testing is usually initially intact	• Attention and orientation are generally preserved • Patients may have delusions, auditory hallucinations, and may have difficulty reasoning • Symptoms may interfere with the ability to function in society • Initial onset in late teens or 20s. If symptoms are acute or present after the age of 40 years, consider a general medical or substance-related cause

CNS, central nervous system; HIV, human immunodeficiency virus.

TABLE 11-7 Selected Medications and Legal and Illicit Substances That Can Cause Psychosis

Medications	Corticosteroids, adrenergics, antiarrhythmics, antibiotics, anticholinergics, antihistamines, antimalarials, antituberculars, dopamine agonists, lithium (at supratherapeutic levels)
Herbal supplements	St John's wort, Valerian root
Controlled substances	Stimulants (e.g., Adderall, Ritalin), dextromethorphan (in cough medicine)
Illicit substances	Cannabis, ketamine, bath salts, cocaine, methamphetamines, opioids, MDMA, LSD, PCP, mescaline, psilocybin, salvia divinorum (legal in some states)
Others	Heavy metals, organophosphates

them to harm themselves. Similarly, in a manic episode, patients may experience grandiose delusions of having a superpower or infinite wealth. The experience of psychosis often intensifies as the mood episode worsens and is present during the active mood episode (see Chapters 8, 9, and 10 for a full discussion on Depressive and Bipolar Disorders). Psychosis or psychotic-like symptoms may also occur in patients who suffer from posttraumatic stress disorder, although this has not been fully characterized.[12] We recommend all patients with even subtle psychotic symptoms be thoroughly assessed for comorbid psychiatric disorders using the AMPS (Anxiety, Mood, Psychotic, Substance) screening tool (see Chapter 2).

Assess for Suicidality and Homicidality

Patients experiencing psychotic symptoms are at an increased risk for suicide. Approximately 30% of patients with schizophrenia attempt suicide and about 10% complete suicide.[13] Although the vast majority of individuals with psychotic disorders are not violent, psychosis is a risk factor for violence, particularly when associated with substance use or specific psychotic symptoms, such as paranoid delusions. Individuals should be screened about the content of delusional beliefs, whether they have command auditory hallucinations to harm others or whether they have homicidal thoughts toward identifiable individuals. Other patients who are experiencing paranoid delusions may feel that they have no way out but to take their own lives or to attack those whom they perceive are threatening them. It is therefore important to assess for suicide and violence risk in all patients with psychosis (see Chapter 22 for a full discussion on Suicide and Violence Risk Assessment).

NOT TO BE MISSED

- Systemic medical conditions
- Delirium
- Neurocognitive disorder
- Mood disorders
- Medication-induced psychosis
- Substance-induced psychosis
- Suicidal and homicidal ideation or intent

BIOPSYCHOSOCIAL TREATMENT
OVERVIEW OF TREATMENT

The treatment of primary psychotic disorders requires a comprehensive biopsychosocial approach to treatment (*Figure 11-3*) The Schizophrenia Patient Outcomes Research Team (PORT) recommends evidenced-based psychosocial interventions as an adjunct to medication treatment.[14] Treatment of co-occurring medical, psychiatric, and substance use disorders is essential for recovery in chronic persistent psychotic disorders. Before treatment can commence, it is important to weigh safety

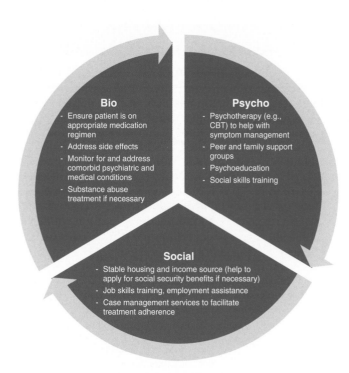

FIGURE 11-3 The biopsychosocial model in the treatment of schizophrenia. CBT, cognitive behavioral therapy.

considerations. If the patient has thoughts of harming himself or herself or others, or if they are too symptomatic to perform their ADLs (e.g., if they are not eating or drinking), they should be referred immediately to the emergency department or psychiatric crisis unit for acute care. Treatment considerations can be weighed once the safety of the individual and others is assured.

Treatment of a primary psychotic disorder typically involves antipsychotic medication. Mood stabilizers or antidepressants are often concurrently initiated with antipsychotics for psychotic symptoms occurring as part of a primary mood disorder. With secondary psychosis, treatment involves addressing the primary medical condition, discontinuing the offending agent, or counseling for substance use cessation. In such situations, an antipsychotic may be needed to treat the psychosis acutely and may be discontinued once the patient's condition improves. For example, patients with delirium may benefit from an antipsychotic to treat their hallucinations while they are treated with antibiotics for sepsis. A patient with major depression with psychotic features should be treated with both an antidepressant and antipsychotic until the psychotic depressive episode fully resolves, but chronic antipsychotic therapy is generally not necessary. In most cases, once the psychosis remits, the antipsychotic can be discontinued, but the patient should continue to be treated with an antidepressant. In contrast, the American Psychiatric Association (APA) recommends lifelong antipsychotic treatment in patients with primary psychotic disorders if two psychotic episodes occur within a 5-year period.[13] In patients with remission of a first break, single- or multi-episode psychosis, clinicians should discuss the risks and benefit of indefinite antipsychotic maintenance medication versus tapering of medications (after at least 1 year of symptom remission) with close follow-up and plan to reinstitute antipsychotic treatment with symptom recurrence. Once a patient is stable, dose reduction to the lowest effective dose is recommended for chronic care.

PSYCHOPHARMACOLOGY

Since the discovery of the first antipsychotics or neuroleptics, there has been great advancement in the number of treatment options available for psychosis with improved side effect profiles. First-generation antipsychotics (FGAs), also known as typical antipsychotics, are more likely to result in short-term and long-term movement disorders such as tardive dyskinesia (TD) particularly when prescribed in high doses (see *Table 11-8*). High-potency FGAs (e.g., haloperidol) have a high potential for inducing extrapyramidal symptoms (EPS) due to high dopamine (DA-2) blockade. Lower potency FGAs (e.g., chlorpromazine) have decreased affinity for the DA-2 receptors and have less potential of causing EPS but cause other side effects (e.g., hypotension, sedation, and anticholinergic effects) through action on other receptors. Use of second-generation antipsychotics (SGAs), also known as atypical antipsychotics, is less likely to cause EPS and TD, but they are often associated with significant metabolic side effects. Although FGAs and SGAs are thought to be equally effective treatments for schizophrenia, SGAs have emerged as a first-line treatment given the lower likelihood for treatment-resistant TD and other EPS.

Table 11-9 provides a summary of different antipsychotics, their side effect profiles, starting doses, titration schedules, and monitoring requirements. Given the adverse effects of SGAs on metabolism, it is important to record baseline weight, BMI, vitals, and fasting glucose and lipid profile. Patients with cardiac risk factors or who are being treated with an antipsychotic with known risks for QTc prolongation should obtain a baseline (ECG). If the baseline QTc is elevated (>450 ms in males and >470 ms in females), providers should consider antipsychotics with the least risk for QTc prolongation. These indices should be monitored longitudinally, along with monitoring for the development of EPS for as long as the patient continues to take antipsychotics.

The choice of an initial antipsychotic often depends on side effect profile, ease of dosing, and adherence strategies. If a patient is known to have diabetes or hyperlipidemia or develops these conditions as a side effect of another SGA, consider the use of aripiprazole, lurasidone, or brexpiprazole, which have lower risk for causing metabolic abnormalities.[15] FGAs such as haloperidol may also be an option for some patients, as many have lower risk of weight gain. Olanzapine and quetiapine have significant sedative effects and may be tried for those patients experiencing activation or comorbid insomnia. Patients themselves may have their own reasons for preferring one antipsychotic over another (e.g., a patient may be partial to a medication that is being used to treat a relative, or vice versa), and their preferences should be taken into account to facilitate medication adherence.

In the medically compromised or elderly patient, it is prudent to start antipsychotics at half the usual starting dose and titrate at a slower rate to decrease the risk of side effects. Such patients are also more sensitive to extrapyramidal side effects and might do better with low-potency DA antagonist, such as quetiapine. Be aware that the Food and Drug Administration (FDA) has issued a black box warning on the use of all antipsychotics in patients with dementia owing to an increased risk of cerebrovascular events and mortality.[16] Moreover, the evidence for behavioral disturbances is lacking, although they may have a role in the treatment of psychosis in dementia. Given the increased risk of death, alternative strategies and avoidance of antipsychotics for patients with dementia should be explored. Primary care providers may receive patients who have been prescribed antipsychotics for delirium; the medication should be tapered off, as such patients should not need prolonged antipsychotic treatment. Patients with dementia should also have trials off the medications to see if they are still indicated.

Most antipsychotics are classified in FDA pregnancy category C except for clozapine and lurasidone, which are category B medications.[18] Because clozapine is reserved for treatment-resistant psychosis due to significant serious side effects, lurasidone would be an appropriate consideration for treatment of psychosis in a pregnant or lactating woman.

Once antipsychotics are administered, psychotic symptom reduction usually occurs within 1 to 2 weeks, although optimal response may take as long as 6 months. For those who adhere to the treatment plan, approximately 50% of patients with schizophrenia respond to an antipsychotic medication, 25% respond partially, and 25% have little to no response.[19] Positive symptoms respond to antipsychotic treatment more readily than negative symptoms. An immediate improvement in behavior may be seen because of the tranquilizing effect of antipsychotics. In primary psychotic disorders, negative symptoms and cognitive deficits will generally be more refractory to medication treatment. In fact, the presence of negative symptoms carries a worse long-term prognosis when compared with someone who has predominantly positive symptoms. Such patients should be ideally reevaluated within 2 to 4 weeks to assess for side effects, improvement, and further medication dose titration and to rule out a parkinsonian syndrome or untreated major depression.

The side effects of antipsychotics are further described in *Table 11-8*. There are short- and long-term side effects that require screening and monitoring at follow-up visits. Short-term side effects usually present within 1 month of initiation or an increase in dose of an antipsychotic. These include akathisia, EPS, anticholinergic effects, orthostatic hypotension, sedation, and a prolonged QT interval on an ECG. EPS occur as a result of DA-2 receptor blockade of regulatory neurons that modulate descending motor neurons and are generally associated with high potency and higher antipsychotic dose. They include akathisia, dyskinesia, dystonic reactions, and parkinsonism (bradyphrenia, tremor, cogwheeling,

TABLE 11-8 Common Side Effects of Antipsychotics			
DESCRIPTION	TIME COURSE	TREATMENT	COMMENT
Akathisia			
A subjective, intolerable feeling of inner restlessness or sensation of the need to move	Transient reaction that may remit spontaneously over a few weeks	May trial propranolol 10 mg PO BID or TID and increase as tolerated. Benzodiazepines may be effective as well	Common side effect of aripiprazole
Dystonia			
Painful, uncontrollable tightening of muscles usually involving neck, back, or ocular muscles	Few hours to days of starting an antipsychotic	IM diphenhydramine (25-50 mg) or benztropine (1-2 mg) is a rapid, effective treatment	The emergence of dystonia can be a frightening experience for the patient, and reassurance coupled with education is critical to maintaining a trusting clinician–patient relationship and ongoing adherence with a treatment plan
Parkinsonian syndrome			
Mimics Parkinson disease, masked facies, limb rigidity, bradykinesia, pill-rolling tremor, micrographia, shuffling gait with postural instability		Oral anticholinergic medications (diphenhydramine 25-50 mg PO TID. Trihexyphenidyl (5-10 BID) or benztropine 1-2 mg BID	May use anticholinergics as a prophylaxis for parkinsonian syndrome when using high-potency antipsychotic such as Haldol. If used for prophylactic treatment, they can generally be tapered and stopped after 10 days. In those who poorly tolerate anticholinergic medications (e.g., patients with dementia), amantadine 100-300 mg BID may be used to treat parkinsonian symptoms, although the lowest effective antipsychotic dose should be used
Neuroleptic malignant syndrome (NMS)			
Rare, life-threatening side effect of all antipsychotics, involving muscle rigidity, autonomic dysregulation, fever, leukocytosis, elevated creatinine phosphokinase (>300 U/mL), and acute confusion	Usually occurs immediately following the initiation or increased dose of antipsychotic medication	Immediate transport to emergency department for IV fluids, supportive treatment. When severe, may require dopaminergic agents (e.g., dantrolene, bromocriptine)	NMS is difficult to evaluate in the outpatient setting and usually requires emergency medical management
Tardive dyskinesia			
Nonrhythmic, quick, choreoathetoid movements of the face, trunk, and extremities characterize TD. Examination for writhing of the tongue, hands, or trunk should be checked every 6-12 months, as this condition is generally permanent with no known treatment	Long-term EPS and can develop at a rate of about 3%-5% per year for FGAs. TD can occur with SGAs at a rate of about 0.8% per year	Discontinuation of offending antipsychotic, consider lower potency agent. Some reported improvement with vitamin E supplementation	TD risk factors include older age, longer use of antipsychotics, brain damage, diabetes mellitus, and comorbid mood disorder[13]

shuffling gait). At its most extreme, EPS can present as neuroleptic malignant syndrome, which is thankfully rare. Long-term side effects include irreversible movement disorders (e.g., TD), metabolic disorders, and idiosyncratic effects of specific antipsychotics. The Abnormal Involuntary Movement Scale (AIMS) is commonly used to monitor for EPS and other movement abnormalities in patients on chronic antipsychotic treatment.

Anticholinergic side effects such as dry mouth, sedation, and transient orthostatic hypotension are common among antipsychotics (e.g., chlorpromazine, olanzapine). Some antipsychotics carry more serious and rare side effects including prolonged QTc, which increases the risk of torsades de pointes (e.g., ziprasidone). The potential for metabolic abnormalities exists for all SGAs, but clozapine and olanzapine carry a higher relative risk.

TABLE 11-9 First-Line Antipsychotic Medications for Schizophrenia[a]								
	STARTING DOSE	TARGET RANGE[a] (mg/day)	PRIMARY CARE TITRATION SCHEDULE	EPS	ORTHOSTATIC HYPOTENSION	METABOLIC SYNDROME[b]	SEDATION	OTHER
Haloperidol (Haldol) (available in long-acting injectable formulations)	2-5 mg PO BID	20-40 mg/day	Increase up to 5 mg daily, as tolerated	+++	+	+/–	+	
Risperidone[c] (Risperdal) (available in long-acting injectable and ODT formulations)	1 mg BID or 2 mg QHS	4-6	Increase up to 2 mg daily, as tolerated	+++	++	++	++	Hyperprolactinemia
Olanzapine[c] (Zyprexa) (available in long-acting injectable and ODT formulations)	5-10 mg QHS	10-30	Increase 5 mg every 3-5 days, as tolerated	+	+	+++	+++	Not to be routinely used for the treatment of insomnia
Quetiapine[d] (Seroquel)	50-100 mg BID	300-800	Increase 50-100 mg every 2 days, as tolerated (monitor for orthostatic hypotension)	+/–	+++	++	+++	
Quetiapine (Seroquel XR)	300 mg QHS	400-800	Increase every 1-2 days, as tolerated	+/–	+++	++	+++	
Ziprasidone[e,f] (Geodon)	40 mg BID (must be taken with meals)[f]	40-160	Increase every other day to target dose, as tolerated	+	+	+	++	QTc prolongation
Aripiprazole[c] (Abilify) (available in long-acting injectable and ODT formulations)	10-15 mg QAM	10-30	Increase dose after 2 days, as tolerated	+/–	+	+	+	
Paliperidone[c,g] (Invega) (available in long-acting injectable formulation)	6 mg QAM	6-12	Increase by increments of 3 mg every 5 days, as tolerated	++	+	++	++	

(continued)

TABLE 11-9 First-Line Antipsychotic Medications for Schizophrenia[a] (continued)

	STARTING DOSE	TARGET RANGE[a] (mg/day)	PRIMARY CARE TITRATION SCHEDULE	EPS	ORTHOSTATIC HYPOTENSION	METABOLIC SYNDROME[b]	SEDATION	OTHER
Asenapine (Saphris) (available in ODT formulation)	5 mg BID	5-20	Increase by increments of 5 mg over one week	+	+	+	++	Dysgeusia
Iloperidone (Fanapt)	1 mg BID	6-24	Increase by 2 mg BID each day	+++	+	+	+++	
Lurasidone[f] (Latuda)	40 mg QAM	40-160	Increase by 20 mg per day	+++	+	+	+++	
Brexpiprazole (Rexulti)	1 mg PO QAM	1-4	Increase to 2 mg per day for three days, then increase to 4 mg per day	+	+	++	+++	
Cariprazine (Vraylar)	1.5 mg PO QAM	6-12	Increase by 1.5 mg per day	+++	+	+	++	

Monitoring

Initial:
Baseline weight and body mass index, waist circumference, vital signs, fasting glucose or Hgb A1C, and lipid profile
Consider doing a pregnancy test and drug toxicology
Neurologic examination (+/– brain imaging) should be performed if psychotic symptoms present after the age of 50 years
An ECG should be performed on patients who have cardiac disease
First 4 weeks: BMI, EPS, vital signs, prolactin (if clinical symptoms of hyperprolactinemia exist)
First 12 weeks: BMI, EPS, vital signs, fasting glucose of Hemoglobin A1C (Hg A1C), a lipid profile
Quarterly: BMI
Annually: BMI, EPS, fasting glucose of Hemoglobin A1C (Hg A1C)
Every 3-5 years: lipid panel
Special populations:
Medically compromised or elderly: Start antipsychotics at half the starting dose. Titrate over longer period, increase by half the recommended dose.
Pregnant/lactating: Most SGAs are categorized under class C. Consider lurasidone (Latuda), which is in Class B. Start at 20 mg BID, increase by 10-20 mg/day up to a maximum of 160 mg/day

[a]Dosing information derived from Lehman AF, Lieberman JA, Dixon LB, et al; American Psychiatric Association. Practice guideline for the treatment of patients with schizophrenia, second edition. Am J Psychiatry. 2004;161(S2):1-56 and the authors' clinical expert opinion. These doses do not apply to geriatric or pediatric patients.
[b]Metabolic effects include hyperglycemia, weight gain, and hyperlipidemia.
[c]Patients may be able to transition to an intramuscular depot formulation of the drug.
[d]Because of its low potency, quetiapine is ideal for patients who are sensitive to dopamine blockade, particularly patients sensitive to EPS.
[e]Contraindications to the use of ziprasidone include persistent QTc >500 ms, recent acute myocardial infarction, and uncompensated heart failure.
[f]Should be taken with food, as it increases bioavailability.
[g]Paliperidone is the active metabolite of risperidone. Relative risks for metabolic syndrome and EPS are similar to risperidone.
BMI, body mass index; ECG, electrocardiogram; EPS, extrapyramidal symptoms.

The American Diabetes Association and APA recommend routine screening and follow-up of metabolic profiles in patients on chronic SGA treatment, as outlined in *Table 11-9*.

There are different approaches one can take if a patient develops a side effect from an antipsychotic. EPS can often be resolved by lowering the dose. If dose decrease is not feasible, adding another medication to mitigate side effects may help. For example, anticholinergic agents, such as benztropine or trihexyphenidyl, can be used to treat parkinsonism or dystonia. Propranolol or benzodiazepines can be helpful to treat akathisia.

TABLE 11-10 Summary of PORT Psychosocial Treatment Recommendations		
DEFINITION	**TARGET POPULATION**	**GOALS, OUTCOMES**
Assertive community treatment		
The patient is supported by a multidisciplinary team with frequent patient contact and outreach to patient in the community	Patients at risk for repeated hospitalizations or who were recently homeless	Reduces hospitalizations and homelessness among patients with schizophrenia
Supportive employment		
Individually tailored program with integrated vocational and mental health services geared toward helping individuals prepare for, find, and maintain employment	Any patient with a desire to be employed	Helps patients obtain and maintains stable employment
Skills training		
Training for skills required for daily activities, to improve social interactions and promote independent living	Patients with skills deficits	Maintains independent living and functioning in society
Cognitive behavioral therapy		
Individual or group therapy to help identify target problem or symptoms and to develop cognitive strategies to address them	Patients with persistent psychotic symptoms while receiving adequate pharmacotherapy	Reduces severity of persistent symptoms
Token economy interventions		
Positive enforcement of adaptive behaviors (e.g., improving personal hygiene, social interactions)	Patients in a long-term inpatient or residential care facility	Improve adaptive behaviors within specific care facility
Family-based services		
Psychoeducation, training, and supportive services for families of patients	Families of patients that are still connected with them	Increased medication adherence, maintain family support, prevent family burnout
Psychosocial interventions for alcohol and substance use disorders		
Psychoeducation, motivational enhancement, coping skills training, and relapse prevention	Patients with co-occurring substance use disorders	Reduce substance use and improve psychiatric symptoms and functioning
Psychosocial interventions for weight management		
Psychoeducation focused on improving nutrition, physical activity	Overweight or obese patients (BMI >25)	Weight loss, prevent onset/worsening of metabolic syndrome

Another approach is to switch to another antipsychotic that has lower DA antagonism. For example, if a patient is experiencing dystonia from a higher potency antipsychotic, consider switching to a lower potency SGA, although the first strategy should be to reduce the current medication dosage by 10% to 25% and monitor for side effect improvement.

For patients with chronic psychotic disorders, the APA recommends at least 1 year of antipsychotic continuation after remission of the psychotic episode.[13] Medication adherence can be problematic particularly in patients with executive functioning deficits, poor insight into their mental illness, significant adverse effects, or stigma about mental illness and treatment. When using oral medications, once-daily medication regimens are optimal to foster adherence. Additionally, long-acting injectable (LAI) formulations exist for haloperidol, fluphenazine, risperidone, paliperidone, aripiprazole, and olanzapine. Long-acting formulations provide consistent blood levels and eliminate the need for a patient to adhere to a daily medication schedule.[17] Moreover, LAIs increase patient contact with their health team as depot medications are administered every 2 to 4 weeks. Emerging evidence now indicates that early initiation or transition to LAI may have a significant positive effect on prognosis.[18] From another perspective, patients often struggle with the diagnosis of schizophrenia (and other severe mental illness) and therefore become discouraged about the indefinite need to take antipsychotic medications. In such scenarios, the provider can highlight the possibility of improved functioning, decreased need for hospitalization, achieving independence, and maintaining relationships and employment with consistent medication adherence.

Clozapine is a highly effective antipsychotic that improves both positive and negative psychotic symptoms. However, it is not used as a first-line treatment in the United States owing to its slow titration schedule, the potential for serious side effects, and the need for frequent blood draws. Patients who are on clozapine receive weekly leukocyte monitoring to monitor the development of agranulocytosis for the first 6 months. Monitoring frequency is then reduced and continued for the duration of clozapine treatment. Other idiosyncratic side effects include frequent development of sialorrhea and rare occurrence of myocarditis. Owing to its anticholinergic, antihistaminic, and anti–alpha-adrenergic effects, clozapine is notorious for its association with delirium in vulnerable populations, sedation, and orthostatic hypotension, respectively. Because of these side effects and the increased risk of seizures, we recommend that clozapine be prescribed by a psychiatrist, at least initially.

Psychopharmacology Pearls for Treating Primary Psychotic Disorders

- Start with an SGA.
- Start low and go slow in the elderly and medically compromised to avoid serious side effects.
- Titrate to the middle dose range and observe for response for 2 to 4 weeks; avoid changing agents prematurely.
- Obtain baseline laboratory tests and periodically monitor for short- and long-term side effects.
- Monitor and treat components of metabolic side effects when they develop. For EPS, consider modest dose reduction, switching to a lower potency antipsychotic or adding an anticholinergic agent to treat EPS.
- Use once-daily dosing or LAI antipsychotics to promote medication adherence.

PSYCHOSOCIAL APPROACHES

Psychosocial interventions are an important part of recovery in schizophrenia and are recommended as an adjunct to medication treatment. A significant percentage of morbidity in schizophrenia is related to problems with relationships, employment status, lack of housing, cognitive function, social deficits, and substance use disorder. Addressing these domains requires a multidisciplinary

approach. There are eight evidence-based psychosocial intervention recommendations by PORT,[14] which are summarized in *Table 11-10*. These include assertive community treatment (ACT), supportive employment, skills training, cognitive behavioral therapy (CBT), token economy interventions, family-based services, and psychosocial interventions for alcohol and substance use disorders as well as for weight management.

The degree and type of psychosocial interventions a patient may require varies widely depending on the etiology, course, and prognosis of their disorder, as well as consideration of the patient's individual resources. For example, a patient with multiple recent hospitalizations will require ACT, an intensive model of case management involving a proactive multidisciplinary team that will tailor support for the patient to prevent relapse and rehospitalization. The ACT team will typically seek the patient out in the community (including homeless shelters), provide medication and outreach services, and, when necessary, facilitate emergency psychiatric hospitalization.

The cognitive deficits and negative symptoms often observed in schizophrenia may lead to difficulty in maintaining employment, relationships, and treatment adherence, leading to further complications including homelessness, hospitalizations, and lack of an ability to independently care for oneself. Supportive employment and skills training can help to prevent or delay the decline in function. Furthermore, family-based interventions such as education and peer support have been found to significantly reduce the rates of relapse and rehospitalization and increase medication adherence.

CBT is an evidence-based intervention for primary psychotic disorders and considered standard of care as part of the National Health Service in the United Kingdom.[20] In CBT, patients learn to identify their cognitive distortions and consequent behaviors. For example, a patient will learn to challenge his own paranoia by examining events that support this belief system and evidence that does not. For example, "I think that someone is watching me right now. But, I haven't seen anyone watching me in the past 5 years, even when I've looked around the corner today. Is someone really watching me?" The patient eventually reconciles his delusions as part of schizophrenia rather than reality. The patient may also be encouraged to design "behavioral experiments" to examine the evidence. There is an emerging movement to adopt CBT and other psychiatric rehabilitation programs in many mental health programs throughout the United States. Cognitive remediation therapy via rehearsal of predesigned cognitive tasks is an additional treatment modality that is actively researched for patients early in the course of a psychotic disorder to improve their cognitive capacity.

Many of the above interventions are outside the scope of a primary care practice. However, a primary care physician can help their patient access these services through a social work or mental health program referral. Interventions that could be started in the primary care setting include initiation of antipsychotic medication, screening and referral for treatment of alcohol and substance use disorders, and monitoring and treatment of metabolic comorbidities. Motivational interviewing can be used in the primary care setting to assess and encourage engagement in a substance abuse treatment program in patients with comorbid substance use disorders (see Chapters 13 and 14 for further details). In addition, given the lower life expectancy and higher rate of mortality in those with schizophrenia, primary care physicians should also address risk factors that contribute to morbidity in schizophrenia, such as smoking. Finally, owing to the increased risk for metabolic syndrome posed by many antipsychotics, providers should address weight management in patients treated with antipsychotics, especially in those who are already overweight or obese. Some primary care settings may already be staffed for psychosocial interventions for weight management, such as counseling services with a dietician.

Patient and Family Education

At the time of initial diagnosis of a psychotic disorder, there may be a lot of confusion about the cause of the psychosis, anxiety about the course of the disorder and its treatment, and hopelessness about the prognosis. It is a time of high stress for patients and their families. For clinicians, presenting the patient with a diagnosis of schizophrenia for the first time is much like the experience of delivering bad news. Patients receiving a first diagnosis of schizophrenia are at a higher risk of suicide compared with other stages of the disorder.[11] Yet, providing education and addressing misconceptions and myths can be very reassuring to patients and families and helps to increase adherence to treatment and decrease the risk of suicide.

It is important to elicit the patient and family's understanding of psychotic disorders and address any questions they may have to dispel any misconceptions. Patients and families may have preconceived ideas about psychosis from popular media and other sources that stigmatize mental illness. Parents experience guilt, feeling as though they "gave" schizophrenia to their child because of something they did in the past. Patients may feel that they had done something wrong and are being punished with the symptoms. There are also many general misconceptions about the effects of antipsychotics. *Table 11-10* summarizes some common questions about schizophrenia with suggestions for how clinicians could respond.

Psychoeducation is an ongoing process and should be addressed as treatment is continued. Patients and families should also be encouraged to better understand the illness by utilizing available education and support networks (see Practical Resources). The impact of hearing about the experiences of other individuals and families on the same journey to recovery cannot be underestimated. Peer support and peer-led family psychoeducation is a growing field and includes evidence-based approaches such as the Wellness Recovery Action Plan (WRAP) and Family-to-Family program by the National Alliance on Mental Illness, both of which are widely available.[11] Primary care physicians play an important role in referring and encouraging patients with schizophrenia to engage in psychoeducation and psychosocial treatments.

Social Services

The prevalence of schizophrenia among homeless persons is around 11%, which is much higher than the prevalence of schizophrenia in the general population.[13] Given the severity of the illness, referral for housing assistance is often needed. Many patients cannot afford to live independently, despite disability income. Some patients live in low-cost hotels (single-room occupancy) or rooming homes (room and boards). Family care and group homes may be options for patients with disability income, although some patients do not have the funding or perceive a loss of autonomy associated with such placements.

Patients with primary psychotic disorders may qualify for general public assistance with food, public housing, social security disability income, and government-sponsored health care insurance. These programs are region specific and administered by different agencies at different levels of government. Therefore, a social work or community mental health program referral is indicated for everyone with serious mental illnesses, such as schizophrenia, and mood disorders with psychotic features.

WHEN TO REFER

- Suicidal or homicidal ideation
- Grave disability or the inability to care for self, due to mental illness
- Persistent psychotic symptoms that are resistant to initial treatment
- Diagnostic uncertainty
- Psychosocial treatments or the need for more intensive case management
- Psychosis in the pregnant or postpartum patient
- Comorbid pathology

PRACTICAL RESOURCES

National Alliance on Mental Illness: http://www.nami.org/
Has complete listings of professional and consumer support with local chapters.

National Institute of Mental Health: http://www.nimh.nih.gov/
Has up-to-date information on diagnosis, prevention, and treatment

Brain & Behavior Research Foundation: http://www.bbrfoundation.org/
Has up-to-date information on research on the etiology, treatment, and prognosis of schizophrenia and other mental illnesses and multimedia resources.

CASES AND QUESTIONS

CASE 1:

Henry is a 19-year-old college student who you have seen in your primary care clinic since he was 10 years old. He has been brought into clinic by his parents who report concern about his declining academic performance after his first semester of freshman year. When he arrives, you are alarmed to observe that Henry has lost a substantial amount of weight since his last annual checkup and appears disheveled, withdrawn, and wearing clothing with noticeable staining. His parents explain that his college counselor called them with concern that Henry had stopped attending classes and missed multiple assignments. His roommate reported that Henry had grown increasingly worried about "the establishment" spying on him, following him, and sending messages to him through his television. Henry's parents add that before leaving for college 5 months ago, he appeared "his normal social self."

1. What additional history would help clarify Henry's diagnosis?

   A. Henry has a medical history of hyperlipidemia.
   B. Henry has been drinking alcohol excessively since leaving for college.
   C. Henry began using marijuana intermittently in high school and has continued to smoke marijuana on occasion over the past semester.
   D. Henry performed within the top 5% of his high school class in academics.
   E. Henry acknowledged that he sometimes hears membersof"theestablishment"callinghisnamewhen they are in close proximity.

   Correct answer: E. *This is an example of auditory hallucinations.*

2. What is Henry's most likely diagnosis?

   A. Schizophrenia
   B. Schizophreniform disorder
   C. Cannabis-induced psychotic disorder
   D. Alcohol-induced psychotic disorder
   E. Psychotic disorder due to general medical condition

   Correct answer: B. *Because the patient has not had symptoms for more than 6 months, he does not meet the diagnostic criteria for schizophrenia.*

3. You refer Henry to a local early intervention and treatment program for new-onset psychosis but learn that there is a 3-month waitlist before he can be seen for consultation. After screening for imminent safety concerns, what is your next best step in management of Henry's condition?

   A. Enroll Henry in a substance abuse treatment program immediately.
   B. Stabilize Henry's cholesterol levels with appropriate medication.

   C. Check Henry's fasting blood glucose level.
   D. Initiate antipsychotic treatment.
   E. Start an antidepressant given Henry's recent social withdrawal.

   Correct answer: E. *The patient has schizophreniform disorder, a condition similar to schizophrenia and may likely develop schizophrenia after sufficient follow-up. Assuming that substance use and medical conditions are not causing the persistent psychotic symptoms, initiating treatment is a reasonable option here. Treating the psychotic symptoms while the workup is in progress is a common practical approach.*

CASE 2:

An 80-year-old man with Parkinson disease and related dementia as well as frequent urinary tract infections presents with concerns of progressive confusion. He reports that the nursing home staff is abusing him and keeping him away from his family. He also believes that his dead wife has been visiting him regularly. The nursing home caregiver says the patient has been more aggressive and confrontational. He has been leaving the nursing home and wandering into the street.

1. Your differential diagnosis includes the following:

   A. Delirium caused by a urinary tract infection
   B. Psychosis related to progression of Parkinson disease
   C. Late-onset schizophrenia
   D. Choices A and B
   E. Choices A, B, and C

   Correct answer: D. *Both A and B are likely causes. Late onset schizophrenia is rare and unlikely the explanation in this patient.*

2. Workup for delirium is negative for acute causes of cognitive decline and psychosis. Given the agitation risk, you decide to order a medication. Which medication is the most appropriate first choice?

   A. Quetiapine 12.5 mg nightly
   B. Fluoxetine 10 mg every morning
   C. Lithium 150 mg nightly
   D. Risperidone 3 mg nightly
   E. Diphenhydramine 25 mg nightly

   Correct answer: A. *Quetiapin is a low-potential SGA that is least likely to cause or worsen parkinsonism and other EPS. Risperidone needs to be used with caution, as it is a high-potency SGA and is likely to worsen Parkinson symptoms. A low dose of 0.25 mg or 0.5 mg twice daily is often recommended as the starting dose, not 3 mg/day.*

3. You determine that the patient lacks capacity to consent to medication treatment and identify a surrogate decision-maker. Informed consent would need to include _____.

   A. a discussion of the poor prognosis associated with late-onset schizophrenia
   B. a discussion that antipsychotic medications are associated with an increased risk of mortality in the elderly, weighed against the benefit or treating psychosis or agitation
   C. potential side effects of antidepressants including headache, GI disturbance, and sexual side effects
   D. the risk of developing a tolerance to antipsychotic medication
   E. the FDA-issued black box warning involving suicidality risk in antipsychotic use

   Correct answer: B. *In this situation, the decision-maker needs to be informed that antipsychotic medications are associated with an increased risk of mortality in the elderly. Therefore, the individual must weigh the benefits against this risk.*

CASE 3:

Joanne is a 33-year-old woman with a history of schizophrenia who you have been treating over the past 5 years since her psychotic symptoms have stabilized with antipsychotic medication and she transferred back to your clinic from her former psychiatrist. She books an urgent appointment and reveals that she is going through a divorce, losing her housing, and on the verge of losing her employment. Although she had previously been able to tolerate occasional auditory hallucinations, she reports that the voices have been getting louder and have been making negative comments toward her. When you ask about her safety, she reluctantly tells you that the voices have been telling her to "grab a knife and get it over with." She adds that she is not certain that she can ignore the voices for much longer.

1. Your next step in management includes _____.

   A. scheduling Joanne for an urgent appointment with her psychiatrist
   B. increasing her dose of antipsychotic medication
   C. arranging emergent evaluation for possible psychiatric hospitalization
   D. sending Joanne to the lab for stat metabolic panel, complete blood count, thyroid function tests, and urine toxicology
   E. initiating treatment with antidepressant medication

   Correct answer: C. *This patient is at acute risk of harming herself. She meets criteria for involuntary psychiatric hospitalization and should be referred to emergency psychiatric services for further treatment and evaluation.*

2. Joanne is stabilized in an acute inpatient facility and returns to your clinic for follow-up. During her hospitalization, she disclosed that she had been drinking alcohol excessively and did not always remember to take her medication. In addition to recommending substance abuse treatment, you should consider _____.

   A. discussion of long-acting injectable antipsychotic medication
   B. switching to an antipsychotic with a longer half-life and lower withdrawal risk
   C. adding a mood stabilizer to target recent depression
   D. discontinuing the antipsychotic owing to the potential adverse interaction with alcohol
   E. administering a cognitive screening test to evaluate for possible alcohol-related cognitive deficits

   Correct answer: A. *Long-acting antipsychotic medication often help improve treatment adherence due to forgetfulness and has been demonstrated in a number of controlled studies to have better outcomes, despite substance abuse and other comorbidities.*

3. Joanne reports that, because her antipsychotic medication was increased during her hospitalization, she has experienced feelings of restlessness, which are at times unbearable. A reasonable next step includes _____.

   A. raising the dose of the antipsychotic to address her new somatic delusions
   B. laboratory screening for heavy metal toxicity
   C. switch her to a new antipsychotic
   D. trial with propranolol to address likely akathisia
   E. discontinue antipsychotic treatment given new-onset tardive dyskinesia

   Correct answer: D. *The restlessness associated with antipsychotic initiation or dose escalation is called akathisia. This may be improved with use of beta-blocker such as propranolol or with reduction of antipsychotic medication dosage.*

4. Joanne eventually loses her employment and you learn that she has been living out of her car since her divorce. What recommendations can you make for further care?

   A. Referral for assertive community treatment
   B. Employment and skills training
   C. Working together with Joanne's family to coordinate care
   D. Referral for cognitive behavioral therapy
   E. All of the above

   Correct answer: E. *All of the options are rational psychosocial treatments that have been proved to be associated with good functional outcomes in chronic psychotic disorders.*

REFERENCES

1. Olfson M, Lewis-Fernandez R, Weissman M, et al. Psychotic symptoms in an urban general medicine practice. *Am J Psychiatry*. 2002;159:1412-1419.

2. Perälä J, Suvisaari J, Saarni SI, et al. Lifetime prevalence of psychotic and bipolar I disorders in a general population. *Arch Gen Psychiatry*. 2007;64:19-28.

3. Anderson KK, Fuhrer R, Wynant W, et al. Patterns of health services use prior to a first diagnosis of psychosis: the importance of primary care. *Soc Psychiatry Psychiatr Epidemiol*. 2013;48:1389-1398.

4. Beng-Choon H, Black DW, Andreasen NC. Schizophrenia and other psychotic disorders. In: Hales RE, Yudofsky S, eds. *Essentials of Clinical Psychiatry*. Washington, DC: American Psychiatric Publishing, Inc.; 2004:189-241.

5. Carton L, Cottencin O, Lapeyre-Mestre M, et al. Off-label prescribing of antipsychotics in adults, children and elderly individuals: a systematic review of recent prescription trends. *Curr Pharm Des*. 2015;23:3280-3297.

6. Kelleher I, Cannon M. Psychotic-like experiences in the general population: characterizing a high-risk group for psychosis. *Psychol Med*. 2011;41:1-6.

7. American Psychiatric Association. *Diagnostic and Statistical Manual of Mental Disorders*. 5th ed. Washington, DC: American Psychiatric Publishing, Inc.; 2013.

8. Courvoisie H, Labellarte MJ, Riddle MA. Psychosis in children: diagnosis and treatment. *Dialogues Clin Neurosci*. 2001;3:79-92.

9. Griswold KS, Del Regno PA, Berger RC. Recognition and differential diagnosis of psychosis in primary care. *Am Fam Physician*. 2015;15:856-863.

10. Thomas H. A community survey of adverse effects of cannabis use. *Drug Alcohol Depend* 1996;42:201-207.

11. Radhakrishnan R, Wilkinson ST, D'Souza DC. Gone to pot—a review of the association between cannabis and psychosis. *Front Psychiatry*. 2014;5:54.

12. OConghaile A, DeLisi LE. Distinguishing schizophrenia from posttraumatic stress disorder with psychosis. *Curr Opin Psychiatry*. 2015;28:249-255.

13. Lehman AF, Lieberman JA, Dixon LB, et al; American Psychiatric Association. Practice guideline for the treatment of patients with schizophrenia, second edition. *Am J Psychiatry*. 2004;161(S2):1-56.

14. Kreyenbuhl J, Buchanan RW, Dickerson FB, et al. Schizophrenia patient outcomes research team (PORT). The schizophrenia patient outcomes research team (PORT): updated treatment recommendations 2009. *Schizophr Bull*. 2010;36:94-103.

15. De Hert M, Yu W, Detraux J, et al. Body weight and metabolic adverse effects of asenapine, iloperidone, lurasidone and paliperidone in the treatment of schizophrenia and bipolar disorder: a systematic review and exploratory meta-analysis. *CNS Drugs*. 2012;9:733-759.

16. Steinberg M, Lyketsos C. Atypical antipsychotic use in patients with dementia: managing safety concerns. *Am J Psychiatry*. 2012;169:900-906.

17. Miyamoto S, Wolfgang Fleischhacker W. The use of long-acting injectable antipsychotics in schizophrenia. *Curr Treat Options Psychiatry*. 2017;4:117-126.

18. Armstrong C. ACOG guidelines on psychiatric medication use during pregnancy and lactation. *Am Fam Physician*. 2008;78:772-778.

19. Lieberman JA, Stroup TS, McEvoy JP, et al. Effectiveness of antipsychotic drugs in patients with chronic schizophrenia. *N Engl J Med*. 2005;353:1209-1223.

20. Turkington D, Kingdon D, Weiden PJ. Cognitive behavior therapy for schizophrenia. *Am J Psychiatry*. 2006;163:365-373.

12

NEUROCOGNITIVE DISORDERS

Amy Newhouse, MD and Sarah Rivelli, MD, FACP

- Delirium, also called altered mental status, acute confusional state, or encephalopathy, is characterized by an acute onset of altered consciousness that fluctuates and is generally reversible.

- In the *Diagnostic and Statistical Manual of Mental Disorders*, Fourth Edition (*DSM-IV*), patients with cognitive deficits on testing without apparent functional impairment were coded as having mild cognitive impairment, whereas per the updated *DSM-5*, they should be coded as mild neurocognitive disorder.

- Dementia, also referred to as mild or major neurocognitive disorder, refers to a progressive and irreversible condition involving impairments in at least two areas of cognitive function, such as memory, language, attention, reasoning, judgment, and visual perception.

- Those who are found to have cognitive impairment, yet retain normal level of functioning, are diagnosed with minor neurocognitive disorder (previously "mild cognitive impairment"), whereas those with a decline from their previous level of functioning have major neurocognitive disorder (previously "dementia").

- There are only four medications approved for the treatment of dementia by the Food and Drug Administration. These are three cholinesterase inhibitors, donepezil, rivastigmine, and galantamine, and a noncompetitive NMDA antagonist, memantine.

- Psychosocial treatment of dementia includes patient and family education, caregiver support, frequent reorientation, reminders, recreational therapy and stimulation, safety measures, advanced care planning, and palliative care.

INTRODUCTION

Neurocognitive disorders (NCDs) encompass a broad range of diagnoses including delirium and the dementias. These disorders are characterized by deficits primarily in cognitive functions, which are acquired, as opposed to being developmental, and therefore represent a decline from previously established baseline functioning. Delirium refers to an acute change in mental status that is generally reversible once the underlying cause is addressed. Dementia refers to chronic and generally progressive NCDs. While dementias are classically thought of as a late-life disease, there is growing knowledge that NCDs are present in many younger patients, such as those with traumatic brain injury (TBI) and human immunodeficiency virus (HIV).

DELIRIUM

Delirium, also called altered mental status, acute confusional state, or encephalopathy, is characterized by an acute onset of altered consciousness that fluctuates and is generally reversible. Impaired attention that waxes and wanes over a short period is the hallmark of delirium. Communication and language may be impaired. Thought processes may be disorganized. Hallucinations, illusions, and delusions may be present. Emotional dysregulation may also be present. Sleep disturbances are common; these can begin with insomnia and frequent napping and progress to complete reversal of the day–night cycle.

Delirium can be classified as hypoactive, hyperactive, or mixed with regard to the level of activity. Those with hyperactive delirium may be agitated and at increased risk of harm to self or others. Those with hypoactive delirium often appear more withdrawn or apathetic, often with a paucity of speech. Delirium is a clinical diagnosis; the recommended workup is outlined below; however, there is no specific test that rules it in or out.

Delirium is most often the result of an acute medical condition; however, it may also be due to medications, substance intoxication, substance withdrawal, or a combination of factors. The pathophysiology of delirium is complex and not clearly delineated. Inflammation and dysregulation of the following neurotransmitter systems are thought to be involved: acetylcholine, serotonin, gamma-aminobutyric acid (GABA), and dopamine. It is likely that delirium represents a downstream, phenotypic display of central nervous system (CNS) impairment that can be reached via multiple pathways.

DEMENTIA (ALSO KNOWN AS MAJOR OR MILD NEUROCOGNITIVE DISORDER)

In contrast to delirium, dementias are chronic, persistent, generally irreversibly, and often progressive. The *DSM-5* dropped the term "dementia" and replaced it with "neurocognitive disorder" with a subclassification of mild or major. This was done to acknowledge that someone may have cognitive deficits noted on testing, but these may or may not cause functional impairment. In the *DSM-IV*, patients with cognitive deficits on testing without apparent functional impairment were coded as having mild cognitive impairment, whereas in the updated *DSM-5*, they should be coded as mild NCD.

Cognitive deficits may span a range of functions that include not only memory but also the ability to communicate, plan, use abstract reasoning, focus, and pay attention and visual perception. Individuals generally have impairment in at least two cognitive functions. Moreover, NCDs are often accompanied by other neuropsychiatric symptoms, including mood changes, apathy, anxiety, impulsivity, sleep disturbances, hallucinations, delusions, restlessness, and sometimes findings on the neurologic examination, such as abnormal tone, abnormal movements, gait changes, and frontal release signs. Dementia is a progressive disorder that leads to increasing loss of independence over its course.

The following are types of NCDs:

- Alzheimer disease (AD)
- Vascular
- Lewy body (ABD)
- Parkinson disease
- Frontotemporal dementia (FTD)
- HIV disease
- Prion disease
- Substance or medication induced
- Multiple etiologies

It is important to note that these disorders may co-occur and patients may present with mixed clinical pictures.

CLINICAL SIGNIFICANCE

Delirium is common, particularly in acute care settings, and confers significant health care burden, risk for debility, and mortality. The prevalence in primary care is unknown largely due to a paucity of studies looking at delirium in this setting. One retrospective review of 785 patients seen over the course of a year found a 1.1% rate of newly diagnosed delirium in the primary care setting based on ICD-10 codes.[7] In contrast, another study found an incidence of 13% when looking at delirium superimposed on those with dementia in a community dwelling setting.[3] Given that different primary care settings have different populations, the rates likely vary based on the population served.

While delirium is often considered to be more of an inpatient diagnosis, it often develops before patients are even brought to a hospital. Of community dwelling elderly patients, 17% presenting to the emergency department and up to 40% of those living in nursing homes have delirium.[12] Rates of delirium on inpatient general medicine services range from 30% to 40%, and up to 80% of patients in the ICU will have delirium.

The presence of delirium has clinical significance both acutely and in the long term, to the individual, the family, and health care system. In the acute period, it is associated with poor outcomes such as falls, prolonged hospital stay, increased likelihood of restraints, increased likelihood of antipsychotic medication use, and death. In the postdischarge period, it is associated with diagnosis of dementia[6], need for a higher level of care (such as a skilled nursing facility), and 1-year mortality. This should be considered when discussing prognosis with families. The heightened inpatient needs followed by increased longer term debility (and care needs) place a significant cost burden on the health system, cited as $164 billion annually in the United States.[5]

Dementia impacts about 13% of Americans 65 years and older, and the prevalence rises with age; about 30% of patients 85 years old have dementia.[8] Appropriate care for dementia may be extensive, including a multidisciplinary team of doctors, pharmacists, and social workers in addition to medications and daily assistance. Levels of assistance need range from in-home care to short-term nursing home stays up to long-term placement. The estimated annual cost is $259 billion annually in the United States.[1] In addition to the direct care burden and costs of dementia, this condition frequently impacts the morbidity associated with other concurrent diseases.

Caring for such patients is often challenging, with a need for close supervision to promote safety, prevention of falls, and maintain independence. NCDs pose a burden on families and caregivers, and many patients end up cared for in long-term care facilities. For the primary care provider (PCP), ensuring patient safety at home, helping transition into higher levels of care, and dealing with end-of-life issues all present challenges.

DIAGNOSIS
DELIRIUM

Delirium generally presents as an acute change in mental status, characterized mostly by impaired attention and fluctuating levels of consciousness. Disorientation is common, although not necessary for diagnosis; in other words, being oriented does not rule out this condition. Patients often cannot stay awake for long periods, and when they are, they appear easily distracted and unable to focus. Patients may have difficulty providing a clear history and require prompting to cooperate with interview. They may be unable to complete simple, common tasks. Their language may be vague and perseverative. Emotional regulation may also be impaired; patients may present with a dysphoric, euphoric, or labile affect.

These symptoms may prompt the practitioner to consider a diagnosis of depression or mania; however, unless there is a clear history of this, delirium is the more likely culprit, especially in the context of fluctuating levels of consciousness.

If hallucinations are present, they tend to be visual; however, auditory, tactile, or olfactory are possible as well. Illusions, misperception of surrounding stimuli, are common. They are often influenced by external stimuli, such as nearby noises or intravenous access lines. At times patients may appear to have psychotic symptoms, and delusions, such as paranoia, may be present. Patients without a history of psychosis who present with new-onset hallucinations or psychosis are more likely to have delirium than a primary psychotic disorder, such as schizophrenia, especially when these symptoms co-occur with confusion and inattention. The differential diagnosis between dementia, delirium, and other psychiatric conditions is presented in *Table 12-1*.

Disturbances in sleep–wake cycle, including complete reversal of the sleep–wake cycle, are common. Sensorium disturbances can progress to the point of stupor in extreme cases.

Delirium is typically due to an underlying condition and, therefore, often reversible. Common causes include infections, metabolic derangements, stroke, recent surgeries, trauma, indwelling urinary catheters, pain, medication side effects, urinary retention, changes in environment, and restraints. Risk factors for the development of delirium include advanced age, cognitive impairment (such as dementia), functional impairment (such as physical debility), sensory impairment (such as hearing or visual loss), prior CNS insults (such as cerebrovascular events), substance abuse, depression, and increased comorbid complexity. Those with a history of delirium are more likely to develop it again. More vulnerable patients, such as the frail elderly with dementia, may become easily delirious from relatively minor insults, such as metabolic derangements or a urinary tract infection.

Evaluation of the Patient with Delirium

Delirium occurs due to interactions between patient factors, the environment, and one or more insults to the brain. Delirium is diagnosed clinically. It is important to consider predisposing factors in addition to any recent environmental changes. History may reveal risk factors, medical conditions, or medications that might cause delirium. There are many common risk factors between delirium and dementia. Moreover, delirium is a risk factor for a future diagnosis of dementia, and patients with dementia are at increased risk of developing delirium. An acute change in mental status, presenting with inattention and fluctuation in sensorium, is the hallmark of delirium and not dementia. Screening tests may prove useful in detecting delirium. A thorough medical workup is key to identify both the cause of delirium and guide treatment.

Predisposing Patient Factors to Delirium

- Advanced age
- Cognitive impairment
- Functional impairment, frailty
- Malnutrition

TABLE 12-1 Differential Diagnosis of Selected Syndromes				
	DEMENTIA	**DELIRIUM**	**DEPRESSION**	**PSYCHOSIS**
Onset	Gradual	Acute	Varies	Varies
Course	Progressive	Fluctuates	Variable	Variable
Sensorium	Clear	Altered, clouded, fluctuates	Clear	Clear
Memory	Impaired	Impaired	Largely conserved	Conserved
Attention	Intact	Impaired	Intact	Impaired
Psychomotor	May be agitated, can be retarded in late stages	Hypoactive, hyperactive, or mixed	Retarded	May be agitated
Hallucinations	Visual or auditory	Visual, tactile, auditory; misperceptions and illusions	Auditory	Auditory, sometimes command
Delusions	Usually persecutory	Often paranoid	Classically mood congruent	Complex, often bizarre, paranoid
Mood	May be apathetic	Labile, fearful	Sad, dysphoric	Varies
Sleep	"Sundowning"—brief periods of confusion in the evening	Fragmented, day/night confusion	Insomnia, Early awakening	Varies

- Sensory impairment—hearing and visual loss
- Substance use disorders
- Depression
- Multimorbidity, comorbidity
- Anticholinergic medications
- Benzodiazepines
- Polypharmacy

Environmental Factors

- Lack of sunlight, lack of windows
- Excessive noise, stimulation
- Sensory deprivation
- Sleep interruption
- Urinary catheters, lines, restraints
- Intensive care unit

Screening Tools

Multiple screening tools have been developed to help identify delirium. These are most often performed by nursing staff on inpatient units; however, certain ones can be implemented in the clinic to aid in the diagnosis of delirium. Some common screening tests are the Nursing Delirium Screening Scale (Nu-DESC), Delirium Observational Screening (DOS) scale, Confusion Assessment Method (CAM), and the 4AT. The CAM is a valid and reliable screening tool that is commonly used in the United States. It can be downloaded from the website www.hospitaledlerlifeprogram. org. Another tool that takes only a few minutes to administer, which is used internationally and available in multiple languages, is the 4AT (download from www. the4at.com; *Figure 12-1*).

A **thorough medical workup** including physical examination should be undertaken to seek underlying causes of delirium. Collateral from a caregiver or someone who knows the patient can be useful to determine if there is a change from baseline. Review of medications, especially any recent additions, is generally high yield. Medication classes such as anticholinergics, benzodiazepines, and opioids are common culprits (see *Table 12-2*). Some frequent examples of specific medications in these classes are diphenhydramine, oxybutynin alprazolam, and oxycodone. It is also important, even in the elderly, to assess for use of alcohol or drug and the possibility of a withdrawal syndrome. Common causes or contributors to delirium are listed in *Table 12-3*.

The physical examination should start with assessment of the patient's attention, thought processes, and level of consciousness. Attention can be assessed via forward and backward digit spans, spelling W-O-R-L-D backward, and naming days of the week in reverse order. Thought processes can generally be assessed via intentional observation of the patient's interaction with the interviewer; however, for a more concrete assessment, one can use a picture of a scene and have the patient describe what's happening. It is helpful when the practitioner uses more descriptive terms than simply "altered" to describe a patient's mental status; some examples include somnolent, drowsy, awake, and alert.

There are certain classic neuropsychiatric findings that may suggest etiology. Asterixis may suggest the presence of hepatic or uremic encephalopathy. Tremor, hyperreflexia, and mydriasis may be seen in an alcohol or sedative withdrawal. Myoclonus is seen in many toxic-metabolic syndromes, including drug toxicities such as lithium toxicity. The presence of altered mental status, hyperreflexia, diarrhea, and flushing is consistent with serotonin syndrome. Altered mental status, rigidity, and fever in the setting of antipsychotic medication use is concerning for neuroleptic malignant syndrome. A focused neurologic examination is necessary to assess for aphasia, focal weakness, or sensory deficits that could be indicative of a CNS lesion such as a stroke or tumor.

DEMENTIA

Dementia, also referred to as mild or major NCD, refers to a progressive and irreversible condition involving impairments in at least two areas of cognitive function, such as memory, language, attention, reasoning, judgment, and visual perception. These are often associated with personality changes, behavioral disturbances, psychiatric syndromes, and motor findings. Importantly, these symptoms represent a change from the previous level of functioning. Those who are found to have cognitive impairment, yet retain normal level of functioning, are diagnosed with minor NCD, whereas those whose symptoms affect their previous level of functioning have major NCD.

Mild NCD is not the same as "normal aging." This constellation of symptoms often leads to individuals developing compensatory strategies to assist in continuing their prior level of functioning. Earlier identification of this syndrome allows for earlier intervention, possible slower progression of disease, and a more appropriate, gradual initiation of care assistance.

As mentioned, a key component to diagnosis of any type of dementia is establishing a prior cognitive and functional baseline. Collateral information is often important in determining if there has been a decline in these arenas. Activities of daily living (ADLs) and instrumental activities of daily living (IADLs) are two categories of skills that can be assessed when determining someone's baseline. ADLs include bathing, dressing, grooming, self-feeding, and transferring. IADLs include managing finances, maintaining the home, shopping for groceries, preparing meals, navigating around one's community, and taking prescription medications.

The most important risk factor for dementia is advanced age. As mentioned earlier, the prevalence of dementia at age 65 years is 1% to 2%, and this increases to 30% by age 85 years.[1] Gender is also relevant, as the overall prevalence of dementia is higher in women than in men; however, this is likely attributed to longer average life span in women. Certain types of dementia are more common in men, such as Parkinson disease and dementia with Lewy bodies.[4] Genetic predisposition is thought to be implicated, but the clinical relevance of genetic screening is still quite limited unless an autosomal dominant inheritance pattern

4AT

Assessment test for delirium & cognitive impairment

Patient name:

Date of birth:

Patient number:

Date: Time:

Tester:

	Circle

[1] Alertness
This includes patients who may be markedly drowsy (eg. difficult to rouse and/or obviously sleepy during assessment) or agitated/hyperactive. Observe the patient. If asleep, attempt to wake with speech or gentle touch on shoulder. Ask the patient to state their name and address to assist rating.

Normal (fully alert, but not agitated,throughout assessment)	0
Mild sleepiness for <10 seconds after waking, then normal	0
Clearly abnormal	4

[2] AMT4
Age, date of birth, place (name of the hospital or building), current year.

No mistakes	0
1 mistake	1
2 or more mistakes/untestable	2

[3] Attention
Ask the patient: "Please tell me the months of the year in backwards order, starting at December."
To assist initial understanding one prompt of "what is the month before December?" is permitted.

Months of the year backwards	Achieves 7 months or more correctly	0
	Starts but scores <7 months / refuses to start	1
	Untestable (cannot start because unwell, drowsy, inattentive)	2

[4] Acute change or fluctuating course
Evidence of significant change or fluctuation in: alertness, cognition, other mental function (eg. paranoia, hallucinations) arising over the last 2 weeks and still evident in last 24hrs

No	0
Yes	4

4 or above: possible delirium +/- cognitive impairment
1-3: possible cognitive impairment
0: delirium or severe cognitive impairment unlikely (but delirium still possible if [4] information incomplete)

4AT score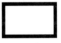

Guidance notes
Version 1.2. Information and download: **www.the4AT.com**

The 4AT is a screening instrument designed for rapid initial assessment of delirium and cognitive impairment. A score of 4 or more *suggests* delirium but is not diagnostic: more detailed assessment of mental status may be required to reach a diagnosis. A score of 1-3 suggests cognitive impairment and more detailed cognitive testing and informant history-taking are required. A score of 0 does not definitively exclude delirium or cognitive impairment: more detailed testing may be required depending on the clinical context. Items 1-3 are rated *solely on observation of the patient at the time of assessment*. Item 4 requires information from one or more source(s), eg. your own knowledge of the patient, other staff who know the patient (eg. ward nurses), GP letter, case notes, carers. The tester should take account of communication difficulties (hearing impairment, dysphasia, lack of common language) when carrying out the test and interpreting the score.

Alertness: Altered level of alertness is very likely to be delirium in general hospital settings. If the patient shows significant altered alertness during the bedside assessment, score 4 for this item. **AMT4 (Abbreviated Mental Test - 4):** This score can be extracted from items in the AMT10 if the latter is done immediately before. **Acute Change or Fluctuating Course:** Fluctuation can occur without delirium in some cases of dementia, but marked fluctuation usually indicates delirium. To help elicit any hallucinations and/or paranoid thoughts ask the patient questions such as, "Are you concerned about anything going on here?"; "Do you feel frightened by anything or anyone?"; "Have you been seeing or hearing anything unusual?"

FIGURE 12-1 The 4AT is a rapid clinical instrument for delirium detection. Reprinted with permission from https://www.the4at.com/. Copyright © Alasdair MacLullich.

is suspected. There are environmental risk factors as well, such as head trauma, sedentary lifestyle, smoking, poor diet, low mental activity, social isolation, and poor control of comorbid medical conditions.[2] Thus, dementia occurs owing to multifactorial processes, including genetic predisposition, medical comorbidities, and toxic exposures, including smoking. Specifically, poorly controlled diabetes, hypertension, and hyperlipidemia confer increased risk for NCDs. It is important to note that many of these risk factors are modifiable; however, data showing the positive impact of doing so are limited.

In addition to establishing a cognitive and functional baseline and reviewing risk factors, it is important to consider potential medical and psychiatric confounders. Cross-sectional evaluation risks the misdiagnosis of dementia, when in fact something more acute or potentially reversible is at play, as in delirium. A careful screening for fluctuating attention and consciousness, which would point to a diagnosis of delirium, is crucial (see *Table 12-1*). A thorough physical examination, including a neurologic examination, should reveal if there is a potential medical contributor to cognitive changes. Polypharmacy is again a frequent culprit to cognitive deficits; therefore a thorough review of medications is key. Dementia refers to an acquired deficit in cognitive functioning and cannot

TABLE 12-2 Common Medications Associated with Delirium

Antispasmodics	Hyoscine, Dicylcomine, Oxybutynin
Antihistamines	Diphenhydramine
Benzodiazepines	Alprazolam, Lorazepam, Clonazepam, Diazepam
Hypnotics	Zolpidem, Zaleplon
Opioids	Oxycodone, Hydrocodone, Morphine, Hydromorphone, Fentanyl
Barbiturates	Phenobarbital, Butalbital
Muscle relaxants	Tizanidine, Cyclobenzaprine, Baclofen
Stimulants	Amphetamine, Methylphenidate
Drugs of abuse	Heroin, Cocaine, Phencyclidine (PCP), MDMA ("Ectasy"), Hallucinogens
Antiemetics	Scopolamine, Metoclopramide, Promethazine
Dopamine agonists	Carbidopa/levodopa, Selegiline, Ropinirole
Dopamine antagonists	Olanzapine, Quetiapine

TABLE 12-3 Common Causes or Contributors to Delirium

Intracranial	Tumors, Subdural hematomas, Subarachnoid hemorrhages, Cerebrovascular events, Seizures, CNS vasculitis, Autoimmune encephalitis
Metabolic	Uremia, Liver failure, hyperammonemia, Hypernatremia, hyponatremia, Hypocalcemia, hypercalcemia, Hypoglycemia, hyperglycemia, Acid/base disturbances
Malnutrition	Thiamine deficiency
Endocrinopathies	Hypothyroidism/hyperthyroidism, Adrenal insufficiency, Hypercortisolemia, Hyperparathyroidism
Infections	Sepsis, Influenza, Urinary tract infection, Pneumonia, HIV, Tertiary syphilis, Meningitis, Encephalitis
Medications	Anticholinergic agents, Sedatives, benzodiazepines, Hypnotics, Opioids, Antipsychotics
Withdrawal	Alcohol withdrawal, Sedative-hypnotic withdrawal
Intoxication	Alcohol, Drugs of abuse
Drugs of abuse	Hallucinogens, PCP, MDMA
Low O_2 states	Hypoxia, hypercapnia, Respiratory failure, heart failure, Ischemia

TABLE 12-4 Cognitive Screening Tests

COGNITIVE SCREENING TEST	DESCRIPTION	TIME TO ADMINISTER
Verbal fluency test	Naming as many animals as possible in 60 seconds	1 minute
Minicognitive assessment instrument	3-item recall combined with clock-drawing test	2-4 minutes
Mini-Mental State Examination (MMSE)	30-question test assessing 5 cognitive domains	7-10 minutes
Montreal Cognitive Assessment (MoCA)	1-page exercise assessing 7 cognitive domains	10-12 minutes

be due to other mental conditions, even those that may include comorbid cognitive deficits, such as developmental delay, major depressive disorder, or schizophrenia. Therefore obtaining a thorough psychiatric history, including current assessment of mood, anxiety, and psychotic symptoms in addition to sleep disturbances and substance use, is important as well.

There are multiple rapid cognitive screening tests that can be used in a primary care setting (*Table 12-4*).

Asking caregivers or family members to assess how the patient is functioning now compared with 5 years ago in a structured fashion can be helpful. A toolkit of screening instruments, including a brief informant interview, is provided by the Alzheimer's organization to assist in screening as part of Medicare Annual Wellness visits: https://www.alz.org/documents_custom/141209-CognitiveAssessmentToo-kit-final.pdf.

High educational attainment can result in false negatives, and low education, in false positives.

More extensive neuropsychological testing can be useful to characterize the nature and extent of deficits to inform diagnosis, although it is not always available. Testing should not be reserved for patients older than 65 years, or any other specific age, but rather implemented whenever any patient shares any cognitive concerns or shows functional decline.

After a thorough physical examination and at least a brief cognitive assessment, there are several next steps for further workup. This is largely to evaluate for medical (or

nondegenerative) causes of cognitive or functional decline. These include many conditions, many of which overlap with potential causes of delirium listed earlier (*Table 12-5*).

Brain imaging should be performed for new-onset confusion or sudden cognitive impairment, particularly if focal neurologic signs are present. Noncontrast head CT is accessible and does not require prolonged cooperation from the patient and is particularly sensitive for detecting blood, such as seen in subdural hematomas, subarachnoid hemorrhage, or hemorrhagic stroke. MRI may provide more detail of white matter disease and regional volume loss, such as showing decreased volume of the hippocampi in AD or decreased frontal lobe volume in FTD. Positron emission tomography (PET) has been shown to distinguish between AD and FTD.

Electroencephalography (EEG) is useful for the evaluation of seizure or nonconvulsive status epilepticus, which can lead to the clouded sensorium seen in delirium. EEG shows diffuse slowing in delirium but is generally normal in mild to moderate dementia and psychiatric disorders. As dementia progresses, EEG tends to show increased slow-wave activity and does not help discriminate from delirium.

The term "reversible causes of dementia" while commonly cited is unfortunately clinically rare. While completely reversible dementias are uncommon, addressing certain issues can improve symptoms. Correcting and mitigating heavy alcohol use and vitamin deficiencies may lead to benefits. Supplementing vitamin B12 when

TABLE 12-5 Workup for Neurocognitive Disorders

	STRONG RECOMMENDATION	IF CLINICALLY SUSPECTED	NOT RECOMMENDED
Laboratory tests	Complete blood count Serum electrolytes Glucose BUN/creatinine Liver function Thyroid function Vitamin B12, methylmalonic acid	HIV RPR Folate Serum alcohol level Urine drug screen CSF 14-3-3, tau protein	Genetic testing ApoE4
Imaging	Noncontrast head CT Noncontrast MRI	PET (only if attempting to distinguish between AD and FTD) EEG	Volumetric structural analysis of CT or MRI SPECT

the level is less than 450 pmol/L has been shown to have some benefit in cognitive testing.

Once a dementia diagnosis has been established, determining the specific type is important, as this can have treatment and prognostic implications. Unique features of the most common dementia subtypes are shown in *Table 12-6*.

In considering the type of dementia, one approach is to consider whether the symptoms are more cortical or subcortical. Cortical degeneration often manifests as memory loss, language difficulties, executive dysfunction, and poor insight into cognitive deficits. These symptoms are often seen in Alzheimer disease, vascular dementia with cortical strokes, and frontotemporal dementia. Subcortical degeneration can be suspected when there is tremor, shuffled gait, cogwheel rigidity, or chorea. These symptoms are often seen with Huntington disease, Parkinson disease, progressive supranuclear palsy, HIV dementia, and vascular dementia with subcortical strokes. Presentations can overlap, and such overlap increases with time as neurodegeneration progresses. Some classic physical examination findings may point to specific disorders (*Table 12-7*) but may be only partially present or be seen across disorders.

Types of Dementia and Neurocognitive Disorders

Alzheimer disease is the most common form of dementia and frequently co-occurs with vascular dementia. Key features of the most common dementias are shown in

Table 12-4. Short-term memory loss is a prominent feature early in its course; over time, deficits in executive function, language, mood changes, and even psychosis may be present. Social skills and interaction are preserved initially, often leading to a lack of diagnosis and awareness of the onset of the disease.

Vascular

Pure vascular dementia accounts for up to 10% of dementias; however, it often co-occurs with Alzheimer disease. Vascular dementia refers to the cognitive and behavioral symptoms due to strokes and is therefore classically thought of as having a stepwise progression. This often begins with impaired judgment and executive function, such as planning. Depending on the sites of vascular insults, motor symptoms may be present, such as gait disturbance. Because vascular dementia commonly co-occurs with Alzheimer disease, the progression can be a combination of stepwise and gradual. Cardiovascular risk factors, such as hypertension, hyperlipidemia, tobacco use, and diabetes, are typically seen in patients with vascular dementia. A history of stroke or brain imaging, such as MRI or brain CT, that shows ischemic damage helps support a diagnosis of vascular dementia. Patients may not be aware that they have had strokes in the past, yet this does not necessarily exclude the diagnosis.

Lewy Body

Lewy bodies refer to the round, haloed cytoplasmic inclusions comprising synuclein found in the brain. Lewy body disease is characterized by visual hallucinations,

TABLE 12-6 Unique Features of Dementia Subtypes

	ALZHEIMER	VASCULAR	FRONTOTEMPORAL	LEWY BODY
Onset	Gradual	Acute/subacute	Earlier	Variable
Prevalence	Most common, may be part of mixed dementia	Often co-occurs with Alzheimer disease	About 10% of all dementias	
Course	Progressive	Stepwise	Rapidly progressive	Variable
Prominent symptoms	Forgetting, particularly short-term memory loss, difficulty learning new material	Focal neurologic deficits, evidence of CVA or small vessel ischemic changes on imaging	Deficits in planning, impulsivity, personality change, language difficulties	Visual hallucinations, fluctuating cognition, falls, parkinsonism
Associated neurologic symptoms	Paratonia, frontal release signs late	Focal deficits related to stroke(s), such as motor, gait, or speech impairments	Extrapyramidal symptoms in some variants	Parkinson symptoms: resting tremor, rigidity; such symptoms occur after cognitive and psychiatric symptoms
Unique prodrome			Personality change	REM sleep behavior disorder
Neuroimaging—CT or MRI (may be normal)	Global or hippocampal atrophy	Infarcts, lacunes, white matter lesions (basal ganglia, periventricular)	Frontotemporal atrophy	Global or hippocampal atrophy

TABLE 12-7 Classic Physical Examination Findings Pointing to Certain Types of Neurocognitive Disorders

PHYSICAL EXAMINATION FINDINGS	NEUROCOGNITIVE DISORDER
Nystagmus or ophthalmoplegia Ataxia Short-term memory loss, confabulation	Wernicke-Korsakoff syndrome; thiamine deficiency
Pupil that accommodates but does not constrict to light (Argyll Robertson pupil)	Neurosyphilis
Gait apraxia, incontinence	Normal pressure hydrocephalus
Hypophonia Axial rigidity, ataxia, lack of tremor Paralysis of vertical gaze, decreased blinking	Progressive supranuclear palsy
Bradykinesia Shuffling gait Bradyphrenia Masked facies Pill-rolling tremor	Parkinson disease
Choreiform movements	Huntington disease, Wilson disease
Startle myoclonus Ataxia	Prion disease
Lateral extremity weakness Lateral facial weakness Dysarthria	Vascular
Palmomental reflex Grasping Snout reflex	Frontal, any later stage dementia

fluctuating sensorium, and confusion that can present very similarly to delirium. It accounts for approximately 20% of patients with dementia. REM sleep behavior disorder is a classic prodrome of LBD, often present years before cognitive deficits are noted. Parkinsonism may occur only after cognitive deficits but generally within a year or two of each other. Sensitivity to antipsychotics, orthostasis, and falls are typical features of LBD.

Frontotemporal
FTD is a heterogenous group of disorders that tend to have an earlier age of onset, with onset between 45 and 65 years old. It is characterized by changes in behavior such as impulsivity, disinhibition, or apathy. Patients may appear to lose sympathy or empathy for others. Patients may have repetitive or compulsive behavior. Patients show poor insight, poor planning, and lack judgment. Abstract reasoning is decreased on testing as is mental flexibility. Some patients show hyperorality and odd

eating patterns, such as excessive drive to eat sweets. Those with the language variants show difficulty expressing themselves, with decreased fluency, decreased naming, and decreased comprehension, while memory is generally intact. Slower movements and lack of coordination are common. Related disorders include FTD seen in amyotrophic lateral sclerosis, corticobasal degeneration, and progressive supranuclear palsy.

Huntington Disease
Huntington disease is a rare dementia, transmitted in an autosomal dominant fashion. Symptoms often manifest in the mid-40s with changes in mood, anxiety, irritability, and personality changes. Short-term memory deficits and difficulty learning new material are common. Chorea may occur at any stage of the disease and may include movements of the trunk, extremities, and face. Patients may appear restless and fidgety and lack balance. Difficulty with speech and swallowing become more prominent, and weight loss and pneumonia tend to be common issues toward end of life.

Prion disease, also called transmissible spongiform encephalopathy, is believed to be caused by prions, which are proteins that lead to damage in brain tissue. It is rapidly fatal with memory and coordination deficits and behavioral changes. It may occur due to transmission of the prion from infected meat, such as "mad cow disease," and is then called "variant Creuztfeld-Jakob Disease (CJD)." Classic CJD is generally sporadic, although it may be due to genetic causes in some patients and tends to occur later in life, such as around the mid-60s. In either case, the disease is rapidly progressive and patients tend to die within one year of diagnosis.

Human Immunodeficiency Virus–Associated Dementia
This should be suspected in patients with advanced, generally untreated HIV infection or prolonged infection. It presents as a subacute decline in attention and concentration in addition to psychomotor speed and precision.[9] These symptoms are often combined with depressive symptoms, such as apathy. Some of the symptoms may wax and wane, which is different than the progressive decline seen in Alzheimer disease, and may present more like delirium at times. The severity of cognitive deficits tends to correlate with the severity and duration of CD4 nadir and period of untreated HIV. Treatment of HIV will help partially improve and stabilize cognitive symptoms. Treatment of depressive symptoms and sleep disturbances is also beneficial.

Normal Pressure Hydrocephalus
Normal pressure hydrocephalus is relatively uncommon. It presents with cognitive deficits including attentional deficits, gait apraxia and ataxia, and urinary incontinence. Symptoms may be mitigated and progression stopped with the installation of a shunt to drain CSF fluid off the brain.

Traumatic Brain Injury
Prevalence of TBI has been increasing and is the most common cause of NCD in younger adults. The duration

of loss of consciousness at the time of injury is associated with worsening TBI symptoms. Similarly, low Glasgow Coma Scale (GCS) scores at the time of presentation is associated with more severe TBI. In hospital trauma programs, patients presenting with head injury are generally routinely screened for TBI. The PCP should screen for a history of head injury and inquire about loss of consciousness, its duration, and results of any routine screening, such as the GCS, if it was performed.

BIOPSYCHOSOCIAL TREATMENT

DELIRIUM

The main treatment approach in delirium is the search for the underlying cause(s) as described earlier. The following supportive measures may prevent and reduce severity and duration of delirium:

- Frequent reorientation
- Reassurance (including time to resolution)
- Identification and correction of sensory impairments (hearing aid, glasses)
- Sleep hygiene
- Asses and treat pain (preferably with nonopiates)
- Comforting, calm environment, with exposure to sunlight during the day
    - Remove tethers, lines, catheters, restraints as able
- Adequate physical activity (ambulation, gentle exercise)
- Correction of metabolic abnormalities, dehydration, and nutrition support
- Avoidance of sedatives and hypnotics, particularly benzodiazepines

Antipsychotics have been insufficiently studied for the treatment of delirium, with only two small placebo-controlled randomized controlled trials conducted to date, suggesting that quetiapine may reduce the duration and severity of delirium. The current practice is to use antipsychotics for symptoms causing significant distress or danger after careful evaluation of the risks and benefits. In cases where antipsychotics are employed, the dose and duration should be minimized as much as possible. PCPs may receive patients on antipsychotics from inpatient stays where delirium occurred; tapering off such agents with close monitoring is advisable.

DEMENTIA

Pharmacotherapy

Pharmacotherapy has a somewhat limited role in the treatment of dementia. It should be considered in conjunction with psychosocial treatment, within a framework of maintaining safety and maximizing quality of life. Identifying the type of dementia syndrome is important when considering pharmacotherapy.

There are only four medications approved for the treatment of dementia by the Food and Drug Administration. These are three cholinesterase inhibitors, donepezil, rivastigmine, and galantamine, and a noncompetitive NMDA antagonist, memantine (*Table 12-8*). Trials have shown the most benefit for these drugs in Alzheimer disease; however, even in this setting, the benefit is only modest in terms of slowing or reversing cognitive decline. Donepezil has FDA indications for the treatment of mild to severe Alzheimer disease. Rivastigmine and galantamine have indications for the treatment of mild to moderate Alzheimer disease while memantine has FDA indication only for the treatment of moderate to severe disease. Memantine can be used in combination with a cholinesterase inhibitor medication. It is not yet known if memantine has benefit in the earlier stages of Alzheimer dementia. Off-label use of these cholinergic medications for vascular and Lewy body dementia have shown some benefit,

TABLE 12-8 Agents Approved for the Treatment of Dementia					
NAME	FORMULATION	FDA APPROVAL	DOSE RANGE	ADVERSE EFFECTS	COMMENTS
Cholinesterase inhibitors					
Donepezil	Tablet, orally disintegrating tablet	Alzheimer disease, mild to severe	5-23 mg	Nausea, vomiting, muscle cramps, bradycardia, decreased appetite, vivid dreams; effects tend to decrease after 1-2 weeks	May be helpful in LBD and vascular dementia as well
Rivastigmine	Capsule, transdermal patch	Alzheimer disease, mild to moderate; Parkinson dementia	4.6-13.3 mg		
Galantamine	Tablet, extended release capsule, solution	Alzheimer disease, mild to moderate	8-24 mg		
NMDA receptor antagonist					
Memantine	Tablet, extended release capsule, solution	Alzheimer disease, moderate to severe	5-20 mg, in divided doses twice daily XR: 7-28 mg	Transient sedation, generally well tolerated	May be helpful in vascular dementia as well

although evidence is still limited. Similarly, memantine may have some benefit in the treatment of vascular dementia. Realistic expectations should be discussed frankly with patients and their families when prescribing these medications.

A generally accepted approach to prescribing these medications is to "start low and go slow." Making singular small changes at a time is preferred over multiple at once to help determine which have benefit and which may have side effects in an individual. Common side effects include nausea, vomiting, muscle cramps, bradycardia, and vivid dreams for the anticholinergic medications. Memantine is generally well tolerated, although it may cause sedation early on. Side effects typically resolve within 1 to 2 weeks of administration.

Continuing to address other comorbidities is an important part of dementia care. Those with advanced dementia may not be able to communicate their needs, so actively assessing for symptoms such as constipation, urinary retention, and pain is key. Treatment of conditions such as hypertension and diabetes mellitus is important as well, especially in the context of vascular dementia to help prevent further vascular damage. As always, a healthy diet is recommended; however, supplements such as vitamin E, gingko biloba, and hormones are not recommended owing to lack of efficacy and the potential for adverse events. Melatonin, however, is considered to be safe and efficacious in assisting with sleep cycle regulation.

Psychosocial Treatment

Even though dementia is generally irreversible, there are still many factors to consider in the treatment of this disease. Safety should be considered from the patient and caregiver's perspective. Some common environmental hazards, especially for those living alone, are household appliances that have risks of fire (stoves, ovens) and surfaces with increased risk of falls (bathroom floors, steps, steep driveways). Certain behaviors, such as wandering or agitation, can place the patient and others in danger. Whether or not the patient can drive safely should be considered as well. A multidisciplinary approach, which includes assessment by physical and occupational therapy and social work, can help assess needs and mitigate these risks.

Frequent PCP visits with the family or caregivers is recommended to allow for frequent assessment, education, and planning. Early discussions regarding prognosis and expectations can help a patient and his or her family prepare for things such as transition to a higher level of care, health care, and financial power of attorney and code status. Involving palliative care, even at early stages, can help individuals be involved in their own care planning before they are unable to do so. In addition to code status, having specific discussions about topics such as nasogastric tubes, longer term feeding tubes, and dialysis can promote autonomy in decision-making and improve quality of life. Anticipatory planning can be of benefit once the patient with dementia gets admitted to an inpatient unit.

Key strategies in psychosocial treatment of dementia:

- Education of the patient and family
- Caregiver support (support groups, respite care)
- Frequent reorientation, reminders (calendars, journals, blister packs for medications)
- Recreational therapy and stimulation (art therapy, music therapy, pet therapy)
- Physical and occupational therapy (promote safe ambulation and independence)
- Environmental safety measures: elevated toilet seat, bars in bathroom, remove loose rugs, minimize wandering, caution against driving
- Advanced care planning with healthcare power of attorney (HPOA) and/or family
- Legal issues: plan for patient's eventual incapacity (advanced directives, power of attorney, will and testament)
- Palliative care, symptom treatment

Behavioral Disturbances in Dementia

Agitation, aggression, hallucinations, and delusions are frequent in patients with dementia and are a common reason for placement in nursing homes. When such symptoms occur, careful evaluation for medical, environmental, and psychosocial problems should first be undertaken. Evaluation and treatment of pain, constipation, and infections may all be useful approaches. Patients may make statements that appear to be delusions related to memory loss, such as believing things from the past are still true. Hallucinations that are well defined, vivid, and often visual are more commonly seen in NCD due to Lewy bodies. However, such patients do not tolerate antipsychotic medication well, and thus such should only be used if hallucinations are disturbing and at low dose. In general, interventions should primarily be family education, reassurance, and redirection.

Nonpharmacologic intervention with redirection, reassurance, and correction of any unmet needs is indicated. There are no medications specifically approved for use in behavioral disturbances associated with dementia. If such symptoms cause significant distress or danger, antipsychotics may be prescribed, but careful monitoring for effect and the evaluation of the risks and benefits is necessary.[10] It should be noted that no medication has been shown to be significantly efficacious in reducing overall behavioral problems in dementia, despite at least 17 placebo-controlled randomized trials examining 4 different second-generation antipsychotics (risperidone, olanzapine, quetiapine, aripiprazole) among patients primarily with Alzheimer disease. Moreover, these agents are associated with significantly increased risk of mortality in this setting and carry a black box warning because of this. One meta-analysis showed a 65% increased risk of mortality among patients prescribed SGAs for agitation in dementia compared with placebo in short (8-week long) trials.[11] Risperidone does appear to be helpful for psychosis in dementia and thus might be considered for such an indication, thought the effect size is modest and is associated with metabolic and motor adverse events, in addition to the increased risk of mortality.

First-generation antipsychotics, such as haloperidol, appear to carry an even higher risk of mortality in demented patients. Such antipsychotics may also be more poorly tolerated by the elderly, who are more sensitive to extrapyramidal symptoms, in particular. The APA practice guidelines recommend against haloperidol as a first-line agent among such patients. If antipsychotics are used, trials off the medication should be undertaken to see if they are still indicated.

Benzodiazepines should be avoided altogether owing to the risk of impaired cognition, delirium, and falls. Moreover, these agents tend to be disinhibiting, leading to worsened emotional dysregulation and impulsivity.

Common Pitfalls

- Dementia is generally underdiagnosed in primary care, and many providers do not perform routine screening.
  - Early diagnosis of dementia may allow the patient and family to complete advanced directives and discuss end-of-life planning with the patient involved.
- Delirium and dementia are likely to co-occur in elderly.
- Don't miss information from friends and family, which can help determine if a patient is "at his or her baseline."
- Psychosocial and environmental approaches are often overlooked, despite limited evidence for pharmacologic treatments of dementia and delirium.

CASES AND QUESTIONS

CASE 1:

Ms. A is a 76-year-old woman with hypertension, stress incontinence, and anxiety who presents for a blood pressure check at her PCP's office. She is found asleep in the room when the provider enters. She wakes easily although appears to have difficulty staying awake. She stares ahead when the provider greets her. When then asked how her BP has been running at home, she starts to answer but then starts talking about her son's recent trip to Mexico. The provider has never seen her like this before and is quite concerned by this change.

1. What is the most appropriate mental status screening test to do at this time?

   A. Verbal fluency test
   B. Confusion Assessment Method (CAM)
   C. Montreal Cognitive Assessment (MoCA)
   D. Mini-Mental State Examination (MMSE)

   Correct answer: C. *The patient presents with an acute change in her cognition, has an altered and fluctuating sensorium characterized by difficulty staying awake. She is unable to stay focused enough to answer questions appropriately. This presentation suggests delirium.*

2. You review any recent additions to her medical history. She shares that last week she went to the emergency department for a panic attack. She was

prescribed a medicine, but she can't remember the name. Which of the following is the most likely to have been prescribed for anxiety and be contributing to her current altered mental status?

   A. Alprazolam
   B. Hydrocodone
   C. Citalopram
   D. Mirtazapine
   E. Zolpidem

   Correct answer: A. *Alprazolam is a benzodiazepine and an agent that might be prescribed in an acute setting, such as an emergency department, for anxiety. Such agents are associated with confusion and delirium, however, particularly among vulnerable patients, such as the elderly.*

3. In addition to the above, you remember that at her last visit, she requested to try a medication for her stress incontinence. You had prescribed oxybutynin. She shares that over the past few days, she has had trouble initiating urination, notes burning on urination, and has noticed a foul smell to her urine. Which of the following is the best next step in her workup?

   A. Head CT
   B. Ammonia
   C. Urinalysis
   D. Urine drug screen
   E. Oxybutynin level

   Correct answer: C. *The patient describes urinary symptoms and presents with confusion. A urinary tract infection sounds likely and should be evaluated with a urinalysis.*

4. You suspect that this patient has delirium; which of the following diagnostic tests can be used to confirm this diagnosis?

   A. Vital signs
   B. Orientation questions
   C. Complete blood count
   D. Brain MRI
   E. None of the above

   Correct answer E: *Delirium is a clinical diagnosis, and there is no single test that may confirm its presence. A diagnosis is given based on the presence of a disturbance in attention and awareness, and the presence of other cognitive deficits, which tend to fluctuate and are generally of acute onset.*

CASE 2:

Mr. B is a 72-year-old man with hypertension, hyperlipidemia, and coronary artery disease. He presents for a routine clinic visit accompanied by his daughter. He reports no complaints, although she reports recent forgetfulness, irritability, and difficulty in the grocery store when she takes him out to do errands. She recalls noticing memory impairment 5 years ago and she had to help him with his bills, but afterward he seemed stable to her. She notes recent worsening over the past month.

1. Which of the following types of dementia classically follows a stepwise progression of decline?

   A. Frontotemporal dementia
   B. Alzheimer disease
   C. Lewy body dementia
   D. HIV dementia
   E. Vascular dementia

   > **Correct answer: E.** *This patient presents with progressive cognitive and functional decline that is consistent with dementia, with a recent stepwise decline. He has risk factors for vascular dementia (hypertension, hyperlipidemia, and coronary artery disease), making this the most likely type of dementia in this patient.*

2. Which of the following types of dementia most commonly co-occurs with vascular dementia?

   A. Frontotemporal dementia
   B. Alzheimer disease
   C. Lewy body dementia
   D. HIV dementia
   E. Vascular dementia

   > **Correct answer: B.** *Postmortem brain studies have shown that Alzheimer disease and vascular disease co-occur.*

3. Which of the following CNS imaging modalities would be the most appropriate to include in the workup of this patient?

   A. MRI
   B. PET scan
   C. EEG
   D. SPECT
   E. CT with volumetric analysis

   > **Correct answer: A.** *An MRI may provide information on acute and chronic vascular insults in the brain. PET scan has been shown to be helpful in differentiating Alzheimer disease from frontotemporal dementia, but this more expensive and involved test is not needed in this case where the suspicion of vascular dementia is high. SPECT is not used routinely clinically. EEG would be helpful if seizures were suspected.*

4. Which of the following are important to inquire about when treating a patient with an NCD?

   A. Whether or not they live alone
   B. Whether or not they drive
   C. Who manages their finances
   D. Whether or not they have access to firearms
   E. All of the above

   > **Correct answer: E.** *A full safety assessment should include exploration of the patient's living situation and help he or she might have to manage finances and get to appointments or the store. Firearms may pose a hazard in terms of intentional or accidental harm and should be discussed.*

CASE 3:

Mr. C is an 85-year-old man who resides in a nursing home owing to his advanced Alzheimer dementia. He is brought in to clinic by staff at the nursing home for agitated behavior. He refuses to change into a gown for his examination yelling that he knows the nurses will steal his clothes. He demands to be taken home and uses profanities when the nursing home staff say they will bring him back to the facility after the visit. He swings at the doctor while she is listening to his lungs. This behavior has been gradually getting worse over the past 6 months. The accompanying staff asks if there is any medication that will treat this condition.

1. Which of the following is a FDA-approved medication for treatment of agitation in dementia?

   A. Haloperidol
   B. Risperidone
   C. Quetiapine
   D. Aripiprazole
   E. There are none

   > **Correct answer: E.** *There are no medications approved for this indication, although antipsychotics are often prescribed. Randomized, placebo-controlled trials have failed to provide much evidence for any significant benefit for risperidone, quetiapine, or aripiprazole for agitation in dementia and are not FDA approved for this indication. Haloperidol has not been studied for this indication.*

2. What does the black box warning cite as the primary risk associated with using antipsychotics for treatment of agitation in those with dementia?

   A. Increased risk of delirium
   B. Increased risk of extrapyramidal symptoms
   C. Increased risk of death
   D. Increased risk of metabolic syndrome

   > **Correct answer: C.** *Randomized, placebo-controlled trials have shown statistically significant increased short-term risk of death among patients randomized to receive a second-generation antipsychotic, compared with placebo. When these studies were pooled together in meta-analyses, the signal of increased risk of death over an 8-week period became evident, leading to the FDA warning.*

3. After a careful discussion with staff and with the patient's HPOA, it is decided that the risk of prescribing an antipsychotic is worth the potential benefit of reducing paranoia and agitation. While the evidence is limited, which of the following is the best choice?

   A. Haloperidol
   B. Olanzapine
   C. Thioridazine
   D. Quetiapine
   E. Risperidone

continued

Correct answer: E. *Moderate-quality evidence has shown that risperidone is one of the agents studied that confers a modest improvement in psychosis and agitation, compared with placebo. Thioridazine and haloperidol have not been studied for the treatment of agitation in randomized placebo-controlled trials.*

4. Nursing staff shares that his sleep cycle has been irregular for several months now. Which of the following is the best first-line treatment to help right his sleep cycle?

   A. Temazepam
   B. Lorazepam
   C. Melatonin
   D. Quetiapine
   E. Diphenhydramine

   Correct answer: C. *Melatonin levels decline with age and are low in dementia, thus correcting this by prescribing a melatonin supplement may be helpful. It is not a hypnotic, however, but may help restore a more normal circadian rhythm. Lorazepam and temazepam would be unwise, as they are benzodiazepines and thus more likely to cause confusion and falls, particularly in patients with dementia. Diphenhydramine is anticholinergic and thus likely to cause confusion and has a negative side effect profile. Given that quetiapine is an antipsychotic, which may cause orthostasis and metabolic abnormalities, it should not be used first line to treat insomnia.*

5. Which of the following medications is not FDA approved for the treatment of Alzheimer dementia?

   A. Amantadine
   B. Donepezil
   C. Memantine
   D. Rivastigmine
   E. Galantamine

   Correct answer: A. *There are only four medications approved for the treatment of dementia by the Food and Drug Administration. These are three cholinesterase inhibitors, donepezil, rivastigmine, and galantamine, and a noncompetitive NMDA antagonist, memantine. Trials have shown the most benefit for these drugs in Alzheimer disease; however, even in this setting, the benefit is only modest in terms of slowing or reversing cognitive decline. Donepezil has FDA indications for the treatment of mild to severe Alzheimer disease. Rivastigmine and galantamine have indications for the treatment of mild to moderate Alzheimer disease while memantine has FDA indication only for the treatment of moderate to severe disease. Memantine can be used in combination with a cholinesterase inhibitor medication.*

REFERENCES

1. Alzheimer's Association. 2017 Alzheimer's disease facts and figures. *Alzheimers Dement.* 2017;13(4):325-374.
2. Daviglus ML, Plassman BL, Pirzada A, et al. Risk factors and preventive interventions for Alzheimer disease: state of the science. *Arch Neurol.* 2011;68(9):1185-1190.
3. Fick DM, Kolanowski AM, Waller JL, Inouye SK. Delirium superimposed on dementia in a community-dwelling managed care population: a 3-year retrospective study of occurrence, costs, and utilization. *J Gerontol.* 2005;60A(6):748-753.
4. Knopman DS, DeKosky ST, Cummings JL, et al. Practice parameter: diagnosis of dementia (an evidence-based review). Report of the Quality Standards Subcommittee of the American Academy of Neurology. *Neurology.* 2001;56(9):1143-1153.
5. Leslie DL, Marcantionio ER, Zhang Y, et al. One-year health care costs associated with delirium in the elderly population. *Arch Intern Med.* 2008;168(1):27-32.
6. Lundstrom M, Edlund A, Bucht G, Karlsson S, Gustafson Y. Dementia after delirium in patients with femoral neck fractures. *JAGS.* 2003;51:1002-1006.
7. Lixouriotis C, Peritogiannis V. Delirium in the primary care setting. *Psychiatry Clin Neurosci.* 2011;65:102-104. doi:10.1111/j.1440-1819.2010.02165.x.
8. Moga DC, Roberts M, Jicha M. Dementia for the primary care provider. *Prim Care Clin Office Pract.* 2017;44:439-456. doi:10.1016/j.pop.2017.04.005.
9. Price RW. HIV-associated neurocognitive disorders: epidemiology, clinical manifestations, and diagnosis. In: Bartlett JG, Bloom A, eds. *UpToDate.* Feb 2017. https://www.uptodate.com/contents/hiv-associated-neurocognitive-disorders-epidemiology-clinical-manifestations-and-diagnosis.
10. Reus VI, FOchtmann LJ, Eyler AE, et al. The American Psychiatric Association Practice Guideline on the use of antipsychotics to treat agitation or psychosis in patients with dementia. *Am J Psychiatry.* 2016;173(5):543-544.
11. Schneider LS, Dagerman KS, Insel P. Risk of death with atypical antipsychotic drug treatment for dementia. *JAMA.* 2005;294(15):1934-1943.
12. Setters B, Solberg L. Delirium. *Prim Care Clin Office Pract.* 2017;44:541-559. doi:10.1016/j.pop.2017.04.010.

13

SUBSTANCE USE DISORDERS—ALCOHOL

Eleasa A. Sokolski, MD, Simone T. Lew, MD, MS, Craig R. Keenan, MD, and Martin H. Leamon, MD

CLINICAL HIGHLIGHTS

- Problematic alcohol use is widespread, costly, and under-recognized by primary care providers.
- Screening tools such as the NIAAA Single Question Screen, AUDIT, or AUDIT-C questionnaires should be used in the primary care setting, as they are efficient in identifying patients with risky alcohol use.
- Management strategies for alcohol use disorders (AUDs) share similarities with those of other chronic illnesses and treatment should be individually tailored in a stepwise fashion.
- The mainstays of AUD treatment are behavioral interventions, but effective adjunctive medications are underutilized in primary care settings.
- Brief intervention for at-risk alcohol use has been extensively studied. It is effective in primary care settings and can be delivered in as little as four 15-minute sessions.
- Benzodiazepines are not effective treatment for AUD and can undermine treatment goals. Benzodiazepines do have an important role in alcohol withdrawal management.

CLINICAL SIGNIFICANCE

Alcohol use disorder (AUD) is one of the most common psychiatric disorders in the United States with a prevalence of 29% in adults 18 years and older.[1] AUD is associated with significant morbidity and mortality and has social, economic, and personal consequences for patients, their families, and society. The rate of AUD is similar to that of other primary care conditions such as hypertension and diabetes mellitus; however, it is identified and treated at only one-fourth the rate of similarly prevalent illnesses.[2] Alcohol use is responsible for almost 100,000 deaths and nearly $249 billion in direct and indirect costs each year.[3,4]

DIAGNOSIS

Alcohol use can be described along a heuristic spectrum from moderate drinking, to at-risk drinking, to AUD. According to the National Institute on Alcohol Abuse and Alcoholism (NIAAA), the standard drink (1.5 oz liquor, 12 oz beer, or 5 oz table wine) contains 12 to 14 g of ethanol, raising blood ethanol levels to about 0.08 gm/dL in a typical 150-lb. man.[5] "Moderate drinking" is no more than 7 drinks per week or 1 drink per occasion for all persons aged 65 years or older; no more than 7 drinks per week or 3 drinks per occasion for younger women; and no more than 14 drinks per week or 4 drinks per occasion for younger men. For pregnant women, no level of alcohol use is considered healthy. Drinking that exceeds the NIAAA guidelines is "at-risk" or "heavy" drinking and puts patients at risk for multiple alcohol-related health problems, including cardiovascular disease and several forms of cancer.[4]

ALCOHOL USE DISORDER

As with the other substance use disorders (SUDs), the 2013 *Diagnostic and Statistical Manual of Mental Disorders, Fifth Edition* (DSM-5), changed the classification of alcohol-use disorders from the mutually exclusive diagnoses of alcohol dependence and alcohol abuse to a single, continuous AUD rated as mild, moderate, or severe (*Table 13-1*).[6] One in four persons who are "at-risk" drinkers will meet criteria for AUD. Diagnosis of AUD is not based on the specific amount or pattern of a patient's drinking, but on the resulting multidimensional behavioral impairment and emotional distress. Of note, because of differences in classification systems, alcohol use that does not reach the threshold for DSM-5 AUD, but exceeds NIAAA guidelines, can be classified in the World Health Organization's International Classification of Diseases, 10th edition (ICD-10), as "alcohol use, unspecified" (code F10.9).

TABLE 13-1 DSM-5 Criteria for Alcohol Use Disorder

Diagnostic criteria for alcohol use disorder include:

A. A problematic pattern of alcohol use leading to clinically significant impairment or distress, as manifested by at least two of the following, occurring within a 12-month period:

  1. Alcohol is often taken in larger amounts or over a longer period than was intended.
  2. There is a persistent desire or unsuccessful efforts to cut down or control alcohol use.
  3. A great deal of time is spent in activities necessary to obtain alcohol, use alcohol, or recover from its effects.
  4. Craving, or a strong desire or urge, to use alcohol.
  5. Recurrent alcohol use resulting in a failure to fulfill major role obligations at work, school, or home.
  6. Continued alcohol use despite having persistent or recurrent social or interpersonal problems caused or exacerbated by the effects of alcohol.
  7. Important social, occupational, or recreational activities are given up or reduced because of alcohol use.
  8. Recurrent alcohol use in situations in which it is physically hazardous.
  9. Alcohol use is continued despite knowledge of having a persistent or recurrent physical or psychological problem that is likely to have been caused or exacerbated by alcohol.
  10. Tolerance, as defined by either of the following:
      a. A need for markedly increased amounts of alcohol to achieve intoxication or desired effect.
      b. A markedly diminished effect with continued use of the same amount of alcohol.
  11. Withdrawal, as manifested by either of the following:
      a. The characteristic withdrawal syndrome for alcohol.
      b. Alcohol (or a closely related substance, such as a benzodiazepine) is taken to relieve or avoid withdrawal symptoms.

Specify if:

In early remission: After full criteria for alcohol use disorder were previously met, none of the criteria for alcohol use disorder have been met for at least 3 months but for less than 12 months (with the exception that criterion A4, craving, or a strong desire or urge to use alcohol, may be met).

In sustained remission: After full criteria for alcohol use disorder were previously met, none of the criteria for alcohol use disorder have been met at any time during a period of 12 months or longer (with the exception that criterion A4, craving, or a strong desire or urge to use alcohol, may be met).

Specify current severity:

Mild: Presence of two to three symptoms.
Moderate: Presence of four to five symptoms.
Severe: Presence of six or more symptoms.

Reprinted with permission from American Psychiatric Association. Diagnostic and Statistical Manual of Mental Disorders. 5th ed. Arlington, VA: American Psychiatric Association; 2013:490-491. Copyright ©2013 American Psychiatric Association. All Rights Reserved.

ALCOHOL WITHDRAWAL

Alcohol withdrawal, while usually mild, can be life-threatening. Withdrawal typically begins 6 to 12 hours after stopping or reducing alcohol use, peaks at 48 to 72 hours, and resolves by the 5 to 7th day (*Table 13-2*).[7] Alcohol withdrawal symptoms stem from unsuppressed excitatory neuronal activity and may include diaphoresis, tachycardia, peripheral tremor, anxiety, insomnia, nausea, vomiting, restlessness, and transient hallucinations or illusions. Although patients with mild symptoms of alcohol withdrawal may be managed as outpatients, patients at risk for developing severe withdrawal symptoms such as seizures or alcohol withdrawal delirium (delirium tremens, DTs) should be managed in the hospital.[8]

ALCOHOL WITHDRAWAL SEIZURES

Withdrawal seizures are generally tonic–clonic and, other than the temporal relationship to alcohol cessation, are clinically indistinguishable from other tonic–clonic seizures. They appear 6 to 48 hours after the last drink and are caused by central neuronal rebound hyperactivity. Patients typically have a single seizure, but can have

TABLE 13-2 Timing of Alcohol Withdrawal

SYNDROME	TIME SINCE LAST DRINK (H)
Mild withdrawal symptoms	6-36
Seizures	6-48
Alcoholic hallucinosis	12-48
Delirium tremens	48-96

Reprinted from Long D , Long B, Koyfman A. The emergency medicine management of severe alcohol withdrawal. Am J Emerg Med. 2017;35(7):1005-1011. Copyright © 2017 Elsevier. With permission.

multiple. Up to 3% develop status epilepticus. Recurrent or prolonged seizures should prompt an investigation for other potential causes. The risk of developing alcohol withdrawal seizures increases with number of times a patient has experienced symptomatic alcohol withdrawal. Once alcohol withdrawal seizures resolve, ongoing prophylaxis is rarely required apart from treatment of the AUD itself.

ALCOHOLIC HALLUCINOSIS

In alcoholic hallucinosis, hallucinations develop within 12 to 24 hours of abstinence and resolve within 24 to 48 hours. These are typically visual hallucinations, but tactile and auditory hallucinations can occur. Reality-testing may remain intact. The patient's sensorium is otherwise clear, which differentiates hallucinosis from DTs, which occur later and include global clouding of the sensorium.

ALCOHOL WITHDRAWAL DELIRIUM/DELIRIUM TREMENS

DTs occur in about 5% of alcohol withdrawals with a mortality rate of up to 5%.[8] DTs are characterized by altered consciousness that includes disorientation, confusion, agitation, hallucinations, and signs of severe autonomic instability (including tremor, hypertension, diaphoresis, tachycardia, and fever). Symptoms may appear within 2 weeks of abstinence, but usually 48 to 96 hours after the last drink. Risk factors for DTs include concurrent acute medical illness, daily heavy drinking, a previous history of DTs or withdrawal seizures, and age over 30 years.[9] Patients at high risk for alcohol withdrawal seizures or DTs require immediate triage at an emergency department. Those with DTs need fluid and electrolyte replacement and intravenous benzodiazepine therapy and often require close monitoring in an intensive care unit.

SCREENING AND ASSESSMENT

Primary care providers are well poised to detect at-risk drinking and AUD. The U.S. Preventive Services Task Force recommends alcohol use screening for all adults aged 18 years or older.[10] Although there are many validated screening tools available, the NIAAA Single Question screen, the AUDIT, and the abbreviated AUDIT-Consumption (AUDIT-C) have been shown to have good sensitivity and specificity for detecting at-risk drinking and AUDs across varied populations.

The NIAAA Single-Question Screen (*Table 13-3*) is the simplest. The patient is asked, "How many times in the past year have you had X or more drinks in a day?" (X = 5 for men, 4 for women, irrespective of age.) A response of 1 or more is a positive screen. In the primary care setting, the Single Question was found to be 81% sensitive and 79.3% specific for either of risky drinking or AUD and was 87.9% sensitive and 66.8% specific for current AUD.[11] For the busy clinician, it provides an effective, efficient screen.

The AUDIT is a 10-question screening test developed by the World Health Organization and takes about 5 minutes to complete (*Table 13-4*). Patients can complete the AUDIT in the waiting room. In primary care settings, the AUDIT has a sensitivity of 84% to 85% and specificity of 77% to 84% for detecting both at-risk drinking and AUD.[12] The AUDIT-C (*Table 13-3*) uses only the first three "consumption" questions of the AUDIT and

TABLE 13-3 Brief Screening Instruments

NIAAA SINGLE QUESTION SCREENING

Question	"How many times in the past year have you had X or more drinks in a day?" (X = 5 for men, 4 for women)
Scoring	More than 1 instance is a positive screen

AUDIT-C

	POINTS				
Questions	**0**	**1**	**2**	**3**	**4**
1. How often did you have a drink containing alcohol in the past year?	Never	Monthly or less	2-4 times a month	2-3 times a week	4 or more times a week
2. How many drinks did you have on a typical day when you were drinking in the past year?	None, or 1-2	3-4	5-6	7-9	10 or more
3. How often did you have five or more drinks on one occasion in the past year?	Never	Less than monthly	Monthly	Weekly	Daily or almost daily
Scoring	A score of ≥6 for men and ≥4 for women is considered positive and warrants further investigation.				

National Institute on Alcohol Abuse and Alcoholism. Helping Patients Who Drink Too Much: A Clinician's Guide; 2008. https://www.niaaa.nih.gov/guide. Accessed January 10, 2017. This questionnaire (the AUDIT) is reprinted with permission from the World Health Organization.

TABLE 13-4 AUDIT

QUESTIONS	POINTS				
	0	1	2	3	4
1. How often do you have a drink containing alcohol in the past year?	Never	Monthly or less	2-4 times a month	2-3 times a week	4 or more times a week
2. How many drinks containing alcohol do you have on a typical day when you are drinking?	1-2	3-4	5-6	7-9	10 or more
3. How often do you have five or more drinks on one occasion?	Never	Less than monthly	Monthly	Weekly	Daily or almost daily
4. How often during the last year have you found that you were not able to stop drinking once you started?	Never	Less than monthly	Monthly	Weekly	Daily or almost daily
5. How often during the last year have you failed to do what was normally expected of you because of drinking?	Never	Less than monthly	Monthly	Weekly	Daily or almost daily
6. How often during the last year have you needed a first drink in the morning to get yourself going after a heavy drinking session?	Never	Less than monthly	Monthly	Weekly	Daily or almost daily
7. How often during the last year have you had a feeling of guilt or remorse after drinking?	Never	Less than monthly	Monthly	Weekly	Daily or almost daily
8. How often during the last year have you been unable to remember what happened the night before because of your drinking?	Never	Less than monthly	Monthly	Weekly	Daily or almost daily
9. Have you or someone else been injured because of your drinking?	No		Yes, but not in the last year		Yes, during the last year
10. Has a relative, friend, doctor, or other health care worker been concerned about your drinking or suggested you cut down?	No		Yes, but not in the last year		Yes, during the last year
Scoring	Add up points from all 10 items. A total score ≥8 for men younger than 60 years, and ≥4 for women, adolescents, and men older than 60 years is positive, warranting further investigation.				

National Institute on Alcohol Abuse and Alcoholism. Helping Patients Who Drink Too Much: A Clinician's Guide; 2008. https://www.niaaa.nih.gov/guide. Accessed January 10, 2017. This questionnaire (the AUDIT) is reprinted with permission from the World Health Organization.

takes 1 to 2 minutes to complete. It has a sensitivity of 74% to 76% and specificity of 64% to 83% for detecting both at-risk drinking and AUD.

Although the CAGE questionnaire has historically been used in primary care settings to screen for alcohol-related problems, it has a lower sensitivity and specificity compared with the above-mentioned methods and is no longer recommended.

Without using screening tools, AUDs are often overlooked in clinical settings, and even so, detection requires a high index of suspicion.[10] Certain clinical conditions and findings should trigger further assessment (*Table 13-5*). Typical clues may include co-occurring psychiatric symptoms such as anxiety, depression, irritability, panic attacks, impaired concentration, and persistent insomnia. There is a high prevalence of co-occurrence with other SUDs, including tobacco use disorders. Physical symptoms may include malaise, fatigue, headaches, loss of consciousness, amnesia, heartburn, hematemesis, jaundice, erectile dysfunction, hemorrhoids, and paresthesias or neuropathic pain. Several medical conditions are commonly associated with alcohol use: gastroesophageal reflux disease, peripheral neuropathy, hypertension, and pancreatitis.[9] Alcohol use is also implicated as a factor in a large percentage of sexually transmitted infections and unintended pregnancies.

TABLE 13-5 Clinical Clues for Alcohol Use Disorders

Commonly associated conditions	Dilated cardiomyopathy Erectile dysfunction Alcohol-related hepatitis Hepatic encephalopathy Hepatitis B and C Hypertension Malnutrition states Neuropathy Pancreatitis Pneumonia (especially Legionnaire Disease) Tuberculosis Sexually transmitted infections Unintended pregnancy
Social history	Multiple traumatic injuries Recent arrest for driving while intoxicated Arrests for property damage Sudden change in behavior Erratic occupational history Domestic violence
Physical examination findings	Weight changes with muscle atrophy Shrunken, firm liver Hepatomegaly Splenomegaly Jaundice, scleral icterus Ascites Hemorrhoids Spider angiomata Caput medusa Palmar erythema Cognitive impairment

Asking how a patient deals with life's challenges or emotional distress may uncover alcohol use as a maladaptive coping mechanism. Unstable interpersonal relationships or work history is common in AUD. Lack of response of general medical problems to usual therapies or chronic difficulties with medication adherence should alert the provider to screen for problematic alcohol use. Skillful interviewing with confidence, empathy, expectancy and a nonjudgmental stance will normalize questions about alcohol use and facilitate soliciting open and more complete information from the patient.[5] The provider may ask about the overall role and function of alcohol for the patient (e.g., "How has alcohol benefited or harmed you"? or "Has alcohol affected your relationships with family and close friends?"). There may also be a history of alcohol-related problems in first-degree relatives. The mental status examination of someone who is suspected of suffering from AUD may reveal anxious, depressed, or irritable moods; psychomotor changes; cognitive slowing; defensiveness or suspiciousness; and impaired insight and judgment. Slurred speech, mood/affect lability, or the characteristic smell of exhaled partly metabolized alcohol may indicate current intoxication. Tachycardia, hypertension, tremulousness, and/or diaphoresis may be signs of withdrawal.

In addition to the history and physical examination, laboratory studies may suggest an AUD via association with heavy prolonged alcohol consumption but are usually not diagnostic because of lack of specificity. One exception is ethyl glucuronide, an ethanol conjugate that can be detected in the urine for up to 5 days following drinking, depending on amount consumed and individual factors. It is readily detected in the lab or via point-of-care testing and its presence is indicative of recent alcohol use. It is both more sensitive and specific than either the older carbohydrate-deficient transferrin or gamma-glutamyl transferase (GGT) tests, so it can be useful in monitoring sobriety.[9]

DIFFERENTIAL DIAGNOSIS

Alcohol use symptoms may mimic mood or anxiety disorders and those of alcohol withdrawal may resemble anxiety or psychotic disorders. Although alcohol use is far more common than illicit drug use, there is a high rate of co-occurring use, so the presence of one should trigger screening for the other. Moreover, co-occurring substance use and other psychiatric disorders are so common as to be considered "the rule rather than the exception." After adjustment for sociodemographic variables, the National Epidemiological Survey found that AUD is most highly associated with bipolar disorders, major depressive disorder, antisocial and borderline personality disorders.[1] Alcohol-related mood or anxiety disorders typically resolve within 3 to 4 weeks following cessation of alcohol use, although a lower level dysphoria and malaise can be longer lasting. An independent, co-occurring psychiatric disorder may be diagnosed based on a clear history of its presence during earlier sustained periods of sobriety, or diagnosis may require serial observations of mood and behavior for 3 to 4 weeks after cessation of substance use.[13]

BIOPSYCHOSOCIAL TREATMENT

Although individual disease course can vary widely, AUD, at least when moderate to severe, is probably best conceptualized as a chronic medical disorder, and a biopsychosocial treatment approach should be utilized. Although long-term cessation of alcohol use may be the best long-term therapeutic goal, a patient's stage of readiness to change may indicate the need for other interim goals, such as increasing awareness, enhancing motivation for change, supporting self-efficacy, and realistic treatment planning based on availability of resources. Biological treatment includes withdrawal management for patients who are at high risk for moderate to severe withdrawal symptoms. Subsequently, pharmacologic agents may be added for maintenance treatment and relapse prevention as an adjunct to psychosocial treatment. Psychosocial interventions include community self-help programs, supportive therapy, brief intervention, cognitive behavioral therapy (CBT), motivation-based treatments, family therapy, residential or vocational rehabilitation, and sober living community homes.[13]

PHARMACOTHERAPY

Withdrawal Management

Medication can be used to reduce the more severe symptoms of alcohol withdrawal and to prevent withdrawal seizures or DTs. It is much more difficult to treat severe withdrawal than it is to initiate treatment to prevent it. Although other options are available, the benzodiazepines are most commonly used.[7-9] A benzodiazepine is substituted for the alcohol and the dose is gradually tapered. Although longer-acting agents such as chlordiazepoxide or diazepam are generally preferred because of a smoother withdrawal course, lorazepam or oxazepam may be indicated in patients with advanced liver disease as there is less risk of serum accumulation and resultant sedation or delirium. For patients under close monitoring, such an inpatient setting, the well-validated revised Clinical Institute Withdrawal Assessment for Alcohol (CIWA-Ar) may be used to monitor and treat withdrawal. Provider and staff training are required to ensure proper use of the instrument, which guides benzodiazepine dosing based on signs and symptom severity. Other treatment protocols call for a benzodiazepine loading dose to completely suppress withdrawal signs and symptoms, with the dose reduced on a scheduled taper over 4 to 7 days. The dose and duration of the benzodiazepine treatment generally correlates with a patient's tolerance to alcohol.

For a patient with a history of withdrawal seizures or comorbid seizure disorders, anticonvulsants such as phenytoin, carbamazepine, or valproic acid may be added. All patients with heavy alcohol use should be closely monitored for volume and electrolyte abnormalities and given multivitamin, thiamine, and folate supplements.

Stable, motivated patients with mild-to-moderate withdrawal symptoms can be managed in the outpatient setting as long as there is available support at home to monitor progress, ready access to an outpatient provider to supervise the care, and no history of severe alcohol withdrawal or seizures.[14] A growing body of evidence demonstrates that gabapentin can be used for outpatient treatment of mild-to-moderate acute alcohol withdrawal. A randomized double-blind trial of gabapentin versus lorazepam found that a 4-day gabapentin taper effectively treated mild-to-moderate alcohol withdrawal, and that the patients treated with gabapentin versus lorazepam had a lower risk of drinking during the 12-day study.[15] However, complicated cases of alcohol withdrawal that involve progressively worsening symptoms must be treated in an inpatient setting equipped to manage severe complications.

Maintenance Therapy

Maintenance medication to reduce relapse should always be combined adjunctively with psychosocial interventions (*Table 13-6*). Drugs approved by the FDA for AUDs include the opioid antagonist naltrexone, the glutamate and NMDA receptor antagonist acamprosate, and the acetaldehyde dehydrogenase inhibitor disulfiram.

Naltrexone is available in an oral form (Revia) and a long-acting injectable form (Vivitrol) but cannot be used in patients receiving opioids or in severe liver disease. Acamprosate does not have drug–drug interactions with alcohol, diazepam, or naltrexone but may require dose adjustment in patients with severe kidney impairment. Disulfiram blocks the normal metabolism of alcohol, leading to the accumulation of a toxic alcohol metabolite that causes severe discomfort (e.g., nausea, vomiting, flushing, hypotension, and tachycardia), so the medication must be used with caution in patients with cardiovascular or advanced liver disease.

In several clinical trials, both naltrexone and acamprosate have shown modest efficacy for maintaining abstinence or reducing heavy drinking, but their effectiveness is more variable when translated into clinical practice.[13] In 2006, a large trial of nearly 1,400 patients compared 16 weeks of naltrexone and acamprosate, alone or in combination, and with or without specialist behavioral treatments. All groups were compared with a control group that received specialist behavioral treatment alone. In this study, naltrexone monotherapy and behavioral monotherapy were shown to have the most robust success in achieving abstinence at 16 weeks and were equivalent to combined naltrexone and specialist behavioral therapy.[16] At 1 year, however, even the best treatment had over 75% rate of return to heavy drinking, perhaps illustrating the notion that most chronic conditions usually worsen if treatment is discontinued.

Antidepressants, anticonvulsants, and antipsychotics have also been studied for the prevention of alcohol relapse in patients with and without co-occurring psychiatric disorders. For example, topiramate titrated to 300 mg/day has been shown to be effective in reducing alcohol relapse (as measured by percentage of heavy drinking days and serum GGT) in a 14-week randomized, placebo-controlled study. Topiramate may be used off-label, at 200 or 300 mg total daily dose, with a slow titration generally over several weeks to reduce the risk of cognitive side effects.[13]

Gabapentin, which modulates γ-aminobutyric acid (GABA) and glutamate neurotransmitters, titrated to divided doses of 900 to 1,800 mg per day can reduce relapse and may be combined with naltrexone to improve outcomes such as longer time to relapse, increased time to first heavy drinking day, decreased drinks per drinking day, and decreased craving. Gabapentin may also reduce postwithdrawal insomnia, which has been associated with increased risk of relapse.

As in other chronic illnesses, medication adherence is a major obstacle to the long-term efficacy of pharmacologic treatment. In addition, limited access to and experience with these medications by primary care providers have delayed their widespread use. We recommend naltrexone or acamprosate as first-line treatment for moderate/severe AUD, because of their evidence base, safety profile, and efficacy. The injectable form of naltrexone can be considered in patients with problems adhering to daily oral medications. Gabapentin, which is well-known to primary care providers and has few

TABLE 13-6 Medications for Maintenance Treatment of Alcohol Use Disorders

MEDICATION	DOSAGE AND ADVERSE EFFECTS	SIDE EFFECTS/CAUTION/COMMENTS
Naltrexone (Revia, Vivitrol) • FDA approved	50-100 mg daily, may start 25 mg daily for several days 380 mg IM q4 weeks (intramuscular) Side effects: nausea, headache, insomnia, decreased hedonic drive	• Must be opioid free (opiates, semisynthetics and synthetics) with negative urine opioid test, otherwise may induce full opioid withdrawal. Consider naloxone challenge • Contraindication: active opioid use, pregnancy • Caution in patients with depression, suicidal ideation, thrombocytopenia, acute hepatitis, or liver failure • Baseline evaluation: liver transaminases, opioid urine drug screen, pregnancy test • Pregnancy Category C
Acamprosate (Campral) • FDA approved	666 mg TID, preferably with meals Avoid if creatinine clearance less than 30 mL/minute Side effects: diarrhea, anxiety, asthenia, insomnia	• Pretreatment abstinence may improve response. May be continued despite alcohol relapse • Requires dose adjustment in renal failure • Caution in patients with depression, anxiety. Monitor for suicidal ideation • Baseline evaluation: renal function • Pregnancy Category C
Disulfiram (Antabuse) • FDA approved	250 mg/day, range 125-500 mg daily Side effects: metallic taste, headache, hepatotoxicity, peripheral neuropathy, psychosis, delirium Must avoid alcohol-containing medications and foods	• Must be abstinent from alcohol at least 12 hours and have zero blood alcohol • Toxic reaction of headache, vomiting, malaise, and generalized distress when used with alcohol • Drug interactions with isoniazid and metronidazole, phenytoin, warfarin, oral hypoglycemics • Baseline evaluation: liver transaminases, then monthly ×3, then periodically • Pregnancy Category C
Topiramate (Topamax, Qudexy) • Off-label	50 mg/day, titrate 25-50 mg daily each week to maximum 150 mg BID, to minimize side effects. Taper off if no response in 3 months Side effects: cognitive dysfunction, paresthesia, nervousness, fatigue, ataxia, abdominal pain, decreased effectiveness of oral contraceptives, increased risk of cleft lip/palate during first trimester	• May be continued despite alcohol relapse • Caution in patients with depression, seizure disorder, or pregnancy • Do not suddenly discontinue because of risk of rebound seizures • Baseline evaluation: renal function, pregnancy • Pregnancy Class C
Gabapentin (Neurontin, Horizant, Gralise) • Off-label	*Mild–moderate alcohol withdrawal:* 400 mg TID × 3 days, then 400 mg BID ×1 day, then 400 mg once ×1 day, with additional prn dosing *Maintenance.* Day 1, 300 mg, increase by 300 mg a day to 600 mg TID as tolerated Side effects: dizziness, sedation, nightmares, diarrhea	• Requires dose adjustment in renal failure • Caution in patients with depression and suicidal ideation • Abuse potential at supratherapeutic doses. Monitor usage/prescribing patterns • Baseline evaluation: renal function • Pregnancy Category C

Modified from Department of Veterans Affairs. Management of substance use disorder (SUD) (2015)—VA/DoD clinical practice guidelines; 2015. https://www.healthquality.va.gov/guidelines/mh/sud/. Accessed October 1, 2017.
BID, twice daily; IM, intramuscular; TID, three times daily.

drug–drug interactions and serious side effects, has also been shown to be safe and effective for alcohol maintenance therapy, although there are some case reports of it being misused itself. Topiramate requires a long initial titration but may be useful where the medication will also address co-occurring disorders or where medication adherence is sound. Finally, psychosocial treatments are widely regarded as foundational for long-term relapse prevention. Therefore, even with provision of medication, the primary care provider should encourage and facilitate a patient's participation in psychosocial treatment.[13]

PSYCHOSOCIAL TREATMENT

The evidence base for the impact of psychosocial interventions and the psychotherapies in the reduction of at-risk drinking and in the treatment of AUDs is robust and well-established.

Brief Intervention

Brief intervention, in 10 to 15-minute repeated sessions in the primary care setting, is effective for reducing at-risk drinking, although probably not for treatment of

TABLE 13-7 Brief Intervention for Alcohol Use Disorders (AUDs)

STEPS	COMMENTS	SAMPLE STATEMENTS
1. Assessment and direct feedback	• Ask about alcohol use (screen) • Provide education and feedback on connections between alcohol use and legal, occupational, or relationship problems	• Your liver disease is probably related to alcohol use. Would you like some information about hepatitis and alcohol? • I am concerned about your drinking and how it's affecting your health
2. Goal setting	• Individually tailored goals based on collaboration between the patient and the provider • Goals may change depending on readiness for change • Goals should be realistic and include psychotherapy, social support, and use of medications when indicated	• What are your thoughts about alcohol use? • Although I would advise sobriety, how realistic is that? • Although medications are important in your recovery, it is critical to attend AA and to learn how to avoid relapse triggers
3. Behavioral modification	• Identify situational triggers, finding other enjoyable activities and adaptive coping skills • Includes relapse prevention	• What triggers your drinking? • What else can you do when you feel alone, stressed, or frustrated? • Who can you talk to for support in cutting down?
4. Self-help	• Encourage self-discipline and increased self-awareness about AUD	• Would you like the following information booklet about alcohol addiction? • Do you know where you can get help for your drinking problem?
5. Follow-up and reinforcement	• Often considered most important aspect of treatment plan • Provide praise, reassurance, and encouragement during periods of sobriety • Returning to appointment is a sign of patient motivation and effort, even if relapse occurs	• I'm very glad to see you come back to talk more about your alcohol use • How did your plan to stop or reduce your drinking work?

Adapted from National Institute on Alcohol Abuse and Alcoholism. *Helping Patients Who Drink Too Much: A Clinician's Guide; 2008. https://www.niaaa.nih.gov/guide.* Accessed January 10, 2017.

full AUD. Despite the evidence, it remains to be widely disseminated and consistently implemented. The key elements of brief intervention include nonjudgmental assessment and the provision of ongoing education and feedback using a patient-specific motivational approach (*Table 13-7*).[5] Once the patient's personal goals are identified (e.g., cession or reduction of drinking), then the provider may help the patient identify a plan of action. Further feedback and refinement of goals and action plans are then addressed on follow-up, either telephonically or at the next visit. The screening and brief intervention can be coupled with referral to treatment for patients with diagnosed AUDs, although this may be less effective than initiating medication management with one of the aforementioned maintenance medications.[17]

Motivational Interventions Combined with Pharmacotherapy

Motivational interventions are adapted from motivational interviewing, a caring, nonconfrontational, persuasive counseling style that elicits long-standing behavioral change. Although there are formal psychotherapies for AUD based on motivational principles such as motivational enhancement therapy, motivational techniques can be incorporated into routine medication management of AUD. Nonjudgmental medication management has been shown to be effective in patients with only AUD and in those with combined AUD and opioid use disorders.

Self-help and 12-Step Programs

A variety of self-help, patient initiated programs employ learning, acceptance, change, and support when combating alcohol and substance dependence with the eventual goal of achieving abstinence. The oldest and most well-known of these programs is Alcoholics Anonymous (AA), and more frequent attendance at AA has been shown to be associated with improved outcomes.[18] AA is a fellowship of men and women where the primary purpose is for members to help other members stay sober.[19] The only requirement for membership is "the desire to stay sober." AA regards alcoholism as an irreversible lifelong disease with physical, psychological, and spiritual aspects and regards total abstinence as part of more comprehensive personal and social recovery. The Twelve Steps of AA describe one possible sequence for the process. In the first step, members admit that they are "powerless over alcohol" and that their lives had become "unmanageable."[20] Subsequent steps include acknowledging and making amends for past harms, and admitting to new mistakes when they occur. The twelfth step encourages members to pass on lessons learned to other individuals who have AUD. Although AA emphasizes spirituality, this focus can vary from group to group, and the factors responsible for therapeutic change in members are similar to those active in other nonspiritually based interventions.[21] Other self-help groups that are less widespread include Life Ring and Smart Recovery (both have a more cognitive approach), Celebrate Recovery (explicitly Christian), and Refuge Recovery (explicitly Buddhist). Most groups have Internet resources that link to local meeting schedules.

Family and Community Programs

Social stability, such as full-time employment and supportive networks of friends and family, is associated with good overall outcomes in those with AUDs. With the patient's consent, family and friends can help facilitate access to community resources and act as chaperones or "sponsors" to whom the patient must be accountable. Moreover, family and friends often serve as the key source of support and motivation to maintain sobriety and will usually prompt their loved one to consider treatment after a relapse. When maladaptive family dynamics precede or contribute to AUDs, couples and family therapy should be considered to address issues of anger, guilt, and shame that often interfere with sobriety. Family and loved ones often struggle alone and would benefit from involvement in support groups such as Al-Anon. For a patient who is unemployed or has minimal psychosocial support, it is reasonable to encourage participation in a therapeutic community or a substance use disorder treatment program that provides a supportive environment, housing, and vocational rehabilitation.

OTHER TREATMENT CONSIDERATIONS

Preventing and Addressing Relapse

Although often stigmatized and misunderstood by patients and support networks alike, relapse of alcohol use after cessation is not unexpected in long-term management. Common precipitants of relapse include use of other substances, a return to substance-using friends, substance-associated sexual behavior, depression, anxiety, and craving for alcohol.[13] These triggers need to be discussed openly and directly with patients early in treatment. Ideally, the clinician and patient collaboratively identify patient-specific triggers and create a prevention plan to address such situations when they arise. The plan may encourage the patient to use proactive strategies such as self-imposed alcohol reduction or cessation while in a supportive environment, calling a "sponsor" or similarly knowledgeable and supportive person, acknowledging relapse in the treatment setting, and staying away from people, places, and things that have been tied to past alcohol use. If a relapse does occur, patients should be encouraged to use it as an opportunity for self-evaluation of treatment goals, evaluation of

the efficacy of treatment, identification and recognition of triggers associated with misuse, and reassessment of comorbid medical and psychiatric disorders.

Treatment of Comorbid Psychiatric Disorders (Co-occurring Disorders)

Studies have shown that other nonsubstance-induced psychiatric disorders frequently co-occur with alcohol and SUDs.[1] Co-occurring disorders can create serious morbidities and complications for treatment. For patients with comorbid psychiatric disorders, simultaneous treatment of both the AUD and the co-occurring psychiatric disorder will produce better outcomes than either sequential or split treatment.[13] Treatment of the co-occurring disorder should not be delayed because of concerns about therapeutic futility, and while not advised and each patient must be individually considered, there are often only limited interactions between alcohol and major psychiatric medications such as antidepressants, antipsychotics, or mood stabilizers. In more difficult cases where diagnostic uncertainty is high, consultation with a psychiatrist or an addiction medicine specialist should be considered.

WHEN TO REFER

- Continued alcohol use despite a reasonable primary care intervention (e.g., failure to respond in 3 to 4 months)
- Need for specific psychosocial treatments (AA, CBT, MET, support groups, couples and family therapy, or a therapeutic community)
- Diagnosis and treatment of complex comorbid psychiatric disorders
- Suicidal intent or worsening psychiatric symptoms

CASES AND QUESTIONS

CASE 1:

Mary is a 43-year-old software engineer with a history of hepatitis C and hypertension who presents for a blood pressure check and to discuss treatment options for hepatitis C. She divorced 1 year ago and has one adult son who is estranged from her. She reports a history of intravenous heroin use ending more than 8 years ago (and still attends an occasional Narcotics Anonymous meeting), smokes two packs of cigarettes per day, and drinks 3 to 4 12 oz beers each evening, but not more than that. Her physical examination is unremarkable except for a blood pressure of 165/95 mm Hg, heart rate of 108 beats per minute, a moderate bilateral hand tremor. Alanine aminotransferase (ALT) and aspartate aminotransferase (AST) are mildly elevated at 100 units/liter and 80 units/liter respectively, which worries her.

continued

1. What is Mary's AUDIT-C score?

   A. 1
   B. 2
   C. 3
   D. 5
   E. 7

   Correct answer: D. *She drinks nightly (4 points), 3 to 4 drinks (1 point), never 5 or more (0 points). Because the cutoff score for women is 4 points, her alcohol use bears further assessment.*

2. What is the significance of her elevation in transaminase levels?

   A. It is because of her alcohol use.
   B. It is because of her Hepatitis C.
   C. Her concern about it may help motivate her to change her alcohol use.
   D. It is because of hypertensive nephropathy.
   E. It is an incidental finding and is not relevant.

   Correct answer: C. *The transaminase pattern of AST/ALT >1 would be consistent with alcohol-related problems, but in the presence of Hepatitis C, is too nonspecific to be useful diagnostically. In delivering a Brief Intervention, it's best to link patient findings and concerns to alcohol (or substance) use, so the physician could say something like, "You're right to be worried. While it's nonspecific, the blood tests indicate that the combination of hepatitis and your drinking may not be good for your liver. Have you considered drinking less?"*

3. What is the significance of her presumptive heroin use disorder in full sustained remission?

   A. It puts her at increased risk for other SUDs.
   B. It puts her at risk for return to heroin use.
   C. She may be able to use similar coping skills to help change her drinking.
   D. She may be able to utilize existing sobriety social supports to help change her drinking.
   E. All of the above.

   Correct answer: E. *The presence of one SUD (even tobacco use disorder) puts one at increased risk for other SUDs, and because SUDs are best conceptualized as chronic diseases, the possibility of relapse should always be kept in mind, even after years of recovery, if relapse triggers and stressors arrive. Although some 12-Step groups will be monosubstance focused, most groups would encourage discussion of other substances, so Mary should be asked if she's brought up her drinking in her NA group, and, if appropriate, encouraged to do so or to increase her involvement in NA if she wants to reduce her drinking. One of the amethystic medications could be recommended as well.*

CASE 2:

Michael is a 55-year-old accountant who presents to his primary care provider complaining of depression. He has a long history of heavy alcohol use resulting in poor work performance and a recent arrest for driving under the influence of alcohol. He used to drink five to seven 20-oz beers per night (heavier over the last 5 years) including drinking in the morning before work. His last drink was 2 weeks ago before the traffic stop. He is ashamed of his arrest has begun attending AA groups by court mandate, although he doesn't like going. He also has to provide random urine samples for drug and ethyl glucuronide testing. Since then he's had increased depressed mood, low energy and poor concentration at home and at work, restlessness, insomnia, and increasing anxiety without any provocations. He denies any suicidal ideation. He reports that his relationship with his wife and three children are improving as they are very glad and supportive of his resolution to stop drinking. His was able to tell his boss who was similarly supportive.

The AMPS screening for psychiatric symptoms is negative for any history of hypomania, mania, psychotic symptoms, or anxiety. He smokes about one pack per day of tobacco and notices that his smoking habit may be getting worse since he has stopped drinking. He was sober for 9 years in his 30s, and in the middle of that, had an episode of major depression, successfully treated with psychotherapy and fluoxetine. Family history is significant for AUD in his father and his mother has been treated since his childhood for recurrent depression. His vials are normal and there is no evidence of alcohol withdrawal or intoxication. His mental status examination is notable for a depressed mood and a fully reactive affect.

1. Which of the following are relevant to deciding on an approach to Michael's depressive symptoms?

   A. His symptoms have worsened since he's been sober.
   B. He has a family history of mood disorder.
   C. He has a history of a depressive episode during a period of sobriety.
   D. There is no history of abnormal mood elevation.
   E. All of the above.

   Correct answer: E. *An alcohol-induced depressive disorder would be expected to improve with sobriety, not worsen. A family history of mood disorder increases his risk for mood disorder. The occurrence of a depressive episode during a period of sobriety and the absence of any history of mania or hypomania suggest the diagnosis of major depressive disorder, recurrent.*

2. Which medication would be best to treat the AUD?

   A. Fluoxetine
   B. Naltrexone
   C. Aripiprazole
   D. Clonazepam
   E. Lithium

   Correct answer: B. *Although fluoxetine or aripiprazole may be useful for his depression, they are not indicated for AUD. Lithium might be appropriate if a bipolar disorder were present, but again, for the mood disorder, not the SUD. Benzodiazepines are rarely helpful outside of treating moderate/severe alcohol withdrawal and may trigger cravings and increase relapse risk.*

3. Which type of psychotherapy would be best for Michael at this time?

   A. Twelve-step facilitation therapy (TFT)
   B. Motivational enhancement therapy (MET)
   C. Contingency management (CM)
   D. Interpersonal psychotherapy (IPT)
   E. CBT

   Correct answer: A. *IPT has a good evidence base for the treatment of depression, but not for AUD. CM relies on providing randomized rewards on an escalating reinforcement schedule based on urine drug screens, and with the court-ordered testing, Michael already has another contingency riding on those results. Michael is court-ordered to attend AA but is having difficulty doing so, and TFT is specifically designed to address such issues. Although MET could be an option, as it has been shown to be effective in treating AUD, the ready issue of AA attendance makes TFT a better choice.*

CASE 3:

Robert is a 29-year-old graduate student who asks to have his sertraline renewed, which he's taken for the past 4 years for social anxiety disorder. He reports that the medication works very well for him and he has no side effects. He filled out the AUDIT-C in the clinic waiting room before the appointment, in accordance with usual clinic protocol. He drinks two to three times per week, usually three to four drinks, and will drink five or more drinks per occasion at monthly department social gatherings. He doesn't really keep track of how much he drinks and hasn't had any alcohol-related problems. His other history and examination are unremarkable.

1. What is Robert's AUDIT-C score?

   A. 2
   B. 3
   C. 4
   D. 6
   E. 8

   Correct answer: D. *He drinks three to four drinks two to three times/week (1 point + 3 pints) and binges monthly (2 points). His score of 6 puts him at the cutoff for further assessment of his alcohol use.*

2. What is the best way to characterize Robert's alcohol use?

   A. No characterization is recommended
   B. Alcohol use, unspecified
   C. AUD, mild
   D. AUD, moderate
   E. AUD, severe

   Correct answer: B. *The absence of any other alcohol-related problems rules out an AUD, but he would be classified as a heavy drinker, which should be addressed, and so is worth characterizing in his medical record as the ICD-10 category of alcohol use, unspecified.*

3. What is the next best step in addressing Robert's alcohol use?

   A. Refer to an intensive outpatient program.
   B. Encourage him to attend AA.
   C. Begin acamprosate therapy.
   D. Provide education about drinking norms and ask about motivation to change.
   E. No further intervention at this point, but order blood test for liver transaminases.

   Correct answer: D. *Options A, B, or C might be appropriate if he did have an AUD. Because he does not, he is an ideal candidate for Brief Intervention, which would include providing education about drinking norms and asking about his motivation to decrease his risky alcohol use.*

PRACTICAL RESOURCES

- http://www.niaaa.nih.gov/
- https://www.asam.org/
- https://findtreatment.samhsa.gov
- http://www.aa.org/
- https://al-anon.org/
- http://www.lifering.org
- http://www.smartrecovery.org/

REFERENCES

1. Grant BF, Goldstein RB, Saha TD, et al. Epidemiology of DSM-5 alcohol use disorder: results from the national epidemiologic Survey on alcohol and related conditions III. *JAMA Psychiatry*. 2015;72(8):757-766.

2. National Center for Health Statistics. *Health, United States, 2016, with Chartbook on Long-term Trends in Health*. Hyattsville, MD: US Department of Health and Human Services; 2017.

3. Sacks J, Gonzales K, Bouchery E, et al. 2010 national and state costs of excessive alcohol consumption. *Am J Prev Med*. 2015;49(5):73-79.

4. Centers for Disease Control and Prevention. Alcohol and public health: alcohol-related disease impact (ARDI), average for United States 2006–2010, alcohol-attributable deaths due to excessive alcohol use; 2013. https://nccd. cdc.gov/DPH_ARDI/Default/Report.aspx?T=AAM&P=f-6d7eda7-036e-4553-9968-9b17ffad620e&R=d7a9b303-48e9-4440-bf47-070a4827e1fd&M=8E1C5233-5640-4EE8-9247-1ECA7DA325B9&F=&D=. Accessed October 11, 2017.

5. National Institute on Alcohol Abuse and Alcoholism. Helping patients who drink too much: a clinician's guide; 2008. https://www.niaaa.nih.gov/guide. Accessed January 10, 2017.

6. American Psychiatric Association. *Diagnostic and Statistical Manual of Mental Disorders*. 5th ed. Arlington, VA: American Psychiatric Association; 2013.

7. Long D, Long B, Koyfman A. The emergency medicine management of severe alcohol withdrawal. *Am J Emerg Med*. 2017;35(7):1005-1011.

8. Simpson SA, Wilson MP, Nordstrom K. Psychiatric emergencies for clinicians: emergency department management of alcohol withdrawal. *J Emerg Med*. 2016;51(3):269-273.

9. Jesse S, Bråthen G, Ferrara M, et al. Alcohol withdrawal syndrome: mechanisms, manifestations, and management. *Acta Neurol Scand*. 2017;135(1):4-16.

10. Centers for Disease Control and Prevention. *Planning and Implementing Screening and Brief Intervention for Risky Alcohol Use: A Step-by-step Guide for Primary Care Practices*. Atlanta, Georgia: Centers for Disease Control and Prevention, National Center on Birth Defects and Developmental Disabilities; 2014.

11. Smith PC, Schmidt SM, Allensworth-Davies D, Saitz R. Primary care validation of a single-question alcohol screening test. *J Gen Intern Med*. 2009;24(7):783-788.

12. Babor TF, Higgins-Biddle JC, Saunders JB, Montiero MG. AUDIT: alcohol use disorders identification test. *Guidelines for Use in Primary Care*. 2nd ed. Geneva: World Health Organization; 2001.

13. Department of Veterans Affairs. Management of substance use disorder (SUD) (2015)—VA/DoD clinical practice guidelines; 2015. https://www.healthquality.va.gov/guidelines/mh/sud/. Accessed October 1, 2017.

14. Edelman E, Fiellin DA. Alcohol use. *Ann Intern Med*. 2016;164(1):ITC1-ITC16.

15. Myrick H, Malcolm R, Randall PK, et al. A double-blind trial of gabapentin versus lorazepam in the treatment of alcohol withdrawal. *Alcohol Clin Exp Res*. 2009;33(9):1582-1588.

16. Anton RF, O'Malley SS, Ciraulo DA, et al. Combined pharmacotherapies and behavioral interventions for alcohol dependence: the combine study: a randomized controlled trial. *J Am Med Assoc*. 2006;295(17):2003-2017.

17. Jonas DE, Garbutt JC, Amick HR, et al. Behavioral counseling after screening for alcohol misuse in primary care: a systematic review and meta-analysis for the U.S. preventive services task force. *Ann Intern Med*. 2012;157(9):645-654.

18. Humphreys K, Blodgett JC, Wagner TH. Estimating the efficacy of alcoholics anonymous without self-selection bias: an instrumental variables re-analysis of randomized clinical trials. *Alcohol Clin Exp Res*. 2014;38(11):2688-2694.

19. Alcoholics Anonymous World Services, Inc. *Alcoholics Anonymous*. New York: Alcoholics Anonymous World Services, Inc.; 2001.

20. Alcoholics Anonymous World Services, Inc. *Twelve Steps and Twelve Traditions*. New York: Alcoholics Anonymous World Services, Inc.; 1981.

21. Kelly JF. Is alcoholics anonymous religious, spiritual, neither? Findings from 25 years of mechanisms of behavior change research. *Addiction*. 2017;112(6):929-936.

14

SUBSTANCE USE DISORDERS—ILLICIT AND PRESCRIPTION DRUGS

Anna Lembke, MD and Chinyere I. Ogbonna, MD, MPH

CLINICAL HIGHLIGHTS

- Addiction is a chronic, relapsing, and remitting disorder. The natural history of addictive disorders is similar to that of other chronic diseases with a behavioral component (e.g., type 2 diabetes, asthma, hypertension).
- "Recovery" from addictive behaviors is akin to remission from a cancer diagnosis—there is always a chance the behavior will recur or manifest in a new form.
- Drug dependence, risky drug use, and drug use disorder (addiction) are distinct categories of drug use problems. Although they often co-occur, they can occur independently of the other.
- Primary care providers are in prime positions to identify harmful substance use patterns in their patients.
- Brief intervention often involves physician–patient contacts of 10 to 15 minutes and a limited number of session, with the goal of reducing harm to the patient—whether that means reduction in use or cessation in use based on the patient's readiness to change.
- The risk–benefit calculator is a way to compare the side effects, pain relief, and functional benefits incurred from chronic opioid therapy, to determine if the relative benefits outweigh the risks, and if a decrease in dose or full taper is indicated.
- Primary care providers need to be aware of available treatment resources for their patients, including community-based mutual support groups.

CLINICAL SIGNIFICANCE

PREVALENCE

According to the National Survey on Drug Use and Health (2016), approximately 20.1 million people aged 12 years or older (7.5%, or 1 in 13 people aged 12 years or older) met criteria for a substance use disorder (SUD), excluding tobacco, within the past year. This number includes 15.1 million people with an alcohol use disorder (74.9%, or nearly 3 in 4 people with SUD), 7.4 million people with an illicit drug use disorder (36.7%, or about 1 in 3 people with SUD), and 2.3 million people with both an alcohol and illicit drug use disorder (11.6%, or about 1 in 9 people with SUD). Among the 7.4 million people with an illicit drug use disorder, 4 million had a past year disorder related to their use of marijuana, and 1.8 million people had a disorder related to prescription pain relievers (opioids).[1]

Thirty-five percent of those misusing prescription drugs get those drugs from a single prescriber. Less than 10% gets them from a drug dealer. The majority gets them indirectly from friends and family, who often obtained them from health care providers.[1] Although opioid prescribing has decreased by 18% since its peak in 2012, U.S. prescribers still write over 200 million opioid prescriptions annually, more than three times what they wrote at the end of the 1990s.[2] By volume, primary care providers (family practice, internal medicine, nurse practitioners, and physician assistants) write more opioid prescriptions than other medical specialties.[3]

DISEASE BURDEN AND ECONOMIC COSTS

Alcohol, tobacco, and illicit substance use are included among the top nine external (nongenetic) factors that contribute to death in the United States.[4] In the 12 months leading up to August 2017, there were 67,344 drug overdose deaths in the United States, a 13% increase from the preceding 12 months, and more deaths annually than caused by AIDS at the height of the HIV epidemic.[5] Two-thirds of drug overdose deaths involve opioids, and at least half of those involve prescription opioids. When considering disease burden (e.g., substantial comorbid health costs resulting from substance use, lost wages and productivity, etc.), addressing the impact of substance use alone is expected to cost Americans more than $600 billion each year.[6]

It is imperative for the primary care physician to have a basic understanding of how to screen and intervene for substance use problems and to identify the type of substance use problem the patient has, because the most effective interventions are tailored to the specific problem type. We discuss here patients struggling with a spectrum of drug use problems, focusing on illicit and prescription drugs. Alcohol and tobacco are covered in chapter 13.

DIAGNOSIS

The *Diagnostic and Statistical Manual of Mental Disorders* (*DSM*)—an imperfect but nonetheless useful catalog of behaviors the medical profession relies upon to diagnose psychopathology—uses 11 different criteria to diagnose SUDs (addiction). The diagnostic criteria in the newest edition of the *DSM* (i.e., *DSM-5*) can be remembered simply as the "**four C's**": **C**ontrol, **C**ompulsion, **C**raving, and **C**ontinued use despite consequences.

Control refers to out-of-control use, for example using more than intended.

Compulsion refers to mental preoccupation with using a substance, and using the substance against a conscious desire to abstain.

Craving refers to physiologic and/or mental states of wanting.

Continued use despite consequences refers to the social, legal, economic, interpersonal, and other problems that arise as a result of use, yet which still do not deter use.

If the patient endorses two to three items on the *DSM* diagnostic list, then the patient has a *mild* SUD. Four to five items signifies a *moderate* SUD, and six or more items indicates a *severe* SUD. For example, the patient who describes "a persistent desire ... to control substance use," "important ... activities given up because of substance use," "the substance taken in larger amounts than was intended," and "tolerance" (needing more of the substance to get the same effect) has a moderate SUD (four criteria met).

Note that older versions of the *DSM* before the *DSM-5* used the terms *substance abuse* and *substance dependence* to denote an SUD. These terms have been phased out in recognition of the existence of physiologic dependence in the absence of a use disorder and because the term *abuse* is increasingly viewed as stigmatizing. Also, note that the term *addiction*, the commonly accepted term for SUD, is not recognized as *DSM* terminology. Nonetheless, we use the terms SUD and addiction interchangeably here.

While tolerance and withdrawal are part of the *DSM* criteria for an SUD, the diagnosis of SUD cannot be based solely on the patient meeting criteria for tolerance and withdrawal. Similarly, tolerance and withdrawal do not need to be present to make a diagnosis of an SUD (see section on Differential Diagnosis for more details).

According to neuroscientists, addiction is a disorder of the brain's reward circuitry.[7] Survival of the species depends on maximizing pleasure (finding food when hungry, for example) and minimizing pain (avoiding noxious stimuli). Seeking out pleasure and avoiding pain

is adaptive and healthy; but the individual with a severe SUD will commit all available resources toward obtaining and consuming the drug of choice, and forgo natural rewards such as food, finding a mate, or raising children. Over time, the substance itself is mistaken as necessary for survival.

Addiction is a chronic relapsing and remitting disorder. When a patient "relapses" from the state of being in recovery to "using" again, the appropriate response is compassion and a more aggressive treatment intervention, just as would occur for a patient with any other type of chronic illness. Evidence shows that when addiction is treated like any other chronic illness with a behavioral component, such as type 2 diabetes, asthma, or certain types of heart disease, patients show similar rates of remission, recurrence, and adherence to treatment.[8]

DIFFERENTIAL DIAGNOSIS

SUDs and psychiatric illness often co-occur, and symptoms of substance intoxication or withdrawal may mimic common psychiatric symptoms seen in mood, anxiety, and psychotic disorders. It's important to obtain a full psychiatric history and family history to help distinguish underlying psychiatric illness versus a substance-induced psychiatric presentation. A urine drug screen, complete metabolic panel, and a complete blood count can be helpful objective measures of recent substance use, in addition to collateral information obtained from family members or close friends.

It's also important for the clinician to determine whether the substance use meets criteria for risky substance use, SUD, or physiologic substance dependence, as the correct diagnosis will determine the next appropriate step in further assessment and recommended treatment interventions. Risky substance use, SUDs, and substance dependence can occur independently and can also co-occur (see *Figure 14-1*).

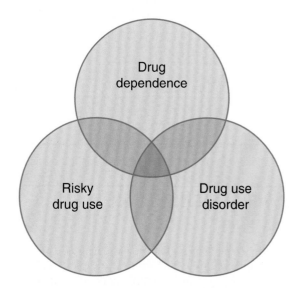

FIGURE 14-1 Categories of drug use problems.

RISKY DRUG USE (DRUG MISUSE)

Risky drug use is defined as engaging in drug use that is harmful to self and/or others. Risky drug use can occur within the context of a drug use disorder (addiction) but need not necessarily do so. According to the Surgeon General's Report "Facing Addiction in America," risky drug use "can be of low severity and temporary, but it can also result in serious, enduring, and costly consequences due to motor vehicle crashes, intimate partner and sexual violence, child abuse and neglect, suicide attempts and fatalities, overdose deaths, various forms of cancer (e.g.,

breast cancer in women), heart and liver diseases, HIV/AIDS, and problems related to drinking or using drugs during pregnancy, such as fetal alcohol spectrum disorders (FASDs) or neonatal abstinence syndrome (NAS)."[9]

The public health burden of drug misuse necessitates increased efforts to identify patients who exhibit risky drug use and offer early interventions to reduce the risk of long-term medical, psychiatric, and social consequences.[9]

See *Table 14-1* for trends in current (past month) substance use among adults age 12 years or older in the United States, 2016.

TABLE 14-1 Current (Past Month) Substance Use Trends among Adults Aged 12 Years or Older in 2016		
SUBSTANCE	**PREVALENCE**	**TRENDS**
Marijuana	Total: 24 million (8.9%) • 12 to 17 years: 1.6 million (6.5%) • 18 to 25 years: 7.2 million (20.8%) • 26 years or older: 15.2 million (7.2%)	• 2016 estimates were higher than those from 2002 to 2015, reflecting an increase in marijuana use by adults aged 26 years or older, and to a lesser extent, increases in use among young adults aged 18 to 25 years old
Prescription drugs	Total: 6.2 million (2.3%) • 12 to 17 years: 389,000 (1.6%) • 18 to 25 years: 1.6 million (4.6%) • 26 years or older: 4.2 million (2%)	• New baseline started in 2015 for all prescription drug measures
• *Pain relievers*	*Total: 3.3 million (1.2%)* • *12 to 17 years: 239,000 (1%)* • *18 to 25 years: 631,000 (1.8%)* • *26 years or older: 2.5 million (1.2%)*	
• *Stimulants*	*Total: 1.7 million (0.6%)* • *12 to 17 years: 92,000 (0.4%)* • *18 to 25 years: 767,000 (2.2%)* • *26 years or older: 876,000 (0.4%)*	
• *Sedatives*	*Total: 497,000 (0.2%)* • *12 to 17 years: 23,000 (0.1%)* • *18 to 25 years: 50,000 (0.1%)* • *26 years or older: 425,000 (0.2%)*	
Cocaine	Total: 1.9 million (0.7%) • 12 to 17 years: 28,000 (0.1%) • 18 to 25 years: 552,000 (1.6%) • 26 years or older: 1.3 million (0.6%)	• 2016 estimates of cocaine use were similar to estimates between 2007 and 2015, but lower than the estimates in 2002 to 2006.
Heroin	Total: 475,000 (0.2%) • 12 to 17 years: 3,000 (<0.1%) • 18 to 25 years: 88,000 (0.3%) • 26 years or older: 383,000 (0.2%)	• 2016 estimates of heroin use were higher than those for most years between 2002 and 2013, but similar to estimates between 2014 and 2015
Methamphetamines	Total: 667,000 (0.2%) • 12 to 17 years: 9,000 (<0.1%) • 18 to 25 years: 65,000 (0.2%) • 26 years or older: 594,000 (0.3%)	• New baseline started in 2015, as most methamphetamines now used in the United States are produced and distributed illicitly rather than through the pharmaceutical industry

Adapted from Substance Abuse and Mental Health Services Administration. Key Substance Use and Mental Health Indicators in the United States: Results from the 2016 National Survey on Drug Use and Health (HHS Publication No. SMA 17-5044, NSDUH Series H-52). Rockville, MD: Center for Behavioral Health Statistics and Quality, Substance Abuse and Mental Health Services Administration; 2017.

Physiologic Dependence, Tolerance, and Withdrawal

Physiologic drug dependence is the process whereby the body biochemically adapts to the continual presence of a drug. In the context of dependence, tolerance and withdrawal can occur. Tolerance is the need for increasing doses to get the same effects and/or the loss of efficacy at a given dose. Withdrawal refers to signs and symptoms related to lowering or stopping the drug.

Drug dependence, tolerance, and withdrawal, independent of addiction, are important clinical syndromes that the primary care provider should recognize and address, especially today, as we face a national opioid epidemic, spurred in part by opioid analgesic overprescribing.

Although physical dependence, withdrawal, and tolerance are part of the *DSM-5* diagnostic criteria for SUD, they cannot be the sole criteria for making a diagnosis of an SUD. An individual can be physically dependent on and tolerant to a substance or behavior without being addicted. For example, someone who takes an opioid pill daily for pain as prescribed by a doctor may be dependent on opioids, need more and more medication to get the same effect (tolerance), and experience opioid withdrawal when cutting back or discontinuing use but is not addicted to opioids by virtue of taking them as prescribed. This individual would meet criteria for a diagnosis of "opioid dependence, physiologic," but not "opioid use disorder."

Likewise, an individual can be addicted to opioid pain pills (i.e., using them in a way that is out of control, compulsive, and leads to consequences) without necessarily being dependent on opioids. For example, someone who binges on opioids to the point of respiratory suppression, risking death, but doesn't take opioids daily, will not develop the tolerance and withdrawal symptoms (i.e., physical dependence) that arise with daily use. This individual would meet criteria for a diagnosis of "opioid use disorder," but not "opioid dependence, physiologic."

For guidance on when and how to taper opioid-dependent patients down and off of opioids, including how to intervene when prescription drug misuse and addiction is detected, see the section Prescription Drug Dependence, Misuse, and Addiction.

BIOPSYCHOSOCIAL TREATMENT
PHARMACOLOGIC TREATMENT

Medications to treat SUDs should, when possible, be prescribed in combination with behavioral therapies (e.g., cognitive behavioral therapy, motivational enhancement therapy, contingency management) and psychosocial interventions (12-step facilitation therapy) targeted to the complex behaviors that characterize addictive substance use. Psychosocial interventions are crucial for improving skills to cope with stress and environmental cues that may trigger cravings and put the patient at risk for relapse.[10]

Psychopharmacology for Substance Use Disorders, with a Focus on Drug Use Disorders

Medication can be a useful tool for treating SUDs, as they can help to address acute symptoms of withdrawal, reduce cravings, and help stabilize patients during recovery. Medications to treat SUDs work through four basic mechanisms: agonism, partial-agonism, deterrence, and craving reduction. We focus here on FDA-approved medications to treat drug use disorders. We will also briefly address evidence-based off-label medication usage. We make a distinction between medications to treat substance withdrawal and medications to treat the use disorder. Medically assisted withdrawal does not by itself constitute treatment for an SUD and should be followed by ongoing treatment for the "four C's" (control, compulsion, craving, and continued use despite consequences) that define SUDs.[10,11]

Opioids
Medications for Opioid Withdrawal

Opioid withdrawal consists of a wide range of symptoms that occur after a significant reduction or abrupt discontinuation of opioid use after a period of heavy or prolonged use. The onset of withdrawal symptoms varies based on the half-life of the opioids used. For short-acting opioids (e.g., oxycodone, hydrocodone, heroin), withdrawal symptoms typically start 12 to 24 hours after the last use, with peak symptoms around 24 to 48 hours, lasting an average of 3 to 5 days. For long-acting opioids (e.g., buprenorphine, methadone), withdrawal symptoms typically start around 30 hours from the last use, lasting an average of 10 to 14 days. Symptoms of opioid withdrawal include muscle aches, runny nose, dilated pupils, goose bumps, agitation, anxiety, nausea, vomiting, diarrhea, sweats, chills, and yawning. The Clinical Opioid Withdrawal Scale (COWS) can be helpful for providers to clinically assess signs and symptoms of opioid withdrawal objectively.[12-14]

Opioid withdrawal can be extremely distressing and uncomfortable but is rarely life-threatening. Providing anticipatory guidance and reassurance that withdrawal symptoms are often time limited can help reduce anticipatory anxiety that many patients have based on previous experiences with cessation of use, often in the context of abrupt discontinuation of opioids. While medication-assisted withdrawal management can help reduce the discomfort of opioid withdrawal, patients should be counseled that it is common to still experience mild symptoms of withdrawal while taking these medications. Use of anesthesia to avoid discomfort associated with opioid withdrawal has not been shown to be safe or cost-effective and may result in serious adverse events including cardiac arrest and death.[12-14] Medications for management of acute opioid withdrawal management are summarized in *Figure 14-2*. In addition, off-label gabapentin 1,600 mg/day has been shown to be effective in decreasing some symptoms of opioid withdrawal and may be an effective adjunctive therapy when added to opioid agonist therapy, resulting in reduced daily and cumulative doses of opioid agonist medications.[15]

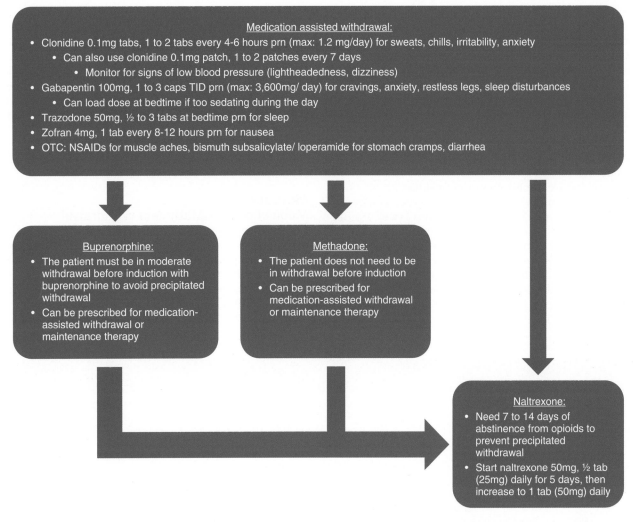

FIGURE 14-2 Management of opioid use disorder in primary care setting. (Adapted from Stine SM, Kosten TR. Pharmacologic interventions for opioid depedence. In: Ries RK, Fiellin DA, Miller SC, Saltz R, eds. *The ASAM Principles of Addiction Medicine.* 5th ed. Philadelphia, PA: Wolters Kluwer; 2014:735-777.)

Medications for Opioid Use Disorder

There are three FDA-approved medications for opioid use disorders: methadone, buprenorphine, and naltrexone. Methadone is a full agonist at the μ-opioid receptor, buprenorphine is a partial agonist at the μ-opioid receptor, and naltrexone is an antagonist at the μ-opioid receptor. Buprenorphine is often prescribed in a combination pill, buprenorphine–naloxone, in which the naloxone serves as a deterrent for misuse of the medication. Naloxone has low bioavailability when this medication is taken as prescribed (sublingual absorption) and will only become bioavailable if the medication is crushed or altered and administered by other routes (i.e., snorting, injecting).[10,14]

Both methadone and buprenorphine are themselves opioids and work by activating the μ-opioid receptor in a way that is similar to other opioids, with methadone as a full agonist and buprenorphine as a partial agonist. Both methadone and buprenorphine have a long half-life (methadone: 8 to 59 hours, buprenorphine: 20 to 44 hours), which creates a steady opioid level in the patient's bloodstream that typically lasts at least a day (can vary according to individual metabolism). This long half-life allows the patient to get out of the cycle of intoxication and withdrawal/drug-seeking, which is so destructive to their lives. Instead, with methadone or buprenorphine maintenance therapy, patients achieve a mental and physical stability that allows them to engage in activities of daily living, including in psychosocial and behavioral treatments targeting addiction.[10,14]

Buprenorphine has several other properties, which make it effective in the treatment of opioid addiction, and also a potentially safer medication than methadone. Buprenorphine has a ceiling effect on respiratory suppression, which means even at very high doses, the risk of slowing breathing and heart rate, and hence overdose death, is much lower than other opioids. This ceiling effect on respiratory suppression is due to the partial agonist effect of buprenorphine on the μ-opioid receptor, meaning when it binds to the μ-opioid receptor, it does not elicit the full response that would be elicited by a full agonist. Buprenorphine also has a partial agonist effect for euphoria, producing less euphoria than other opioids (although in an opioid naïve person, buprenorphine can produce euphoria). Finally, buprenorphine has a high binding affinity on the µ-opioid receptor, which means that once buprenorphine is on a receptor, other opioids, such as heroin, cannot bind. This property can also make it difficult to get patients started on buprenorphine. As a partial agonist, buprenorphine can cause precipitated withdrawal if taken by a patient who has recently used opioids, as the administration of buprenorphine will displace most opioids from the opioid receptor. For this reason, patients need to be in active and moderate opioid withdrawal before initiating buprenorphine.[10,14]

As part of a comprehensive treatment plan, which may include medical, psychiatric, and social services, opioid agonist therapy (buprenorphine and methadone) have been shown to reduce the risk of transmission of HIV and hepatitis, substance use relapse rates, involvement in crime, and morbidity and mortality related to SUDs. Patients stabilized on these medications are better able to engage in other behavioral interventions to support sustained recovery.[10,14]

Naltrexone is the third FDA-approved medication for opioid use disorders. It works as a deterrent by blocking the µ-opioid receptor, negating the effects of other opioids taken simultaneously. Naltrexone may also help to reduce cravings for opioids; however, the mechanism of opioid craving reduction is not well understood. To avoid precipitated withdrawal, naltrexone should be given at least 7 days after the last dose of opioids. It may be necessary to wait up to 14 days or longer to initiate naltrexone if the patient has been using a long-acting opioid, such as methadone.[10,14]

FDA-approved medications for opioid use disorder are summarized in *Table 14-2*.

Marijuana
Medications for Marijuana Withdrawal
Common symptoms of marijuana withdrawal include weakness, sweating, chills, restlessness, dysphoria, body aches, sleep problems, vivid dreams, anxiety, headaches, hallucinations, difficulty concentrating, tremor, nausea, stomach cramps, weight loss, irritability, and cravings. Onset of withdrawal symptoms typically present after 1 to 3 days from the last use, with peak severity of symptoms

TABLE 14-2 FDA-Approved Medications for Opioid Use Disorder

	METHADONE	BUPRENORPHINE	NALTREXONE PO/VIVITROL IM
Mechanism of action	• Synthetic µ-opioid receptor antagonist	• Partial opioid agonist with high affinity at µ-opioid receptor	• Long-acting opioid antagonist
Prescribing	• Federally regulated for treatment of opioid use disorder • Can only be prescribed at an opioid treatment program (OTP) • Withdrawal management, reduces cravings	• Can be prescribed in primary care setting • Prescribers need to have DATA 2000 waiver from the DEA (SAMHSA) • Withdrawal management, reduces cravings	• Can be prescribed in primary care setting • Naltrexone PO—administered daily • Vivitrol IM—extended release injectable Naltrexone, administered every 4 weeks • No effect on withdrawals, reduces cravings • No addictive potential
Dosing	• Administered daily as an oral dose • Individualized therapeutic dose is determined to maintain an asymptomatic state (no withdrawal symptoms, or signs/symptoms of overmedication)	• Sublingual absorption, with poor oral bioavailability • Owing to its unique pharmacologic properties, it can cause acute opioid withdrawal taken while on a full opioid agonist • Formulated as a combination pill with naloxone (Suboxone) as a deterrent for abuse—if taken correctly naloxone is not absorbed	• Most effective when utilized following detoxification from opioids—need 7 to 10 days abstinent from opioids • Naltrexone PO—can start 25 mg daily for 5 days, then increase to 50 mg daily for maintenance • Vivitrol IM—380 mg injected intramuscularly every 4 weeks
Common adverse effects	• Cardiac: prolonged QTc • GI: constipation, abdominal pain • Endocrine: hormonal dysregulation, sexual dysfunction	• Headaches • GI: constipation, nausea • Endocrine: hormonal dysregulation, sexual dysfunction	• Headache • Nausea/vomiting • Dysphoria • Myalgia • Insomnia

Adapted from Lee J, Kresina TF, Campopiano M., et al. Use of pharmacotherapies in the treatment of alcohol use disorders and opioid dependence in primary care. Biomed Res. *2015:1-11. Stine SM, Kosten TR. Pharmacologic interventions for opioid dependence. In: Ries RK, Fiellin DA, Miller SC, Saitz R, eds. The ASAM Principles of Addiction Medicine. 5th ed. Philadelphia, PA: Wolters Kluwer; 2014:735-777. American Society of Addiction Medicine. National practice guidelines for the use of medications in the treatment of addiction involving opioid use. American Society of Addiction Medicine. Published June 1, 2015. https://www.asam.org/docs/default-source/practice-support/guidelines-and-consensus-docs/asam-national-practice-guideline-supplement.pdf?sfvrsn=24. Accessed July 3, 2017.*

within 10 days from the last use. Physical symptoms typically present before psychological symptoms and will generally resolve sooner than psychological symptoms (average 2 to 19 days vs. 5 weeks to greater than 1 year, respectively). The severity of withdrawal symptoms is correlated with frequency and amount of use.[16]

Off-label gabapentin (1,200 mg/day) and N-acetylcysteine (1,200 mg/day) may help in managing symptoms of marijuana withdrawal. Mirtazapine may be helpful in addressing sleep disturbance during marijuana withdrawal.[15,16]

Medications for Marijuana Use Disorder

There are no FDA-approved medications for treatment of marijuana use disorder.

Cocaine and Amphetamines (Stimulants)
Medications for Stimulant Withdrawal

Cocaine withdrawal is often characterized by an initial "crash" that can occur within hours or days from the last use. Common symptoms of withdrawal include anhedonia, dysphoria, anxiety, irritability, fatigue, sleep disturbance, increased appetite, psychomotor retardation, and cravings.[11]

Propranolol may be effective for cocaine withdrawal only if the patient remains adherent to the medication. Progesterone, tiagabine, topiramate, and gabapentin have also been shown to decrease cocaine use in patients with low withdrawal severity. Modafinil may work as "agonist substitution" therapy; however, the replacement approach for stimulant use disorder is not recommended owing to concern for misuse or diversion and lack of clear evidence of efficacy from clinical trials.[11]

Like cocaine, abrupt discontinuation of methamphetamine use typically results in a time-limited withdrawal syndrome characterized by dysphoria, fatigue, vivid dreams, insomnia or hypersomnia, increased appetite, psychomotor agitation or retardation, fatigue, anxiety, irritability, agitation, paranoia, and cravings. Most withdrawal symptoms resolve in a week. Treatment of withdrawal symptoms should begin as soon as possible following the last dose of methamphetamines and can be continued for up to 2 weeks to allow for sufficient symptomatic relief.[17]

Mirtazapine has been shown to improve suicidal ideation and may be helpful in addressing mood and sleep symptoms during acute methamphetamine withdrawal.[17]

Medications for Stimulant Use Disorders

There are no FDA-approved medications for treatment of cocaine or methamphetamine use disorder.

Studies have not shown consistent efficacy of antidepressants (e.g., SSRIs/SNRIs), dopamine agonists (e.g., modafinil), or antagonists (e.g., quetiapine) in the treatment of cocaine use disorder. Patients with co-occurring SUD and attention deficit hyperactivity disorder should be treated with nonstimulant medications or long-acting stimulant formulations with close monitoring to limit the risk of risky use and use disorders in this patient group. Bupropion may be helpful adjunctive treatment to behavioral interventions for methamphetamine use disorders.[11,17,18]

PSYCHOSOCIAL TREATMENT

Behavioral therapies have been shown to be effective in helping patients with SUDs develop healthy coping skills for managing life stressors, identify triggers and manage cravings, and modify attitudes and behaviors related to substance abuse.[17,18]

Table 14-3 summarizes evidence-based psychosocial interventions for SUDs.

What Are Some Brief Behavioral Interventions the Primary Care Provider Can Try in a 20- to 30-Minute Patient Visit to Help Patients with Risky Substance Use (Screening, Brief Intervention, and Referral to Treatment or SBIRT)?

Primary care providers are in prime positions to identify harmful substance use patterns in their patients, as they are able to establish continuity of care and therapeutic alliances with their patients. Studies have shown the impact that primary care providers can have on changing patient behaviors through providing empathetic feedback and brief interventions once problematic substance use patterns are identified with routine screening during health maintenance visits. Many primary care providers may already feel overwhelmed due to increased demands of managed care and may be reluctant to discuss substance use behaviors with patients for fear of the time constraints and limited access to patient resources. Approaching screening and brief interventions as a series of graduated approaches that can be incorporated into a normal clinic or office routine can lessen the burden on the physician by emphasizing a team approach to help patients decrease harmful patterns of substance use, thereby reducing the risk of harmful health consequences related to their substance use.[19]

General guidelines for primary care providers are summarized in *Figure 14-3*.

The goal of screening for problematic substance use behaviors is to identify patients who are at risk for health consequences related to their pattern of substance use. These patients with high-risk substance use/behaviors may benefit from early intervention with the goal of reducing harmful consequences and/or further assessment to diagnose their SUD and receive the appropriate level of treatment. As visual examination alone is insufficient to detect the subtle signs of intoxication or drug-affected behavior, it is recommended that primary care providers routinely screen all patients for SUDs as part of the ongoing care process. Screening can be seamlessly incorporated into clinic workflow utilizing brief written, oral, or computerized questionnaires. Patients with negative screens (abstinence or no harmful use) should be given positive reinforcement about the benefits of abstaining from illicit drug use and abstinence/low-risk alcohol use.[19]

While a positive screen does not constitute a diagnosis, it should warrant further discussion with the patient clarifying quantity, frequency, duration of substance use pattern, as well as the severity of substance-related health, legal, and social consequences in the past 12 months.

TABLE 14-3 Evidence-Based Behavioral Therapy Interventions

BEHAVIORAL THERAPY	OPIOIDS	MARIJUANA	COCAINE	METHAMPHETAMINES
Cognitive behavioral therapy				
• *Theory: learning processes play a critical role in the development of maladaptive patterns* ◦ Explores the positive and negative consequences of continued use ◦ Self-monitoring to recognize cravings and identifying triggering situations ◦ Develop strategies for coping with cravings and triggers		✓	✓	✓
Contingency management interventions/motivational incentives				
• *Theory: giving patients tangible rewards to reinforce positive behaviors (e.g., abstinence)* ◦ *Voucher-based reinforcement (VBR)*—the patient receives a voucher for every drug-free urine sample provided, which can be exchanged for goods or services consistent with a drug-free lifestyle ◦ *Prize incentive contingency management*—uses chances to win cash prizes instead of vouchers	✓	✓	✓	✓
Community reinforcement approach (CRA) plus vouchers				
• *Theory: intensive 24-week outpatient therapy using a range of reinforcers and material incentives to make drug-free lifestyle more rewarding than substance use* ◦ Maintain abstinence for patients to help patients learn new skills for sustained abstinence ◦ Reduce polysubstance use	✓		✓	
Motivational enhancement therapy (MET)				
• *Theory: helps individuals resolve their ambivalence about stopping their use and engaging in treatment* ◦ Aims to evoke rapid and internally motivated change ◦ Motivational interviewing principles are used to strengthen motivation and build a plan for change ◦ Therapist monitors change, reviews strategies for cessation, and encourages commitment to change or sustained abstinence	✓	✓		
Matrix model				
• *Theory: provides a framework for engaging patients with stimulant use disorder* ◦ Patients learn about substance use disorders and relapse, receive direction and support from a trained therapist, and become familiar with self-help programs ◦ Therapist functions as a teacher and coach—authentic and direct, but not confrontational or parental ◦ Includes elements of relapse prevention, family and group therapies, drug education, and self-help participation			✓	✓
12-step facilitation therapy				
• *Theory: an active engagement strategy designed to increase likelihood of the patient becoming actively involved in 12-step self-help groups* ◦ Three key ideas: acceptance, surrender, and active involvement in 12-step meetings and related activities	✓		✓	✓
Family behavior therapy (FBT)				
• *Theory: addresses substance use problems and co-occurring problems such as conduct disorders, child mistreatment, depression, family conflict, and unemployment* ◦ Combines behavioral contracting with contingency management ◦ Involves the patient with at least one significant other (i.e., parent, cohabiting partner) ◦ Patients participate in treatment planning, choosing from a menu of evidence-based options	✓	✓	✓	✓

Adapted from National Institute on Drug Abuse. Principles of Drug Addiction Treatment: A Research-Based Guide (Third Edition). Retrieved July 3, 2016, from United States, National Institute on Drug Abuse. Principles of Drug Addiction Treatment: A Research-Based Guide (Third Edition). 2012, December.

Screening

- Routinely screen all patients for harmful substance use
  - Ask questions about substance use in the context of other lifestyle questions or use a validated screening tool (e.g., AUDIT, ASSIST, DAST-10, CAGE-AID, CRAFFT, TWEAK)
- Screen adolescents for substance abuse every time they seek medical services
- Present results of positive screen and discussions about substance use in a nonjudgmental manner

Brief intervention

- Appropriate for patients with a positive screen result, but most effective for patients with less severe substance use problems
- Includes feedback about screening results, risks of use, information about safe consumption limits, advice about change, assessment of patient's readiness to change, negotiated goals and strategies for change, and arrange follow-up visit to monitor patient progress

Assessment and treatment

- Become familiar with available assessment and treatment options
- Refer high-risk patients to a specialist if possible
- Encourage reluctant patients to accept treatment of some kind

Confidentiality

- Set up reminders about the need to screen and reassess patients for harmful substance use
- Do not perform screening or laboratory tests (i.e., blood or urine tests) without the patient's consent
- Consult the patient before discussing his or her substance use with anyone else

FIGURE 14-3 General recommendations for primary care providers. (Adapted from Center for Substance Abuse Treatment. *A Guide to Substance Abuse Services for Primary Care Physicians. Treatment Improvement Protocol (TIP) Series, No. 24.* DHS Publication No. (SMA) 08-4075. Rockville, MD: Substance Abuse and Mental Health Services Administration; 1997.)

Primary care physicians should also ask patients how the drug was obtained and the route of ingestion. This information can point toward any additional testing or medical interventions. For example, a patient who trades sex for drugs will need testing for sexually transmitted disease and access to condoms; a patient who smokes a drug should be advised of the risk of oropharyngeal and lung disease; and a person who injects drugs needs access to clean needles and testing for HIV and hepatitis C.

Patients who meet criteria for mild or moderate risk for harmful consequences related to their current pattern of substance use may benefit from brief, office-based intervention. This may be done immediately during the initial visit or scheduled for a subsequent visit based on the severity of the problem and possible risk to the patient.[3] Brief intervention often involves physician–patient contacts of 10 to 15 minutes and a limited number of sessions. At minimum, one follow-up visit is recommended, but the frequency and duration of sessions may depend on the severity of the problem, the patient's willingness to discuss their current substance use pattern, and the physician's available time. FRAMES (**F**eedback about personal risk or impairment; patient **R**esponsibility to change; **A**dvice to change; **M**enu of alternative self-help or treatment options; **E**mpathetic style of counseling; highlighting patient **S**elf-efficacy) is a common acronym highlighting the six critical elements of brief intervention for patients with positive screening results for harmful substance use behaviors.[19,20]

The goal of brief intervention is to reduce harm to the patient; whether that means a reduction in substance use or cessation of substance use will depend on the patient and his or her readiness to change. Specific goals during these sessions will vary based on the patient's stage of change but should be individualized to the patient and SMART (**S**pecific, **M**easurable, **A**ttainable, **R**elevant, and **T**ime limited). Patients should be encouraged to set limited, incremental goals and reminded that it may take several tries before achieving their goals. Repeated interventions or treatment may be needed before the patient being able to stabilize their progress. The physician can play a vital role in motivating patients to move toward the "action" stage of change, or even accept referral to more specialized care, by encouraging them to view difficulties in achieving goals set during brief interventions as a learning experience and evidence that their substance use problem may be more serious than previously acknowledged.[19,20]

Tips for interview approaches based on the patient's stage of change are summarized in *Figure 14-4.*

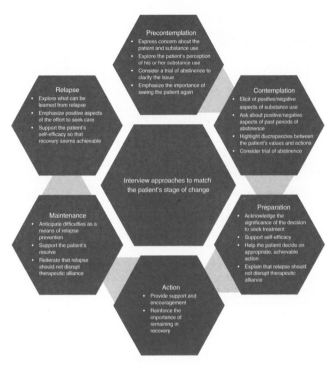

FIGURE 14-4 Interview approaches to match the patient's stage of change. (Adapted from Center for Substance Abuse Treatment. *A Guide to Substance Abuse Services for Primary Care Physicians. Treatment Improvement Protocol (TIP) Series, No. 24. DHS Publcation No. (SMA) 08-4075*. Rockville, MD: Substance Abuse and Mental Health Services Administration; 1997.)

PRESCRIPTION DRUG MISUSE, DEPENDENCE, AND ADDICTION

Health care providers should be able to recognize the phenomena of dependence, tolerance, and withdrawal and work with patients to initiate a taper when risks outweigh benefits. Yet, providers receive little training in this area. According to a 2016 Washington Post-Kaiser Family Foundation survey of patients prescribed opioids for chronic pain, 1 in 5 said doctors provided insufficient information about the risk of side effects, and more than 6 in 10 said doctors offered no advice on how or when to stop taking the drugs.[21] "BRAVO" provides an overview of how to taper patients down and off chronic opioid therapy.

"BRAVO" is an apt rejoinder to patients and doctors who take on the difficult challenge of addressing problematic prescription opioid use, including opioid dependence (see *Figure 14-5*). We will focus here on opioid medication, but the same principles apply with any drug that can create dependence, tolerance, and withdrawal, such as benzodiazepines or benzodiazepine-like medications (e.g., Ambien).

Broaching the Subject

In this initial conversation, even suggesting an opioid taper can trigger extreme anxiety in some patients, to the point where patients may temporarily lose their ability to fully attend to the conversation. To mitigate the anxiety, the primary care provider can try identifying this feeling for patients, normalizing it, and expressing empathy. For example, the provider might say:

> *"Hi Mrs. Smith, I scheduled some extra time for us today because I want to discuss a very important topic with you. I've been thinking a lot about your chronic pain and how to help you with that, and would like to suggest that we taper you down and maybe even off your opioid medication. Now, I know the very thought of an opioid taper is terrifying for you, and you're not alone in that ... it's totally normal to feel afraid about going down on your dose, especially after you've been taking opioids for so long. But, please hear me out, and let me tell you the reasons why I think it's a good plan for you."*

Note here how the provider tells the patient *"I've been thinking a lot about your chronic pain...."* This is an important and multilayered communication. With this phraseology, the provider is communicating to the patient that the opioid taper was carefully considered and not an impulse or some form of retaliation. The provider communicates to the patient that he or she is in the provider's mind even when the patient is not immediately in front of them; the patient exists for the provider outside of the clinic environment. As the famous psychoanalyst, Donald Winnicott says, the provider, like the "good enough mother," creates a "holding environment" for the patient to feel safe. By arranging for enough time to discuss this delicate topic and anticipating the patient's strong emotional reaction to the topic, the provider increases the chances of preserving a good therapeutic alliance and hence a more successful taper experience.

Risk–Benefit Calculator

The risk–benefit calculation is a way to compare the side effects, pain relief, and functional benefits incurred from chronic opioid therapy, to determine if the relative benefits outweigh the risks, and if a decrease in dose or full taper is indicated.[22] In many cases, the adverse effects of chronic opioid therapy often exceeded its medical utility.

Once the primary care provider determines that the adverse effects of the opioids for a given patient outweigh the benefits, the provider should take time to discuss his or her reasoning with the patient. The provider might say something like:

> *"I think we need to get you off opioids because they're doing more harm than good. Your pain is no better than before you started on opioids, and may even be worse. More importantly, you're less functional than you used to be, spending most of the day in bed. Your husband reports you are detached from family life. Opioids can do that, even when we're not aware of them doing that. For all of those reasons, we're going to work together to slowly taper you off these medications."*

Invariably, many patients will protest the taper and endorse all the ways the opioids are helping them, even with clear evidence to the contrary. The provider's job is to remain empathic, yet resolute, and communicate to patients that a careful risk–benefit assessment informed

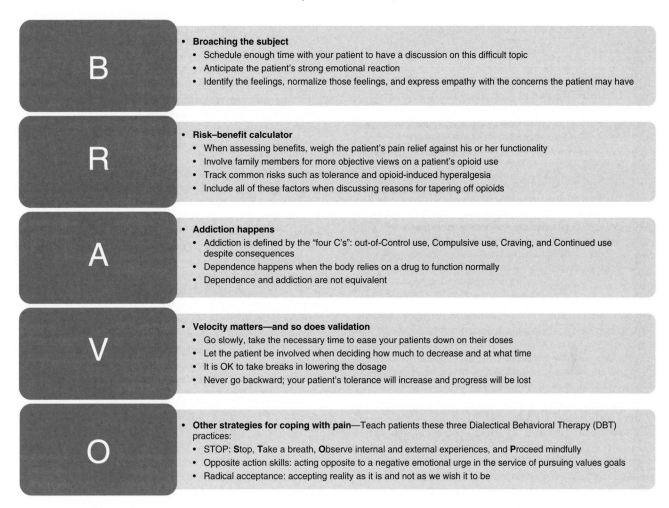

B
- **Broaching the subject**
  - Schedule enough time with your patient to have a discussion on this difficult topic
  - Anticipate the patient's strong emotional reaction
  - Identify the feelings, normalize those feelings, and express empathy with the concerns the patient may have

R
- **Risk–benefit calculator**
  - When assessing benefits, weigh the patient's pain relief against his or her functionality
  - Involve family members for more objective views on a patient's opioid use
  - Track common risks such as tolerance and opioid-induced hyperalgesia
  - Include all of these factors when discussing reasons for tapering off opioids

A
- **Addiction happens**
  - Addiction is defined by the "four C's": out-of-Control use, Compulsive use, Craving, and Continued use despite consequences
  - Dependence happens when the body relies on a drug to function normally
  - Dependence and addiction are not equivalent

V
- **Velocity matters—and so does validation**
  - Go slowly, take the necessary time to ease your patients down on their doses
  - Let the patient be involved when deciding how much to decrease and at what time
  - It is OK to take breaks in lowering the dosage
  - Never go backward; your patient's tolerance will increase and progress will be lost

O
- **Other strategies for coping with pain**—Teach patients these three Dialectical Behavioral Therapy (DBT) practices:
  - STOP: **S**top, **T**ake a breath, **O**bserve internal and external experiences, and **P**roceed mindfully
  - Opposite action skills: acting opposite to a negative emotional urge in the service of pursuing values goals
  - Radical acceptance: accepting reality as it is and not as we wish it to be

FIGURE 14-5 Discussing prescription opioid dependence with patients in the primary care setting.

by experience and compassion has led to this treatment plan. Providers should communicate to patients that to continue opioids under these circumstances would be to cause the patient further harm.

Addiction Happens

Patients who become addicted to prescription opioids do things like take more of the medication than directed, hoard the medication and take a lot at once to change the way they feel, take the medication to improve mood and energy rather than to treat pain, spend a lot of time and effort trying to get more medication, crave the medicine, or get into trouble at work or in their personal lives owing to use of the medication. Recent studies suggest that as many as 25% of patients taking daily opioid medications long term will misuse those medications, a harbinger of addiction. Quite an increase from the 1% risk of addiction doctors were taught in the 1990s.[23]

When talking to patients about addiction to prescription opioids, providers should begin by normalizing the process of becoming addicted to opioids prescribed for pain and reassuring patients that there is effective treatment for opioid use disorders/addiction, as follows:

"When we [doctors] first started prescribing opioids more liberally for chronic pain in the 1980s, we believed the risk of becoming addicted, as long as we were prescribing them for a medical condition, was very low. Since then, we have learned a lot and now know that even when patients are being prescribed opioids for a legitimate pain condition, and take them as prescribed, they can become addicted to those opioids. So, if in the process of a slow and medically supervised taper, you are unable to come off opioids, it is possible that you too have become addicted. If that's true for you, you're not alone. Millions of people have become addicted to prescription opioids through a doctors' prescription. The good news is there's treatment for addiction, which may even help your pain."

By being transparent about the ways in which the health care field has contributed to the opioid epidemic, and discussing treatment for opioid use disorders upfront, providers minimize the shame patients experience in admitting to themselves and others that they have become addicted and provide hope in the form of treatment if the opioid use disorder is a problem. It is also helpful to talk to patients about the difference between "opioid dependence, physiologic" and "opioid use disorder/addiction" and share with patients what their diagnosis is and why the diagnosis is appropriate.

Velocity Matters (And So Does Validation)

The mechanics of getting patients off chronic opioid therapy are relatively easy—definitely not rocket science. However, managing the speed of the rocket, and understanding the extent to which the astronauts inside the rocket are prepared for takeoff, makes all the difference in facilitating a smooth and successful launch. The biggest mistake providers make in tapering patients off chronic opioid therapy is tapering too fast. The standard recommendation to decrease by 5% to 10% of the starting dose every 1 to 2 weeks is intolerable for some patients, especially those on high doses long term. Some patients may need to decrease by as little as 5% or less every 2 to 3 months, with even smaller decrements toward the end of the taper. It is not unreasonable to take many months to years to wean some patients off chronic opioid therapy, especially those who have been taking opioids daily for decades. So, go slowly.

It's also important to keep the same dosing schedule. When it comes to addictive substances, brains are like little alarm clocks that sound whenever they're used to getting a dose. If the patient is on a twice-daily or thrice-daily regimen, keep him or her on that schedule as they taper, decreasing by increments at a given dose.

Patient involvement, and to some extent autonomy, in the taper process, is vital to success. If the patient is on several different opioids, let the patient decide which medication to taper first unless there is an immediate safety issue, which demands tapering a specific medication first (e.g., concern for overdose with methadone, which because of unpredictable metabolism, has been shown to contribute to overdose in some cases). Involve the patient in the decision of how much to taper and when. It's okay to take breaks in the taper, waiting at a given dose for some period before continuing. For example, if the patient has an important event coming up (e.g., wedding, family reunion, professional presentation) and doesn't want to be in low-grade withdrawal, it would be reasonable to defer the next decrement in dose until after that event. Most importantly, never go backward during the taper (i.e., increase the dose), lest the hard work of withdrawal from the last dose reduction is lost.

If the patient who is opioid dependent isn't tolerating the taper well, despite going slowly, or if the patient is discovered in the course of the taper to have an opioid use disorder/addiction, consider switching to buprenorphine/buprenorphine naloxone (see section on Medications for opioid use disorder) to taper the patient off opioids or for maintenance therapy. Additionally, the use of nonaddictive medications to ameliorate the symptoms of withdrawal can be helpful (see section on Medications for opioid withdrawal).

The second most common reason opioid tapers fail is because the provider doesn't validate the patient's experience about opioid withdrawal before and during the taper. Most patients on chronic opioid therapy have already experienced varying degrees of opioid withdrawal and are frightened to experience it again, with many misconceptions about withdrawal and what it means for their underlying disease process. Even people without chronic pain have body pain when going through opioid withdrawal. Indeed, patients should be told once opioid withdrawal is over, their pain may improve, due to a resetting of the pain threshold.

To prepare patients for opioid withdrawal, the provider should be honest with patients: they will feel worse before they feel better. The "feeling worse" will include all the typical symptoms of opioid withdrawal, as well as softer symptoms of opioid withdrawal, namely: irritability, insomnia, anxiety, and dysphoria (or low mood). Most importantly, many patients on chronic opioid therapy for chronic pain believe the physical pain they experience during withdrawal is evidence of their need for medication. The provider needs to explain to patients that the opioid is probably no longer treating the underlying pain condition but merely withdrawal from the last dose. Furthermore, the pain during opioid withdrawal is not an indication of progression of their underlying pain condition and not the pain they will have to live with off opioids. It is opioid withdrawal-mediated pain.

To validate and reassure patients through this process, the provider may want to consider using a cancer treatment analogy when talking to patients about the process of the opioid taper. For example:

> *"What we're asking you to do is very difficult, but it's a little bit like going through chemotherapy for cancer treatment. The treatment can be uncomfortable, and at times unbearable, but when it's over, there is hope that you will be in a better place and feel better than before the treatment."*

Be generous with accolades for patients going through this process.

Other Strategies for Coping with Pain

Consider some brief office-based interventions to help patients cope with pain, as an alternative to opioids. The following interventions are adapted from Dialectical Behavioral Therapy.

First, teach patients *mindfulness practices*. An example would be asking them to acknowledge pain and notice if something in the environment is making it worse at the moment, then remember the top three reasons why they want to stay off opioids (e.g., "my kids, I don't want to feel dependent on something, my health").

Second, teach patients *opposite action skills*: acting opposite to the emotional urge in the service of pursing values or goals. Many patients with chronic pain become obsessively focused on their pain and let it limit their participation in many activities. By contrast, providers can encourage patients to do the opposite and engage in activities, within reason, despite pain being present. This does not mean asking patients to go bungee jumping. This means asking them to engage in physical and mental activities as tolerated, despite being in pain, instead of spending the day in bed focused on their pain. By engaging in other activities, patients are promoting blood flow and neural engagement in areas of the brain that are unrelated to their chronic pain condition. This may even have the added benefit of reducing their pain.

Third, teach patients *radical acceptance*: accepting reality as it is, not as we wish it would be. For chronic pain patients, this often means accepting that their pain may likely never go away, but life can still be worth living even if it includes pain.

PRESCRIPTION AND DRUG MONITORING

The Prescription Drug Monitoring Database (PDMD) offers vital data on whether patients may be overusing, misusing, or becoming addicted to prescription drugs (e.g., getting the same or similar prescriptions from other providers). It also offers information on dangerous drug–drug interactions, like combining opioids with benzodiazepines. A recent cohort study in North Carolina showed a 10-time greater risk of accidental overdose in patients receiving both opioids and benzodiazepines compared with those only receiving opioids.[24] PDMDs collect data from pharmacies on dispensed controlled substance prescriptions and make those data available to authorized users through a secure, electronic database. As of 2018, all states have a PDMP, although they vary in quality state to state. Concerning patterns to look for on the PDMD include early refills, the same or similar prescriptions from multiple providers simultaneously (doctor shopping), dangerous drug–drug interactions (opioids and benzodiazepines), total morphine milligram equivalents (MMEs) exceeding 100 mg daily, an amount which has been shown to increase risk of adverse consequences of opioids, including addiction.[22]

While PDMDs can provide useful information about patient behaviors in obtaining and filling prescriptions for controlled substances, the physician must be careful when reviewing the data. Don't confuse doctors covering for each other or working in a group practice or an academic teaching hospital with doctor shopping. Also don't confuse prescriptions for limited quantities (2 weeks) with early refills. Inconsistencies noted on PDMDs should be addressed with the patient for clarification, and if appropriate, collateral information may be obtained from pharmacists or previous providers with a release of information from the patient.[22]

A urine drug screen (UDS) provides information on whether the patient is taking the medication the doctor is prescribing or taking other substances not prescribed.[14] Most government agencies and private employers typically utilize a 5-panel urine drug screen that will detect recent use of cocaine, marijuana (tetrahydrocannabinol, THC), amphetamines/methamphetamines, opiates, and phencyclidine. A 7-panel drug test may additionally screen for benzodiazepines/barbiturates and alcohol. Urine drug screen panels can be tailored for specific practice needs. Most urine drug screens utilize two-step confirmation, in that if the initial screening test is positive, the sample is sent for gas chromatography/mass spectrometry (GC/MS) or immunoassay testing for confirmation. A urine adulteration panel should be included as part of urine testing to provide additional information about possible dilution of use of an adulteration agent. A urine creatinine level less than 20 mg/dL is evidence of dilution, and a urine creatinine level less than 5 ng/dL is not consistent with human urine. Urine specific gravity and pH tests can also be helpful in assessing for possible adulteration of the urine sample. When tracking THC levels, it's important to normalize the sample by dividing the THC quantification by the urine creatinine levels. The resulting ratio (THC quantification/urine creatinine) can be trended over time to monitor for abstinence of marijuana use. Cannabodiol (CBD), one of many cannabinoids found in the marijuana plant, is not routinely tested for in most standard urine drug screen panels but may be available if requested from the laboratory.

Family members are an excellent source of information regarding functionality. Patients on chronic opioid therapy often lose the ability to assess their own response to opioids, because of the effects of opioids on the pleasure pathways in the brain. Patients often overestimate the efficacy of these drugs and underestimate their adverse effects. According to a 2016 Washington Post-Kaiser Family Foundation survey of people on opioids long term for chronic pain, only one-third of users said they were worried about being addicted to their prescribed opioid, whereas more than half of people living with them suspected addiction. Family members were also far more likely to say the drugs damaged the users' physical and mental health, finances, and personal relationships.[21]

CASES AND QUESTIONS

CASE 1:

Tom has suffered from low-back pain for a decade. He has been taking opioids prescribed by a doctor, for 3 years. Over that period, he has been escalating his dose owing to tolerance but denies any aberrant behavior, such as taking more than prescribed, crushing and snorting his pills, or crushing and injecting his pills. However, when the primary care doctor, who recently inherited his care, checks the prescription drug monitoring database, she discovers that Tom has been going to multiple doctors for more opioid prescriptions, as well as for prescriptions of benzodiazepines. A urine drug screen is positive for the opioids being prescribed, as well as for other opioids his primary care doctor is not prescribing. The urine toxicology is also positive for benzodiazepines and marijuana. The primary care doctor carves out time to discuss these findings with the patient.

At first, Tom denies getting prescriptions from other doctors. "That must be someone else impersonating me," he says. But when the primary care doctor shows him the database, and approaches him in a nonjudgmental way, including assuring him that he is not alone in having become addicted to opioids through a doctor's prescription, he admits to spending part of most days going around to different doctors' offices to get opioids and crushing and snorting the pills on occasion as a way to overcome his increasing tolerance. He has tried to cut back his use, but has been unable to, despite problems in his family and at work owing to his opioid use.

continued

1. What is the most likely diagnosis?
   A. Risky substance use
   B. Normal substance use
   C. Substance use disorder
   D. Major depressive disorder
   E. Anxiety disorder
   Correct answer: C. *Tom meets DSM-5 criteria for an opioid use disorder: he demonstrates compulsivity, out-of-control use, and continued use despite consequences, as well as tolerance and dependence. The most important intervention the primary care doctor can do in this context is to make the diagnosis of an opioid use disorder and assure the patient that she will partner with him to get him treatment for his opioid use disorder. Unfortunately, patients who are found to be misusing or addicted to the opioids a doctor is prescribing are often fired from that practice for engaging in "malingering" and other manipulative behavior. Malingering, manipulation, and denial are part of the disease of addiction. Although these behaviors can't be condoned, when conceptualized as signs and symptoms of a disease process, the primary care doctor is able to preserve compassion toward these patients and help them get the treatment that they need.*

2. What should the primary care doctor do next?
   A. Fire the patient
   B. Report the patient to the authorities
   C. Continue to prescribe opioids at a higher dose to provide better pain control
   D. Plan for a slow opioid taper while providing or referring for treatment of opioid use disorder
   E. Refer the patient to psychiatry
   Correct answer: D. *The primary care doctor should create a doctor–patient agreement with Tom that includes a slow opioid taper and treatment for opioid use disorder with one of the three FDA-approved medications for opioid use disorder: methadone, buprenorphine, or naltrexone. If the prescriber cannot provide treatment for opioid use disorder, Tom should be referred to an opioid treatment program (OTP) for methadone or to someone who can provide office-based addiction treatment. Given Tom's high-risk level, the doctor should prescribe no more than a week's worth of opioids at time, with follow-up weekly visits, including a urine drug screen and a check of the prescription drug monitoring database at each visit. With permission from the patient, the prescriber should contact the other prescribers and inform them that Tom has developed an opioid use disorder, which now needs treatment.*

3. What other treatment options should be offered to the patient?
   A. Opioid taper with plans to transition to opioid maintenance therapy or naltrexone
   B. Individual and/or group psychotherapy
   C. Education about naloxone followed by a prescription for naloxone

   D. Discussion about the risks of concurrent use of opioids and benzodiazepines, followed by a detailed plan for benzodiazepine taper
   E. All of the above
   Correct answer: E. *Tom should be educated about overdose risk, naloxone, and how to use it and then given a prescription for naloxone. He should be offered one of the three FDA-approved medications to treat opioid use disorder. Tom's benzodiazepine prescription should be tapered slowly as well. Tom would benefit from psychosocial interventions to address his substance use disorder.*

CASE 2:

Tiffany is a junior in college when she first presents to the primary care doctor, asking about a pregnancy test and tests for sexually transmitted diseases. Tiffany's questions naturally lead to a discussion of her recent sexual practices, at which time she shamefully admits to attending a party on campus a month ago with friends, where a bowl of pills and marijuana gummy bears was passed around. Tiffany does not drink alcohol or use tobacco and has never used drugs recreationally, but she was encouraged to try a pill or a gummy bear by a boy she has a crush on, the one who invited her to the party. With his encouragement, and because everyone else was doing it, she tried a gummy bear. It had no effect, so 10 minutes later she ate two more. By the end of the hour, she had ingested an unknown quantity of gummy bears, as well as a pill with a peace sign carved into it. She does not know what was in the pill. She woke up alone 6 hours later in a bedroom of the house where the party took place. She was no longer wearing underwear and had no memories of what had happened to her. She gathered herself together and went back to her own dorm room, walking back in the dark in the early hours of the morning.

Since that time, she has distanced herself from that group of friends, and no longer has a crush on that boy, whom she feels betrayed her by pressuring her to use drugs. Indeed, she has not spoken to anyone who was at that party since, preferring to distance herself from the whole experience, which she regrets and feels deeply embarrassed about. She presents today because she is concerned she may have, unbeknownst to her, been sexually assaulted.

1. What is the best way for the provider to approach a discussion about the patient's drug use?
   A. Confront the patient in a direct manner about the risks of substance use
   B. Approach the topic in a nonjudgmental way utilizing the FRAMES approach to provide education and intervention
   C. Refer the patient to a drug and alcohol counselor

D. Avoid discussing substance use to limit retraumatization of the patient

E. Encourage the patient to experiment further to better understand her limits

Correct answer: B. *The primary care doctor can approach a discussion with Tiffany in a nonjudgmental way by making a distinction between recreational drug use, risky drug use, and a drug use disorder. The primary care provider can utilize the FRAMES approach to provide brief intervention and education.*

2. What is the most likely diagnosis regarding this patient's substance use?

A. Risky substance use

B. Substance use disorder

C. Physiologic substance dependence

D. Substance abuse

E. Substance dependence

Correct answer: A. *Tiffany was experimenting with recreational drug use, which many teens and young adults do (see Table 14-1 for prevalence rates of past month drug use by drug type in the United States). She does not meet criteria for a drug use disorder. She has no history of drug use. She has not used habitually or compulsively since the party, and she has no cravings to use again. Indeed, she feels an aversion to the entire experience with no desire to repeat it. But, Tiffany did engage in risky drug use: she took a large quantity of marijuana and ingested a pill without knowing what was in it; she lost memory for the events directly after ingesting drugs; and she may have been involved in a nonconsensual sexual encounter, which carries its own risks.*

3. What is the provider's goal in providing education about substance use?

A. Convince the patient to go to a residential rehabilitation program

B. Encourage the patient to start attending Narcotics Anonymous

C. Reduce harm associated with substance use

D. Encourage continued substance use

E. Reduce medical liability

Correct answer: C. *Although Tiffany says she plans never to use drugs again, the primary care doctor can nonetheless educate Tiffany about harm reduction approaches regarding recreational drug use. Educating patients about harm reduction approaches should not be misconstrued as encouragement of continued drug use; indeed, Tiffany's resolve not to repeat her experiences should be reinforced. The goal of providing education is to build up Tiffany's sense of self-efficacy and empower her to make the decision to avoid repeating risky behaviors.*

4. What screening tests should the provider order during this encounter?

A. Pregnancy test

B. Chlamydia/gonorrhea

C. Hepatitis B and C Ab tests

D. HIV and RPR

E. All of the above

Correct answer: E. *For the possible nonconsensual sexual encounter, the primary care doctor should order a pregnancy test and offer to screen Tiffany for sexually transmitted diseases (HIV, hepatitis, syphilis, gonorrhea, chlamydia). The provider should also refer Tiffany to Student Mental Health or other campus resources to help the patient understand her rights and options in addressing a possible sexual assault.*

CASE 3:

Laura is a patient who struggled with inexplicable chronic pain for much of her life. She sought out help from multiple physicians over the years, many of whom treated her unkindly and without compassion. She was started on opioid pain-relieving medication and experienced immediate relief of her pain; however, what followed was a half-decade of increasing opioid doses, which did little in the long term to relieve pain and contributed to poorer function. Attempts at lowering her opioid dose often resulted in Laura experiencing body aches, abdominal cramping, poor appetite, nausea, vomiting, chills, sweats, and tremors. She described this constellation of symptoms as similar to the time she caught the flu. The doctor who increased her opioids to the highest doses had encouraged Laura to take them liberally whenever she had pain. She reports a history of taking her medication as prescribed for pain and denies aberrant behaviors of requesting early refills, losing prescriptions, or alternative routes of administration (i.e., crushing, snorting, injecting).

Laura relocated with her family to a new area and started over with a new primary care doctor. Her new primary care doctor was appropriately alarmed by her opioid dosage and told her abruptly that her dose was too high and he would start a rapid taper that very day. He did not provide an explanation or a detailed plan. Laura became so anxious after the visit that she had a panic attack and needed to be taken to an emergency room and hospitalized on a psychiatric ward, something that had never happened to her.

Following discharge, she was able to establish care with a primary care physician who recommended a slow taper off opioids. It took her almost 24 months to come down off 150 MMEs per day of opioids. Nearly 2 years after her last dose of an opioid, Laura remains opioid free. She still has pain, but overall it is more manageable, and she is far more functional than she was on chronic opioid therapy.

1. What was Laura's most likely diagnosis?

A. Substance use disorder

B. Risky substance use

continued

C. Physiologic dependence
D. Malingering
E. Somatization disorder

Correct answer: C. *Laura developed a physiologic dependence to opioid medications as manifested by the development of tolerance and emergence of withdrawal symptoms with attempts to lower or discontinue the substance. Laura's experience illustrates how failure to have an effective initial discussion about the plan for a taper leaves patients feeling anxious and desperate. This scenario can be addressed in the primary care setting by following the acronym "BRAVO." When first broaching the subject of problematic prescription opioid use with patients on chronic opioid therapy, the primary care provider should make sure to schedule extra time with patients. When providers attempt to hurry through this important initial conversation, patients are liable to feel angry and abandoned, which in turn adversely affects the therapeutic alliance. Maintaining an effective and compassionate therapeutic alliance between providers and patients is critical to success.*

2. What are the risk associated with chronic opioid therapy?
   A. The development of tolerance, dependence, and opioid-induced hyperalgesia
   B. Cognitive deficits, such as memory impairment
   C. Alterations in mood and anxiety
   D. Hormonal dysfunction (i.e., low testosterone, low estrogen)
   E. All of the above

Correct answer: E. *A risk of chronic opioid therapy that often goes ignored is simple tolerance. Tolerance is the state of needing more and more of the opioid to get the same results. Once a patient develops tolerance, the primary care provider may want to consider tapering the patient off of opioids, as further dose escalation will result in further tolerance over time, leading to very high opioid doses with no significant improvement in pain or functioning. Opioid rotation is not a long-term strategy to address the development of tolerance. Perhaps the most beguiling side effect of long-term opioid use is an increase in pain, also known as "opioid-induced hyperalgesia." Some patients on opioids will experience an increase in pain over time, including experiencing pain in areas of the body where they originally had no pain. This phenomenon is not well understood but has been clinically appreciated and validated in human and animal experimental conditions.*[21]

3. What are some objective ways of monitoring risks associated with chronic opioid therapy?
   A. Urine drug screen results
   B. Discussing patient's functional status with family members
   C. Physician drug monitoring database
   D. Eliciting observations from the significant other
   E. All of the above

Correct answer: E. *No risk–benefit calculation is complete without objective data points. These include checking the Prescription Drug Monitoring Database (PDMD) (or similarly database depending on the state), urine drug screens, and talking with family members or significant others (after a release of information has been signed by the patient owing to privacy laws).*

4. What is the most common pitfall for providers in tapering a chronic opioid therapy patient?
   A. Tapering too slowly
   B. Tapering too quickly
   C. Converting long-acting medication to an equivalent dose of a short-acting medication
   D. Utilizing nonaddictive medication to help mitigate symptoms of opioid withdrawal
   E. Validating the patient's experience while tapering

Correct answer: B. *The biggest mistake providers make in tapering patients off chronic opioid therapy is tapering too fast. It is not unreasonable to take many months to years to wean some patients off chronic opioid therapy, especially those who have been taking opioids daily for decades. Other helpful strategies include maintaining the same dosing schedule (so if the patient is on a twice-daily or thrice-daily regimen, keep him or her on that schedule as he or she taper, decreasing by increments at a given dose); involving the patient in the taper process (let the patient decide which medication to taper first, unless there is an immediate safety issue, which demands tapering that medication first); taking breaks in the taper when appropriate (waiting at a given dose for some period before continuing to avoid patient discomfort during important events—weddings, family reunions, professional presentation); and most importantly maintaining a unidirectional taper plan (never go backward during the taper by increasing the dose, lest all the hard work of the last dose reduction is lost).*

5. What are some strategies for patients to learn to manage chronic pain without the use of opioids?
   A. Mindfulness practices
   B. DBT skills: "radical acceptance" and "opposite action"
   C. Acupuncture, massage, physical therapy
   D. Psychotherapy
   E. All of the above

Correct answer: E. *As providers work with patients to get them off opioids for the treatment of pain, they can encourage other strategies for dealing with pain: physical therapy, massage, psychotherapy, acupuncture, etc. But many providers work in resource-poor settings with limited access to other forms of pain treatment, and/or insurance companies won't pay for nonopioid alternatives. See "O" part of BRAVO.*

PRACTICAL RESOURCES

- TIP 24: A Guide to Substance Abuse Services for Primary Care Physicians https://www.ncbi.nlm.nih.gov/books/NBK64827/pdf/Bookshelf NBK64827.pdf
- TIP 34: Brief Interventions and Brief Therapies for Substance Abuse https://www.ncbi.nlm.nih.gov/books/NBK64947/pdf/Bookshelf NBK64947.pdf
- American Society of Addiction Medicine (ASAM): www.asam.org
  - National Practice Guidelines for the Use of Medications in the Treatment of Addiction Involving Opioid Use: https://www.asam.org/docs/default-source/practice-support/guidelines-and-consensus-docs/asam- national-practice-guideline-supplement.pdf?sfvrsn=24
- Substance Abuse and Mental Health Services Administration (SAMHSA): www.samhsa.gov
  - Directory of substance abuse treatment centers: https://www.findtreatment.samhsa.gov/
  - Buprenorphine training for physicians: https://www.samhsa.gov/medication-assisted-treatment/training- resources/buprenorphine-phvsician-training
- National Institute of Drug Abuse: www.nida.gov
  - *Principles of Drug Addiction Treatment: A Research-Based Guide (Third Edition):* https://www.drugabuse.gov/publications/principles-drug-addiction-treatment-research-based-guide-third-edition/acknowledgments
- U.S. Department of Health and Human Services (HHS), Office of the Surgeon General: Facing Addiction in America: The Surgeon General's Report on Alcohol, Drugs, and Health: https://www.surgeongeneral.gov/librarv/2016alcoholdrugshealth/index.html
- 12-Step Programs:
  - Narcotics Anonymous: www.na.org
  - Cocaine Anonymous: www.ca.org
  - Marijuana Anonymous: www.mariiuana-anonvmous.org
  - Crystal Meth Anonymous: www.crvstalmeth.org

REFERENCES

1. Substance Abuse and Mental Health Services Administration. *Key Substance Use and Mental Health Indicators in the United States: Results From the 2016 National Survey on Drug Use and Health (HHS Publication No. SMA 17-5044, NSDUH Series H-52).* Rockville, MD: Center for Behavioral Health Statistics and Quality, Substance Abuse and Mental Health Services Administration; 2017. Retrieved from: https://www.samhsa.gov/data/.Accessed April 1, 2018.

2. Centers for Disease Control and Prevention. *Annual Surveillance Report of Drug-related Risks and Outcomes—United States, 2017. Surveillance Special Report 1.* Centers for Disease Control and Prevention, U.S. Department of Health and Human Services. Published August 31, 2017. Accessed April 1, 2018 from https://www.cdc.gov/drugoverdose/pdf/pubs/2017cdc-drug-surveillance-report.pdf.

3. Chen JH, Humphreys K, Shah NH, et al. Distribution of opioids by different types of medicare prescribers. *JAMA Intern Med.* 2016;176(2):259-261.

4. National Center for Health Statistics. *Health, United States, 2015: In Brief.* Hyattsville, MD; 2016.

5. Ahmad FB, Rossen LM, Spencer MR, Warner M, Sutton P. Provisional Drug Overdose Death Counts. National Center for Health Statistics. 2018. Designed by Rossen LM, Lipphardt A, Ahmad FB, Keralis JM, Chong Y. National Center for Health Statistics. Accessed from: https://www.cdc.gov/nchs/nvss/vsrr/drug-overdose-data.htm on April 2, 2018.

6. Center for Behavioral Health Statistics and Quality. *Behavioral Health Trends in the United States: Results from the 2014 National Survey on Drug Use and Health (HHS Publication No. SMA 15-4927, NSDUH Series H-50);* 2015. http://www.samhsa.gov/data/. Accessed June 3, 2017.

7. Volkow ND, Li T. Science and society: drug addiction: the neurobiology of behaviour gone awry. *Nat Rev Neurosci.* 2004;5(12):963-970.

8. McLellan AT, Lewis DC, O'brien CP, et al. Drug dependence, a chronic medical illness. *J Am Med Assoc.* 2000;284(13):1689.

9. U.S. Department of Health and Human Services (HHS). *Office of the Surgeon General: Facing Addiction in America: The Surgeon General's Report on Alcohol, Drugs, and Health.* Washington, DC: HHS; 2016.

10. National Institute on Drug Abuse. *Principles of Drug Addiction Treatment: A Research-Based Guide (Third Edition).* Retrieved July 3, 2016, from United States, National Institute on Drug Abuse. *Principles of Drug Addiction Treatment: A Research-Based Guide (Third Edition).* 2012, December. https://www.drugabuse.gov/publications/principles-drug-addiction-treatment-research-based-guide-third-edition/acknowledgments. Accessed July 3, 2017.

11. Diaper AM, Law FD, Melichar JK. Pharmacological strategies for detoxification. *Br J Clin Pharmacol.* 2013;77(2):302-314.

12. Lee J, Kresina TF, Campopiano M, et al. Use of pharmacotherapies in the treatment of alcohol use disorders and opioid dependence in primary care. *Biomed Res.* 2015:1-11.

13. Stine SM, Kosten TR. Pharmacologic interventions for opioid dependence. In: Ries RK, Fiellin DA, Miller SC, Saitz R, eds. *The ASAM Principles of Addiction Medicine.* 5th ed. Philadelphia, PA: Wolters Kluwer; 2014:735-777.

14. American Society of Addiction Medicine. *National practice guidelines for the use of medications in the treatment of addiction involving opioid use.* American Society of Addiction Medicine; Published June 1, 2015. https://www.asam.org/docs/default-source/practice-support/guidelines-and-consensus-docs/asam-national-practice-guideline-supplement.pdf?sfvrsn=24. Accessed July 3, 2017.

15. Berlin RK, Butler PM, Perloff MD. Gabapentin therapy in psychiatric disorders: a systemic review. *Prim Care Companion CNS Disord.* 2015;17(5).

16. Bonnet U, Preuss UW. The cannabis withdrawal syndrome: current insights. *Subst Abuse Rehabil.* 2017;8:9-37.

17. Shoptaw SJ, Kao U, Heinzerling K, Ling W. Treatment for amphetamine withdrawal. *Cochrane Database Syst Rev.* 2009;(2):CD003021.

18. Quednow BB, Herdener M. Human pharmacology for addiction medicine: from evidence to clinical recommendations. *Prog Brain Res.* 2016;224:227-250.

19. Center for Substance Abuse Treatment. *A Guide to Substance Abuse Services for Primary Care Physicians. Treatment Improvement Protocol (TIP) Series, No. 24. DHS Publication No. (SMA) 08-4075.* Rockville, MD: Substance Abuse and Mental Health Services Administration; 1997.

20. Center for Substance Abuse Treatment. *Brief Interventions and Brief Therapies for Substance Abuse. Treatment Improvement Protocol (TIP) Series, No. 34. HHS Publication No. (SMA) 12-3952.* Rockville, MD: Substance Abuse and Mental Health Services Administration; 1999.

21. The Washington Post. *Post-kaiser survey of long-term prescription opioid painkiller users poll, Oct. 3-Nov. 9, 2016. The Washington post.* Published December 14, 2016. https://www.washingtonpost.com/politics/polling/postkaiser-survey-longterm-prescription-opioid-painkiller/2016/12/09/dc981ebc-be3b-11e6-ae79-bec72d34f8c9_page.html. Accessed April 3, 2017.

22. Lembke A, Humphreys K, Newmark J. Weighing the risks and benefits of chronic opioid therapy. *Am Fam Physician.* 2016;93(12):982-990.

23. National Institute of Drug Abuse. *Prescription drugs: abuse and addiction. National Institute of Drug Abuse.* Published July 2001. Updated October 2011. https://www.drugabuse.gov/sites/default/files/rrprescription.pdf. Accessed July 7, 2017.

24. Dasgupta N, Funk MJ, Proescholdbell S, Hirsch A, Ribisl KM, Marshall S. Cohort study of the impact of high-dose opioid analgesics on overdose mortality. *Pain Med.* 2016;17(1):85-98. Accessed April 1, 2018.

15

PERSONALITY DISORDERS

Shannon Suo, MD, Puja L. Chadha, MD, and Philippe T. Lévy, MD

A 67-year-old woman with diabetes, hypertension, and gastroesophageal reflux disease presents to clinic for a routine follow-up evaluation. She is typically seen by your colleague, who is on vacation. The patient appears to have a good general understanding of her ongoing medical issues. However, throughout the interview, she seems anxious and asks you several times to clarify the dose and frequency of her medications. She is accompanied by a close family friend who frequently helps the patient organize her weekly pill box at home, a process that can take up to an hour despite being only on five medications, each once per day. While charting in the room, you review your colleague's electronic medical record inbox, which demonstrates near daily emails and calls to the clinic advice line for guidance on how to take her medications. These messages, sometimes sent in the middle of the night, also ask for advice about a variety of common and seemingly unrelated symptoms ranging from rash, palpitations, bloating, tinnitus, and hip pain. Several of these conversations seem almost identical in nature. She appears reassured only after you gently remind her that her regular clinician will return in time for her next appointment that she has already scheduled for the following week.

CLINICAL HIGHLIGHTS

- Personality disorders are commonly encountered in primary care settings and may disrupt the patient–provider relationship and compromise the quality of care.
- Primary care clinicians should be aware of their own feelings toward patients with personality disorders and ensure that treatment is not adversely influenced by emotionally charged and negative feelings.
- Treating individuals who struggle with personality disorders and/or other diagnoses can be challenging, and our reactions to those patients can blur the focus and treatment goals in primary care settings. Keep interventions and treatment goals focused on improving the quality of life.

- Personality disorders are frequently associated with other psychiatric conditions. Utilize the "AMPS" screening tool to assess for anxiety, mood, psychotic, and substance abuse disorders.
- Personality disorders share many characteristics with other psychiatric conditions but can readily be distinguished by the presence of longstanding inflexible and maladaptive coping styles.
- Collateral information from family, friends, and other providers can be helpful when considering a personality disorder diagnosis.
- As a general rule, long-term treatment goals include elimination of maladaptive coping strategies (e.g., denial, splitting, somatization) and the development of healthy coping skills (e.g., humor, anticipation of stressors).

CLINICAL SIGNIFICANCE

Patients with personality disorders often present challenges to clinicians. As defined by the *Diagnostic and Statistical Manual of Mental Disorders*, Fifth Edition (*DSM-5*), personality disorders begin in adolescence or early adulthood and consist of consistent, problematic patterns of behavior that affect the ways that people think, express emotion, relate with others, and/or control their own impulses.[1] These disorders result in significant dysfunction that often plays out in the clinical encounter in similar ways to how it presents in the individual's day-to-day life. Clinicians should be careful to explain to patients that the "personality" in personality disorders is defined by psychiatry as the way that people think and feel about themselves and interact with the world around them, rather than the colloquial term, "personality."

In the general population, personality disorders have a prevalence of 9.1%.[2,3] They are more frequently encountered in primary care settings with an average prevalence of 20% to 30%.[4,5] Patients with histrionic and dependent personality disorders are more likely to have increased outpatient, emergency, and inpatient visits.[6] Other studies have found higher levels of dissatisfaction with care, lower scores on functioning scales, and increased antidepressant prescriptions in patients who have a personality disorder.[6,7]

Primary care providers rarely receive sufficient training in psychiatry, and what training they receive typically focuses on other common disorders such as major depression or anxiety. However, it is often the person with personality disorder or "traits" that fill us with angst and make us question our skills. The medical literature has historically labeled personality-disordered patients as "difficult" or even "hateful" rather than identifying the specific disorders, which lead to the difficult patient–provider interactions.[8] Given the increased risk for alcohol- and drug use-related disorders, depression, bipolar disorder, and somatic symptom disorders, clinicians should identify these problematic behaviors to offer appropriate intervention to avoid potentially serious consequences.[9-11]

The cluster A personality disorders include paranoid, schizoid, and schizotypal personality disorders, which are characterized by odd or eccentric thinking and behaviors. Such individuals are more prone to substance use and social isolation. Cluster B disorders are antisocial, borderline, histrionic, or narcissistic personality disorders, which are characterized by high emotions and dramatic and unpredictable thinking and behaviors. These patients may engage in deliberate self-injury and high-risk physical and sexual behaviors, with consequent increased risk of injury, disease, and infection. Approximately 75% of people with borderline personality disorder (BPD) have suicidal ideation and up to 10% of BPD patients complete suicide, a rate about 50 times higher than the general population.[12,13] These patients are also more sensitive to perceived "abandonment" and may act in inappropriate ways to retain contact with their providers. Patients with cluster C pathology (i.e., avoidant, dependent, or obsessive-compulsive personality disorders) tend to be anxious and fearful; they may be less compliant with treatment.

DIAGNOSIS

Primary care providers may not feel comfortable making a formal diagnosis of personality disorder owing to lack of training, time, or certainty. Mental health professionals often note "traits" of personality disorders if they are unable or unwilling to make a diagnosis of the full personality disorder. Primary care clinicians can do the same to provide clinically meaningful interpretation to behaviors and patterns that they observe in patients. Noting traits in progress note assessments avoids the commitment to an ICD or *DSM* diagnosis that has implications for insurance and "chart lore" but can convey to other providers important information regarding potential areas of conflict or vulnerability. Features that distinguish "normal" personality traits from pathologic ones include inflexibility and maladaptive behavior that exceed the ethnic, cultural, or social expectations for the individual. Noting these traits or including a personality disorder on the differential diagnosis for a patient can assist the clinician in determining appropriate treatment and boundaries that are more likely to achieve better outcomes for their patients.

Common characteristics of personality disorders and the clusters to which they belong are listed in *Table 15-1*. Although personality disorder diagnoses are intended to be made based on enduring patterns of behavior, patients can have waxing and waning courses; they may also only display their more severe symptoms under stress. The NIMH Collaborative Longitudinal Personality Disorders Study found that only 44% of patients diagnosed with BPD retained the diagnosis 2 years later.[14] This highlights the dimensionality of the diagnosis of personality disorders and gives greater hope to individuals suffering with a disorder. For primary care providers, it may take several encounters with a patient to accurately recognize long-standing and pervasive character pathology versus poor coping mechanisms on a "bad day." As such, providers are encouraged to obtain collateral history and see patients several times before definitively giving a personality disorder diagnosis.

Our visceral response or feelings about a patient encounter can often be helpful when considering the possibility of personality pathology. *Transference* is defined as the unconscious reenactment of feelings or behaviors toward the provider based on the patient's previous experiences with significant others or caretakers. By contrast, *countertransference* is based on the provider's thoughts and feelings about the patient in response to how the patient behaves or acts. Countertransference can be a useful clue that the patient is acting outside of cultural norms. Providers must objectively review their own feelings before assigning personality traits or disorder to a patient, to ensure that the reaction is not one based on the provider's unique experiences and feelings. For example, a patient may remind one of someone he or she dislikes based on appearance, leading to a sense of irritation and dislike, but would not evoke the same response in all people. *Table 15-2* identifies feelings that may arise in health care providers and the disorders with which they are typically associated. Feelings of anger, leading to retaliation against or punishment of the patient, may be particularly problematic. This contrasts with clearly defined consequences, which *should* follow inappropriate behavior by the patient, including termination of care following repeated breaches of clinic rules or laws, despite explanations of limits and consistent responses to violations of those limits. Equally dangerous are feelings of attraction to patients that lead to indiscretions of a sexual or romantic nature. Peer discussions, such as Balint groups, provide a forum for health care professionals to discuss the emotional content of the patient–provider relationship and can be helpful in processing the strong feelings evoked by patients with a personality disorder. These groups are led by health care professionals with psychological training and provide guidance to the members about countertransferential feelings to ensure the preservation of healthy clinical relationships.

DSM-5 UPDATES AND CHANGES

In the latest version of the *DSM-5*, there have been minor changes and evolution for the overall understanding of personality disorders. Psychiatric conditions are no

TABLE 15-1 *DMS-5* Personality Clusters, Specific Types, Clinical Features, and Clinical Significance

CLUSTER	TYPE	CHARACTERISTIC FEATURES	CLINICAL SIGNIFICANCE
A	**Odd, eccentric behavior**		
	Paranoid	General distrust and suspicion of others; interpretation that others' motives are malevolent	Preoccupation with rules and suspiciousness, leading to litigiousness
	Schizoid	Detachment from relationships with others; decreased expression of emotions, little/no interest in social relationships	Disinterest in care or relationships
	Schizotypal	Interpersonally uncomfortable with close relationships, associated with distortions of thought (e.g., "magical thinking") and eccentric behavior	Unusual health beliefs/practices leading to rare complications or presentations
B	**Dramatic, emotional, or erratic behavior**		
	Antisocial	Must have history of conduct disorder before age 15 years; disregard for others' rights; at least 18 years old at the time of diagnosis	Increased risk for theft, aggression, even in clinical setting
	Borderline	Chaotic and intense interpersonal relationships, poor self-image, affective instability, and impulsivity	Self-injury, sexually-transmitted infections (STIs), domestic violence
	Histrionic	Increased emotional lability, constantly seeking attention	Self-injury, STIs, seductive behavior with clinician
	Narcissistic	Grandiosity, needs to be admired, lacks empathy	Tendency to insult clinician or compare with self or other "important" people
C	**Anxious or fearful**		
	Avoidant	Socially inhibited, feels inadequate, and oversensitive to perceived criticism	Reluctance to disclose potentially "disappointing" information to clinician
	Dependent	Excessive need to be cared for, associated with submissive behavior and separation anxiety	Help seeking, help rejection, lack of follow-through
	Obsessive-compulsive	Preoccupation with order, perfection, and control	Intolerance of flexibility, tardiness, or unclear plans

longer placed in a specific axis (previously axis II for personality disorders) and are considered potentially primary issues for patients. There are now two approaches to the conceptualization of personality disorders. The first describes moderate adaptations to how personality disorders were formulated in *DSM-IV-TR*.[15] The second is an area still undergoing research, which explores a transition to a spectral approach to personality disorders.[16] The latter incorporates dimensions of function including identity, self-direction, empathy, and intimacy;

defenses used maladaptively; and levels of functioning. It also explores the concept that personality disorders exist on a spectrum with other mental illness diagnoses, and there is overlap between personality disorders. One proposed model of overlap is shown here (*Figure 15-1*). This diagram illustrates one potential model of looking at how personality disorders may exist in synchrony with overlapping characteristics. On one end of the spectrum are disorders considered to be more psychotic in origin (i.e., schizotypal and schizoid), whereas others are

TABLE 15-2 Feelings of Countertransference and Reactions to Avoid

PROVIDER'S FEELING	PERSONALITY DISORDER	POTENTIAL PROVIDER PITFALLS	SUGGESTED ACTION
Anger (patient is viewed as manipulative)	• Borderline • Antisocial • Narcissistic	Overreaction to provocation, retaliation (e.g., verbal/physical abuse of patient, substandard care, inappropriate comments in charting)	• Be aware of feelings and unconscious bias • Process with peers, such as in Balint groups • Strict adherence to evidence-based standard of care
Fear of patient (physical or legal threat)	• Antisocial • Paranoid	Immediate emotional or physical overresponse (out of proportion to threat)	• Maintain personal safety • Thorough documentation • Appropriate familiarity with clinic policy and procedure
Sympathy	• Borderline (sympathy by some providers associated with negative views by other providers may represent *splitting* by the patient) • Dependent	Overindulgence or desire to "rescue" the patient	• Regular, structured, and scheduled visits with the same provider that do not run over scheduled time • Splitting should be dealt with by interdisciplinary meetings to make sure all members of team are acting in accordance with treatment plan and not providing "special" treatment
Anger, self-doubt	• Narcissistic • Paranoid	Putting down the patient; questioning your own abilities in a nonrealistic way	• Examine your abilities in a realistic way • Seek peer support, process in Balint groups
Frustration	• Borderline • Avoidant • Dependent	Patients do not follow-through with treatment recommendations or rely heavily on providers	• Set clear expectations • Ally yourself with patient's family/friends to assist (as permitted by privacy restrictions) • Treat patient with a consistent team approach so that no single provider burns out
Attraction	• Histrionic • Borderline	Inappropriate relationship with patient	• Consider using a chaperone for examinations requiring examination of genitalia, even in gender-matched provider–patient situations • Do not see the patient after-hours or in social settings

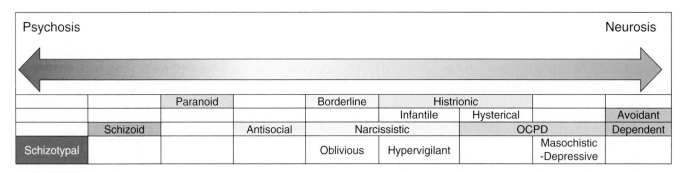

FIGURE 15-1 Personality disorders spectral organization. OCPD, obsessive-compulsive personality disorder.

considered more neurotic (i.e., avoidant, dependent and obsessive-compulsive). Exploring personality disorders in this light can be helpful when individuals have multiple traits and to explore similarities between the disorders. This novel approach is still undergoing research, but it is expected that the next revision of *DSM* will describe personality disorders with this different perspective from the traditional categorical descriptors.

Physical examination should be guided by complaints and review of systems in patients thought to have a personality disorder, as with any patient. Providers should ask about and check for self-inflicted injuries in patients with borderline pathology, including cuts, burns, or other forms of self-mutilation. Patients who self-inflict injuries may hide their wounds by wearing long sleeves or pants. Patients with borderline or dependent personality disorders are at increased risk for domestic violence, emotional abuse, and sexual victimization and should be carefully screened and assessed for history of and signs of abuse. Providers should always use chaperones when performing genital examinations but should consider incorporating a chaperone into physical examinations with people with borderline or histrionic traits owing to their possible sexual transference, rejection hypersensitivity, and impulsivity. For those same reasons, these patients are at increased risk for sexually transmitted infections (STIs) and should be screened regularly and counseled on contraception and STI prevention. All patients with a suspected personality disorder should be asked about alcohol and other substance use. Obtaining collateral information from other care providers as well as family members and friends can help establish a diagnosis or confirm the presence of traits.

BORDERLINE PERSONALITY DISORDER— SPECIAL DIAGNOSTIC CONSIDERATIONS

Of the personality disorders, BPD has received the most attention in terms of epidemiologic research and evidence-based treatment approaches. When asked which personality disorders prove most challenging, providers frequently respond with "borderline personality disorder." People with BPD present challenges to our patience, risk tolerance, and even self-esteem. The suicidal and parasuicidal behavior of patients with BPD frequently leaves primary care providers in fear for the patients' safety and their own liability. These experiences with patients with BPD lead to stigmatization of the disorder within the medical field and a reluctance to reveal the diagnosis to the patient. Keep in mind that the individual with BPD is suffering, and often the angst that providers experience in their care of patients with BPD is caused by the patients' subconscious attempt to recreate the suffering which they regularly experience, providing an opportunity to develop empathy. Exploring empathy for their suffering may be critical in clinical settings to establishing good rapport and treatment planning.

When considering a diagnosis of BPD, we recommend a stepwise approach to ascertain if the patient has the following typical features: an enduring pattern of unstable identity, intense relationships, emotional dysregulation, and self-harm. First, summarize the emotional, behavioral, and interpersonal difficulties the patient seems to be having. Second, inquire about the patient's understanding of his or her difficulties and what role they play in the problems. Third, introduce BPD as a possible, but not definitive, explanation. Last, recommend the patient learn about BPD either through reading or consultation with a mental health professional. Upon follow-up, the provider can reassess the patient's understanding of BPD. If significant conflicts arise, primary care providers should refer to a mental health professional for ongoing assessment and treatment.

An open discussion with patients about a possible diagnosis of BPD can be both therapeutic and rewarding. Patients are often relieved when someone can explain why they behave the way they do, especially when informed that effective treatment options are available. Not every patient with BPD or borderline traits requires an in-depth discussion of BPD. Such discussions should be limited to when they are clinically indicated, such as when referring for specific treatments (especially psychotherapy) or when reflecting on maladaptive patterns of behavior.

DIFFERENTIAL DIAGNOSIS

There can be considerable overlap between symptoms of personality disorders and other psychiatric diagnoses; appropriately differentiating the condition is important to develop the optimal treatment plan. The AMPS screening tool may be used to systematically screen for comorbid psychiatric conditions (see Chapter 1). Anxiety disorders, mood disorders (e.g., bipolar disorder, depressive disorders, and substance-induced mood disorders), and behavioral changes induced by general medical conditions are important to consider as either alternate or co-occurring conditions. BPD and bipolar disorder, in particular, can be difficult to differentiate owing to the overlap of symptoms of impulsivity and affective lability. Some distinguishing features between bipolar disorder and BPD include decreased *need* for sleep with mania and episodic mood swings lasting days to weeks, both found in the former. Keep in mind that borderline personality and bipolar disorder can coexist; bipolar disorder has been found to be more prevalent in people with BPD than in people with other personality disorders.[17] *Table 15-3* highlights common primary care complaints and comorbid conditions frequently encountered in patients with personality disorders.

Information about long-standing patterns of behavior, affect, thought disorder, and behavioral lability can help distinguish between personality pathology and other psychiatric disorders. Personality symptoms that only occur during the course of another psychiatric disorder should not be diagnosed as a personality disorder. Personality changes caused by medical conditions (e.g., endocrine disorders, traumatic brain injury, and seizure disorders) can usually be distinguished by the development of symptoms with the onset of the medical condition as opposed to having their development in adolescence or early adulthood.

TABLE 15-3 Differential Diagnosis of Personality Disorders

PERSONALITY DISORDER (PD)	COMMON PRIMARY CARE PRESENTATIONS AND CONCERNS	DIFFERENTIATION FROM OTHER PSYCHIATRIC DISORDERS	COMMON PSYCHIATRIC COMORBIDITY
Paranoid	• Guarded, hypervigilant, anxious, irritable/hostile, businesslike, suspicious of harm from clinicians • Preoccupied with justice and rules	<u>Psychotic disorders</u>, which have overt delusional or psychotic content <u>Posttraumatic stress disorder (PTSD)</u> in which hypervigilance is rooted in previous trauma and consistent with traumatic experience	• Depression • Substance use • Obsessive-compulsive disorder (OCD) • Agoraphobia
Schizoid	• Eager for visits to end • Offers little comment or elaboration • May delay seeking care until conditions are advanced	<u>Avoidant PD</u> in which patients crave intimate relationships	
Schizotypal	• Odd, peculiar behavior, idiosyncratic speech/dress • Difficulty with face-to-face communication • Eccentric beliefs, paranoid tendencies, may appear guarded • Uncomfortable with physical examination, especially gynecologic/rectal examinations	<u>Psychotic disorders</u> in which a fixed and false belief is generally bizarre or paranoid in nature	• Depression
Antisocial	• May be superficially cooperative and charming • Impulsive and manipulative • Lacking guilt or remorse for behavior • Little or no regard for the rights of others • Usually deceitful	<u>Adult antisocial behavior,</u> which consists of purely criminal behavior <u>Substance use disorders</u> are often accompanied by antisocial behavior that resolves with resolution of substance use	• Impulse control disorders • Depression • Substance use • Pathologic gambling • Anxiety • Malingering
Borderline	• Interpersonally intense with superficial sociability and periods of intense anger • Idealization/devaluation • Impulsive self-destructive behavior • Identity disturbance (unstable choices in career, sexual orientation, appearance)	<u>Bipolar disorder</u> in which lability of mood and affect is episodic and occurs days to weeks, not a fixed personality trait	• Substance use • Mood disorders (higher risk of suicide) • Eating disorder • PTSD
Histrionic	• Dramatic, exhibitionistic, attention-seeking • Avoid/forget unpleasant feelings or ideas (such as appointments, seriousness of medical conditions) • Exaggerated displays of emotion to manipulate/seduce.	<u>Borderline PD</u> which includes an unstable self-image and feelings of emptiness	• Depression • Somatic symptom disorder
Narcissistic	• Egocentric, entitled, hypersensitive to criticism and preoccupation with being envied • Seek the "best" clinician and demand special attention • Difficulty accepting diagnoses that are incompatible with their self-image	<u>Antisocial PD</u> The narcissist knows the rules and thinks s/he is above them. The antisocial does not wish to know the rules.	• Depression (especially with "failure") • Substance use

TABLE 15-3 Differential Diagnosis of Personality Disorders   (continued)

Avoidant	• Extreme sensitivity and fear of rejection, shy, anxious about what others think of them • Reluctant to disagree or ask questions • May delay seeking medical care for fear of appearing foolish	<u>Schizoid PD</u> in which people do not have interest in relationships <u>Social phobia</u> experiences less/ no fear in settings with close/ intimate friends/family	• Mood disorders • Social phobia
Dependent	• Excessive reliance on others, trying to get others to be responsible for health care (e.g., a diabetic seeks others to give insulin injections) • Asks many questions to avoid terminating the interview • Brings family or friends to appointments and inappropriately asks them to provide answers or decisions	<u>Histrionic PD</u> patients are flamboyant and/or seductive.	• Mood disorders • Anxiety disorders • Adjustment disorder
Obsessive-compulsive	• Perfectionistic, obsessed with the "right" way • Facts preferable to emotions • Responds negatively to clinician being late • Keeps detailed notes to track her illness • May seek opinions from multiple clinician sources	<u>OCD</u> which has specific obsessions and compulsions and tends to be more severe	• Depression • Anxiety disorders • OCD

NOT TO BE MISSED

- Depression
- Anxiety disorders
- Bipolar disorder
- Posttraumatic stress disorder
- Substance use disorder
- Psychotic disorders (e.g., schizophrenia)
- General medical condition(s)
- Suicidal intent and plan

BIOPSYCHOSOCIAL TREATMENT

The following discussion on the treatment for personality disorders will focus primarily on paranoid, borderline, antisocial, and dependent personality disorders, as they are the most commonly encountered personality disorders in the primary care setting.

PSYCHOTHERAPY

The best long-term treatment for personality-disordered patients is psychotherapy. Several evidence-based studies demonstrate the efficacy of specific psychotherapies

for borderline, narcissistic, and dependent personality-disordered patients.[18,19] In most primary care settings, psychotherapy requires a referral to mental health professionals, although certain techniques of cognitive behavioral therapy (CBT) may be useful in clinical encounters.

Patients with BPD, in particular, benefit from dialectical behavior therapy (DBT), a form of CBT that also utilizes mindfulness meditation techniques and focuses on emotional regulation and distress tolerance. Transference-based psychodynamic psychotherapy can also be helpful for patients with BPD. Other therapy interventions include mentalization-based treatment, which is rooted in attachment theory. Its goal is to improve a patient's ability to "mentalize"—to understand his or her own and others' mental states.[20] Studies of evidence-based psychotherapies show not only greater efficacy, but also cost-savings to the health care systems in the United States, Europe, United Kingdom, and Australia, with a mean savings of over US$2,900 per patient per year.[21]

DBT involves once-weekly group and once-weekly individual therapy focused on optimizing coping skills and modifying maladaptive behaviors. The initial goal of DBT is to reduce "parasuicidal" behaviors such as cutting and self-mutilation, while progressing to the development of behaviors that further improve the quality of life. A firm, detailed, and explicit treatment contract is established with the patient that addresses attendance, vacations, homework, and boundary issues such as limits on extra sessions and telephone and email contact. DBT is highly structured and compels the patient to identify deficits, learn skills, and apply these skills to replace dysfunctional behaviors that the patient has developed in response to intense emotional dysregulation and conflicts in relationships.

Transference-based psychodynamic involves once- or twice-weekly individual therapy that is mainly focused on the patient's internal experiences and relationships.

Patients with dependent personality disorder benefit from individual and group psychotherapy using supportive psychotherapy techniques, which teach, model, and reinforce adaptive coping skills, independence, and discourage behaviors, which rely on others to succeed.

Paranoid personality may respond to CBT, although it can be hard to engage and retain such patients in treatment. Similarly, antisocial personality disorder (ASPD) is considered difficult to treat, and high-quality studies are lacking; there is some limited evidence for group CBT being effective to reduce some behaviors, but such patients tend not to engage in treatment.

PSYCHOSOCIAL INTERVENTIONS

Whenever possible, it is important to include the patient's family and support network as part of the treatment plan. With due diligence to patient privacy, educating the patient and his or her caregivers about the nature of behavioral patterns related to a personality disorder may assist the patient in anticipating and avoiding some of the more harmful consequences. As mentioned previously, it is often an enormous relief to patients when they are informed about a diagnosis of BPD. Caregivers and friends may have greater patience and sympathy for the patient's frustrating behaviors if the nature of the illness is explained for them. Involved family and friends may also need to learn about boundaries and how not to overreact when the patient seems out of control.

Community organizations, such as the National Alliance on Mental Illness (NAMI), offer additional support and education for patients and their families. Other support interventions, known as "peer partner" programs, are available through some organizations. Peer partner programs offer workshops and individual support from other consumers. Another specific support is the Wellness Recovery Action Plan (WRAP), which focuses on navigating crisis in healthier ways (see resource section for more information). Support groups, where a patient can meet others who share similar difficulties, provide the additional advantage of peer-to-peer feedback. For BPD, DBT groups as well as mentalization-based workshops/treatment groups are becoming more popular both in public mental health systems and in the private sector.

Therapeutic Relationship and Reframing Conflict

The management of patients with personality disorders is challenging to even the most experienced clinicians. BPD is usually associated with intense dependency, maladaptive use of self-destructiveness, and alternating idealization and devaluation of interpersonal relationships, which often generate intense feelings of anger and sometimes attraction in health care providers. Many providers enter their profession owing to a desire to "help people." Thus, the relinquishing of control by people with dependent personality can initially feel fulfilling but can quickly become draining and lead to burnout. The abusive behavior of people with narcissistic or ASPD or traits can leave providers angry and inclined toward retaliation. Acting on any of these feelings is counterproductive and can even be dangerous, as these actions not only jeopardize the therapeutic relationship but also leave the provider vulnerable to possible legal or disciplinary action. The clinician should try to recognize and acknowledge these intense feelings (countertransference), consult with colleagues, actively set limits, and avoid the seduction of idealization.

All patients with personality disorders who make "special" demands should be managed with validation about their concerns yet an explicit explanation of clinic rules (e.g., number and frequency of phone calls, length and frequency of appointments, only seeing the patient in the office) and reasonable expectations for what the clinician can provide.[9] The clinician who tries to meet unreasonable requests may quickly be dealing with escalating demands. Reframing conflict and limit setting may be challenged, and the clinician should remain calm and demonstrate concern, while repeatedly reinforcing clear boundaries. Consistency in limit setting and response to the patient by all clinic staff avoids undue burden on one provider alone. The $E = MC^3$ mnemonic can be used to minimize frustration and facilitate the delivery of compassionate and effective care for patients with personality disorders (*Table 15-4*).

Shaping of patient behavior through positive reinforcement is possible, and rewards for desirable behavior should be *clear* and *consistent*. Providers should strive to be empathetic and validating, yet firm with boundaries. Similarly, negative consequences for harmful behaviors should be explicit and enforceable. To prevent impulsive and self-destructive behaviors, the provider should encourage the patient to put feelings into words rather than counterproductive actions. Rage and aggression are common problems in patients with cluster B personality disorders, and the clinician should help the patient identify underlying anger as potential maladaptive defense for underlying vulnerability, tolerate patient outbursts when they are not abusive, and redirect aggression to healthy and adaptive outlets such as hobbies or leisure activities.

DON'T BE THE SLOT MACHINE

Consistency begets consistency. When providers inconsistently enforce boundaries, some patients continue to test them to check if they are still there. Consider the phenomenon of playing a slot machine. You know that the odds of winning are low, but people continue to play coin after coin because they know that it will occasionally pay out. If no one ever won at the slot machine, people would stop playing.

TABLE 15-4 Using E = MC³ as Part of the Treatment for Borderline Personality Disorder

Empathy	Try to fully understand the details of one's turbulent and chaotic life.
"Manage," not "cure"	Personalities are formed early and can be difficult to modify. Improvement may be gradual and temporary with frequent "relapses" of behavior.
Countertransference	Consider why you are feeling a certain way before you respond to a patient.
Comorbidity	Screen for other psychopathology (e.g., mood, anxiety, and substance use disorders).
Consistency	Make consequences clearly known and enforce boundaries every time. Avoid making exceptions or treating some people as "special."

Managing Acute Conflicts in the Clinical Setting

It can be helpful to explore the energy in the room and potential for a power struggle dynamic. The Triangle Method: Reframing Conflict can be used to shift energy to allow better, joint problem-solving (*Figure 15-2*). Medical needs/pain/demands (both provider's and patient's) can be a source of contention in appointments, as it can be a challenge to align goals and expectations around issues. Such conflicts have the potential to become explosive and lead to negative outcomes. An alternative is to approach this by mindfully reframing the conflict: building rapport with the patient, establishing mutual goals, having shared expertise; allowing the individual to be an expert on his or her lived experiences/body; and sharing your limits as a provider can also be helpful. Focusing on better rapport and jointly solving the conflict as separate (or outside of) the provider–patient relationship can be very mobilizing for issues and promote healthier problem-solving with a healthier dynamic. Some helpful dialogues can include the following:

Provider: "I can see how much pain you are in and how it affects your daily life and quality of life. I share your goal in decreasing your pain to improve your ability to function. One of my limits as a prescriber is: *medication xyz* may not be the best for your needs because of *reasons abc.* What I would like to offer is/are options *123.* What are your thoughts on this and how can we help meet your needs with the known limits we have?"

Provider: "<Issue> seems to be causing you a lot of distress. I'd really like to help you with it. I've offered several suggestions for addressing <issue>, but none of them seem to work for you. I have training and expertise on treatments and medication, but I also realize you are the expert on your body and what your experience is. Is there anything that you've tried in the past that was more helpful or something you think may be more doable?"

Provider: "I'm sorry that you don't feel heard. Can we start over and I'll just listen to you for the next few minutes without interrupting and you tell me what you've been trying to say? When you're done, I'll let you know what I understood and make sure we're on the same page." (Note: 3 to 5 minutes is usually plenty of time for most patients, but providers must resist the urge to interrupt or respond until the patient has had their time, even if the patient starts to become redundant. If the patient goes longer than 5 minutes and shows no signs of stopping, a provider may need to interrupt and point out that time is limited but still reflect back what was communicated.)

By using this approach, it can shift the conversation/interaction from oppositional (*Figure 15-2A*) to a team approach with joint problem-solving (*Figure 15-2B*).

PHARMACOTHERAPY: OVERVIEW

While psychotherapy remains the mainstay treatment for personality disorders, medications may facilitate psychotherapy and stabilize a patient to tolerate the process of psychotherapy.[1] No medications have been approved by the Food and Drug Administration (FDA) for the treatment of personality disorders, and therefore, all recommendations for medication management are for off-label use only. Medication should be selected to first target any comorbid identified psychiatric disorder. For *paranoid personality disorder*, low-dose antipsychotics may reduce anxiety and paranoid tendencies, but patients are often reluctant to take medications, especially if they believe medications impair their ability to remain hypervigilant. For *dependent personality disorder,* antidepressants used for comorbid anxiety or depression may need to be used at higher-than-usual doses and with a longer treatment duration to evaluate clinical response. Antidepressants have the potential to improve assertiveness and outgoing behavior in dependent personality disorder.[22,23] ASPD is usually managed by firm limit setting and not with the use of psychiatric medications.

Pharmacotherapy of Borderline Personality Disorder

Pharmacotherapeutic options for BPD have been studied more than any other personality disorder. Despite this, there remains significant controversy regarding the use of pharmacotherapy as an adjunctive treatment to psychotherapy.[24] For example, the UK National Institute for Health and Care Excellence (NICE) recommended in their 2015 quality standard for borderline and antisocial personality disorders against the routine (non-emergent) use of drug treatment for BPD and ASPD and cited concerns regarding lack of evidence and fear of ongoing polypharmacy in such patients.[25] A recent Cochrane review found against routine use of SSRIs but suggested that mood stabilizers had a role in decreasing impulsive–aggressive symptoms and decreasing affective dysregulation.[26]

The American Psychiatric Association Practice Guidelines suggest that SSRIs, mood stabilizers, and antipsychotics provide the greatest effect in treatment of the disorder.[27] Antidepressants may be used to target depression, rejection sensitivity, anger, and self-harm behavior. Mood stabilizers and second-generation antipsychotics may

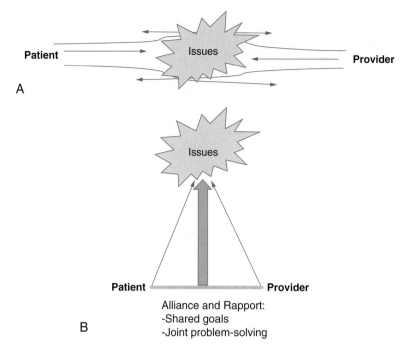

FIGURE 15-2 The Triangle Method: Exploring interpersonal dynamic strategies for navigating conflict versus Oppositional Approach. (A) Oppositional Approach. (B) The Triangle Method: Reframing Conflict Joint Problem-Solving Approach, shifting focus to the relationship and placing the conflict outside of the relationship.

be selected to target affective instability and impulsivity. For paranoia, dissociation, and other psychotic features, secondary generation antipsychotics may be prescribed.[27,28] Further evidence regarding the utility of existing and novel pharmacotherapies are needed, including emerging evidence for the use of omega-3 fatty acids as monotherapy or as supplements to mood stabilizers.[29]

When considering pharmacotherapeutic agents in management of BPD, standard doses for mood stabilizers, antipsychotics, and antidepressants are recommended (see chapter 8 for depression, chapter 10 for bipolar, and chapter 11 for psychotic disorders for dosing protocols). Before prescribing antidepressants, all patients should be thoroughly screened for a history of mania to avoid iatrogenic induction of a manic or mixed episode in a patient with an undiagnosed bipolar spectrum disorder. Patients should also be closely monitored for the presence of suicidal ideation, intent, and plan upon the initiation of an antidepressant.

WHEN TO REFER

- Persistently negative thoughts and feelings (countertransference) causing significant angst or distress in the provider
- Providers who find themselves indulging in behavior outside their norm or outside community standards
- Co-occurring personality disorders with other psychiatric disorders, such as mood or anxiety disorders
- High risk for suicide or self-harm, active intent or plan for self-harm, recent self-harm
- Need for ongoing individual or group CBT, DBT, and other psychotherapies

CASES AND QUESTIONS

CASE 1:

A 67-year-old woman with diabetes, hypertension, and gastroesophageal reflux disease presents to clinic for a routine follow-up evaluation. She is typically seen by your colleague, who is on vacation. The patient appears to have a good general understanding of her ongoing medical issues. However, throughout the interview, she seems anxious and asks you several times to clarify the dose and frequency of her medications. She is accompanied by a close family friend who frequently helps the patient organize her weekly pill box at home, a process that can take up to an hour despite being only on five medications, each once per day. While charting in the room, you review your colleague's electronic medical record inbox, which demonstrates near daily emails and calls to the clinic advice line for guidance on how to take her medications. These messages, sometimes sent in the middle of the night, also ask for advice about a variety of common and seemingly unrelated symptoms ranging from rash, palpitations, bloating, tinnitus, and hip pain. Several of these conversations seem almost identical in nature. She appears reassured only after you gently remind her that her regular clinician will return in time for her next appointment that she has already scheduled for the following week.

1. What type of personality traits should be considered?

   A. Dependent personality
   B. Avoidant personality

C. Borderline personality
D. Schizoid personality

   Correct answer: A. *Overreliance on others is a hallmark of dependent personality disorder. Avoidant personality traits lead people to avoid interactions in which they may be rejected or judged, whereas those with schizoid personality have little to no interest in interactions. People with BPD are often more dramatic than what is demonstrated here.*

2. What kind of interventions are recommended for management? (Select all that apply)

   A. Responding to every request immediately
   B. Regularly scheduled visits, discouraging interval visits between unless medically indicated
   C. Limiting frequency of telephone contact
   D. Confronting patient about her needy behavior and telling her it is interfering with her relationships

   Correct answer: B and C. *People with personality disorders typically respond well to clearly defined limits. Such limits can include the length and frequency of contact and establishing regular appointments and ways of contacting the provider. Responding to every request immediately is likely to escalate the demands and risks burnout of the provider. Unless there is a long-term plan for meeting the patient's needs through behavioral modification/therapy, confrontation is unlikely to be productive.*

3. What conditions would *not* be part of the differential at this point?

   A. Obsessive-compulsive disorder (OCD)
   B. Major neurocognitive disorders
   C. Generalized anxiety disorder
   D. Schizophrenia

   Correct answer: D. *The patient demonstrates obsessiveness with her regimen, which could indicate underlying OCD, or neurocognitive disorder, which is interfering with her comprehension. Her anxiety could be explored further to determine if it is more widespread or interferes with function. However, there is no indication of psychosis and it would be very unusual for someone to present with schizophrenia for the first time in their 60s.*

Discussion

Dependent personality disorder is characterized by a pervading need to be taken care of by others in a maladaptive manner, leading to clinging behavior and a fear of separation. It can be a challenge to care for such patients in a way that is empathic without succumbing to feelings about the patient (termed *countertransference*) that could impede a therapeutic relationship. In particular, feeling frustrated in providing such frequent (and seemingly fruitless) reassurance is common. Setting clear and consistent expectations about clinic visits, scheduling visits at regular intervals while discouraging making

appointments in-between (unless medically indicated), and establishing an alliance with the patient's caregivers are essential in these cases. Limit setting is often required, as people's dependency needs may outpace the ability of a provider to respond and may paradoxically escalate with immediate response on the part of a provider because the person experiences temporary relief.

When suspecting dependent personality disorder, be cautious not to overlook possible underlying or comorbid conditions. In this example, a psychiatric differential diagnosis includes primary anxiety disorders, OCD, or obsessive-compulsive personality disorder, particularly regarding perseverative behaviors around medications and organization. Similarly, a basic cognitive screening tool including the Mini-Mental State Examination and/or the Montreal Cognitive Assessment (MoCA) should be performed to rule out the early presentation of a neurocognitive or neurodegenerative disease including Alzheimer disease or vascular dementia that could also present as confusion, memory loss, and anxiety while not yet having progressed to a global decline of function. This would be distinguished from a personality disorder by its timing of onset/marked *change* in behavior, compared with a personality disorder, which has been present chronically through much of the person's adult life. There is no evidence of psychosis in this woman's presentation that would suggest a diagnosis of schizophrenia be considered. Schizophrenia typically presents first in young adulthood, with a second peak in women in their 30s, but would be highly unlikely to present for the first time in their 60s.

CASE 2:

A 45-year-old female new patient presents to your office with a chief complaint of sore throat and asks for an antibiotic. She denies fevers, endorses cough, and has no sick contacts. On physical examination, she is afebrile with normal blood pressure and pulse and has no tonsillar exudate or lymphadenopathy. You explain that antibiotics are not indicated and attempt to counsel her on care for pharyngitis. Although she initially appeared pleasant and cooperative, her demeanor rapidly changes and she criticizes your care and threatens to go to the emergency department to obtain antibiotics. She denies any alcohol or drug use recently but states that she just got out of jail for amphetamine possession.

1. What behaviors would lead you to suspect ASPD?

   A. Threatening suicide
   B. Initially charming, becoming threatening when she doesn't get her way
   C. Asking for her boyfriend to come into the room to help her talk to you
   D. Accusing the medical establishment of creating the Centor criteria to prevent patients from obtaining the care they need

continued

Correct answer: B. *Although not diagnostic, her history of criminal behavior, immediate reaction with anger/threats, and manipulative behavior is suggestive of ASPD. Threatening suicide is more commonly associated with BPD, while asking for someone else to come in would suggest dependent personality traits, and accusations about the "establishment" are seen in paranoid personality disorder.*

2. What is not an appropriate response to this patient?
   A. Calling her a liar
   B. Referring her to over-the-counter remedies
   C. Offering nonantibiotic prescription medications
   D. Calling security/police if she becomes aggressive

   Correct answer: A. *Providers must always remain professional, even in the face of inappropriate behavior on the part of patients. Name-calling or engaging in a debate will be counterproductive to a therapeutic alliance. Additionally, clinicians may be found negligent if they do not provide care at the community standard unless the patient's behavior has made that care impossible to provide.*

Discussion

This patient presents with symptoms and findings consistent with pharyngitis but not strep throat. While ASPD occurs more commonly in men (5.5% vs. 1.9%), 8.5% of women engage in adult antisocial behavior (compared with 16.5% of men).[30] Providers should not let their unconscious bias affect their consideration of these behaviors in women. Adult antisocial behavior is an ICD-10 diagnosis and is intended to be diagnosed in the absence of another psychiatric condition (including ASPD). We do not have enough information to make a diagnosis of either condition in this patient yet.

An appropriate and empathic response to this patient's distress is an acknowledgment of her discomfort and medical condition. This must be coupled with the provider's transparency about their own willingness (or lack thereof) to meet the patient's needs with antibiotics. The focus should be shifted to common goals: decreased discomfort and recovery time. Interventions focused on those goals should be offered. It can be difficult to engage with individuals that challenge us and do not fit into the clinic flow. It is important for us to be aware of our reactions as well as the patient's struggle. Try to stay connected with the relationship in the room; appreciate that they may not be acting intentionally but may be reacting in the way that was formed in childhood based on a traumatic or unsupportive upbringing. It is critical to appreciate that personality disorders can often arise from a lack of supportive modeling or coping skills learned in childhood. Our consideration of other facets of our patients' histories can help us stay connected with empathy and successfully support patients in accessing resources and getting their needs met.

Behavior that is inappropriate (threats, assault) should not be tolerated, and patients should be redirected or security should be called to escort the patient out. In rare cases of extreme behavior (typically serious assault), law enforcement may be called. Providers must be explicit with boundaries and consistent about enforcement of the boundaries so that patients with antisocial behavior know not to continue to cross them.

CASE 3:

A 14-year-old boy presents to urgent care with a laceration on his thigh that requires stitches. He states that he was cutting his leg with a pocket knife when it slipped and cut deeper than he intended. It would not stop bleeding, so his foster mother brought him to the urgent care. You notice several superficial linear scars on his left arm and legs. He states that his girlfriend just broke up with him and he wanted to feel physical pain instead of emotional pain. He is embarrassed and says he has no suicidal ideation, nor did he intend to try to die. You verify with his foster mother that he has no history of suicide attempt or psychiatric hospitalization/treatment.

1. This patient demonstrates traits of which disorder most prominently?
   A. Obsessive-compulsive personality disorder
   B. Antisocial personality disorder
   C. Borderline personality disorder
   D. Avoidant personality disorder

   Correct answer: C. *Self-injury and impulsive behavior in response to rejection is common with borderline personality disorder. Obsessive-compulsive personality disorder is typically concerned with rules and order, whereas individuals with antisocial personality disorder show little regard for others. Individuals with avoidant personality disorder fear rejection but are less likely to engage in self-injury than those with BPD.*

2. What is the most appropriate management of this patient's behavior?
   A. Assessment of future safety, referral for psychotherapy
   B. Immediate hospitalization
   C. Report to child protective services
   D. Start an antipsychotic

   Correct answer: A. *Intervention should be focused on prevention of serious injury (including unintentional injury such as today) and stabilizing affective dysregulation. The patient should be referred for further evaluation and therapy: ideally DBT or psychodynamic psychotherapy. In the process of referral, it is important to emphasize to the patient that you, as his primary care provider, remain a resource and advocate. Referrals to mental health without clear follow-up or involvement in primary care may result in perceptions of abandonment by the patient. Medication is not indicated at this point.*

3. What type of psychotherapy would be most likely to be helpful for this young man's behavior?

    A. Long-term psychoanalysis
    B. Self-psychology
    C. Hypnotherapy
    D. DBT

        Correct answer: D. *DBT, a form of CBT, has been shown to be effective in reducing self-harmful behavior and distress tolerance.*

Discussion

Nonsuicidal self-injury (NSSI) or deliberate self-harm (DSH) is becoming increasingly common in adolescents.[31] NSSI is more common in women/girls than in men, but providers should be vigilant about the phenomenon in both sexes. While the reasons for NSSI are not always grounded in psychopathology, there are several signs that should point toward a consideration for BPD in this young man. Given his placement with a foster family, it is likely that he has had adverse childhood experiences that may predispose him to later psychiatric illness. His reaction to breaking up with his girlfriend warrants exploration of the historical stability of that relationship, which may indicate borderline personality pathology if found to be chronically chaotic. It would be important to elicit symptoms of dissociation as well, as NSSI, affective instability, and dissociation have the strongest correlation with suicide attempts.[32]

Providers should explore more about the cutting behavior itself. This can be a difficult topic to broach but worthwhile to assess safety and motivations/etiology of the behavior as well as to demonstrate empathy.

Provider: "I heard you say that you would rather experience physical pain instead of emotional pain, but can you tell me more about the cutting? ... How long had you been thinking about cutting? ... What did you use to cut? ... What was your intention/what did you hope would happen by cutting? ... How did you feel immediately after you cut? ... How do you feel about it now?"

Patients can often describe behaviors as being impulsive and associated with "escape" or "grounding" from intense emotions or emotional pain. Individuals with BPD may experience senses of relief when they draw blood or feel the pain as a distraction, as it draws them away from other intense feelings/thoughts. People may have a ritual in cutting, use specific tools, and make superficial cuts, often with the intent to draw blood or feel pain rather than ending their lives. These important distinguishing factors can be critical for risk assessment and safety. It is also important to bear in mind that no matter how superficial cuts/self-harm were intended, there is always a risk that cuts/self-inflicted injuries can result in lethal/serious outcomes.

This case illustrates several features that are suspicious for BPD, but clinicians should be aware that the 12-month prevalence for NSSI in adolescents is 19% to 28%, depending on the type of assessment used. Adolescents may also overreport self-injury and even suicide attempts.[33] One clinician even reported a patient describing "cutting" behaviors that were done with a marker!

As multiple other psychiatric conditions may be comorbid with BPD, the AMPS screening tool should be used to assess for anxiety, mood, psychotic, or substance use disorders. Appropriate treatment of all comorbidities in adolescence may avert more serious sequelae in adulthood.

CASE 4:

A 37-year-old man from a rural area presents to your clinic for court-ordered treatment for substance abuse. He was found to be cultivating large quantities of marijuana with other assorted drug paraphernalia in the home, including methamphetamine. He describes himself as always being a "loner" and feeling more comfortable engrossed in books, television, and video games than around other people. He completed high school, attended college for a couple of years, and most recently has been enrolled in online classes in computer science. He wears a long black trench coat, biking gloves, and large reflective sunglasses throughout the encounter. His affect is guarded, but his speech is fluent and spontaneous, and he often changes the subject to assess your understanding of "spirit vortices" and "interdimensional energies" and rumors of "demonic possessions" in the woods. He begins to tell you about his ability to participate in séances with the deceased but stops abruptly saying "you wouldn't understand what it's like to have this power" and changes the subject.

1. What psychiatric disorder seems most likely?

    A. Paranoid personality disorder
    B. Delusional disorder
    C. Paranoid schizophrenia
    D. Schizotypal personality disorder

        Correct answer: D. *The patient in this scenario presents with certain characteristic features of schizotypal personality disorder, which is characterized by interpersonal discomfort with close relations, distortions of thought consistent with "magical thinking," and eccentric dress and behavior. It is considered to be along the spectrum toward psychotic in origin, but individuals do not have the quality of delusion seen in delusional disorder or schizophrenia. People with paranoid personality disorder are generally mistrustful of everyone but do not have the associated eccentricity seen in schizotypal personality disorder.*

2. What part of his presentation leads your differential away from a psychotic disorder?

    A. Educational history
    B. Affect
    C. Speech
    D. Drug use

continued

Correct answer: A. *An appropriate differential diagnosis should also include schizophrenia; however, in this case it is less likely at his age/educational level and without overt evidence of psychotic or negative symptoms. Negative symptoms of schizophrenia can include flattened or blunted affect or disorganized speech, but neither is required for a diagnosis of schizophrenia/psychosis. Drug use is common in people with mental illness, including psychosis.*

3. What other psychiatric illness is commonly comorbid with this personality disorder?

   A. OCD
   B. Bipolar disorder
   C. Major depressive disorder
   D. ADHD

   Correct answer: C. *Major depressive disorder is the most common comorbid psychiatric condition seen with schizotypal personality disorder. Other conditions, such as OCD, bipolar disorder, and ADHD are both less common and less commonly seen with schizotypal personality disorder.*

Discussion

Care should also be taken to distinguish primary psychotic symptoms from those of psychosis in the setting of substance use, in his case both cannabinoids and stimulants. He should also be asked about any alcohol use, depressive symptoms, and symptoms of posttraumatic stress given their concomitant prevalence and other consistencies with his presentation, in particular, his social isolation.

PRACTICAL RESOURCES

- https://www.nimh.nih.gov/health/topics/borderline-personality-disorder/index.shtml
- http://nlm.nih.gov/medlineplus/personalitydisorders.html
- http://mentalhelp.net/poc/center_index.php?id=8&cn+8
- http://www.bpdresourcecenter.org/
- https://www.nami.org/Learn-More/Mental-Health-Conditions/Borderline-Personality-Disorder
- http://mentalhealthrecovery.com/wrap-is/
- http://www.psychiatryonline.com

REFERENCES

1. American Psychiatric Association. *Diagnostic and Statistical Manual of Mental Disorders.* 5th ed. Arlington, VA: American Psychiatric Publishing; 2013:645-781.
2. Lenzenweger MF, Lane MC, Loranger AW, Kessler RC. DSM-IV personality disorders in the national comorbidity survey replication. *Biol Psychiatry.* 2007;62(6):553-564.
3. Trull TJ, Jahng S, Tomko RL, Wood PK, Sher KJ. Revised NESARC personality disorder diagnoses: gender, prevalence, and comorbidity with substance dependence disorders. *J Pers Disord.* 2010;24(4):412-426.
4. Hueston WJ, Werth J, Mainous AG. Personality disorder traits: prevalence and effects on health status in primary care patients. *Int J Psychiatry Med.* 1999;29:63-74.
5. Casey PR, Tyrer P. Personality disorder and psychiatric illness in general practice. *Br J Psychiatry.* 1990;156:261-265.
6. Hueston WJ, Mainous AG, Schilling R. Patients with personality disorders: functional status, health care utilization, and satisfaction with care. *J Fam Pract.* 1996;42(1):54-60.
7. Shea MT, Pilkonis PA, Beckham E, et al. Personality disorders and treatment outcome in the NIMH treatment of depression collaborative research program. *Am J Psychiatry.* 1990;147(6):711-718.
8. Groves JE. Taking care of the hateful patient. *N Engl J Med.* 1978;298(16):883-887.
9. Devens M. Personality disorders. *Prim Care.* 2007;34(3):623-640.
10. Rost KM, Akin RN, Brown FW, et al. The comorbidity of DSM-III-R personality disorders in somatization disorder. *Gen Hosp Psychiatry.* 1992;14(5):322-326.
11. Grant BF, Stintson FS, Dawson DA, et al. Co-occurrence of 12-month alcohol and drug use disorders and personality disorders in the United States. *Arch Gen Psychiatry.* 2004;61:361-368.
12. Gross R, Olfson M, Gameroff M, et al. Borderline personality disorder in primary care. *Arch Intern Med.* 2002;162(1):53-60.
13. American Psychological Association (APA). Practice guideline for the treatment of patients with borderline personality disorder. American Psychiatric Association. *Am J Psychiatry.* 2001;158:1-52.
14. Grilo CM, Shea MT, Sanislow CA, et al. Two-year stability and change of schizotypal, borderline, avoidant, and obsessive-compulsive personality disorders. *J Consult Clin Psychol.* 2004;72(5):767-775.
15. American Psychiatric Association. *Diagnostic and Statistical Manual of Mental Disorders.* 5th ed. Arlington, VA: American Psychiatric Publishing; 2013:645-684.
16. American Psychiatric Association. *Diagnostic and Statistical Manual of Mental Disorders.* 5th ed. Arlington, VA: American Psychiatric Publishing; 2013:676-781.
17. Gunderson JG, Weinberg I, Daversa MT, et al. Descriptive and longitudinal observations on the relationship of borderline personality disorder and bipolar disorder. *Am J Psychiatry.* 2006;163(7):1126-1128.
18. Linehan MM, Comtois KA, Murray AM, et al. Two year randomized controlled trail and follow-up of dialectical behavior therapy vs therapy by experts for suicidal behaviors and borderline personality disorder. *Arch Gen Psychiatry.* 2006;63(7):757-766.
19. Clarkin JF, Levy KN, Lenzenwger MF, Kernberg OF. Evaluating three treatments for borderline personality disorder: a multiwave study. *Am J Psychiatry.* 2007;164(6):922-928.
20. Biskin RS, Paris J. Management of borderline personality disorder. *CMAJ.* 2012;184(17):1897-1902.
21. Meuldijk D, McCarthy A, Bourke ME, Grenyer BF. The value of psychological treatment for borderline personality disorder: systematic review and cost offset analysis of economic evaluations. *PLoS One.* 2017;12(3):e0171592.

22. Gabbard GO, ed. *Gabbard's Treatments of Psychiatric Disorders.* 3rd ed. Washington, DC: American Psychiatric Publishing, Inc.; 2007.

23. Morse JQ, Pilkonis PA, Houck PR, et al. Impact of cluster C personality disorders on outcomes of acute and maintenance treatment of late-life depression. *Am J Geriatr Psychiatry.* 2005;13:808-814.

24. Bateman AW, Gunderson J, Mulder R. Treatment of personality disorder. *Lancet.* 2015;385(9969):735-743.

25. NICE. *Personality Disorders: Borderline and Antisocial;* 2015. https://www.nice.org.uk/guidance/qs88/chapter/Quality-statement-4-Pharmacological-interventions. Accessed July 9, 2018.

26. Nose M, Cipriani A, Biancosino B, Grassi L, Barbui C. Efficacy of pharmacotherapy against core traits of borderline personality disorder: meta-analysis of randomized controlled trials. *Int Clin Psychopharmacol.* 2006; 1;21(6):345-353.

27. NICE. *Borderline Personality Disorder: Treatment and Management;* 2009. https://www.nice.org.uk/guidance/cg78. Accessed June 19, 2017.

28. Lieb K, Völlm B, Rücker G, Timmer A, Stoffers JM. Pharmacotherapy for borderline personality disorder: cochrane systematic review of randomised trials. *Br J Psychiatry.* 2010;196(1):4-12.

29. Stoffers JM, Lieb K. Pharmacotherapy for borderline personality disorder–current evidence and recent trends. *Curr Psychiatry Rep.* 2015;17(1):534.

30. Compton WM, Conway KP, Stinson FS, Colliver JD, Grant BF. Prevalence, correlates, and comorbidity of DSM-IV antisocial personality syndromes and alcohol and specific drug use disorders in the United States: results from the national epidemiologic survey on alcohol and related conditions. *J Clin Psychiatry.* 2005;66:677-685.

31. Peterson J, Freedenthal S, Sheldon C, Andersen R. Nonsuicidal self injury in adolescents. *Psychiatry (Edgmont).* 2008;5(11):20-26.

32. Wedig MM, Silverman MH, Frankenburg FR, Reich DB, Fitzmaurice G, Zanarini MC. Predictors of suicide attempts in patients with borderline personality disorder over 16 Years of prospective follow-up. *Psychol Med.* 2012;42(11):2395-2404.

33. Muehlenkamp JJ, Claes L, Havertape L, Plener PL. International prevalence of adolescent non-suicidal self-injury and deliberate self-harm. *Child Adolesc Psychiatr Ment Health.* 2012;6:10.

FUNDAMENTALS OF PRIMARY CARE PSYCHIATRIC TREATMENT

16

COGNITIVE BEHAVIORAL THERAPY

Rachel J. Ammirati, PhD, D. Brian Haver, MS, and Martha C. Ward, MD

CLINICAL HIGHLIGHTS

- There is strong evidence to support the effectiveness of cognitive behavioral therapy (CBT) for a variety of disorders and problems that are seen commonly in primary care.
- CBT is an umbrella term comprising structured, problem-solving-oriented, time-limited psychotherapies based primarily on Aaron T. Beck's cognitive model and principles and procedures of behavior modification derived from various learning theories.
- Each disorder/problem to which CBT has been applied has its own, distinct formulation (i.e., a set of characteristic maladaptive beliefs and behaviors) but individual case conceptualizations
- Cognitive behavioral therapists work collaboratively with their patients to formulate and test hypotheses about cognitive (e.g., distorted or unhelpful thoughts) and behavioral (e.g., avoidance) mechanisms underlying an individual's problems.
- It is common to acknowledge interactional relations among thoughts, emotions, physical sensations, and behaviors in CBT.
- As is emphasized in nearly all psychotherapies, the formation of a strong, collaborative relationship with patients is considered crucial in CBT.

OVERVIEW

Cognitive behavioral therapy (CBT) is an umbrella term comprising structured, problem-solving, time-limited psychotherapies based primarily on Aaron T. Beck's cognitive model and principles and procedures of behavior modification derived from various learning theories.[1-4] Cognitive behavioral therapists work collaboratively with their patients to formulate and test hypotheses about

cognitive (e.g., distorted thoughts) and behavioral (e.g., avoidance) mechanisms underlying an individual's problems. Patients are encouraged to become more aware of and examine the accuracy or helpfulness of thoughts, try new things, and recognize how situations, thoughts, emotions, physical symptoms, and overt behaviors interact to produce distress. Within this collaborative framework, patients begin to change maladaptive thoughts, beliefs, and behaviors that play key roles in the onset and maintenance of a variety of disorders and problems.[3] Ultimately, patients are expected to become their own therapists by continuing to apply the skills they learn to future problems.

> Although biochemical mechanisms are not explicitly targeted in CBT, cognitive behavioral therapists acknowledge the very important role of such mechanisms in pathology of various kinds and often work alongside medical providers who prescribe medications to patients receiving CBT.

A great deal of empirical evidence supports the effectiveness of CBT for a variety of disorders and problems. For example, two recent reviews of meta-analyses[5,6] indicated that CBT can be used to effectively treat not only mood and anxiety disorders but also physical health conditions such as chronic pain and insomnia. Moreover, empirical data indicate that CBT for depression among adults is at least as effective, and in some cases more effective (especially over the long-term after cessation of treatment), than antidepressant medication.[5] Trained mental health professionals deliver CBT in a variety of formats, including individual, group, and even over the Internet.[7]

Increasingly, behavioral health services are being integrated into primary care settings.[8] In addition to increasing patients' access to behavioral health care, integrated care is often recognized as being superior to either primary or behavioral health care alone because it allows for patients' needs to be addressed more comprehensively and efficiently. Of the various psychotherapies, CBT has been of particular interest to providers in primary care settings for two key reasons: (1) its time-limited, structured, goal-focused nature and (2) myriad high-quality research studies support its effectiveness for a wide range of conditions treated commonly in primary care settings.[9-11] Otto and colleagues have highlighted that "[a]s with pharmacotherapy, disorders are viewed syndromally, and interventions are matched to the underlying disorder."[12] Thus, for primary care providers interested in incorporating psychotherapeutic techniques into their practice, CBT may be an especially good fit.

Although it is far beyond the scope of this chapter to equip readers with the nuanced knowledge, skills, and experience necessary to deliver comprehensive CBT competently, we do hope that the information we provide will facilitate communication and collaboration between primary care and behavioral health providers, particularly those integrated within primary care settings. In addition, we also intend for this chapter to introduce primary care providers to some basic, key CBT concepts and techniques that can be integrated into existing practices. Indeed, the effectiveness and utility of CBT in primary care settings has been reviewed in numerous publications. Many books have been written to provide mental health providers with detailed guidance on the use of CBT in primary care settings.[13] However, guidance on the practical use of basic CBT principles and related techniques by primary care providers who are typically untrained in psychotherapy is less common.[14] In addition to reviewing the information contained in this chapter, primary care providers may also find the book *10-Minute CBT: Integrating Cognitive-Behavioral Strategies into Your Practice* useful.[12] For those providers interested in obtaining a deeper understanding of the nature and application of CBT, we recommend the book *Cognitive Behavior Therapy: Basics and Beyond*, Second Edition.[3] The Academy of Cognitive Therapy (www.academyofct.org) also provides many resources for learning more about CBT, including a required and recommended reading list for individuals applying to obtain certification in CBT.

CONCEPTUAL FRAMEWORK

In CBTs, a great deal of attention is paid to the way individuals think about (i.e., perceive or interpret) situations. Most clinicians have probably experienced the powerful mediating role of thoughts in their everyday lives. For example, whereas one person may feel anxious, nauseated, and stutter while speaking in front of an audience, thinking, "I can't do this," another person in the same situation may feel excited, energetic, and smile frequently, thinking, "this presentation is going to be great!" Within a cognitive behavioral framework, thoughts are crucial because they, rather than the situation directly, give rise to idiosyncratic emotions (e.g., anxiety), physical sensations (e.g., nausea), and behaviors (e.g., stuttering).

As *Figure 16-1* illustrates, thoughts in a given situation—often referred to as automatic thoughts because they arise quickly and outside of awareness—do not develop in a vacuum. Rather, they flow from deeper cognitive structures, often referred to as core beliefs or schemas, which are believed to develop as a result of life experiences. Although people can hold both adaptive and maladaptive core beliefs simultaneously, distress (and in more extreme instances psychopathology) is believed to arise when maladaptive core beliefs (e.g., "I am incompetent") are activated and give rise to distorted/unhelpful thoughts (e.g., "I can't do this"). In a full course of CBT, various strategies (e.g., thought restructuring via Socratic questioning; exposure to feared stimuli) are used to modify situation-specific thoughts and core beliefs. To achieve lasting change, the modification of cognitive distortions or core beliefs is considered essential. Each disorder/problem to which CBT has been applied has its own, distinct formulation (i.e., a set of characteristic maladaptive beliefs and behaviors), but conceptualizations of individual patients may vary to some degree (e.g., not all individuals with obsessive-compulsive disorder will engage in the same compulsive behaviors or report the exact same relevant life experiences).

As *Figure 16-1* illustrates further, it is also common to acknowledge interactional relations among thoughts, emotions, physical sensations, and behaviors in CBT. For example, in panic disorder, misperceptions of physical sensations are considered key to understanding why individuals experience panic attacks. Although thoughts and behaviors are generally the primary targets of intervention, CBT clinicians often directly target the regulation of physical sensations to facilitate adaptive cognitive and behavioral change. Because many patients experiencing clinically significant anxiety do not engage regularly in activities that promote relaxation, teaching a patient how to engage in deep breathing provides them with a coping tool to increase confidence when it comes time to confront the physical symptoms of panic. For an individual who believes "hyperventilation means I will suffocate," the ultimate goal of treatment will be to repeatedly expose that individual to the experience of hyperventilation to promote learning that hyperventilation will not result in suffocation.

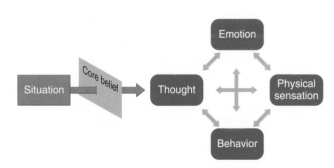

FIGURE 16-1 Basic cognitive behavioral conceptual framework.

CLINICAL INDICATIONS

Health care providers in the primary care setting see a wide variety of physical health conditions. A recent study of more than 600,000 patients across 148 primary care clinics found that around one-third of all the patients met criteria for hypertension and hyperlipidemia, and just less than 12% met criteria for diabetes and obesity.[15] Many of the patients seen in primary care have several comorbid conditions;—nearly two-thirds of patients in that study had more than one chronic condition.

Behavioral health concerns are also common presenting problems in primary care settings. Nearly 70% of patients visit primary care providers to address behavioral health concerns.[16,17] In the primary care setting, roughly 19% of patients meet criteria for major depressive disorder, 15% meet criteria for generalized anxiety disorder, and 8% meet criteria for panic and substance use disorders. Up to 77% of primary care patients may have more than one behavioral health condition. Therefore, it is likely that most primary care providers will see patients with multimorbid physical and mental health concerns.

Research has shown that the cognitive behavioral model can be applied effectively in brief interventions in primary care settings.[10] Furthermore, these brief cognitive behavioral treatments can be applied to many of the physical as well as mental health conditions seen in primary care. Some of the most common medical and psychiatric concerns treated in primary care are depression and generalized anxiety, panic disorder, posttraumatic stress disorder (PTSD), insomnia, chronic pain, tobacco use, obesity, diabetes, and poor treatment adherence.

Depression and generalized anxiety often present in primary care as vague somatic complaints.[17] Without proper identification and treatment of these conditions, primary care providers may struggle to resolve patients' complaints. Even when recognized, depression and anxiety are often treated insufficiently with pharmacologic interventions alone. The combination of CBT and pharmacologic interventions tends to improve patient outcomes.[16]

Panic disorder affects less than 5% of the population, but individuals experiencing panic attacks are often high utilizers of medical services.[16] Patients with panic may present with complaints of shortness of breath, chest pain, racing heartbeat, dizziness, numbness, tingling, or uncontrollable trembling.[17] Identification and treatment of a panic disorder may help reduce overutilization and clarify the focus of primary care visits.

PTSD and other stress reactions are also common in the primary care setting. Treatment of PTSD is often reserved for specialty mental health clinics, as intensive cognitive behavioral treatments such as prolonged exposure require a great deal of training and experience to deliver (see Chapter 7). To date, little evidence exists for the use of CBT to treat PTSD in primary care.[16] However, recent preliminary research suggests that modified protocols that included elements of prolonged exposure and cognitive processing therapy—each of which is a cognitive behavioral treatment—administered by mental health professionals in primary care settings show promise.[18] Use of screening tools, such as the Primary Care PTSD Screen (PC-PTSD-5), can help the primary care provider determine if a referral to more specialized treatment is needed. *Table 16-1* lists this and other useful screening measures for several conditions discussed in this section.

Insomnia and other sleep difficulties are estimated to impact well over half of all primary care patients, including those patients who are prescribed sleep aids.[16] A comprehensive review of research on CBT for primary insomnia suggests that it is an effective treatment strategy and also easily adapted to primary care settings.[19] In addition, more recent research indicates that brief CBT for the management of insomnia (bCBTi) may produce improvements after only three sessions.[20] Small studies have shown superiority of CBTi over medications in the long term.[21]

Pain is a significant patient complaint across a wide range of conditions including cancer, diabetes, fibromyalgia, chronic headaches, and rheumatoid arthritis, among many others. Cognitive behavioral interventions are an important component in the long-term management of chronic pain, helping patients to overcome negative thought patterns about their pain and circumstance, as well as helping them to effectively use relaxation skills and refocus on pleasant activities. The topic of pain and somatic symptom disorders in general is covered in more depth in Chapter 23.

Tobacco use screening is recommended for every patient in primary care.[22] Every patient using tobacco should be informed that quitting may be the most

TABLE 16-1 Mental Health Screening Tools for Primary Care

Depression	• Patient Health Questionnaire (PHQ-2/9) • Geriatric Depression Scale (GDS) • Edinburgh Postnatal Depression Scale (EPDS)
Anxiety	• Generalized Anxiety Disorder Screener (GAD-2/7) • Penn State Worry Questionnaire (PSWQ)
Bipolar disorders	• Mood Disorders Questionnaire (MDQ) • Altman Self-Rating Mania Scale (ASRM)
Posttraumatic stress disorder	• Life Events Checklist (LEC) • Primary Care PTSD Screen (PC-PTSD-5) • The Posttraumatic Stress Disorder Checklist—Civilian Version (PCL-C)/The PTSD Checklist for *DSM-5* (PCL-5)
Panic	• Panic Disorder Severity Scale (PDSS)

From Beidas RS, Stewart RE, Walsh L, et al. Free, brief, and validated: Standardized instruments for low-resource mental health settings. Cogn Behav Pract. 2015;22(1): 5-19. SAMHSA Screening Tools. http://www.integration.samhsa.gov/clinical-practice/screening-tools. Siu A. Screening for depression in adults: US Preventive Services Task Force recommendation statement. JAMA. 2016;315(4):380-387. Sveen J, Bondjers K, Willebrand M. Psychometric properties of the PTSD Checklist for DSM-5: a pilot study. Eur J Psychotraumatol. 2016;7:10.

important change one can make to improve health.[16] However, cessation of tobacco use can be extremely difficult to achieve, and patients often make multiple quit attempts before succeeding. Cognitive and behavioral coping strategies, as well as pharmacologic aids, are likely to increase patient success.[23]

Obesity may be the symptom of, or a precipitating factor in, a number of health conditions. Regardless of etiology, eating behaviors can be modified to reduce the severity of excess weight. CBT can serve as the first step in a stepped-care approach by helping patients to set goals and to plan and execute behavioral change.[16]

Diabetes management often hinges on the patient's own self-management behaviors. Behaviors such as blood glucose monitoring, maintaining a healthy diet, and increased physical activity have significant impacts on the overall health of those with diabetes.[16] Any of these behaviors may serve as targets for CBT-based intervention.

Treatment adherence is a broad concept encompassing medication adherence, self-management behaviors, appointment attendance, as well as open and meaningful communication about needs or questions during appointments. It is often the central factor in almost any intervention. Helping patients to identify barriers, set goals for overcoming them and address any unhelpful thinking patterns that may interfere with adherence can benefit the treatment of almost any disorder.

CLINICAL APPLICATION

In CBT, a variety of techniques are used to assist patients in learning new ways to think, behave, and feel. Moreover, as is emphasized in nearly all psychotherapies, the formation of a strong, collaborative relationship with patients is crucial. In this section, we'll first address some basic strategies that can be used to foster good working relationships with patients. We'll then summarize the basics of some fundamental techniques used to facilitate change in CBT, followed by a more detailed description of the use of such techniques with a handful of disorders and problems that are commonly treated in primary care.

FOSTERING COLLABORATION

To foster a good working relationship, CBT clinicians collaborate with patients on treatment plans and setting session-specific agendas. They also share their thoughts on case conceptualization and elicit feedback to make sure the patient is in agreement with the course of treatment. Although providers in primary care settings often have limited time to spend with patients, the example questions and statements outlined in *Box 16-1* can go a long way to build rapport with a patient. In addition, the questions in *Box 16-1* also provide helpful structure to a meeting. Notice that each question/statement communicates warmth and caring while simultaneously acknowledging the importance of efficiency and focusing on specific goals.

BOX 16-1 EXAMPLE QUESTIONS/ STATEMENTS AIMED AT BUILDING A COLLABORATIVE RELATIONSHIP WITH YOUR PATIENT

1. "Was there anything you wanted to make sure we discuss today?"
2. "It sounds like pain is a big problem for you and that we should make it a focus of our work together. Would it be okay if we review a few additional health-related matters before we begin talking more about the pain you're experiencing?"
3. "From what you tell me it sounds like you may be depressed and that you've stopped doing a lot of things you used to enjoy. I'm concerned that your lack of involvement in pleasant activities is something that may keep you depressed. Would it be okay if we spent a few minutes talking about how we might start to get you reconnected with one or two things you used to enjoy? Then we can see if that has any effect on your mood."

ORIENTING PATIENTS TO A COGNITIVE BEHAVIORAL MODEL

CBT clinicians always begin their work by orienting patients to a cognitive behavioral model of their presenting problems. Showing and describing *Figure 16-1* to patients promotes learning and provides an opportunity for patients to ask questions about concepts they may not understand.

PSYCHOEDUCATION ABOUT DISORDERS AND PROBLEMS

In addition to orienting patients to a cognitive behavioral model, CBT clinicians also provide patients with basic information about the nature of their disorder(s) or problem(s). Often, patients are provided with information related to diagnostic criteria, prevalence rates, risk factors, and even common comorbidities. This helps to facilitate the CBT clinician's goal of teaching patients to eventually become their own therapists and also promotes the setting of realistic goals.

THOUGHT RECORDS

Because one of the primary goals of CBT is to help patients become more aware of how thoughts are related to feelings and behaviors in various situations, thought records are a key cognitive behavioral tool. An example thought record is depicted in *Figure 16-2*. Thought records can be relatively simple (e.g., include three or five columns) or more comprehensive (e.g., include eight columns).

Name: _____

Thought Record

Date	Situation *What was happening at the time? What were you doing?*	Thought(s) *What was going through your mind?* **On a scale from 0 to 100%, how much do you believe what you were thinking?*	Emotion(s) *How were you feeling at the time? Sad? Angry? Another emotion?* **On a scale from 0 to 100, how intense was your emotion?*	Behavior *What did you do in response to, or to cope with, your emotion(s)? Did you yell at somebody or get into bed? Did you take a walk or drink alcohol?*

Name: _____

Thought Record

Date	Situation *What was happening at the time? What were you doing?*	Thought *What was going through your mind?* **On a scale from 0 to 100%, how much do you believe what you were thinking?*	Emotion(s) *How were you feeling at the time? Sad? Angry? Another emotion?* **On a scale from 0 to 100, how intense was your emotion?*	Physical Feeling(s) *How did your body feel?* *For example, shaky, heart racing, tense, pain?*	Behavior(s) *What did you do in response to, or to cope with, your emotion(s)? For example, did you yell at somebody or get into bed? Did you take a walk or drink alcohol?*	Alternative Thought(s) *What is a more helpful or realistic way to think about the situation?*	Alternative Behavior(s), Emotion(s), and Physical Feeling(s) *What might be a more helpful way to respond or cope? Do you think you'd experience different emotions/physical feelings?*

FIGURE 16-2 Sample thought records (five-column and eight-column versions).

When using a thought record, it is common to ask patients to record some or all of the following data elements: (1) date; (2) a description of a situation; (3) the thoughts that went through the patient's mind in that situation and intensity of belief in the thoughts; (4) an associated emotion and intensity of the emotion; (5) an associated physiological sensation; (6) an associated behavior; (7) a potential alternative, more adaptive thought (if the original thought was distorted or unhelpful); and (8) a potential alternative, more adaptive behavior (if the original behavior was maladaptive). When first orienting a patient to thought records, it can be helpful to start with something simpler like the thought record depicted in *Figure 16-2*. If you need to simplify things further, you can remove the last column or the intensity ratings and add those later. As your patient becomes more comfortable with working on thought records and demonstrates understanding of the task, you can add additional columns, including those that ask the patient to identify more adaptive thoughts and behaviors. We recommend completing at least one thought record during the appointment with patients when the task is introduced. We also recommend that providers focus on an in-meeting example

or on something that recently happened to the patient. If a patient is having difficulty identifying thoughts, it can be helpful to start with describing emotions when initiating the process of completing a thought record. An in-meeting example could be "What were you feeling when you first saw me today?" followed by "What kinds of things did you think about when you were feeling _____, no matter how silly the thoughts might sound?" and then help the patient complete the rest of the thought record from there. The patient should be assigned "homework" or an "action plan" to complete at least one thought record on the identified problem before the next appointment.

To further facilitate learning and the completion of thought records, CBT clinicians also often provide patients with lists of common cognitive distortions/ unhelpful types of thinking associated with a variety of disorders and problems (e.g., *all-or-nothing thinking* such as "I can't do anything when I'm in pain."). A link to a list of 10 cognitive distortions popularized by Dr. David D. Burns can be found on his website (https://feelinggood. com/tag/cognitive-distortions/). We describe some of these and other distortions/unhelpful types of thinking in *Table 16-2*.

TABLE 16-2 Common Cognitive Distortions/Types of Unhelpful Thinking

DISTORTION	DESCRIPTION	EXAMPLE
All-or-nothing thinking	When you see things in black and white terms; as "either/or."	"I can't do anything when I'm in pain."
Mind reading	When you think you know what someone else is thinking (and usually assume something negative).	"He's thinking I look terrible."
Discounting or ignoring the positive	When you focus on the negative aspects of something and assume the positive aspects don't count.	"It doesn't matter that I used to take my medication every day; I'm a failure because I haven't taken any medication over the past week."
Catastrophizing or magnifying	When you think something is much worse than it actually is; you blow things out of proportion.	"If I have a panic attack at work I'll lose control and everyone will think I'm crazy."
Fortune-telling	When you think you can predict the future.	"If someone offers me a cigarette I won't be able to refuse it."
Overgeneralization	When you perceive an overly negative pattern in something but base this on a single or rare event.	"I always seem to mess up my diet."
Emotional reasoning	When you draw conclusions based on how you're feeling.	"I feel anxious when my partner says she's going to be home late so she must be cheating on me."
Regret focus	When you focus on mistakes you made in the past, rather than on what you can do now.	"I should have never let myself gain so much weight."

Modified from Burns DD. The Feeling Good Handbook: Using the New Mood Therapy in Everyday Life. New York, NY: William Morrow & Co.; 1989. Leahy RL. Cognitive Therapy Techniques: A Practitioner's Guide. New York, NY: Guilford Press; 2003.

FACILITATING NEW, MORE ADAPTIVE WAYS OF THINKING AND BEHAVING

To help patients examine the accuracy or helpfulness of their thinking (either in the context of reviewing a thought record or after asking a patient, "What's going through your mind right now?"), CBT clinicians often ask patients to consider questions like those listed in *Box 16-2*. In addition, CBT clinicians often use behavioral experiments to test the accuracy of patients' thoughts and beliefs. A behavioral experiment form is depicted in *Figure 16-3*. For example, a depressed patient who has never undergone a sufficient trial of an antidepressant and thinks, "antidepressants don't work" may benefit from a simple behavioral experiment that can be structured using *Figure 16-3*. To evaluate his/her thinking about antidepressants, the patient could commit to a trial of taking the medication for 6 weeks and then record what happened as a result of staying on the medication longer than he or she had in the past. As a result of taking the medication longer, the patient may learn that early unwanted side effects subsided after a week or two and eventually; the patient experienced a boost in energy and appetite. The new, more realistic/adaptive thought/belief that could arise as a result of an experiment of this nature may then be, "antidepressants work to treat some of my symptoms as long as I take them for a sufficient amount of time." If the patient does not experience any benefit as a result of taking the medication for 6 weeks, the new thought/belief before conducting a new behavioral experiment might be, "this antidepressant didn't work for me but there are others I can try that may work as long as I take the medication for a sufficient amount of time."

BOX 16-2 QUESTIONS TO HELP PATIENTS EXAMINE THE ACCURACY OR HELPFULNESS OF THEIR THINKING

Is there any evidence that my thought is true? (What is the evidence?)

Is there any evidence that my thought is not true? (What is the evidence?)

What would I say to a friend who had the same thought?

Is there another way to think about this situation?

If I was a lawyer and had to make a case for the opposite of my thought, what would I say?

If my thought is true, what's the worst that can happen?

If my thought is true, what do I need to do to solve my problem?

Activity charts, such as those depicted in *Figures 16-4* and *16-5*, are also very helpful when the aim is to increase a patient's involvement in pleasant activities, or to assist the patient in developing a sense of accomplishment.

Figure 16-4 depicts an hourly activity chart. Patients can be asked to list activities in which they'd like to engage, as well as to record a mood or sense of accomplishment associated with doing the activity. Ratings can be on a scale from 0 to 10, with 0 equivalent to "worst possible mood/sense of accomplishment" and 10 equivalent to "best possible mood/sense of accomplishment." Scheduling activities, rather than simply talking about them, can increase the chances a patient will actually begin to change his or her behavior. In addition, activity charts can be used to assist a patient in identifying mood-activity patterns (e.g., noticing that one's mood is better when engaged in social activities). If a provider thinks that an hourly activity chart may be too overwhelming for a patient, we recommend starting with a simplified version that replaces specific times with "morning, midday, evening" (*Figure 16-5*).

COGNITIVE BEHAVIORAL THERAPY APPLIED TO DEPRESSION

It is common for depressed individuals to think in overly negative terms with regard to themselves (e.g., "I am a failure"), others (e.g., "nobody likes me"), and the future (e.g., "my life will always be difficult") and to withdraw from pleasant activities. Therefore, CBT for depression tends to focus on helping patients identify and alter problematic patterns of thinking that maintain depressed mood and behavioral avoidance and to slowly increase engagement with activities that have the potential to provide enjoyment or a sense of accomplishment. Patients are asked to use thought records to track their thinking patterns, and activity schedules are used to promote behavioral activation. Behavioral activation involves inquiring about what used to be of interest to patients before they became depressed and helping patients set small, reasonable goals to increase the likelihood of successful activation. For example, if a patient used to enjoy going to the local library, an initial behavioral activation goal may be simply looking up the library's hours of operations.

Antidepressants are not contraindicated when patients are receiving CBT for a depressive disorder. It is not uncommon for patients receiving CBT for depression to also be prescribed an antidepressant.

COGNITIVE BEHAVIORAL THERAPY APPLIED TO PAIN

CBT for chronic pain aims to improve quality of life and functioning in spite of the fact that one is living with pain. Patients are taught to identify and challenge problematic pain-related thoughts (e.g., "I can't do anything when I'm in pain"), with special attention to pain catastrophizing, as this is a particularly common cognitive distortion among patients with chronic pain. Patients are also taught the difference between hurt and harm (i.e., that feeling pain does not necessarily mean one is experiencing tissue damage). Reengagement in pleasant activities and physical exercise is emphasized, and patients are

---

Name: _____   Date: _____

Behavioral Experiment Form

Thought/belief to be evaluated: _____
_____
_____
_____
_____

What will you do to evaluate your thought/belief? _____
_____
_____
_____
_____

What happened as a result of your experiment? What was the outcome and what did you learn?
_____
_____
_____
_____
_____

Now that you've conducted your experiment, how might you change your original thought/belief?
_____
_____
_____
_____
_____

FIGURE 16-3 Behavioral experiment form.

taught how to implement time-based activity pacing to avoid significant pain flares as a result of cycles of over- and underactivity. In addition, techniques for relaxation are taught (e.g., deep breathing and progressive muscle relaxation). Patients are taught that although opiates are appropriate for treating acute pain after an injury or surgery, they are not appropriate for the treatment of chronic pain after the body has healed, and evidence of harm related to unintended overuse or polypharmacy should be stressed with an emphasis on the mutual goal of quality of life (see Chapter 23 for more information about treatment of chronic pain).

COGNITIVE BEHAVIORAL THERAPY APPLIED TO GENERALIZED ANXIETY

Patients with generalized anxiety disorder tend to believe, erroneously, that there is utility in worrying. In addition, they also tend to catastrophize and overestimate danger across a variety of situations. Therefore, in CBT for generalized anxiety, cognitive techniques focus on helping patients to consider the negative consequences of worrying excessively (vs. problem-solving), and the modification of catastrophic thought patterns is emphasized. Patients are taught relaxation exercises to improve regulation of the physiological arousal and muscle tension that often occur with anxiety. Because patients with generalized anxiety disorder also tend to avoid a variety of thoughts and situations that cause anxiety, they are systematically and repeatedly exposed to such thoughts and situations to learn that what they most fear rarely or never occurs. Thus, exposure exercises promote more realistic thinking. Because avoidance behavior is considered a key mechanism in cognitive behavioral formulations of all anxiety disorders, medications, such as benzodiazepines, are generally considered contraindicated.

Name: _____   Date: _____

Hourly Pleasant Activity Schedule (indicate planned activity and then record your mood or sense of accomplishment during/after the activity on a scale from 0 to 10, with 0 = worst possible mood/sense of accomplishment and 10 = best possible mood/sense of accomplishment)

	Monday		Tuesday		Wednesday		Thursday		Friday		Saturday		Sunday	
(Example)	Go to library	7			Call a friend	8	Go for a walk	6			Watch TV	5		
7am-8am														
8am-9am														
9am-10am														
10am-11am														
11am-12pm														
12pm-1pm														
1pm-2pm														
2pm-3pm														
3pm-4pm														
4pm-5pm														
5pm-6pm														
6pm-7pm														
7pm-8pm														
8pm-9pm														
9pm-10pm														

FIGURE 16-4 Hourly pleasant activity schedule.

COGNITIVE BEHAVIORAL THERAPY APPLIED TO PANIC DISORDER

Patients with panic disorder tend to misinterpret physiological symptoms of anxiety as indicative of catastrophic medical problems. In addition, anxiety-provoking situations can also trigger panic attacks. Therefore, as is the case with other anxiety disorders, exposing patients to uncomfortable physiological sensations and situations is a key part of CBT for panic disorder because it teaches patients that what they most fear rarely or never happens. For example, a patient who fears that their shortness of breath means they will suffocate may be instructed to take fast, shallow breaths during an exposure exercise to simulate shortness of breath. Similar to the treatment of generalized anxiety disorder, patients are also taught relaxation techniques and to examine the utility and accuracy of their anxious thoughts. Because avoidance behavior is considered a key mechanism in a cognitive behavioral formulation of panic disorder, sedative-hypnotic anxiolytics such as benzodiazepines are generally considered contraindicated. However, antidepressants are not contraindicated when patients are receiving CBT for panic disorder.

COGNITIVE BEHAVIORAL THERAPY APPLIED TO INSOMNIA

Patients with primary insomnia often hold erroneous beliefs about the causes of their sleep problems, lack knowledge about behaviors that initiate and maintain poor sleep, and worry excessively about the potential consequences of not getting adequate sleep. Therefore, in addition to teaching patients to think differently about sleep, CBT for primary insomnia also focuses on helping patients to slowly change sleep behaviors that interfere with normal sleep processes. Regarding medication considerations, because a major goal of CBT for primary insomnia is to restore natural mechanisms that regulate sleep, fast-acting sleep medications are typically considered to be contraindicated over the long term.

Name: _____				Date: _____		
Pleasant Activity Schedule (indicate planned activity and then record your mood or sense of accomplishment during/after the activity on a scale from 0 to 10, with 0 = worst possible mood/sense of accomplishment and 10 = best possible mood/sense of accomplishment)						
	Monday	Tuesday	Wednesday	Thursday	Friday	Saturday	Sunday
Morning						
Midday						
Evening						

FIGURE 16-5 Pleasant activity schedule.

COGNITIVE BEHAVIORAL THERAPY APPLIED TO POSTTRAUMATIC STRESS DISORDER

CBT for PTSD addresses maladaptive thoughts and associated beliefs (e.g., "I can't trust anybody"), and behaviors that develop, or are worsened, as a result of experiencing or reexperiencing trauma. Because avoidance of internal (e.g., trauma memories) and external (e.g., trauma-related stimuli) trauma reminders is considered a key maintenance factor, efforts are made to repeatedly and systematically expose patients to the very things they are trying to escape. As a result of being exposed repeatedly to situations or objects (in vivo exposure) and memories (imaginal exposure) associated with trauma, patients are able to learn that they can tolerate trauma-related distress, and that the intensity of trauma-related distress will decrease as a result of repeated exposures. In addition, patients learn to distinguish trauma reminders from the actual trauma. Although all forms of CBT for PTSD currently include exposure-based exercises to target avoidance directly (exposure-based techniques are used most heavily in *prolonged exposure therapy* for PTSD), *cognitive processing therapy* focuses additional emphasis on the use of cognitive techniques, such as using thought records and Socratic dialogue to question maladaptive thoughts and beliefs, for the purpose of cognitive restructuring.[24] Similar to anxiety disorders, because avoidance behavior is considered a key mechanism in a cognitive behavioral formulation of PTSD, medications (e.g., anxiolytics) or illicit substances (e.g., marijuana) that prevent patients

from fully engaging in exposure exercises are generally considered contraindicated.

COGNITIVE BEHAVIORAL THERAPY APPLIED TO TOBACCO USE

When using CBT to assist patients with smoking cessation, patients are taught to think of smoking as a learned habit that can be "unlearned." In treatment, emphasis is often placed on the importance of setting realistic, achievable goals for behavioral change, and efforts are made to help patients identify and change cognitive, behavioral, and emotional factors that maintain tobacco use. Patients are encouraged to monitor how often and under what conditions they smoke, and they also are taught new, more adaptive skills that can be substituted for smoking. Typically, a realistic quit date is set early in treatment. Medications such as bupropion, varenicline, and/or nicotine replacement that may also help patients quit smoking are not contraindicated in CBT.

COGNITIVE BEHAVIORAL THERAPY APPLIED TO OBESITY

When applied to obesity, CBT for weight loss teaches patients that in addition to increasing exercise and decreasing caloric intake, other cognitive and behavioral changes must also be made. For example, cognitive restructuring often focuses on helping patients to identify and replace maladaptive thoughts (e.g., "It's ok if I overeat while I'm on this trip; I'll just starting watching what I eat again when I get home") that maintain maladaptive behaviors (e.g., overeating), and lessons in problem-solving focus on helping patients to identify and cope with various external factors that may trigger overeating and avoidance of exercise. Patients are also taught to set realistic goals to increase the chances of success and the development of a sense of accomplishment.[25] Medications such as appetite suppressants, satiety promoters, and/or drugs that interfere with fat absorption that may assist a patient in losing weight are not considered contraindicated when working within a cognitive behavioral framework.

COGNITIVE BEHAVIORAL THERAPY APPLIED TO DIABETES

Diabetes management requires a great deal of self-monitoring. Therefore, when CBT is used to improve compliance with a diabetes treatment regimen, emphasis is often placed on helping patients to identify and correct inaccurate or unhelpful thoughts and beliefs that may be driving maladaptive behaviors. In addition, patients and clinicians work together to set realistic, achievable goals for diabetes care, and activity schedules are often used to help patients track and keep up with adaptive behaviors (e.g., taking medications, monitoring blood glucose levels, and engaging in regular exercise).

COGNITIVE BEHAVIORAL THERAPY APPLIED TO MEDICATION ADHERENCE

When applying CBT to medication adherence challenges, potential cognitive (e.g., erroneous beliefs about the side effects of medication), behavioral (e.g., avoidance of medications because they serve as a reminder of a patient's diagnosis), and situational barriers (e.g., pharmacy too far away) to adherence are first identified. Cognitive techniques, such as evaluating the evidence for and against a belief, are used to assist patients in restructuring maladaptive and inaccurate cognitions about medications, and additional strategies may be used to help patients tolerate distress associated with taking medications (e.g., for a patient who fears swallowing pills, graduated exposure-based exercises may encourage the patient to first practice swallowing a very small item of food, followed by progressively larger items so that the patient learns he or she will not choke or stop breathing).

ADDITIONAL CLINICAL APPLICATION TIPS

Box 16-2 provides guidance on how providers might consider responding to patients when various condition-related concerns arise in conversation. *Table 16-3* includes a selection of conditions commonly discussed and treated in primary care. The cognitive behavioral principle that informs each example provider response is also listed.

TABLE 16-3 Additional Clinical Application Tips

CONDITION	PRINCIPLE	PATIENT STATEMENT	PROVIDER RESPONSE
Posttraumatic stress disorder	Avoidance of trauma-related situations, thoughts, and emotions maintains PTSD symptoms	"I spend so much time trying not to think about what happened to me. It's exhausting and I still can't leave my house."	"It sounds like your attempts to avoid thinking about what happened to you aren't helping you to feel any better. As it turns out, research shows that avoiding memories and feelings related to traumatic events tends to make symptoms worse. Would you be willing to talk with one of our mental health providers about effective treatments that can help you to confront and process what happened to you so you can feel better and improve your functioning?"
Tobacco use	Inaccurate beliefs about smoking often drive smoking behavior	"I need to smoke about one cigarette per hour; if I don't, nobody will want to be around me because I'll be an anxious mess."	"What if you and I conduct an experiment to see what happens when you avoid smoking for at least one hour each day? Collecting these data will help us to see if in fact people avoid you more when you smoke less."

TABLE 16-3 Additional Clinical Application Tips (continued)

CONDITION	PRINCIPLE	PATIENT STATEMENT	PROVIDER RESPONSE
Obesity	Unrealistic expectations related to exercise cause avoidance of exercise	"I know I should be exercising but it just seems like too much."	"It sounds like it's been hard for you to get started with exercise. This can happen to any of us when we try to take on too much at once. What if you and I come up with a few small exercise goals for the next few weeks just to get you started?"
Diabetes	Overly negative, unhelpful thoughts about diabetes can interfere with self-monitoring activities	"It's not that I forget to monitor my blood sugar; I just don't want to do it."	"What goes through your mind just before you consider checking your blood sugar?"

CASES AND QUESTIONS

CASE 1:

Mr. Rao is a 68-year-old man with obesity and type 2 diabetes who is returning to primary care for follow-up. He has been forgetting to check his blood glucose at home and more recently has been coming to clinic with blood glucose readings in the 400s. When asked about recent changes in his adherence, Mr. Rao reports having had difficulty remembering to check his glucose since a car accident two months ago. He did not sustain any head trauma in his car accident. Mr. Rao adds that he has been feeling detached and is not sleeping well and has had repeated, intrusive thoughts and nightmares about his car accident, despite trying not to think about the event.

1. Based on Mr. Rao's psychiatric symptoms, which of the following would be an appropriate screening test to administer to help make a diagnosis?
   A. Patient Health Questionnaire (PHQ-2/9)
   B. Panic Disorder Severity Scale (PDSS)
   C. Mood Disorders Questionnaire (MDQ)
   D. Primary Care PTSD Screen (PC-PTSD-5)
   E. Generalized Anxiety Disorder Screener (GAD-2/7)

   Correct answer: D. *Mr. Rao has had a recent traumatic event, occurring more than one month ago, and describes reexperiencing of the trauma (intrusive thoughts and nightmares), avoidance (trying not to think about the trauma), negative thoughts (feeling detached), and hyperarousal (difficulty sleeping). Such symptoms should make the clinician suspect that the patient has PTSD, and thus, the PTSD screen should be used to elicit further symptoms and a probable diagnosis. Panic disorder and generalized anxiety disorder*

are less likely conditions given the nature of his reported symptoms. The PHQ-2/9 can be helpful in uncovering depressive symptoms in addition to PTSD but would not be the first screening tool given the presenting complaints. He does not endorse any symptoms suggestive of mania, so the MDQ is not indicated, although screening for symptoms of mania if considering antidepressant medication is advised.

2. The next best step in treating Mr. Rao's PTSD may be (choose one of the following answers)

   _____

   A. encouraging the patient to avoid thinking about the distressing event
   B. prescribing benzodiazepines to help with sleep and anxiety
   C. Referring the patient to a colocated primary care mental health provider or mental health specialist for evaluation and treatment
   D. scheduling the patient for a six-month follow-up to begin prolonged exposure therapy for his trauma
   E. admitting the patient involuntarily to the hospital for failure to care for himself

   Correct answer: C. *Treatment of PTSD is often reserved for specialty mental health clinics, as intensive cognitive behavioral treatments such as prolonged exposure require a great deal of training and usually at least more than 10 to 15 hour-long sessions. Avoidance is a key maintenance factor in a cognitive behavioral formulation of PTSD, so efforts are made to repeatedly and systematically expose patients to the very things they are trying to escape. Benzodiazepines are not recommended as a first-line therapy for PTSD and may decrease efficacy of prolonged exposure therapy. The patient does*

continued

not meet criteria for involuntary hospitalization and needs more immediate follow-up given his distress and morbidity. Although prolonged exposure therapy is indicated for PTSD, it is important to collaborate with patients on treatment plans. Therefore, scheduling a patient for treatment without his agreement would not be consistent with a cognitive behavioral framework.

3. The CBT intervention most likely to be efficacious in the long term for treating Mr. Rao's PTSD is
_____

  A. prolonged exposure therapy
  B. scheduling of pleasurable activities
  C. identifying automatic negative thoughts
  D. relaxation techniques
  E. keeping a diet log

  Correct answer: A. *A great deal of evidence supports the effectiveness of prolonged exposure therapy for PTSD, a specific kind of CBT delivered by a trained mental health professional. Answer options B through D are helpful components of more comprehensive cognitive behavioral treatments for PTSD, such as prolonged exposure therapy and cognitive processing therapy. Answer option E is a useful CBT technique used in the treatment of obesity.*

CASE 2:

Ms. Lee is a 36-year-old, Asian-American woman with a history of essential hypertension who has had multiple walk-in and emergency room visits for "chest pain and shortness of breath" over the last year. Workups, including cardiac enzymes, ECG, chest X-ray, CT PE protocol, and a nuclear cardiac stress test, have all been negative. Ms. Lee has become increasingly anxious about the meaning of her symptoms and has begun to worry that they may mean she either has some undiagnosed underlying cardiac problem or that she may be "going crazy."

1. Which of the following patient history items would help you to make a diagnosis of panic disorder?

  A. Syncopal episodes associated with the chest pain and shortness of breath
  B. Perioral paresthesias occurring along with chest pain and shortness of breath
  C. A history of hyperthyroidism
  D. Symptoms peaking for 6 to 7 hours
  E. Symptoms occurring when seeing spiders, which Ms. Lee admits she has always been afraid of

  Correct answer: B. *Panic disorder consists of recurrent, unprovoked panic attacks (paroxysmal onset of intense fear or discomfort, associated with four or more of the following: palpitations,*

pounding heart, or accelerated heart rate; sweating; trembling or shaking; sensations of shortness of breath or smothering; feeling of choking; chest pain or discomfort; nausea or abdominal distress; feeling dizzy, unsteady, lightheaded, or faint; chills or heat sensations; paresthesias; derealization or depersonalization; fear of losing control or going crazy; fear of dying), combined with at least one month of persistent worry about the meaning of the attacks or maladaptive behavior concerning the attacks. Answer options A and C indicate that another medical condition may be responsible for the patient's presentation. In panic attacks, symptoms peak within minutes, although total duration may be hours. Answer option E describes specific phobia with panic attacks.

2. Of the following, which is a maladaptive thought pattern associated with panic disorder?

  A. Excessive worry about the potential consequences of not getting adequate sleep
  B. Misinterpretation of physiological symptoms of anxiety as indicative of catastrophic medical problems
  C. Believing that there is utility in worrying
  D. Underestimating one's self-worth
  E. Overestimating danger across a variety of situations

  Correct answer: B. *People with panic disorder frequently misinterpret physical signs to mean that there is something physically wrong and catastrophize the consequences of that problem. Answer option A is consistent with insomnia. Answer options C and E are consistent with generalized anxiety disorder. Answer option D is associated with depression.*

3. Regarding the treatment of panic disorder, which of the following statements is NOT true?

  A. Antidepressants can be used with CBT.
  B. Exposing patients to uncomfortable physiological sensations and situations is a useful CBT technique.
  C. Benzodiazepines are contraindicated.
  D. Relaxation techniques may help patients to cope with the symptoms of panic attacks.
  E. Examination of the utility and accuracy of thoughts may lead to increased anxiety and should be avoided.

  Correct answer: E. *Answers A through D are true. Answer E is false—examination of the utility and accuracy of anxious thoughts may allow patients to become conscious of maladaptive assumptions and substitute more accurate, adaptive thoughts.*

CASE 3:

Ms. Lincoln is a 45-year-old, African-American woman with a diagnosis of fibromyalgia. She attends almost every one of her appointments with the stated goal of finding an end to her pain and returning to her life before pain. Ms. Lincoln rates her pain as at least a 10/10. The pain is worsened by increased activity of any sort, including shopping or walking to the bus stop. Because of how easily her pain is triggered, Ms. Lincoln reports having cut back on all of her activities outside of the home, and as a result, many of her relationships with friends and family have suffered. She reports that most medication "doesn't work" for her pain, and she is angry at you for not prescribing her narcotics. She describes poor sleep and appetite "due to pain," and she states that she finds very little enjoyment in life.

1. Given Ms. Lincoln's description of her symptoms, which of the following rating scales may assist the physician in making a psychiatric diagnosis?

   A. Altman Self-Rating Mania Scale (ASRM)
   B. Primary Care PTSD Screen (PC-PTSD-5)
   C. Panic Disorder Severity Scale (PDSS)
   D. Patient Health Questionnaire (PHQ-2/9)
   E. Life Events Checklist (LEC)

   Correct answer: D. *Major depressive disorder is commonly comorbid with pain syndromes, particularly fibromyalgia; additionally, patients presenting to primary care with mood or anxiety disorders often present with somatic complaints alone. Ms. Lincoln also describes many of the symptoms of a major depressive episode, including poor sleep, poor appetite, and anhedonia. The PHQ-2/9 are validated rating scales for assessing depression in primary care settings. The ASRM is used to evaluate for bipolar disorder. The PC-PTSD-5 and LEC are used to screen for PTSD. PDSS is used to evaluate for panic disorder.*

2. The following are statements or questions that may assist in establishing a collaborative therapeutic relationship with your patient, Ms. Lincoln, EXCEPT which one of the following?

   A. "It sounds like pain is a big problem for you and that we should make it a focus of our work together. Would it be okay if we review a few additional health-related matters before we begin talking more about the pain you're experiencing?"
   B. "Tell me a little bit about the strategies that you are using for your pain. What has worked and what has not worked for you in the past?"
   C. "Narcotics are just not going to work for you, and I'm not giving them to you. If that's what you were hoping for, I'm sorry."
   D. "From what you tell me, it sounds like you may be depressed. Would you mind if I asked you a few more questions to help me understand how you have been feeling?"

   E. "I hear that you want to end your pain, and that this is a goal for you in treatment. Would you like to come up a with a few short-term goals that may improve your quality of life, while we also think about how to decrease your pain?"

   Correct answer: C. *Although narcotics are often not indicated in the treatment of chronic pain, the patient has already set up an adversarial and confrontational relationship with the physician regarding her desire to obtain this medication. Direct confrontation, without offering alternatives or another treatment plan, perpetuates this confrontational relationship and can lead to a therapeutic rift.*

3. The following statements are all examples of maladaptive thoughts that may be associated with chronic pain, EXCEPT which one of the following?

   A. "My pain will never get any better."
   B. "I can't do anything anymore because of my pain."
   C. "Well, I'll never go to sleep tonight since I'm in so much pain this afternoon."
   D. "Limiting the duration of my physical activity can help with decreasing my pain, though it may not make it go away completely."
   E. "If you can't make my pain go away, you can't help me at all."

   Correct answer: D. *Answer options A, B, C, and E are all examples of maladaptive automatic negative thoughts. Answer options A, B, and E show catastrophic, all-or-nothing thinking. Answer option C displays fortune-telling. In contrast, answer option D shows a reasonable thought about limitation of physical activity. Time-based pacing (limiting physical and other activities by duration, to prevent overuse or exhaustion) is a CBT strategy used in treating chronic pain. Additionally, the patient is being realistic about the expected outcome of an intervention.*

4. Which of the following should NOT be advised when treating chronic pain?

   A. Use of relaxation techniques, such as deep breathing
   B. Realistic goal setting
   C. Psychoeducation about the pain cycle and the difference between hurt and harm
   D. Increasing physical activity to "push through" the pain
   E. Examining catastrophic pain-related thoughts

   Correct answer: D. *"Pushing through" pain is the opposite of the idea of time-based pacing (limiting physical and other activities by duration, to prevent overuse or exhaustion) is a CBT strategy used in treating chronic pain.*

PRACTICAL RESOURCES

- Therapist Aid: http://www.therapistaid.com/
  A free collection of worksheets, informational hand-outs, and videos. Resources can be filtered by topic (e.g., CBT).
- Psychology Tools: http://psychologytools.com/
  A free collection of professional and self-help materials. Resources can be filtered by topic (e.g., CBT).
- VISN 2 Center for Integrated Healthcare: https://www.mirecc.va.gov/cih-visn2/clinical_resources.asp
  Clinical resources developed by the VA to aid in the operation and management of integrated primary care. The site includes patient and provider education information. Whereas some materials are veteran specific, others are not. Nearly all materials are cognitive behavioral in nature.
- Association for Behavioral and Cognitive Therapies: http://www.abct.org/Home/
  A professional organization devoted to the scientific study and clinical practice of CBT. Their website has student, teaching, resource, and clinical resources. Members have access to further resources, networking opportunities, and three regularly published journals.
- CBT-i Coach: Found in the app store for all major devices
  Free app developed by U.S. Department of Veterans Affairs rooted in CBT for insomnia. It is a structured program that provides education, exercises designed to improve sleep, and recording tools to track sleep.

REFERENCES

1. Beck AT. Cognitive therapy: nature and relation to behavior therapy. *Behav Ther.* 1970;1:184-200.
2. Beck AT. The current state of cognitive therapy: a 40 year retrospective. *Arch Gen Psychiatry.* 2005;62:953-959.
3. Beck JS. *Cognitive Behavior Therapy: Basics and Beyond.* 2nd ed. New York, NY: Guilford Press; 2011.
4. Persons JB. *The Case Formulation Approach to Cognitive-behavior Therapy.* New York, NY: Guilford Press; 2008.
5. Butler AC, Chapman JE, Forman EM, Beck AT. The empirical status of cognitive-behavioral therapy: a review of meta-analyses. *Clin Psychol Rev.* 2006;26(1):17-31.
6. Hofmann SG, Asnaani A, Vonk IJ, Sawyer AT, Fang A. The efficacy of cognitive behavioral therapy: a review of meta-analyses. *Cognit Ther Res.* 2012;36(5): 427-440.
7. Cuijpers P, Van Straten A, Andersson G. Internet-administered cognitive behavior therapy for health problems: a systematic review. *J Behav Med.* 2008;31(2):169-177.
8. Weisberg RB, Magidson JF. Integrating cognitive behavioral therapy into primary care settings. *Cognit Behav Pract.* 2014;21(3):247-251.
9. Bower P, Rowland N, Hardy R. The clinical effectiveness of counselling in primary care: a systematic review and meta-analysis. *Psychol Med.* 2003;33(2):203-215.
10. Cape J, Whittington C, Buszewicz M, et al. Brief psychological therapies for anxiety and depression in primary care: meta-analysis and meta-regression. *BMC Med.* 2010;8:38.
11. Høifødt RS, Strøm C, Kolstrup N, et al. Effectiveness of cognitive behavioural therapy in primary health care: a review. *Fam Pract.* 2011;28(5):489-504.
12. Otto MW, Simon N, Olatunji B, et al. *10-Minute CBT: Integrating Cognitive-behavioral Strategies into Your Practice.* New York, NY: Oxford University Press; 2011.
13. DiTomasso RA, Golden BA, Morris H. *Handbook of Cognitive Behavioral Approaches in Primary Care.* New York, NY: Springer Publishing Co; 2010.
14. Dorflinger LM, Fortin AH, Foran-Tuller KA. Training primary care physicians in cognitive behavioral therapy: a review of the literature. *Patient Educ Counsel.* 2016;99(8):1285-1292.
15. Ornstein SM, Nietert PJ, Jenkins RG, Litvin CB. The prevalence of chronic diseases and multimorbidity in primary care practice: a PPRNet report. *J Am Board Fam Med.* 2013;26(5):518-524.
16. Hunter CL, Goodie JL, Oordt MS, Dobmeyer AC. *Integrated Behavioral Health in Primary Care: Step-by-Step Guidance for Assessment and Intervention.* 2nd ed. American Psychological Association; 2017.
17. Robinson PJ, Reiter JT. *Behavioral Consultation and Primary Care: A Guide to Integrating Services.* Springer Science & Business Media; 2007.
18. Cigrang JA, Rauch SAM, Avila LL, et al. Treatment of active-duty military with PTSD in primary care: early findings. *Psychol Serv.* 2011;8(2):104-113.
19. Edinger JD, Means MK. Cognitive-behavioral therapy for primary insomnia. *Clin Psychol Rev.* 2005;25(5):539-558.
20. McCrae CS, Bramoweth AD, Williams J, et al. Impact of brief cognitive behavioral treatment for insomnia on health care utilization and costs. *J Clin Sleep Med.* 2014;10(2):127-135.
21. Mitchell MD, Gehrman P, Perlis M, Umscheid CA. Comparative effectiveness of cognitive behavioral therapy for insomnia: a systematic review. *BMC Fam Pract.* 2012;13(1):40.
22. Fiore MC, Bailey WC, Cohen SJ, et al. *Treating Tobacco Use and Dependence: Clinical Practice Guideline.* Rockville, MD: US Dept of Health and Human Services, Public Health Service; 2000.
23. Wittchen H, Hoch E, Klotsche J, et al. Smoking cessation in primary care: a randomized controlled trial of bupropione, nicotine replacements, CBT and a minimal intervention. *Int J Methods Psychiatr Res.* 2011;20(1):28-39.
24. Zayfert C, Becker CB. *Cognitive-behavioral Therapy for PTSD: A Case Formulation Approach.* New York, NY: Guilford Press; 2007.
25. Beck JS, Busis DB. *The Diet Trap Solution: Train Your Brain to Lose Weight and Keep it off for Good.* London: Hay House, Inc.; 2015.

17

SUPPORTIVE PSYCHOTHERAPY IN PRIMARY CARE

Lindsey Enoch, MD, Christine E. Kho, MD, and Robert M. McCarron, DO, DFAPA

CLINICAL HIGHLIGHTS

- Supportive psychotherapy is incredibly useful for patients with mental illness who refuse, fail, or have contraindications to psychotropic medications.
- Supportive therapy works by helping patients increase healthy coping skills and decrease unhealthy coping skills. Providers can help patients self-identify and utilize existing healthy coping strategies, while encouraging patients to recognize maladaptive coping mechanisms and replace with new strategies to address life stressors.
- Two of the most common distortions you will be working to adjust are patient's beliefs that their problems are unique and that their problems cannot be fixed.
- The acronym "PARENTS" will help you remember the core principles and skills needed to provide effective supportive therapy: **P**roblem focused, **A**lly with patient, **R**ecognize emotions, **E**nhance coping, **N**ormalize, **T**each, and **S**elf-esteem.

OVERVIEW

Patients present to their primary care doctors with many complex problems. Among the most challenging patient encounters include those with psychiatric and psychosocial concerns. Many providers feel they lack the resources, time, or skills necessary to address these kinds of issues. Yet with so many patients unable to access mental health specialty care, primary care doctors are often first line in treating mental illness and guiding their patients through everyday conflict and distress.

In this chapter, we will introduce the principles and techniques used in supportive therapy. These techniques, which can be learned and applied over just a few appointments, are effective in managing a variety of complex issues seen in primary care. By learning these skills, primary care providers can provide substantial and effective

treatment to patients unable to access other forms of mental health care or social support. They are also incredibly useful for patients with mental illness who refuse, fail, or have contraindications to psychotropic medications. Moreover, supportive psychotherapeutic techniques can also be utilized in the busy primary care setting.

Conditions that can be addressed with supportive therapy techniques include the following:

- Depression
- Anxiety
- Chronic pain
- Problems with relationships, employment, housing, and other social stressors
- Grief
- Substance abuse
- Recurrent hospitalizations or noncompliance
- Stress related to general medical problems
- Difficulties adhering to the treatment of general medical problems

First we will review the evidence and core principles in supportive therapy, with particular focus on building coping skills. Next, we'll provide a practical approach, showing how to structure appointments so that you can use these tools effectively in just two to four visits. Lastly, we will go over a case vignette, which illustrates how and when to use supportive psychotherapy.

EVIDENCE

Historically, supportive therapy has been considered a nonstandardized form of therapy, making it difficult to reproduce and study against other forms of treatment. Although large randomized trials are lacking, there is evidence that supportive therapy can be effective for a variety of patients. In a recent meta-analysis by Cuijpers et al., authors found that supportive therapy was as effective for treating depression as medications and other types of therapy.[3] In another study looking at treatment of depression in primary care, authors found that problem-solving therapy and interpersonal therapy, which use many of the same techniques and principles as supportive therapy, were more effective for treating depression than medications and other types of therapy.[8]

There is also evidence that some of these therapeutic techniques can benefit patients after just a few visits, and even when provided by non–mental health professionals. In a systematic review by Nieuwsma et al., authors found that even brief therapy was effective for the treatment of depression in primary care. Many studies included used protocols with only six 30-minute sessions provided by non–mental health professionals.[6] **Although this study excluded supportive therapy, these findings suggest that primary care doctors can effectively learn and use therapeutic techniques to treat depression, even when delivered in a busy general medical setting.**

CORE PRINCIPLES

Broadly speaking, supportive therapy works by helping patients increase healthy coping skills and decrease unhealthy coping skills. Put another way, providers can help patients self-identify and utilize existing healthy coping strategies, while encouraging patients to recognize maladaptive coping mechanisms and replace with new strategies to address life stressors. By learning and applying healthier coping skills, patients can manage problems more effectively and with greater sense of control. This leads to increases in function and higher self-esteem. Also, these valuable skills can be used for a lifetime.

The acronym "PARENTS" will help you remember the core principles and skills needed to provide effective supportive therapy:

Problem focused
Ally with patient
Recognize emotions
Enhance coping
Normalize
Teach
Self-esteem

First, we describe the theory behind each core principle, followed by the tools you will need to apply them.

PROBLEM FOCUSED

In supportive therapy, it's important to first identify a specific problem to treat. When patients come in with broad complaints such as, "life is awful," it's important to identify a more specific problem contributing to this belief. When there are numerous or large, complex problems, break things into smaller pieces and address whatever is most pressing. Focus on the details on the *specific* problem, noting any contributing factors, associated symptoms, etc. In addition to understanding the problem better, asking for details like this will help patients "connect the dots" between symptoms, problems, or other key factors. Be sure to ask for the patients' goals for addressing the problem, which is what your supportive therapy and their coping skills will be working toward. Help them identify a goal, making sure it's realistic and could be achieved after the next few visits.

Tools to Use

Socratic Questioning

- Ask open-ended questions
- Identify triggers, symptoms, and associated dysfunctions

Example of provider response: "You're really struggling with your anxiety. Tell me how that's impacted your life?"

Determine a Goal

- Make it realistic, concrete, and time limited

Example: If a patient says the goal is to be "pain free" (which may be unrealistic), it's better to identify a functional goal, like getting back to work (concrete). You might say, "Getting your pain under control is really important. What would you like to do if you could be pain free? It sounds like work is important to you, and something we could work toward accomplishing over the next few visits. I think that would help you feel better in a lot of ways. What do you think?"

Summarize

- Confirm your understanding.
- Make connections they may not have seen.
- Use as redirection when the patient is getting off topic.

Example of provider response: "You're having a lot of pain and trouble just getting through the day. There are a lot of different stressors weighing on you, and you'd like better pain control so you can go back work."

ALLY WITH PATIENT

Supportive techniques are most akin to being a "good parent." Listen, empathize, and advise when necessary but without directly providing an answer or solution. It is usually more effective to lead the patient to self-discovery of a workable solution. Ask about the problem, and try to listen to the patient without initial interruption. Although listening can sometimes seem too passive to be effective, many patients lack a safe place to express their feelings and concerns. In many clinical situations, silence on the part of the provider is therapeutic and, although likely foreign to patients, will often be welcome and evidence of genuine interest and investment of time for the patient by the provider. Building rapport and expression of interest in a patient with high levels of psychosocial stress will take time but will most often yield positive results, including improved adherence to mutually agreed upon treatment plans.

Tools to Use

2 Ears, 1 Mouth Rule

- For at least 5 minutes, try to listen without interruption.

Show Support

- Show interest with engaging body language (such as nodding in agreement, making eye contact, and avoiding crossing arms).

Be Empathic

- "Become the patient" or understand the emotional state and life circumstances as best you can.
- Demonstrate genuine empathic remarks.

Example of provider response: "You've endured a lot with your husband, and you've really tried your best. I'm glad you're telling me this."

RECOGNIZE EMOTION

Oftentimes, when people are distressed, they disconnect and misidentify their feelings. In almost every condition we listed earlier, patients have trouble recognizing, accepting, or articulating their emotions. Any emotion can become debilitating and difficult to manage when not clearly understood. In supportive therapy, the task is to help patients recognize and understand their emotions and connect them to the problem being discussed. With better emotional awareness, patients can cope more effectively and appropriately, which will lessen their distress. You can help patients develop this valuable skill by inviting them to reflect on their emotions in the specific problem being discussed.

Tools to Use

"And How Did That Make You Feel?"

- Ask and ask again. People have lots of emotions and often need a few chances to recognize them.
- Use this approach when patients get overly focused on what happened (rather than why it's bothering them).

Example of provider response: "Did you have other feelings about this? Like what? What else?"

Name the Emotion

- Suggest a "normal" emotional response when applicable (e.g., grief reaction).
- Ask patients to identify the emotion when challenging for them to do so.
- Use this approach to clarify and simplify complicated experiences.

Example of provider response: "Wow, it sounds like you were really scared!"

Objective Interpretation

- Suggest a more accurate emotion or interpretation when applicable.
- Use when
  - patients' feeling/interpretations differ significantly from your understanding of the problem and
  - their "misinterpretation" is interfering with resolution of the problem.

Example of provider response: "You feel lonely and like nobody cares about you, but from what you're telling me, multiple people have reached out to you in the past week. You mentioned 6 people called you and asked how you were doing. It seems like people do care about you."

Summarize

- Connect emotions to the problem being discussed.
- Use diagrams and list of key emotions and problems; provide them to the patient as a reference.

Example: The patient wants to address her chronic pain with opiates but has agreed to work with you in learning more about triggers and possible treatments. You might summarize: "Your pain is very severe, and it's making it hard for you to do many things, including exercise, sleep, and take care of your kids. You're feeling pretty angry, sad, and disappointed. This seems like important stuff to discuss. Can we talk a bit more about how you're handling all this?"

E COPING

One of the main goals of supportive therapy is to increase patients' use of healthy coping skills. It's important to explain this concept to patients, and that together, you will be coming up with ways (coping skills) for them to improve their problem or relieve symptoms. Emphasize that everyone needs ways to manage problems, and healthier coping skills are simply skills that are more effective ways of reaching goals and controlling symptoms.

Start by learning about which coping skills patients already have. Ask about how they've managed difficult situations in the past. As their provider, you may know of some qualities and strengths they've used to overcome previous conflicts or illnesses. Point these out. The goal is to help them utilize and expand on these to help them cope with the problem at hand.

Because patients usually can't articulate how they cope, it's important to be able to identify healthy and unhealthy coping skills in the various ways they come up. This requires a bit more understanding about defense mechanisms. Coping skills and "defense mechanisms" are essentially the same thing: They're the way people handle problems. Once you're able to pick out a few of the patient's coping strategies, you can use your supportive techniques to help them build their healthy skills and decrease their unhealthy coping skills. Because this is such an essential part of supportive therapy, we've included detailed tables at the end of this section. These describe common unhealthy and healthy coping skills and the scenarios where they often present. *Table 17-1* includes "unhealthy" skills, examples, and tools you can use to develop healthier coping. *Table 17-2* includes "healthy" skills, examples, and ways to help patient utilizes these skills. These tables will be useful to reference throughout your visits with patients.

NORMALIZE

Patients who are struggling with the common conditions listed at the beginning of this chapter often share similar cognitive distortions or, fixed, false beliefs. Two of the most common distortions you will be working to adjust are patient's beliefs that their problems are unique and that their problems cannot be fixed. In dealing with difficult issues, patients feel alone and hopeless, which leads to additional suffering and interferes with coping.

TABLE 17-1 Unhealthy Coping Skills and Defense Mechanisms

PROBLEM	UNHEALTHY COPING SKILL/ DEFENSE	EXAMPLE OF PATIENT RESPONSE	EXAMPLES OF PROVIDER RESPONSE	SUPPORTIVE TOOL USED	HEALTHIER COPING
Frequent readmissions	Denial	"It's not my fault my blood sugar is so high—I'm doing everything I can. If the pharmacy could remember to fill my insulin, I'd basically be healthy!"	I know it's been tough to manage your diabetes. It's a difficult disease but I think we can do this. What would you like to focus on? How are you managing the stress? Tell me about how you're feeling through this?	Validation Instill hope Problem focus Identifying emotions	Identify a specific goal Identify positives and rewards associated with achieving goal
Housing issues	Projecting *Uncomfortable feeling is believed to come from someone else rather than oneself* (here: anger)	"My sister threw me out onto the streets. She's just an angry and hateful person. I don't need her."	I can see why you might be angry with your sister as well. Do you think that has anything to do it your housing problems? How would you express that feeling to your sister?	Normalizing Problem focus Identifying emotion Role play	Express problems to friend, provider hotline, sister when ready Channel anger: music, art, activity
Substance abuse	Rationalization	"My wife is so annoying, I have to drink just so I can deal with her!"	It sounds like you and your wife are having some problems and that you're looking for a way to deal with that. But your drinking is also causing problems, and maybe we can address that first. What else could you do when you feel annoyed with your wife?	Problem focus Summarizing Confrontation Socratic questioning	Support groups (AA) Alternative hobbies for stress reduction Reducing triggers to drink
Pain	Externalization *Problems attributed to others or external factors*	"I gained 30 pounds since you stopped my opiates. I can't move with all this pain. It's impossible to be healthy now!"	I see your point, but what do you think your role is in all this? What sorts of things have you done to be healthy in the past?	Validation Socratic Questioning Identifying coping skills already present	Meditation Deep breathing Exercise/PT

TABLE 17-2 Healthy Coping Skills and Defense Mechanisms

PROBLEM	HEALTHY COPING SKILL/ DEFENSE	EXAMPLE OF PATIENT RESPONSE	EXAMPLE OF PROVIDER RESPONSE	SUPPORTIVE TOOL USED	NEXT STEP
Depression	Humor	"It's like I'm writing a book on 'how to ruin your life by 30.'"	You have a gift for making people laugh. Even you cheered up a bit with that joke.	Praise Naming emotions Identifying strengths	Set goals Increase frequency of coping skill use Teach how coping skill helps in meeting goals
Grief	Emotional reflection	"I'm not sure that I can handle this. I know it's silly, but sometimes I write my mom post it notes and then rip them up. Then I will cry for hours."	You are sad and you cry. How do you feel after you cry? Oftentimes, people feel a huge sense of relief after they let themselves cry. It's okay for everyone to feel sad from time to time.	Naming emotion Acceptance Normalizing	Listen empathically Suggest journaling, letter writing Identify "good" ways to experience grief
Family discord	Distraction	"Things are so bad at home, I've just been trying to stay busy with other things. I'm pretty sick of homework, but at least my grades are better."	It's great you can use your school work as an outlet. Are there other positive ways you can distract yourself? A lot of people feel better when they can take a break. Sometimes just visualizing a calm, pleasant place can feel like getting away. Can you visualize a place like that?	Praise Teach new coping skills Visualization	Educate how healthy coping skills can be used to lessen distress, improve sense of control Practice visualization Identify other distractions to be used for coping, Like exercise, music, hobbies
Anxiety	Channeling	"Sometimes I get so anxious, i feel like I'm going to explode. There's nothing I can do to make it go away."	Anxiety can feel that way! I know that when I feel that nervous, channeling some of those feelings into exercise can really help. Can I give you some at home workouts, or prices on gyms in your area?	Ally with patient Personal advice Role model Educate	Create concrete goals and educate about ability to control symptoms Identify other channeling activities
Recurrent hospitalization	Altruism and commitment to others	"I want to be a better parent. I know I should be healthy for my kids but it's so hard."	I've noticed how committed you are to your family. I'm confident there are ways we can get you healthier. Do you have any specific goals you'd like to work on to start?	Praise Empathy Problem focus	Create specific goals and how you will measure these goals Assign small tasks between visits

Here, the task is to correct these false beliefs by normalizing. Reassure patients that their problems and feelings are not atypical or abnormal. Let them know there are others who share their difficulties and that people often get better. Your optimism will help patients to feel more hopeful and confident about reaching their goals.

Tools to Use

Validate

- Give "permission" to have feelings.

Example of provider response: "Your mother was really hard on you, so it's ok to be angry with her."

Cheerlead

- Encourage patients to keep trying and that setbacks are common.
- Cheerlead toward a different goal if they cannot meet the original.

Example of provider response: "It's not uncommon for people to feel guilty after the loss of a loved one. You're a strong woman, and I know you will get through this."

Acceptance

- Use for emotions that can't be resolved.
- Explain that understanding is helpful, even if "fixing" isn't possible.

TEACH

In supportive therapy, various tools can be used to teach patients and can be a fast way for them to gain insight and coping skills. Teaching can be done during the visit or by "assigning" patients to read, complete, or practice something before the next visit.

Giving advice and sharing personal examples can also be valuable teaching tools, guide learning, and show empathy.[5] Similarly, role modeling healthy ways of dealing with emotions, such as anger and failure, can be very informative. Being relatable improves the alliance and offers the patient a chance to learn from your experience.

Tools to Use

Educate

- Share expertise
- Use handouts to teach about symptoms (anxiety- vs. cardiac-related pain, for example), new coping technique (guide to meditation)

Advice (Personal or Professional)

- Offer it before giving it.
- Use this sparingly, because it is best for patients to work with you and self-discover a healthy solution.

Example of provider response: "Would you like my medical opinion? I know a few things that helped people in similar scenarios."

Role Play

- Ask patients what they would say/do if they were back in the scenario right now.

SELF-ESTEEM

Many patients suffer from low self-esteem, especially those with mood disorders, stress, pain, or loss of functioning. In time, patients with healthier coping strategies experience higher self-esteem but, early in the process, support patients with genuine affirmation and reassurance. Sharing your expertise in treating similar patients will instill confidence and convey optimism.

Tools to Use

Praise

- Point out *any* success.
- Point out use of healthy coping skills.

Example of provider response: "You were worried about using alcohol to cope with arguments with your wife. Instead, I noticed you took a healthier approach to deal with the anger by going to the gym. Good job!"

Instill Hope

- Remain optimistic when they might not be able to do so.

Example of provider response: "You might be surprised how many people have trouble with finances, and most people can learn skills to help them get out of this problem. I know you can as well."

Confrontation

- It's okay to disagree with the patient's choices and behaviors.
- Reinforce your role to support and help, while expressing concern in a nonjudgmental manner.
- Use when patients are engaging in harmful behaviors (such as drugs or alcohol).

Example of provider response: "It sounds like the insomnia could be related to anxiety, but I'm more concerned about the amount you've been drinking, and how that's affecting your sleep."

STRUCTURING THE CLINIC VISITS
CLINIC VISIT 1

Use the entire visit (even if it's only 15 minutes) to do the following:

1. Problem focus—*find a specific problem to address and learn details*
2. Identify emotions
3. Identify coping skills used in the past
4. Determine goals—*specific, realistic, and measurable*
5. Teach—*in appointment or with handout or homework that emphasizes 2, 3, or 4 above*

CLINIC VISIT 2

Things to do:

1. Provider summarizes the problem
2. Ask about emotions—*don't ask about new problems/concerns. Ask about feelings now or from the last visit; summarize if different from the last visit*
3. Define coping skills—*explain that together you'll be coming up with coping skills—ways to manage the problem, lessen symptoms, and meet goals*
4. Identify, educate, and build healthy coping skills (see Tables 17.1 and 17.2)
5. Assign coping skill between visits—*specify when, how often*
6. Teach—*if time permits*

CLINIC VISIT 3 AND ADDITIONAL VISITS

Goals and symptoms can be addressed with as few as three appointments. Additional appointments are structured similar to the third visit.

Things to do:

1. Review progress toward goal
2. Identify coping skills used
3. Connect how coping skills have helped reach goal or improve function and symptom control
4. Teach
5. Plan—*define how patient will continue to work on problem, how often they will use coping skills*
6. Offer additional resources—*yourself, books, support groups, etc.*

PRACTICE CASE

Ms. Olive is a 26-year-old woman who comes to your clinic complaining of 1 month of poor sleep and daytime fatigue. Despite ideal weather, she has not been hiking, kayaking, or rock climbing with friends as she typically loves to do. She has gained 10 lbs, rarely leaves the house, and her blood sugars are significantly higher than before. She tearfully tells you, "I'm a wreck and no one seems to care. I don't want to do anything. I just hate my life right now."

Provider: "I can tell you're really upset. Can you tell me more about what's bothering you?" *Naming emotions and identifying a specific problem.*

Patient: "I'm not myself. I don't want to get out of bed in the morning, but things are so busy at work, and I have to stay late every night. It's not like my friends want to hang out anymore, so I guess it doesn't matter that I'm at work all the time."

Provider: "Hmm. Can you tell me more about what's going on?" *Listens empathically, asks for details about the problem.*

Patient: "People used to call and invite me out to do things, but now I guess I'm not a very fun person. I'm too tired to talk anyway, so I rarely answer when friends call."

Provider: "And how does that make you feel?" *Identifying emotions.*

Patient: "I feel like they don't care. It makes me sad and angry."

Provider: "That's understandable." *Normalizing, empathy.*

Patient: "I wish they cared."

Provider: "It sounds like your friends have reached out and called you, but you've felt pretty down, and your sleep and energy are lousy. Is there anything that's been making you feel more down lately?" *Summarizing, objective interpretation, connecting problems and symptoms.*

Patient: "I've been feeling really stressed at work and at home. And I'm so tired, and I don't want to exercise or be active like I used to. I guess that used to help relieve a lot of stress."

Provider: "You know, oftentimes when people feel depressed, they lose interest in doing things they once enjoyed, and everyday tasks become more difficult. It sounds like depression could be interfering with your ability to keep up your hobbies and friendships. I know that they've always been important to you." *Education, normalizing.*

Patient: "Yes. that's true"

Provider: "What sorts of things do you do when you're feeling down or stressed?" *Identifying coping skills.*

Patient: "Going outside has always helped me clear my head. But I'm so tired—I can't exercise like I used to."

Provider: "Sometimes, even a small amount of a good thing can really help our mood and sleep. What could you do to get outside more, and how often do you think you could do it in the next two weeks? Do you think this would help?" *More education, surveying for coping.*

Patient: "It probably would help. I could walk around the park twice a week. Maybe I could do it with friends, and that would help me feel better too. I guess my friends are pretty important to me."

Provider: "I think it's a great start and a good goal. Maybe we can check in again in 2 weeks and talk more about how you're dealing with stress. Everyone deals with challenges differently, and we could come up with some different strategies to help you feel like your old self and get your diabetes under control." *Instilling hope, defining coping skills and aim of future visits.*

Patient: "That sounds good. I feel better now that we have a plan. I'm glad I brought this up."

Provider: "Before our next visit, can you write down any other emotions you're struggling with? I can give you a hand out on some common emotions. It sounds silly, but a lot of people find it helpful as they try to identify their feelings." *Setting goals, expectations, and education.*

Patient: "Sure, if you think it will help. I'll write some things down before our next visit."

CONCLUSION

Supportive therapy techniques can be used in primary care to address common and complex issues. The acronym PARENTS will help providers remember core principles and skills, which can be learned quickly and applied effectively in just three visits. This type of treatment can offer substantial relief to many complex patients, particularly those with limited access to care and those who cannot tolerate medications. By learning these skills, providers will be more equipped and more comfortable addressing the needs of their patients.

CASES AND QUESTIONS

CASE 1:

A 36-year-old woman comes into your office to follow up on her hypertension (HTN). Upon walking in the room, she bursts into tears telling you her brother just passed away, and she's felt "hopeless" and "lost." She admits that she's completely neglected her own health, and when you check her blood pressure, it's 166/90. She doesn't think there's any reason to continue medications, when "I'll probably die soon anyway."

1. Which of the following supportive therapy techniques would be most appropriate?
   A. Ask her to list the evidence for and against the belief "I might die at any minute."
   B. Provide her with the phone number of a grief support group.
   C. Validate her feelings about being lost.
   D. Educate her about the importance of blood pressure management and the sequelae of uncontrolled HTN.

   Correct answer: C. *Supportive therapy techniques can be helpful for patients experiencing and processing acute grief. In this setting, it's important to listen empathically, convey concern, and give the patient permission to feel whatever they're feeling. This can be done by validating an emotion, which conveys understanding and acceptance without trying to change it.*

   Asking a patient to list the evidence for and against her cognitive distortion "I'll probably die soon anyway" is a technique used in cognitive behavioral therapy (CBT) and does not address the emotions that she's experiencing in the here and now. While you may give the patient the phone number of a grief support group, this would not be appropriate to do before you validated and explored her grief. Given her degree of distress, she's unlikely to process or benefit from education on better blood pressure management. This also dismisses the problem she's attempting to address, and supportive therapy should be focused on problems identified by the patient. The patient's more pressing concern is her grief, and should be the focus of the visit.

CASE 2:

You are seeing a patient for follow-up on chronic pain. You have successfully tapered her hydrocodone dose by 50%, but she is resistant to further lowering the dose. You suggest that she stops her nighttime PRN Norco; however, she is worried that her pain will be so severe, she won't be able to function.

1. Which of the following is a healthy coping skill the patient could use to manage pain?
   A. Snapping a rubber band against her wrist to distract from pain
   B. Engaging in one of her hobbies every evening around the time she'd normally take her PRN Norco
   C. Repeating "my pain does not exist" 5 to 10 times every night
   D. Channeling her pain by inflicting pain on something else

   Correct answer: B. *Distraction can be a valuable coping skill, especially when the patient is worried about becoming fixated on something. While distractions themselves can be both healthy and unhealthy, most people can identify and commit to use of some sort of positive distraction. Hobbies, leisure activity, and calling friends are all forms of healthy distraction that can help people cope.*

   Snapping a rubber band against one's wrist is a type of harm reduction technique often used in dialectical behavior therapy (DBT) but not supportive therapy. Repeating positive endorsements about oneself is sometimes used to address cognitive distortions in CBT, but this technique will likely make the patient more fixated on her pain and less able to cope. And while channeling can be used as a positive coping skill, it does not involve transferring one's own negative experience into something else. Rather, an unpleasant experience is channeled into something benign or healthy (like anger being channeled and released through exercise).

CASE 3:

You are establishing care with a new patient who was discharged from the hospital last week with a new diagnosis of heart failure. As he begins to tell you how scary it was when he developed difficulty breathing, you look up from your computer screen and ask, "Any paroxysmal dyspnea, orthopnea, peripheral edema, or angina?" Not knowing what those terms mean, the patient shakes his head, "No." Sensing his anxiety, you tell him that with the right diet, limited fluid intake, and medication he can prevent heart failure from getting worse. You tell him that your father-in-law has gained control over heart failure with some hard work.

1. What did the provider do to help build a therapeutic alliance?

  A. Allow the patient to vent his feelings.

  B. Speak to the patient in a conversational manner, avoiding medical jargon.

  C. Ask clarifying questions and summarizing statements.

  D. Self-disclose a personal example where appropriate.

  Correct answer: D. *The provider in the scenario appropriately utilizes self-disclosure through the example of his father-in-law to help reassure the patient that his disease is manageable. This tiny gesture shows the patient that the provider is willing to share part of themselves for the overall benefit of the patient. Unfortunately, the visit is off to a rough start. The provider interrupts the patient with a review of symptoms, as he is trying to share his emotions and prevents the patient from venting his fears about losing his breath. The provider also uses a review of systems for heart failure symptoms with medical jargon that the patient may find unfamiliar and intimidating. Without clarification or summary statements about what the patient has stated, the patient does not feel like he is being heard by the provider.*

PRACTICAL RESOURCES

- Psychology Today: https://www.psychologytoday.com/blog/fighting-fear/201306/supportive-psychotherapy
- Addiction.com: https://www.addiction.com/a-z/supportive-psychotherapy/
- NAMI: https://www.nami.org/Learn-More/Treatment/Psychotherapy

REFERENCES

1. Battaglia J. 5 Keys to good results with supportive psychotherapy. *Curr Psychiatry.* 2007;6(6).
2. Brenner AM. Teaching supportive psychotherapy in the twenty-first century. *Harvard Rev Psychiatry.* 2012;20(5):259-267.
3. Cuijpers P, Driessen E, Hollon SD, van Oppen P, Barth J, Andersson G. The efficacy of non-directive supportive therapy for adult depression: a meta-analysis. *Clin Psychol Rev.* 2012;32(4):280-291.
4. Hellerstein D, Rosenthal RN, Pinsker H, Samstag LW, Muran JC, Winston A. A randomized prospective study comparing supportive and dynamic therapies: outcome and alliance. *J Psychother Pract Res.* 1998;7(4):261-271.
5. Misch DA. Basic strategies of dynamic supportive therapy. *J Psychother Pract Res.* 2000;9(4):173-189.
6. Nieuwsma JA, Trivedi RB, McDuffie J, Kronish I, Benjamin D, Williams JW. Brief psychotherapy for depression: a systematic review and meta-analysis. *Int J Psychiatry Med.* 2012;43(2):129-151.
7. Wallerstein RS. Psychoanalysis and psychotherapy: a historical perspective. *Int J Psychoanal.* 1989;70:563-591.
8. Wolf NJ, Hopko DR. Psychosocial and pharmacological interventions for depressed adults in primary care: a critical review. *Clin Psychol Rev.* 2008;28(1):131-161.

18

MOTIVATIONAL INTERVIEWING

Shelly L. Henderson, PhD

OVERVIEW

Primary care providers are on the front lines of treating chronic lifestyle-related diseases. Health-related behaviors such as diet, physical activity level, and tobacco and alcohol use account for about half of all deaths in the United States.[1] This chapter describes an effective approach to communication, motivational interviewing (MI), that can be used in brief format and is focused on helping individuals change problematic behaviors.

MI is a form of therapy that originated out of substance abuse treatment and is noted to be an effective tool for eliciting behavior change.[2] Miller and Rollnick (2002) describe MI as a "directive, patient-centered counseling style for enhancing intrinsic motivation to change by exploring and resolving ambivalence."[3] MI is more than the use of a set of techniques or strategies. It is characterized by a particular "spirit" or clinical "way of being" which is the context or interpersonal relationship within which the techniques are employed. That is, the effectiveness of MI depends on the fundamental aspect of how the provider relates to the patient.

MI, with its roots in the addiction field, offers an evidence-based approach to address the behaviors related to chronic disease and comorbid psychiatric conditions.

MI has been shown to outperform traditional advice giving in the treatment of behavioral problems and diseases related to alcohol abuse, drug addiction, smoking cessation, weight loss, poor treatment adherence, physical inactivity, asthma, and diabetes.[2] Furthermore, it has been suggested that adapted forms of MI can be brief in nature[4] and implemented into existing primary care initiatives.[5]

SPIRIT OF MOTIVATIONAL INTERVIEWING

The spirit of MI is based on three key elements: collaboration between the provider and the patient; evoking or drawing out the patient's ideas about change; and emphasizing the autonomy of the patient.

Collaboration (vs. confrontation) is a partnership between the provider and the patient, grounded in the point of view and experiences of the patient. This contrasts with the traditional biomedical approach where the physician is the expert and the patient is passive. Collaboration builds rapport and facilitates trust in the helping relationship, which can be challenging in a more hierarchical relationship. This does not mean that the provider automatically agrees with the patient about the nature of the problem or the changes that may be most appropriate. Although the provider and patient may see things differently, the therapeutic process is focused on mutual understanding, not the provider being right or the patient dictating treatment.

Using MI, the provider draws out the individual's own thoughts and ideas, rather than imposing his or her opinion. This tends to increase the patient's motivation, as commitment to change is most powerful and sustainable when it comes from the patient. Lasting change occurs when the patient discovers his or her own reasons and determination to change. The provider's job is to "draw out" the person's own motivations and skills for change, not to tell them what to do or why they should do it, no matter how scientifically valid or clinically convincing the provider's reasons may be.

The final element is based on the bioethical principle of autonomy. Unlike the traditional biomedical model that emphasizes the clinician as an authority figure, MI recognizes that the true power for change rests within the patient. Ultimately, the patient is responsible for making a behavioral change that improves his or her health and chronic disease management. This empowers the patient and increases his or her sense of responsibility to take action in the chronic disease management. Providers reinforce that there is no single "right way" to change and that there are multiple ways that change can occur. In addition to deciding whether they will make a change, patients are encouraged to take the lead in developing a "menu of options" as to how to achieve the desired change.

PRINCIPLES OF MOTIVATIONAL INTERVIEWING

There are four principles (*Table 18-1*) that guide the practice of MI: (1) Express Empathy, (2) Support Self-efficacy, (3) Roll with Resistance, and (4) Develop Discrepancy. Empathy involves seeing the world through the patient's eyes, thinking about things as the patient thinks about them, and feeling things as the patient feels them to share in the patient's experiences. This approach provides the basis for patients to be heard and understood, and in turn, patients are more likely to honestly share their experiences in depth.

For example, a patient tells the primary care provider that he cannot go to work because of his pain and is worried about his finances. The provider mentally places herself in the patient's life and states the following:

- "I imagine not being able to work and worrying about finances is scary."

- "I would feel sad if I could no longer do the things I use to do, particularly at work."

In the above responses, the provider communicates to the patient the core emotion that another would feel if they "put himself/herself in their shoes." Ultimately, the patient feels emotionally heard. This opens the door to the initial stages of building mutual trust.

Regarding Self-efficacy, MI promotes a strengths-based approach. This means that patients have within themselves the capabilities to change successfully. A patient's belief that change is possible (i.e., self-efficacy) is needed to instill hope about making those difficult changes. Patients often have previously tried and been unable to achieve or maintain the desired change, creating doubt about their ability to succeed. In MI, providers support self-efficacy by focusing on previous successes and highlighting skills and strengths that the patient already has. For example, the provider may state the following to promote self-efficacy:

- "You were successful in coming here today and voicing how you want to improve your health."
- "You have made positive changes in your life."
- "Managing depression takes time and energy just like you dedicated time and energy in the past when you stopped your alcohol use."
- "Your value of living a healthy life with your daughter helped you to stop drinking alcohol in the past; I can see you really care for your daughter. Let's keep this value in mind as we discuss cutting back on smoking."

"Rolling with resistance" means slowing down and reflecting back the patient's concerns. From an MI perspective, resistance in treatment occurs when then the patient experiences a conflict between his or her view of the "problem" or the "solution" and that of the clinician

TABLE 18-1 Motivational Interviewing Principles

MI PRINCIPLE	RATIONALE	SKILLS/TOOLS	AS COMPARED WITH …
Express empathy	• Demonstrate acceptance and understanding of patient ambivalence	• Reflective listening • Open-ended questions • Summary	• Providing data and statistics to convince patient of need for change
Support self-efficacy	• Build patient's confidence in their ability to change	• Affirmations • Reflect change talk • Identify patient's strengths	• Getting too far ahead of patient (misalignment with stage of change) • Focusing on what's going wrong rather than patient's attempts to change
Roll with resistance	• Refrain from confronting or arguing about patient's behavior • Use as opportunity to learn about patient's experience	• Reflective listening • Open-ended questions	• Engaging in power struggle • Arguing with patient about why they should change • Giving ultimatums
Develop discrepancy	• Evoke/illuminate discrepancy between patient behavior and patient's beliefs/values	• Use decisional balance • Use change rulers • Reflective listening • Open-ended questions • Summary	• Arguing for healthy behavior based on provider's values • Pointing out inconsistencies in patient behavior

or when the patient experiences his or her freedom or autonomy being impinged on. These experiences are often based on the patient's ambivalence about change, which is a normal part of the change process. In MI, providers avoid eliciting resistance by not confronting the patient and when resistance occurs, they work to de-escalate and avoid a negative interaction, instead of "rolling with it." Actions and statements that demonstrate resistance remain unchallenged especially early in the treatment relationship. The MI value on having the patient define the problem and develop his or her own solutions leaves little for the patient to resist. A frequently used metaphor is "dancing" rather than "wrestling" with the patient. In exploring patient concerns, health care providers invite patients to examine new points of view and are careful not to impose their own ways of thinking. A key concept is that providers avoid the "righting reflex," a tendency born from concern, to ensure that the patient understands and agrees with the need to change and to solve the problem for the patient. An example of rolling with resistance includes the following:

A primary care provider wants to lower the patient's opioids because she is feeling sedated with oxycodone.

- Patient: "I need my medication, I don't want to stop it. It helps me go to work!"
- Provider: "It's stressful to even think about changing the oxycodone. You need it to go to work" (Complex Reflection). "I wonder if we can brain storm some solutions? How do you think we can provide you with pain relief at work but with less sedating effects of the oxycodone?"

This empathetic and reflective response builds rapport and trust between the patient and provider allowing for further conversation:

If resistance continues, the provider may respond, "I see that work and pain relief are important to you. Can I have your permission to return to opioid medications at later time? I really want for us to spend a good amount of time thinking about pain management options that are right for you and that I feel comfortable with."

Motivation for change occurs when people perceive a mismatch between "where they are and where they want to be." Providers practicing MI work to develop this by helping patients examine the discrepancies between their current behavior and their values and future goals. When patients recognize that their current behaviors place them in conflict with their values or interfere with accomplishment of self-identified goals, they are more likely to experience increased motivation to make important life changes. It is important that the provider using MI does not use strategies to develop discrepancy at the expense of the other principles (such as empathy and self-efficacy). The provider aims to gradually help patients to become aware of how current behaviors may lead them away from, rather than toward, their important goals. For example, providers may highlight the discrepancy in the following ways:

- For the patient who is ambivalent about taking antidepressants: "You mentioned that your goal is to have a healthy delivery for your baby. How does your current drug use fit into that plan?"
- For the patient who is ambivalent about physical therapy: "Your goal is to wean off pain pills. How does physical therapy fit in with that goal?"
- For the patient who is ambivalent about dietary changes for weight loss: "You mentioned that you want to lose weight as a way to manage your back pain. How does your soda intake fit with that goal?"

The practice of MI involves the skillful use of certain techniques for bringing to life the "MI spirit," demonstrating the MI principles and guiding the process toward eliciting patient change talk and commitment for change. Change talk involves statements or nonverbal communications indicating the patient may be considering the possibility of change. We will return to change talk and go through specific examples in an upcoming section of this chapter.

SKILLS OF MOTIVATIONAL INTERVIEWING

Often called microcounseling skills, OARS is a brief way to remember the basic approach used in MI: **O**pen-ended questions, **A**ffirmations, **R**eflections, and **S**ummaries are core provider behaviors employed to move the process forward by establishing a therapeutic alliance and eliciting discussion about change.

Open-ended questions are not easily answered with a "yes/no" or short answer containing only a specific, limited piece of information. Open-ended questions invite elaboration and thinking more deeply about an issue. Although closed-ended questions have their place and are at times valuable (e.g., when collecting specific information in an assessment), open-ended questions create forward momentum used to help the patient explore the reasons for and possibility of change. The following are examples of open-ended questions that are directed at understanding the behaviors in questions and help guide the patient toward self-reflection:

- "What role does alcohol play in the way you feel emotionally?"
- "How does stress impact your pain?"
- "How are you currently coping with depression and pain?"
- "What are the advantages of treating depression when it comes to managing pain?"
- "What are the things you would do in your life if anxiety and depression were not in the picture?"

Affirmations are statements that recognize patient strengths. They assist in building rapport and in helping the patient see themselves in a different, more positive light. To be effective they must be congruent and genuine. The use of affirmations can help patients feel that change is possible even when previous efforts have been unsuccessful. Affirmations often involve reframing behaviors or concerns as evidence of positive patient qualities. Affirmations are a key element in facilitating the MI principle of Supporting Self-efficacy. The following are examples of short, simple affirmations:

- "I appreciate you being honest with me and yourself about how much physical therapy you actually did last week."
- "I want to thank you for your openness and trust in me to talk about the sadness you are experiencing. This helps me to better address all aspects of your life."
- "You showed courage and strength when you stopped smoking in the past. I can see your courage and strength now, too, as we work together to help you with pain and opioid management."
- "I can see that your concern about how anxiety interferes with work and finances reflect how much you care about your family."

Reflecting, or reflective listening, is perhaps the most crucial skill in MI. It has two primary purposes. First is to bring to life the principle of Expressing Empathy. By careful listening and reflecting responses, the patient comes to feel that the provider understands the issues from his or her perspective. Beyond this, strategic use of reflective listening is a core intervention toward guiding the patient toward change, supporting the goal-directed aspect of MI. In this use of reflections, the provider guides the patient toward resolving ambivalence by a focus on the negative aspects of the status quo and the positives of making change. There are several levels of reflection ranging from simple to more complex. Different types of reflections are skillfully used as patients demonstrate different levels of readiness for change. For example, some types of reflections are more helpful when the patient seems resistant and others more appropriate when the patient offers statements more indicative of commitment to change. Examples of reflections were noted when discussing the principle of developing discrepancies.

Summaries are a special type of reflection where the provider recaps what has occurred in all or part of a health care visit. Summaries communicate interest, understanding, and call attention to important elements of the discussion. They may be used to shift attention or direction and prepare the patient to "move on." Summaries can highlight both sides of a patient's ambivalence about change and promote the development of discrepancy by strategically selecting what information should be included and what can be minimized or excluded.

CHANGE TALK

Change talk is defined as statements by the patient revealing consideration of, motivation for, or commitment to change. In MI, the provider seeks to guide the patient to expressions of change talk as the pathway to change. Research indicates a clear correlation between patient statements about change and outcomes. This means that the more someone talks about change, the more likely they are to change. Different types of change talk can be described using the mnemonic DARN-CAT.

- Desire (I want to change)
- Ability (I can change)
- Reason (It's important to change)
- Need (I should change)

And most predictive of positive outcome is Implementing Change Talk.

- Commitment (I will make changes)
- Activation (I am ready, prepared, willing to change)
- Taking Steps (I am taking specific actions to change)

STRATEGIES FOR EVOKING CHANGE TALK

There are specific therapeutic strategies that are likely to elicit and support change talk in MI. These ten tools can be used in any given patient encounter.

1. Ask Evocative Questions: Ask an open-ended question, the answer to which is likely to be change talk.
2. Explore Decisional Balance: Ask for the pros and cons of both changing and staying the same.
3. Good Things/Not-So-Good Things: Ask about the positives and negatives of the target behavior.
4. Ask for Elaboration/Examples: When a change talk theme emerges, ask for more details. "In what ways?" "Tell me more?" "What does that look like?" "When was the last time that happened?"
5. Look Back: Ask about a time before the target behavior emerged. How were things better, different?
6. Look Forward: Ask what may happen if things continue as they are (status quo). Try the miracle question: If you were 100% successful in making the changes you want, what would be different? How would you like your life to be 5 years from now?
7. Query Extremes: What are the worst things that might happen if you don't make this change? What are the best things that might happen if you do make this change?
8. Use Change Rulers: Ask: "On a scale from 1 to 10, how important is it to you to change [the specific target behavior] where 1 is not at all important, and a 10 is extremely important? Follow-up: "And why are you at ___ and not _____ [a lower number than stated]?" "What might happen that could move you from ___ to _____ [a higher number]?" Alternatively, you could also ask "How confident are that you could make the change if you decided to do it?"
9. Explore Goals and Values: Ask what the person's guiding values are. What do they want in life? Ask how the continuation of target behavior fits in with the person's goals or values. Does it help realize an important goal or value, interfere with it, or is it irrelevant?
10. Come Along side: Explicitly side with the negative (status quo) side of ambivalence. "Perhaps _____ is so important to you that you won't give it up, no matter what the cost."

STAGES OF CHANGE

Assessing readiness to change is a critical aspect of MI. Motivation, which is considered a state not a trait, is not static and thus can change rapidly from day to day. If providers know where patients are in terms of their readiness to change, they will be better prepared to recognize and deal with a patient's motivation to change. The Stages of Change model[6] (*Table 18-2*) shows that, for most people, a change in behavior occurs gradually, with the patient moving from being uninterested, unaware, or unwilling to make a change (precontemplation), to considering a change (contemplation), to deciding and preparing to make a change (preparation). Genuine, determined action is then taken (action) and, over time, attempts to maintain the new behavior occur (maintenance). Relapses are almost inevitable and become part of the process of working toward life-long change.

TABLE 18-2 Intervention for Stage of Change	
STAGE OF CHANGE	**MI INTERVENTION**
Precontemplation	
The patient is not yet considering change or is unwilling or unable to change.	• Establish rapport, ask permission, and build trust. • Elicit the patient's perceptions of the problem. • Provide personalized feedback about assessment findings. • Express concern and keep the door open.
Contemplation	

The patient acknowledges concerns and is considering the possibility of change but is ambivalent and uncertain.	• Normalize ambivalence.
	• Help the patient "tip the decisional balance scales" toward change by:
	  ◦ Eliciting and weighing pros and cons of behavior
	  ◦ Examining the patient's personal values in relation to change
	  ◦ Emphasizing patient autonomy

Preparation	
The patient is committed to and planning to make a change in the near future but is still considering what to do.	• Clarify the patient's own goals and strategies for change. • Offer a menu of options for change or treatment. • With permission, offer expertise and advice. • Consider and problem-solve barriers to change. • Explore treatment expectancies and the patient's role. • Elicit from the patient what has worked in the past.
Action	
The patient is actively taking steps to change but has not yet reached a stable stat.	• Support a realistic view of change through small steps. • Normalize difficulties for the patient in early stages of change. • Help the patient identify high-risk situations and develop appropriate coping strategies to overcome these. • Assist the patient in finding new support for positive change.
Maintenance	
The patient has achieved initial goals such and is now working to maintain gains.	• Affirm the patient's resolve and self-efficacy. • Affirm the use of new coping strategies to avoid a return to old behavior. • Maintain supportive contact • Develop a "fire escape" plan if the patient resumes old behavior.
Relapse	
The patient has experienced a recurrence of symptoms and must now cope with consequences and decide what to do next.	• Help the patient reenter the change cycle and commend any willingness to reconsider positive change. • Explore the meaning and reality of the relapse as a learning opportunity. • Assist the patient in finding alternative coping strategies. • Maintain supportive contact.

MI, motivational interviewing.

A simple and quick way to assess stage of change is to use a Readiness to Change Ruler. This scaling strategy conceptualizes readiness or motivation to change along a continuum and asks patients to give voice to how ready they are to change using a ruler with a 10-point scale where 1 = definitely not ready to change and 10 = definitely ready to change. Depending on where the patient is, the subsequent conversation may take different directions.

The central dilemma for most people who are confronting health behavior change is ambivalence. Ambivalence is a state of having simultaneous, conflicting feelings toward both a current behavior and a new behavior. Ambivalence is most prominent during the contemplative stage.

BRIEF MOTIVATIONAL INTERVIEWING IN THE OFFICE

When using MI in the primary care setting, it is essential to focus on one behavior at a time. Once the provider and patient have agreed on an agenda for the visit and the patient has identified a behavior of concern, the provider can use a three-step process to frame the conversation. Elicit-Provide-Elicit is a simple approach that is congruent with MI. The steps are as follows: (1) Determine what the patient already knows; (2) Reflect what they know and add information to help them understand more fully; and (3) Ask what they want to know more about. For example, after determining that a patient is ambivalent about exercise, the provider may elicit from the patient:

- "Tell me what you know about the impact of exercise on depression?"
- "What do you think would be the benefits of more regular exercise?"
- "What would you be most interested in knowing about exercise for depression?"

After listing to the patient's perspective and understanding, the clinician asks for permission before offering advice. This increases the likelihood that the patient will not be resistant to the suggestions offered. The clinician provides information:

- "I am aware of some strategies other people have found helpful. Would you like to hear about some of these?"
- "I wonder what you will think about this…."
- "See which of these you think might apply to you…."

Lastly, the provider follows with open-ended questions to check in with the patient and elicit their feedback:

- "What else would you like to know?"
- "What do you think is the next step for you?"
- "So what do you make of that?"
- "What do you think about that?"
- "What does all of this mean to you?"
- "How does that apply to you?"

CLINICAL INDICATIONS

Several meta-analyses of MI in the medical setting suggest that MI is more effective at achieving targeted outcomes than control conditions.[7-10] These results spanned a wide range of behavioral outcomes, such as substance use (self-report and objective GGT levels), household passive smoke exposure, low-impact physical activity time, blood pressure, weight, self-reported smoking cessation rate, self-monitoring, sedentary behavior, patient confidence, intention to change, and engagement in treatment.

MI has been found to be effective in as little as one 15- to 20-minute session, when delivered either entirely over the phone, or when "boosted" by intermittent phone calls after in-person meetings.[11] *Table 18-3* summarizes the most common medical conditions and health behaviors that are responsive to MI interventions in the primary care setting.

Common psychiatric problems encountered in primary care include depression, anxiety, trauma, and addiction. Regardless of the treatment prescribed there remains the clinical challenge of effectively engaging the patient in steps that will lead to behavior change, whether that be taking a medication consistently, seeing a therapist, or some other agreed-on treatment. Ambivalence about treatment and change is common in clinical practice. This ambivalence may give rise to resistance, noncompliance, or limited and reluctant engagement with taking action to change. Acknowledging this ambivalence, and discussing the pros and cons of behavior change while abstaining from imposing one's own agenda, preferences, values, and desires, is a key part of MI. *Table 18-4* offers examples of how providers can use the principles of MI to respond in the moment to patients who are confronting the myriad challenges that accompany the most common psychiatric problems in primary care.

The following vignettes showcase how the tools of MI can be used to address the health behaviors that underlie many of the chronic lifestyle diseases and psychiatric conditions seen in primary care.

PRACTICE CASE

CASE 1: Karina

Karina, a 48-year-old woman comes to you with a chief complaint of low mood, low energy, increased appetite, and loss of interest in previously enjoyed activities for the past 2 months. Her Patient Health Questionnaire-9 (PHQ-9) score is 14, indicating depressive symptoms of moderate severity.[18] She has noticed her symptoms but questions the validity of a diagnosis of depression, wondering instead if it isn't "just menopause." For this reason, she is hesitant to begin medication.

TABLE 18-3 Common Medical Conditions and Health Behaviors Responsive to Motivational Interviewing (MI) as Shown in Randomized Clinical Trials

COMMON MEDICAL CONDITION	INTERVENTION	COMPARISON	OUTCOME
Alcohol addiction	Motivational enhancement therapy (MET)	Twelve-step facilitation or cognitive behavioral coping skills training	On all measures (self-report, collateral, and biochemistry) MET was found to be more effective than the two longer (12 sessions) outpatient treatments.[12]
Alcohol use during pregnancy	1 hour MI session	Prenatal care as usual	Women who reported the highest blood alcohol concentration (BAC) levels in early pregnancy showed significantly greater reduction in their estimated BAC later in pregnancy if assigned to the MI group rather than the control group.[13]
Smoking during pregnancy	MET	Prenatal care as usual	43% of the women who received the full MI intervention ($n = 175$) were not smoking at the 34th week of gestation compared to 34% of the control group. Six weeks postpartum 27.1% of the full intervention group reported to be either abstinent or light smokers, compared with only 14.6% of the control group.[14]
Second-hand smoke in the home of young children (under 3)	One MI session in the home, followed by four follow-up telephone calls	Self-help group received information on quitting smoking in the mail	6-month nicotine levels significantly lower in the MI households compared to the self-help households.[15]
Hypertension/obesity	Low level or high level MI counseling conducted by nurse practitioners	Care as usual	Significant decreases in both weight and blood pressure over 18 weeks.[16]
Physical inactivity	Brief (one session) or intensive (six sessions over 12 weeks) MI, with or without financial incentive (vouchers for free access to gym facilities)	No intervention	Intensive MI intervention (six sessions plus vouchers) was the most effective for promoting the adoption of exercise at 12 weeks.[17]

TABLE 18-4 Motivational Interviewing (MI)-Guided Responses to Common Psychiatric Conditions

CONDITION	PATIENT STATEMENT	MI PRINCIPLE	PROVIDER RESPONSE
Depression	"I feel lost, like I've lost who I used to be."	Express empathy	"I can see how much pain you're in."
Anxiety	"Even though I was promoted, I can't help but worry that I'm going to fail and disappoint my boss."	Support self-efficacy	"It's hard for you to imagine being successful. What does your boss know about you that allowed her to promote you?"
Substance use disorders	"I know I need to quit, but with the holidays coming up, I don't think that's possible right now."	Roll with resistance	"Now doesn't seem like the right time. How would you know it's the right time?"
Trauma	"Sure it's not a perfect relationship, but it works for me right now."	Develop discrepancy	"You mentioned wanting to regain custody of your children. How does this relationship help you achieve that?"

Discussion

Provide Clinical Feedback

The conversation from the point of assessment to establishing the first step in treatment is important. The skill of providing clinical feedback in an objective, nonjudgmental manner includes the following:

* Use a visual graphic to represent the patient score/value and what is expected (e.g., PHQ-9).
* Explain the number in a simple, matter-of-fact manner.
* Ask the patient what he or she thinks or feels about the information. This allows the patient to disclose current thoughts and feelings about the information without any judgment or interpretation by the provider.

Provider: "Based on your PHQ-9, your score is a 14. Looking at this scale here, that score is in the range of a moderate depressive disorder. What are your thoughts or reactions to that?"

Patient: "Really? I've been feeling pretty low lately. But I thought it was just menopause coming on."

Provider: "You're wondering if this is hormonal (Reflection). What else have you noticed that might help us differentiate between depression and menopause?"

Patient: "Well I guess it is kind of strange that I just don't feel like doing anything. I used to get up in the morning and exercise right away. Now I have to force myself to get out of bed."

Elicit-Provide-Elicit

When treating mental health disorders, it is essential to first explore patient preferences[19] and to establish what the patient already knows (including existing beliefs and practices) about depression and treatment options. Once the extent of the patient's existing knowledge is established, the provider asks permission to provide additional information (responsive to what has been said by the patient). After sharing brief, concise information, the provider then explores the patient's thoughts and feelings about what has been shared. The following dialogue provides an example:

Provider (elicit): "What are some of the things you already know about that can help with depression."

Patient: "I know people who take medication, but I really don't think that's for me."

Provider: "What concerns you about taking medication?"

Patient: "I guess I just think I should be able to handle this on my own. Everyone goes through menopause."

Provider (provide): "It's possible that there is some hormonal component to what you're experiencing. And we know that the brain chemicals that are involved in depression interact with hormones. Often the way we treat depression can help us manage menopause. What else have you heard or know about treating depression? (elicit)"

Patient: "I don't know, 'fake it till you make it' I guess."

Provider (provide): "Research and my own clinical experience have shown that different treatments have different degrees or levels of evidence and effectiveness for helping depression. Would you be interested in learning more about some of these? (get permission)"

Patient: "Sure."

The provider gives brief, concise information about options for treatment.

Provider (elicit): "From what I've explained, what are your thoughts at this point?"

Patient: "Just thinking about what used to work for me, I think exercise is something I'd like to start doing again."

In this scenario, the patient is hesitant to call her symptoms "depression," preferring instead to think of it as related to a hormonal change. By partnering with the patient in this belief system, the provider negotiates a treatment plan as a beginning step to treating depression. From here, the provider can help the patient develop an action plan that specifically targets exercise, a behavior identified by the patient. If on follow-up, the patient's depression has not improved, the provider can refer back to this conversation and suggest trying a new approach, possibly medication or psychotherapy. Taking the time to establish a collaborative relationship, even if it means postponing medication, will increase the chances that the patient will return for further treatment.

CASE 2: Huong

Huong is a 35-year-old man who has a chief concern of insomnia and feeling anxious. Part of your clinic's workflow is to have all patients complete the Alcohol Use Disorders Identification Test (AUDIT) before seeing the provider. The AUDIT questionnaire is designed to help in the self-assessment of alcohol consumption and to point out any implications for the person's health. It consists of 10 questions on alcohol use.[20] The total score prompts feedback to the patient. Huong's AUDIT score places him in "zone 2," the "risky" category of use.

Discussion

Raise the Subject

Provider: Before we're done with our visit today I wonder if it's ok for us to talk about your drinking.

Patient: Um, ok.

Provider: You filled out this survey, thank you! I just want to review a couple things. I noticed you said you drink two to three times a week, drink three or four drinks at a time when you do drink, and weekly have more drinks than that, six or more. Does that sound right?

Patient: Yes, on the weekends.

Provider: I just want to let you know I'm a little concerned about your level of drinking. We know that excessive drinking can make problems worse or can cause health problems at times. I wonder if you've thought about the connection between drinking and the anxiety and insomnia you came in with today?

Patient: No, I guess I haven't really thought much of it. I don't think I drink that much in the first place. I have a hard time believing it's causing my anxiety. In fact, the nights when I don't drink, I have a harder time going to sleep.

Provider: Well, you're not alone. A lot of people think that drinking helps them sleep better. And in reality, drinking might make you fall asleep faster but it has what's called this rebound effect and this rebound effect means that you might wake up in the middle of the night or early morning and have a harder time falling back asleep.

Patient: I guess I do wake up about 2 AM on the nights I drink too much.

Provide Feedback

Provider: I wanted to show you this chart. For your age as a male you're drinking more than those at a low risk level. The low risk level for men under 65 is no more than 14 drinks a week and no more than 4 a day. You're right, you're not drinking as much as some people out there. The way you answered the questions, however, put you in the high-risk category.

Patient: I didn't think I was that bad.

Enhance Motivation

Provider: On a scale of 1 to 10 what is your readiness to change, with 1 being not all and 10 being I really want to change.

Patient: I don't know this is all news to me. I don't want to do anything to put myself at risk. I've always thought of myself as a pretty healthy guy. I guess in the middle at a 5.

Provider: That's great, that's half way there. What kept you from giving a lower number, a 1 or a 2?

Patient: Well you know I'm training for the marathon and I want to get my sleep back on track. But I also don't think of myself as "hazardous drinker" and certainly not an alcoholic. So that's why the middle ground.

Provider: Ok, that's a good place to start. I heard you say that your health is important, you're getting ready to run a marathon and you want to do what you can to make that successful. And you also were a little surprised that you fall into this risky category.

Patient: Yes

Negotiate a Plan

Provider: Based on all this information, what are you willing to think about doing to change right now?

Patient: I think the natural thing would be to cut back on my drinking.

Provider: What would that look like to you?

Patient: No more than three to four times a week and on the weekends cut back to no more than five or six beers.

Provider: That's an improvement. You're headed in the right direction. It's my recommendation that at some point you would fall below this level of no more than 14 drinks per week. I really commend you for your willingness to take a look at this and try to make some improvements.

In this scenario, the provider raises the subject and obtains permission to talk about drinking. Using a standardized screening measure, the provider gives specific feedback to the patient and then checks his understanding and reaction. The provider then uses the readiness to change ruler to assess the patient's stage of change. From there, they negotiate a plan for harm reduction.

SUMMARY

For many of the conditions seen in primary care, pharmacologic treatment is a first-line approach in conjunction with nonpharmacologic means (e.g., CBT, exercise, meditation). Many of these disorders are chronic and require life-long, day-to-day management and monitoring. MI, rather than a treatment itself, is a communication tool to engage patients and help them successfully implement treatment regiments in their daily lives.

Repeatedly educating our patients about the importance of health behavior change for chronic diseases is not always successful and can become frustrating for the primary care provider and patient. A feeling of failure, especially when repeated, may cause patients to give up and avoid contact with their provider or avoid treatment altogether. Patients who fail are often labeled "noncompliant" or "unmotivated." Labeling a patient in this way places responsibility for failure on the patient's character and ignores the complexity of the behavior change process.

MI is an evidence-based communication style that brings patients and their primary care providers into a partnership and prevents the stalemate that so often plagues difficult interactions around chronic disease management and health behavior change. These principles and techniques are foundational concepts that are at the root of any therapeutic relationship that intends to bring about change in health-related behaviors.[21]

CASES AND QUESTIONS

CASE:

A 25-year-old woman presents to your office for a 1-month follow-up of low back pain. In your previous visit, you determined that the back pain could be alleviated by weight loss. You and the patient developed a plan that entailed exercise and dietary changes. At today's visit, the patient reports having gained 3 lbs. despite her efforts to make behavior changes. She is tearful and states, "I just don't think it's possible for me to lose weight."

1. Which of the following is the most likely explanation for her statement?

A. She is not capable of making changes to lose weight.

B. She is not confident in her ability to lose weight.

C. She does not think it is important to lose weight.

D. She does not understand how to lose weight.

Correct answer: B. *The patient's use of language "it's not possible" suggests that the patient is lacking in confidence, or self-efficacy, which is one of two (the other being importance) necessary components for change to occur.*

2. You respond to your patient using a MI counseling style. Which of the following communication techniques are you most likely to use at this point in the visit?

A. Confront

B. Give advice

C. Reflect

D. Summarize

Correct answer: C. *Given this patient's tearfulness, reflection is the most empathetic and appropriate response.*

PRACTICAL RESOURCES

- https://www.integration.samhsa.gov/clinical-practice/motivational-interviewing
- www.motivationalinterviewing.org

REFERENCES

1. McGinnis JM, Foege WH. Actual causes of death in the United States. *J Am Med Assoc.* 1993;270(18):2207-2212.

2. Rubak S, Sandbaek A, Lauritzen T, Christensen B. Motivational interviewing: a systematic review and meta-analysis. *Br J Gen Pract.* 2005;55(513):305-312.

3. Miller WR, Rollnick S. *Motivational Interviewing: Preparing People for Change.* 2nd ed. New York: Guilford Press; 2002.

4. Dunn C, Deroo L, Rivara FP. The use of brief interventions adapted from motivational interviewing across behavioral domains: a systematic review. *Addiction.* 2001;96:1725-1742.

5. Burke BL, Arkowitz H, Menchola M. The efficacy of motivational interviewing: a meta-analysis of controlled clinical trials. *J Consult Clin Psychol.* 2003;71:843-861.

6. Prochaska JO, DiClemente CC, Norcross JC. In search of how people change. *Am Psychol.* 1992;47:1102-1104.

7. Lundahl B, Moleni T, Burke BL, et al. Motivational interviewing in medical care settings: a systematic review and meta-analysis of randomized controlled trials. *Patient Educ Couns.* 2013;93(2):157-168.

8. Knight KM, McGowan L, Dickens C, Bundy C. A systematic review of motivational interviewing in physical health care settings. *Br J Health Psychol.* 2006;11:319-332.

9. Martins RK, McNeil DW. Review of motivational interviewing in promoting health behaviors. *Clin Psychol Rev.* 2009;29:283-293.

10. VanWormer JJ, Boucher JL. Motivational interviewing and diet modification: a review of the evidence. *Diabetes Educ.* 2004;30:404-419.

11. VanBuskirk KA, Wetherell JL. Motivational interviewing used in primary care a systematic review and meta-analysis. *J Behav Med.* 2014;37(4):768-780.

12. Project MATCH Research Group. Project MATCH: rationale and methods for a multi-site clinical trial matching patients to alcoholism treatment. *Alcohol.* 1993;17:1130-1145.

13. Handmaker NS, Miller WR, Manicke M. Findings of a pilot study of motivational interviewing with pregnant drinkers. *J Stud Alcohol.* 1999;60:285-287.

14. Stotts AL, DiClemente CC, Dolan-Mullan P. A motivational intervention for resistant pregnant smokers. *Addict Behav.* 2002;27:275-292.

15. Emmons KM, Hammond SK, Velicer JL, Evans WF, Monroe AD. A randomized trial to reduce passive smoking exposure in low-income households with young children. *Pediatrics.* 2001;108:18-24.

16. Woollard J, Beilin L, Lord T, Puddey I, MacAdam D, Rouse I. A controlled trial of nurse counseling on lifestyle change for hypertensives treated in general practice: preliminary results. *Clin Exp Pharmacol Physiol.* 1995;22:466-468.

17. Harland J, White M, Drinkwater C, Chinn D, Farr L, Howel D. The newcastle exercise project: a randomized controlled trial of methods to promote physical activity in primary care. *BMJ.* 1999;25:828-832.

18. Kroenke K, Spitzer R, Williams J. The PHQ-9: validity of a brief depression severity measure. *J Gen Intern Med.* 2001;16(9):606-613.

19. Guadagnoli E, Ward P. Patient participation in decision-making. *Soc Sci Med.* 1998;47(3):329-339.

20. Babor TF, Higgins-Biddle JC, Saunders JB, Monteiro M. *AUDIT. The Alcohol Use Disorders Identification Test: Guidelines for Use in Primary Care.* 3rd ed. Geneva: World Health Organization; 2001.

21. Ramezani A, Rockers DM, Wanlass RL, McCarron RM. Teaching behavioral medicine professionals and trainees an elaborated version of the Y-Model: implications for the integration of cognitive-behavioral therapy (CBT), psychodynamic therapy, and motivational interviewing. *J Psychother Integrat.* 2016;26(4):407-424.

19

FUNDAMENTALS OF PSYCHOPHARMACOLOGY

Lawrence Adler, MD and Shannon Suo, MD

CLINICAL HIGHLIGHTS

- Pharmacokinetics is the study of the time course of drug absorption, distribution, metabolism, and excretion.
- Pharmacodynamics refers to the relation between drug concentration at the site of action and the resulting biologic effects.
- Understanding pharmacokinetics and pharmacodynamics is critical for understanding therapeutic actions, adverse effects, and drug–drug interactions.
- Almost all antidepressant medications have mechanisms of action involving inhibition of serotonin reuptake via the serotonin transporter.
- Mood stabilizers are utilized in the treatment of bipolar disorders and target the acute episode and prevention of future episodes in a disorder characterized by cyclical recurrence.
- Second-generation antipsychotic medications exert their pharmacodynamic effects through postsynaptic D2 blockade in mesolimbic pathways and are used to treat psychotic symptoms and as mood stabilizers.
- Most medications used to treat anxiety and insomnia exert their action at GABA receptors by enhancing the inhibitory actions of the widespread GABAergic projections.
- Novel medications for sleep disorders act at melatonin or orexin systems.

PSYCHOPHARMACOLOGY OVERVIEW
INDICATIONS AND USE OF PSYCHOPHARMACOLOGY

Clinical psychopharmacology is the study of the use of medications in treating people with mental disorders. Over the last 60 years, substantial progress has been made in developing and obtaining approval for medications to treat the symptoms of major psychiatric disorders. Appropriate utilization of these medications requires an understanding of the indications for their use, their mechanism of action, side effects, and the safety of the medications as well as their impact on patients to whom they are prescribed.

The indications for specific medications are embedded in the Food and Drug Administration approval of those medications in the United States. In Europe, the European Medicines Agency serves a similar function. Currently, medications are approved for use in specific psychiatric illness or for domains of psychopathology in those illnesses. Discussion of indications in this chapter will be limited to US-approved medications. Such approval requires at a minimum two clinical trials in which the drug is superior in efficacy to placebo and in which the drug demonstrates safety in the population under study. The pharmacokinetic and pharmacodynamic properties of the drug are evaluated in the preclinical and registration studies to obtain approval.[1]

PHARMACOKINETICS

Pharmacokinetics is the study of the time course of drug *absorption, distribution, metabolism,* and *excretion* (ADME). *Clinical pharmacokinetics* is the application of pharmacokinetic principles to the safe and effective therapeutic management of drugs in an individual patient. This application has important implications regarding both the efficacy of the drug and its potential toxicity.

Drug *absorption* requires consideration of the route of administration. Almost all psychiatric medications are administered orally, although a small group are administered intramuscularly, transdermally, or sublingually. For oral medications, absorption takes place through the mucosa of the stomach or small intestine, and then they enter the hepatic portal circulation. In the liver, and to a smaller extent the bowel wall, drugs may undergo first-pass metabolisms before entering the systemic circulation. Metabolites are excreted into the bile and small bowel and are then reabsorbed into the portal circulation and then the systemic circulation.

Drug *distribution* to the organs is affected by the systemic circulation. The rate of accumulation is largely a function of the organ's vascularity; the concentration of accumulated drug is determined by protein binding and fat content. Most psychotropic medications are highly protein bound and highly lipophilic. Under steady-state conditions, there is a proportional relationship between concentrations in the tissue and plasma compartments; the latter thus may provide an indirect measurement of the former, permitting therapeutic drug monitoring.

Metabolism of drugs serves several purposes. The process may transform an inactive chemical into one which is biologically active, may convert the parent active drug to one which has reduced toxicity, may convert the parent drug to one with less biologic activity, or may transform the parent drug to polar metabolites, which are then excreted in the urine. Whereas most psychotropic drugs undergo extensive oxidative biotransformation (phase I metabolism), others undergo simple conjugation such as glucuronidation (phase II metabolism), and others are excreted unmetabolized.

Cytochrome P450 enzymes in the liver (CYPs) are responsible for about 75% of the metabolism of psychotropic medications. The CYP activity has important implications for efficacy and for safety (*Table 19-1*). Psychotropics may be substrates for CYPs, inducers/ inhibitors of the enzymes, or both. For example, fluoxetine is a CYP 2D6 substrate and an inhibitor of the same enzyme and thereby inhibits its own metabolism. Conversely, some drugs are both substrates and inducers of the same CYP (e.g., carbamazepine at CYP 3A) and thereby increase their own metabolism, necessitating dosage increases.

There are significant safety issues related to CYP blockade. For example, nortriptyline is metabolized by CYP 2D6 and has a narrow therapeutic index. If a potent 2D6 inhibitor such as fluoxetine is coadministered, the nortriptyline levels may increase to levels which are toxic and can lead to potentially fatal cardiac arrhythmias.

The final step in drug clearance is *excretion*; for most psychotropic drugs, this occurs via the kidneys. By this point, most compounds have been converted to more polar compounds whose increased water solubility facilitates renal clearance. Clearance will be reduced in patients with renal insufficiency. For lithium, which is directly excreted by the kidney without undergoing metabolism, this a major safety issue because of lithium's narrow therapeutic index. Additionally, care must be taken regarding drug interactions. For example, coadministration of loop diuretics or NSAIDs can reduce the ability of the kidney to clear lithium.[1]

PHARMACODYNAMICS

Pharmacodynamics refers to the relationship between drug concentration at its sites of action and the resulting biologic effects including the intensity and the time course of its desired effects as well as its adverse effects. For most psychotropic medications, the sites of actions are receptor sites, which are intrinsically activated by neurotransmitters. That said, actions of a psychotropic drug at a neurotransmitter receptor site may promote a dynamic cascade of subsequent actions such as stimulation or inhibition of G-proteins, effects on second messenger systems, enhancement of neurotrophic factors, and changes in genetic transcription and translation processes.

In addition, many drugs have pharmacodynamic effects at several different sites. For example, amitriptyline inhibits serotonin reuptake, norepinephrine reuptake, blocks α1- and α2-noradrenergic receptors, H_1 and H_2 receptors, central cholinergic receptors, and 5-HT_2 receptors. Thus the ultimate biologic effects may be complex and may be both beneficial and deleterious. Furthermore, this provides for the possibility that one medication may target two different illnesses by its actions at different sites. One example of this is with depressive disorders and anxiety disorders. On the other hand, the possibility for untoward drug interactions is greater as well[1] (*Table 19-2*).

Antidepressants

Indications for Use

In primary care practice, antidepressant medications are primarily prescribed as treatments for major depressive disorder, generalized anxiety disorder, panic disorder, and obsessive-compulsive disorder. Although monoamine oxidase inhibitors and tricyclic antidepressants were effective medications, their side effects, lethality in overdose, and drug interactions rendered their use in primary care settings problematic. In the mid- to late 1980s, bupropion and fluoxetine were approved; these drugs were regarded as safer and more tolerable. This section will focus on these and other drugs subsequently developed.[3,4]

Mechanism of Action

Most antidepressant medications inhibit serotonin reuptake via the serotonin transporter; it is assumed that this action results in increased serotonergic throughput and altered regulation of serotonin transporters. Some antidepressants have actions in addition to serotonin reuptake inhibition, which include postsynaptic serotonin receptor antagonism, inhibition of norepinephrine reuptake, or inhibition of norepinephrine autoreceptors on serotonergic neurons. In addition to medications that affect serotonin reuptake, there are medications that inhibit norepinephrine and dopamine reuptake and that inhibit metabolism of monoamines via monoamine oxidase inhibition.[3] The most commonly encountered drugs are as follows:

- **Selective serotonin reuptake inhibitors (SSRIs):** fluoxetine, sertraline, paroxetine, fluvoxamine, citalopram, escitalopram, vilazodone, vortioxetine
- **Noradrenergic and specific serotonergic antidepressants (NaSSAs):** mirtazapine
- **Serotonin norepinephrine reuptake inhibitors (SNRIs):** venlafaxine, duloxetine, desvenlafaxine, levomilnacipran
- **Serotonin antagonist/reuptake inhibitors (SARIs):** trazodone, nefazodone
- **Norepinephrine–dopamine reuptake inhibitors (NDRIs):** bupropion
- **Monoamine oxidase inhibitors (MAOIs):** transdermal selegiline

TABLE 19-1 Cytochrome P450 Activities of Psychotropics and Commonly Used Medications in Primary care

	1A2	2B6	2C8	2C9	2C19	2D6	2E1	3A4,5,7
Strong inhibitors	Fluvoxamine		Gemfibrozil	Fluconazole		Bupropion		Indinavir
	Ciprofloxacin		Trimethoprim			Fluoxetine		Nelfinavir
						Paroxetine		Ritonavir
						Quinidine		Clarithromycin
								Itraconazole
								Ketoconazole
								Nefazodone
								Saquinavir
								Suboxone
								Telithromycin
Moderate inhibitors				Amiodarone		Duloxetine		Aprepitant
						Sertraline		Erythromycin
						Terbinafine		Fluconazole
								Grapefruit juice
								Verapamil
								Diltiazem
Weak inhibitors	Cimetidine					Amiodarone		Cimetidine
						Cimetidine		
Inducers	Carbamazepine	Artemisinin		Carbamazepine	Enzalutamide		Ethanol	Efavirenz
	Char-grilled meat	Carbamazepine		Nevirapine	Rifampin		Isoniazid	Nevirapine
	Rifampin	Efavirenz		Phenobarbital	Ritonavir			Carbamazepine
	Tobacco	Nevirapine		Rifampin	St. John's wort			Phenobarbital
		Phenobarbital		St. John's wort				Phenytoin
		Phenytoin						Rifabutin
		Rifampin						Rifampin
								St. John's wort
								Troglitazone
								Pioglitazone

Adapted from The Flockhart Table. ©2016 by The Trustees of Indiana University.[2]

TABLE 19-2 Monitoring Guidelines for Psychiatric Medications for Primary Care

	BASELINE VS/PE	FOLLOW-UP VS/PE	BASELINE LABORATORY TESTS	FOLLOW-UP LABORATORY TESTS	ECG	THERAPEUTIC DRUG MONITORING
Antidepressants						
All	Pulse, BP, weight/BMI	Pulse, BP, weight/BMI each visit	TSH	As clinically indicated	No	N/A
Mood stabilizers						
Lithium	Pulse, BP, weight/BMI	Pulse, BP, weight/BMI each visit	CBC, BMP, TSH, UPT	CBC, BMP +/– UPT q3-6 months, TSH q6-12 months	Recommended >40 years of age	Lithium level after increases; q3 months ×2; q6-12 months
Divalproex	Pulse, BP, weight/BMI	Pulse, BP, weight/BMI each visit	CBC, LFTs, TSH, UPT	CBC, LFTs +/– UPT q3 months ×3, then q12 months	No	Valproic acid level after increases; annually
Carbamazepine	Pulse, BP, weight/BMI	Pulse, BP, weight/BMI each visit	CBC, CMP, TSH, UPT	CBC, CMP q3 months ×3, then q12 months	No	Carbamazepine level after increases; q3 months ×2; q12 months
Lamotrigine	Pulse, BP, weight/BMI	Pulse, BP, weight/BMI each visit	TSH	As clinically indicated	No	N/A
Atypical antipsychotics						
All, including ziprasidone and clozapine	Pulse, BP, weight/BMI, AIMS	Pulse, BP, weight/BMI each visit, AIMS q6-12 months	Glucose or hemoglobin A1c, lipids	Glucose or hemoglobin A1c, lipids at 3 months, then q12 months	No	N/A
Ziprasidone					If risk factors, after increases	N/A
Clozapine		Refer to psychiatrist	CBC	Per REMS protocol		

AIMS, Abnormal Involuntary Movement Scale.

There is no clear evidence of superior efficacy of one class over another, although meta-analyses suggest a small advantage of SNRIs over SSRIs.[5,6]

Common Side Effects
Across all classes, it appears that there is a small risk of treatment-emergent increases in suicidal ideation in certain subgroups of patients early in the course of treatment. In 2004 the U.S. FDA issued a "black box warning" related to concerns over the risk of suicidal ideation and behavior in children and adolescents. In 2007, this warning was expanded to include young adults. It should be noted that there has been little

evidence that avoiding treatment with antidepressants even in younger individuals will decrease the risk of suicide or suicidal ideation owing to the inherent risks of suicidal thoughts in conditions such as major depression. Providers should weigh the risks and benefits of antidepressant treatment, inform patients/parents of the risks, and remain vigilant to signs and symptoms of suicidality.

Other class-specific side effects are described below:[4,7-10]

SSRIs: drowsiness; nausea; dry mouth; insomnia; diarrhea; constipation; nervousness, agitation, or restlessness; dizziness; reduced sexual desire, erectile dysfunction, or anorgasmia; headache; blurred vision; extrapyramidal symptoms (including parkinsonism and dystonia)

NaSSAs: sleepiness[*]; increased appetite; weight gain; dry mouth; constipation; dizziness; strange dreams

SNRIs: dizziness; nausea; dry mouth; sweating; tiredness; insomnia; anxiety or agitation; constipation; difficulty urinating; headache; loss of appetite; reduced sexual desire, arousal, or orgasm

SARIs: nausea; diarrhea; constipation; dizziness, drowsiness, weakness; dry mouth; headache; increased appetite; decreased sexual desire, erectile dysfunction; confusion; blurred vision; tinnitus; sweating

NDRIs: agitation; dry mouth; insomnia; headache; nausea; vomiting; constipation; stomach pain; dizziness; ringing in the ears; vision problems or blurred vision; loss of interest in sex; increased interest in sex; sore throat; muscle pain; itching or skin rash; sweating; frequent urination; tremor; decreased appetite; weight loss or gain; joint aches; strange taste in the mouth; diarrhea

MAOIs: redness or itching where the selegiline patch is worn; mild headache; muscle pain; diarrhea; constipation; upset stomach; dry mouth; insomnia; mild bruising, itching or rash; cough, sore throat, sinus pain, or stuffy nose

General Medical Concerns and Warnings

As noted earlier, treatment-emergent suicidal ideation or increased severity of suicidal ideation is a concern for all antidepressant medications. All medications may elicit an allergic reaction. All antidepressant medications may lead to a switch to mania in patients with bipolar disorder.[4]

SSRIs: serotonin syndrome (in combination with other medications); increased risk of bleeding especially in conjunction with anticoagulants; hyponatremia (may result in seizures)/SIADH; QTc prolongation; lowered seizure threshold

NaSSAs: orthostatic hypotension

SNRIs: hyponatremia; increases in blood pressure; serotonin syndrome (in combination with other medications at higher doses); lowered seizure threshold

SARIs: priapism (primarily trazodone); orthostatic hypotension; sinus bradycardia; hepatotoxicity (nefazodone)

NDRIs: seizures; hypertension

Selective MAO-B inhibitors (MAOI): serotonin syndrome; tyramine sensitivity/hypertensive crisis

Pregnancy and lactation: Antidepressants are largely regarded as nonteratogenic in pregnancy. Conflicting studies regarding paroxetine and persistent pulmonary hypertension of the newborn resulted in the FDA issuing a statement that there was insufficient evidence of causation in 2011. SSRIs have been associated with lower birth weight and preterm delivery (usually by 3 to 4 days).[11] Package labels warn of possible serotonin

syndrome, drug withdrawal, or drug toxicity causing jitteriness, irritability, hypotonia, and even respiratory distress in newborns. Findings of recent studies citing increased risk of autism associated with SSRI use have been inconsistent. There are no contraindications to breastfeeding with antidepressants, although infants may experience side effects associated with antidepressants, including increased risk of seizure, particularly with bupropion.

Mood Stabilizers

There is ongoing controversy regarding the definition of "mood stabilizers." This class of medications is used in the treatment of bipolar disorders. One definition of a mood stabilizer is a drug that prevents recurrence of manic/mixed and depressive episodes. There is a subtlety in this definition, which centers on the term "recurrence." Many medications will treat acute manic episodes; these medications are considered to be antimanic but are not mood stabilizers unless they have efficacy in preventing subsequent episodes of mania *and* depression. Fewer medications have demonstrated efficacy in treating acute depressive episodes; these medications are referred to here as bipolar depression antidepressant medications. To be classified as mood stabilizers, they must demonstrate efficacy in *preventing* subsequent episodes of mania *and* depression. Except as noted, "indications" refers to FDA-approved indications.[1,4]

Indications for Use

Acute manic and mixed episodes: lithium, divalproex, carbamazepine, and most second-generation (atypical) antipsychotic (SGA) medications. Although the atypical antipsychotics are often effective as monotherapy, their use in combination with lithium or anticonvulsants (particularly divalproex) is prudent

Acute episodes of bipolar depression: lurasidone, quetiapine, olanzapine–fluoxetine combination. Lamotrigine monotherapy does not carry FDA approval, although there is a single quality randomized trial demonstrating superiority to placebo[12]

Prevention of recurrence of manic and depressive episodes: lithium and lamotrigine. Divalproex lacks FDA approval, but is widely used in psychiatry

Classifications

As described earlier, mood stabilizers are most readily classified by considering the indication for which they are prescribed.

Mechanism of Action

Although lithium is clearly effective in treating acute mania, its mechanism of action is less clear and is complex. Lithium downregulates dopaminergic activity, downregulates N-methyl-D-aspartate (NMDA) receptors, and upregulates GABAergic neurotransmission. Thus excitatory neurotransmission is decreased and inhibitory neurotransmission is increased. At the cellular level, lithium inhibits inositol monophosphatase, glycogen synthase kinase-3β, and protein kinase C; it is unclear whether these actions underlie its regulatory actions.

---

[*]Inverse dose relationship.

Valproate and carbamazepine block voltage-sensitive sodium channels. Valproate increases brain GABA, whereas carbamazepine inhibits glutamate release.

Lamotrigine blocks voltage-sensitive sodium channels and inhibits release of glutamate and aspartate.

Atypical antipsychotic medications block postsynaptic dopamine D2 receptors and are presumed to work by decreasing elevated dopaminergic throughput. Atypical antipsychotics also have multiple other actions at serotonergic sites (5-HT2A antagonism, 5-HT1A agonism), muscarinic, histamine, and α1-receptors.

Olanzapine–fluoxetine combination is believed to elevate synaptic serotonin through fluoxetine's inhibition of serotonin reuptake, which is increased through synergy with olanzapine; also dopaminergic throughput is reduced by D2 receptor blockage. In addition to D2 blockade, lurasidone and quetiapine are antagonists at serotonin-2A receptors and are partial agonists at serotonin 1A receptors; lurasidone also antagonizes ionotropic serotonin 3 receptors.

Common Side Effects

Lithium: weight gain; tremor; polyuria; polydipsia; acne; sexual dysfunction; subjective cognitive impairment; nausea

Divalproex: nausea; vomiting; dizziness; ataxia; tremors; weight gain; edema; headache

Carbamazepine: nausea; vomiting; dizziness; drowsiness; dry mouth; swollen tongue; loss of balance or coordination; unsteadiness

Lamotrigine: headache; rash; dizziness; tired feeling; blurred vision; loss of coordination; dry mouth; insomnia

General Medical Concerns and Warnings
Lithium

Lithium is a hydrophilic monovalent cation, which is excreted by the kidney. Lithium levels >1.2 mEq/L may result in toxicity. Although its use in patients with renal insufficiency is not absolutely contraindicated, other mood stabilizers may be safer. Dehydration elevates lithium levels; this is a risk because lithium-induced nausea, vomiting, and diarrhea may lead to dehydration. Inadequate fluid intake and elevated ambient temperature may also cause dehydration. In terms of pharmacokinetics, NSAIDs, COX-2 inhibitors, loop diuretics, and ACE inhibitors may decrease renal clearance and lead to toxicity in patients presumed to be at steady state.

Before initiating therapy with lithium, it is important to assess a basic metabolic profile, particularly checking creatinine (creatinine clearance), TSH, and a CBC. An ECG should be obtained in patients over the age of 40 years to rule out ventricular arrhythmia (Brugada syndrome). Trough (8 to 12 hours after last dose) lithium levels should be monitored as well as thyroid function. Target levels for acute mania should be around 1.0 to 1.5 mEq/L; maintenance treatment target levels should be 0.8 to 1.2 mEq/L, although lower levels may be adequate.

Acute toxicity is a medical emergency. Symptoms include mental status changes including delirium, severe nausea and vomiting and diarrhea, ataxia, incoordination, severe tremors, seizures, and coma. Hospitalization is indicated, and hemodialysis may be required.

Other significant medical side effects include hypothyroidism, interstitial nephritis, pseudotumor cerebri, nephrogenic diabetes insipidus, SIADH, and cardiac conduction abnormalities. Lithium may exacerbate psoriasis.

Pregnancy and lactation: Lithium should be used with caution in women of childbearing age owing to its teratogenicity. Specifically, lithium has been associated with fetal cardiac defects, in particular Ebstein anomaly (a right ventricular outflow tract obstruction defect). Providers should be mindful that fluid shifts in the postpartum period may result in significant increases in lithium levels. Lithium concentrations in breastmilk are similar to maternal serum concentrations, and infants who breastfeed can be expected to have serum levels of approximately 10% to 50% that of the mother.[13] Infants should be monitored for toxicity, especially related to hydration status.

Divalproex

Rare, but serious, side effects include fulminant hepatic necrosis, drug reaction with eosinophilia and systemic symptoms (DRESS), hyperammonemia (symptomatic or asymptomatic), cardiac rhythm abnormalities, delirium, severe thrombocytopenia, and hemorrhagic pancreatitis. Valproate has also been associated with polycystic ovarian syndrome/Stein–Leventhal syndrome.

There are numerous pharmacokinetic and pharmacodynamics interactions with other mood stabilizers and other medications. From a practical standpoint, the most significant is inhibition of lamotrigine metabolism resulting in too rapid escalation of blood lamotrigine levels, which is a risk factor for serious rash with lamotrigine.

Pregnancy and lactation: Valproate/divalproex should be used with caution in women of childbearing age owing to its teratogenicity. It is associated with neural tube defects and should be administered with folate in women who may become pregnant. Valproate is expressed in the breastmilk at low levels, but infants should be monitored for signs of jaundice and bruising.

Lamotrigine

Serious rash progressing to Stevens–Johnson syndrome (SJS) or toxic epidermal necrolysis is a potentially life-threatening side effect of lamotrigine. Risk factors include dose titration rates faster than the recommended slow titration schedule and failure to reduce dose titration when coadministered with valproate. The increased serum blood levels of lamotrigine caused by coadministration with valproate/divalproex have been described earlier. Conversely, oral contraceptive pills and anticonvulsants such as carbamazepine, phenobarbital, phenytoin, and primidone may decrease serum levels of lamotrigine and make it less effective. Other serious side effects include rare aseptic meningitis and rare treatment-emergent suicidal ideation.

Pregnancy and lactation: Lamotrigine is not considered contraindicated in pregnancy or lactation. As with other antiepileptics, women are advised to take a prenatal vitamin or supplemental folate. Infants who breastfeed are at risk for serious rash.

Carbamazepine

Serious side effects include blood dyscrasias including agranulocytosis and aplastic anemia, SJS/toxic epidermal necrolysis, SIADH with hyponatremia, and emergent suicidal ideation. For patients of Asian descent, the FDA recommends testing for a specific variant of HLA-B*1502 because of its association with risk of serious rash.

Pregnancy and lactation: Carbamazepine should be used with caution during pregnancy owing to its teratogenicity. The drug has been associated with neural tube defects and development of intellectual disability. Caution should be exercised with breastfeeding, as infants have been shown to have detectable serum levels with concomitant adverse effects.

Second-Generation Antipsychotic Medications

The serious side effects will be discussed fully in the next section. In brief, the major concerns are neuroleptic malignant syndrome, QTc prolongation, metabolic effects (weight gain, insulin resistance, hyperlipidemia, hyperglycemia), and rare severe leukopenia and agranulocytosis.

Antipsychotic Medications

This section will focus on SGA ("atypical") medications. Antipsychotics, whether first or second generation, are also called "neuroleptics." Although controversy persists regarding whether the newer drugs are more efficacious than older antipsychotic medications, they are less likely to cause extrapyramidal symptoms and probably less likely to cause neuroleptic-induced tardive dyskinesia (TD) after long-term use.

The atypical antipsychotics available in the United States are aripiprazole, asenapine, brexpiprazole, cariprazine, clozapine, iloperidone, lurasidone, olanzapine, paliperidone, quetiapine, risperidone, and ziprasidone.

The term "atypical" bears comment. First-generation ("typical") antipsychotic medications were associated with treatment-emergent parkinsonian symptoms. Clozapine and subsequent antipsychotic medications appeared to have low rates of extrapyramidal side effects (EPSs) despite their ability to reduce psychotic symptoms and their affinity for D2 blockade. Subsequently it was observed that the newer drugs did demonstrate EPS at varying rates. Rates of TD appear to be lower with the newer medications, but this should be evaluated over time.

It was hypothesized that the pharmacodynamic explanation for atypicality was 5-HT2A blockade, leading to increased dopamine release in nigrostriatal pathways. However, sulpiride and amisulpride demonstrated atypicality in the absence of activity at 5-HT2 receptors; these medications are not approved in the United States.

Indications for Use

All SGAs are indicated in the treatment of symptoms of schizophrenia (see *Table 19-3*). The best evidence is in treating positive symptoms (delusions, hallucinations, disorganized thinking and behavior, and agitation). Efficacy in treating the negative symptoms (flat affect, social withdrawal, avolition, and reduced content of speech) and in treating neurocognitive impairment (impairments in working memory, attention, and executive functioning) has not been clearly established.[1]

Mechanism of Action

Aripiprazole, brexpiprazole, and cariprazine are D2 and 5-HT2A partial agonists. The remaining atypical antipsychotics primarily antagonize D2 receptors and 5-HT2A receptors. It is believed that efficacy in treatment of positive symptoms of schizophrenia and of mania is based on the results of decreased dopamine activity at D2 receptors.[1,3]

Common Side Effects

As a class, atypical antipsychotic medications may have the following common adverse effects: tremors, drowsiness, restlessness, muscle stiffness, muscle cramping, nausea, diarrhea, loss of appetite, blurred vision, weight gain, breast swelling or discharge, decreased sex drive, impotence, anorgasmia, dry mouth, and constipation.

Akathisia (motor restlessness) may be objective and/or subjective and bears special note because it may be misconstrued as agitation. If the provider attempts to treat the misdiagnosed agitation by increasing the dose, the restlessness will get worse. Objective akathisia is observable and characterized as compulsive motor activity. Subjective akathisia is reported by the patient as internal restlessness or anxiety. The classic description is of "jumping out of one's own skin." Akathisia is so uncomfortable that some patients have taken their lives to escape it.[1,4,14]

General Medical Concerns and Warnings

The atypical antipsychotic medications as a class are associated potentially with weight gain, hyperlipidemia, hyperglycemia, and insulin resistance/type 2 diabetes. Rare fatal ketoacidosis has occurred. Hypertension may occur, probably secondary to weight gain. All these are risk factors for cardiovascular and cerebrovascular disease, and the number of years of life lost attributable to the side effects is significant. Therefore clinicians should obtain baseline weight, blood pressure, lipid panel, and a glucose or hemoglobin A1c, and these should be repeated every 6 months to a year. Because leukopenia (and rarely agranulocytosis) may occur, a baseline CBC may be prudent to obtain.[14-16]

D2 receptor potency varies across this class of drugs. With the more potent drugs, young African-American males are more likely to suffer dystonic reactions. Although it is not currently recommended to initiate benztropine prophylactically, clinicians can advise patients to use over-the-counter diphenhydramine while awaiting response from their office about an adverse effect.

Neuroleptic malignant syndrome, a rare, but life-threatening illness may occur, particularly with higher potency drugs whose dosage is increased rapidly. Symptoms include fever, autonomic instability, rigidity, leukocytosis, increased CPK, and altered mental status. Hospitalization is indicated for supportive care;

TABLE 19-3 Indications for Oral Atypical Antipsychotics as of 2018

	ARIPIPRAZOLE	ASENAPINE	BREXPIPRAZOLE	CARIPRAZINE	CLOZAPINE	ILOPERIDONE	LURASIDONE	OLANZAPINE	PALIPERIDONE	QUETIAPINE IR/XR	RISPERIDONE	ZIPRASIDONE
Schizophrenia	X[a]	X	X	X	X[d]	X	X[a]	X[a]	X[a]	X[a]	X[a]	X
Schizoaffective					[d]				X			
Acute/mixed mania	X[b]	X[b]		X				X[a]		X	X[b]	X
Adjunct to lithium or divalproex, bipolar	X	X					X[b]	X		X(IR only)		X
Bipolar depression							X[b]			X		
Maintenance bipolar		X										
Adjunct to antidepressant, MDD	X		X							X(XR only)		
Irritability in autism[c]	X										X	
Tourette syndrome[c]	X											

[a] Adults and children 13-17 years old
[b] Adults and children 10-17 years old
[c] Children 6-17 years old
[d] Reducing suicidal behavior

dantrolene (a muscle relaxant), bromocriptine (dopamine agonist), and/or electroconvulsive therapy (ECT) are used in severe cases.

Although the risk of TD appears reduced with atypical antipsychotic medications compared with first-generation neuroleptics, once to twice yearly Abnormal Involuntary Movement Scale (AIMS) evaluation is helpful to detect TD in earlier stages. It should be noted that TD does not always resolve with discontinuation of the antipsychotic, and withdrawal-emergent dyskinesia has been seen, particularly in children. Withdrawal-emergent dyskinesia should resolve within a month, whereas TD may take up to 3 years to resolve, and a small proportion of patients may have persistent TD. Consideration of risks and benefits of restarting or continuing antipsychotic medications should be discussed with patients who experience TD or withdrawal-emergent dyskinesia. In 2017, valbenazine, a parent compound of tetrabenazine, was introduced for treatment of TD. The main side effects of valbenazine appear to be somnolence, dry mouth, and akathisia, so iatrogenic harms caused by a medication intended to help with the side effects of another medication need to be carefully weighed before initiation. Valbenazine should not be used during pregnancy or lactating owing to animal studies showing stillbirths and postnatal death in rat pups.

Significant QTc prolongation has been reported with iloperidone and ziprasidone, leading to concern about development of torsades de pointes or other fatal arrhythmias. Baseline ECG should be obtained in individuals with risk factors for QT prolongation (see *Table 19-4*). Do not start the drugs if baseline QTc >450 milliseconds for males or >460 mg for females. If subsequent ECG indicate QTc interval approaching 500 milliseconds, the medication should be discontinued. The risk of torsades de pointes is significantly increased with QTc ≥500 milliseconds. Other atypical antipsychotics have been associated with less pronounced QTc prolongation, but clinicians should always be mindful of the risk, particularly in medically compromised patients.

Clozapine is a highly effective medication, which is currently reserved for patients who are refractory to other antipsychotic medications. It is commonly associated with weight gain and other metabolic derangements seen with antipsychotics, sedation, orthostatic hypotension, and drooling. Severe side effects include agranulocytosis, myocarditis, and seizures, and so it should be used with caution in people with preexisting heart disease or seizures. The FDA has established a Risk Evaluation and Mitigation Strategy (REMS), which includes online provider training and enrollment and requires weekly ANC monitoring for the first 6 months, then every other week for 6 months, then every 4 weeks thereafter. Given that it is a drug reserved for treatment-refractory patients and that it has potentially lethal side effects, the authors recommend that such patients be referred to psychiatrists trained in prescribing. Primary care providers may be called upon to temporarily refill clozapine while patients are awaiting transfer to another psychiatrist and may do so if prepared to enroll in REMS and monitor the ANC. Patients who discontinue for more than 2 days, in addition to risking decompensation of their psychiatric condition, will have to restart titration of dose at 12.5 mg once or twice daily and further risk worsening of their symptoms on a subtherapeutic dose while titrating back up.[3]

Pregnancy and lactation: None of the atypical antipsychotics have been associated with birth defects, but none can be guaranteed "safe" in pregnancy. Women who take antipsychotics during pregnancy should be monitored closely for development of gestational diabetes and hypertension, as some studies have shown increased rates of diabetes, macrosomia, and hypertensive disorders of pregnancy, although these findings are similar among matched controls.[18] Similar to what is seen with antidepressants, preterm delivery is more common in women treated with antipsychotics. Antipsychotics are transmitted in breastmilk at low levels and have been associated with sedation in infants. There are case reports of women taking aripiprazole who had difficulty establishing or maintaining milk supply, although aripiprazole has also been associated with hyperprolactinemia in nonlactating individuals. There are little data on lurasidone or cariprazine, but they are also partial D2 agonists and may have similar effects on lactation.

Benzodiazepines and Sedative Hypnotics

This section will discuss benzodiazepines, which are primarily used for treatment of anxiety, and will discuss the most commonly used sedative hypnotics; the latter group includes some benzodiazepines along with medications which work at the nonbenzodiazepine site of the GABA receptor, medication targeting the melatonin system, and a novel medication targeting the orexin system.[19-21]

TABLE 19-4 Risk Factors for Drug-Induced QT Prolongation

UNMODIFIABLE	MODIFIABLE
Female gender	Hypokalemia/hypomagnesaemia
Age >65	Bradycardia (including recent conversion from AF)
Congenital long QT syndrome	Use of other QT prolonging medication
Family history of sudden death	Use of medications that inhibit metabolism of QT prolonging medication
History of drug-induced QT prolongation	Starvation or obesity
Structural heart disease/LV dysfunction	Overdose or rapid IV administration of QT prolonging medication
Renal or hepatic insufficiency	

Modified from New Zealand Medicines and Medical Devices Safety Authority. Drug-induced QT prolongation and Torsades de Pointes – the facts. Prescriber Update. 2010;31(4):27-29.[17] Reprinted by permission of Medsafe.

The anxiolytic benzodiazepines include chlordiazepoxide, diazepam, clorazepate, oxazepam, lorazepam, clonazepam, and alprazolam. Sedative hypnotic benzodiazepines include flurazepam, temazepam, triazolam, and estazolam. Sedative hypnotic nonbenzodiazepine medications include zolpidem, zaleplon, eszopiclone, ramelteon, and suvorexant.

Indications for Use

Benzodiazepines are primarily indicated for treatment of anxiety and for the short-term treatment of insomnia. There is some specificity for their use in different anxiety disorders and other disorders.

- **Panic disorder:** clonazepam, alprazolam
- **Generalized anxiety disorder:** chlordiazepoxide, diazepam, clorazepate, oxazepam, lorazepam, and alprazolam
- **Treatment of alcohol withdrawal syndrome:** chlordiazepoxide, diazepam, clorazepate, oxazepam
- **Insomnia (short-term):** flurazepam, lorazepam, temazepam, triazolam, estazolam

Nonbenzodiazepine medications
- **Insomnia (short-term):** zolpidem, zaleplon
- **Insomnia (short- and long-term):** eszopiclone, ramelteon, suvorexant

Mechanism of Action
Benzodiazepines
The anxiolytic effects and sedative hypnotics of benzodiazepines are mediated by their action as positive allosteric modulators at the benzodiazepine-binding site of the GABA-A receptor. This action results in increased chloride conductance at GABA-associated Cl– channels and enhanced inhibitory effects of GABA. Inhibitory actions in the amygdala may account for the anxiolytic effects. Inhibitory actions at sleep centers account for the sedative hypnotic effects. That noted, all the medications in this class are both anxiolytic and sedating to some degree.

For the most part, FDA approval for both anxiety and insomnia were for short-term use (<6 weeks). However, many patients use these agents long term. Discontinuation despite nonresolution of symptoms is discussed in other chapters.

Nonbenzodiazepines
Eszopiclone, zolpidem, and zaleplon are thought to bind specifically to the alpha-1 isoform of the GABA-A receptor. Chloride conductance is increased and GABA inhibitory actions that are more selective for sedative hypnotic effect are enhanced.

Ramelteon is a full agonist at melatonin 1 and melatonin 2 receptors. The melatonin system is believed to regulate sleep through on "on–off" switch. It is used for acute and chronic insomnia.

Suvorexant is an antagonist at orexin receptors. The orexin system promotes wakefulness and that action is diminished by suvorexant, which decreases wakefulness, in contrast to other medications, which increase sedation. It is indicated for insomnia characterized by difficulties with sleep onset and/or sleep maintenance.

Common Side Effects
- **Benzodiazepines:** depression, confusion, amnesia, drowsiness, dizziness, impaired coordination/ataxia, trembling
- **Zolpidem:** daytime drowsiness, dizziness, weakness, feeling "drugged" or light-headed; tired feeling, loss of coordination; stuffy nose, dry mouth, nose or throat irritation; nausea, constipation, diarrhea, upset stomach; or headache, muscle pain
- **Zaleplon:** sedation, diarrhea, difficulty with coordination, loss of memory, nightmares, stomach upset
- **Eszopiclone:** daytime drowsiness, dizziness, "hangover" feeling, problems with memory or concentration, loss of appetite, unpleasant taste
- **Ramelteon:** bad taste, daytime sleepiness, decreased sex drive, diarrhea, headache, nausea
- **Suvorexant:** somnolence, headache, dizziness, abnormal dreams, cough, diarrhea, dry mouth, diarrhea, dry mouth, cough

In 2007, the FDA required all manufacturers of sleeping medications to add a warning about unusual behaviors, including sleepwalking and most concerning, sleep driving. Although all medications for sleep carry this warning, the risk is likely highest among the benzodiazepine and benzodiazepine receptor binding medications.

General Medical Concerns and Warnings
Benzodiazepines
Concerns include abuse potential and dependency, ataxia, confusion, withdrawal syndrome including delirium and seizures upon abrupt discontinuation, respiratory depression particularly in combination with other CNS depressants, worsening of suicidal ideation, rare hepatic dysfunction, renal dysfunction, and blood dyscrasias. This class of medications should not be prescribed to patients with a history of substance use disorder or alcohol use disorder. In response to the growing opioid epidemic, the FDA added a boxed warning in 2016 to all opioids and benzodiazepines, warning that concomitant use of opioids and benzodiazepines or other CNS depressants (such as alcohol) may result in profound sedation, respiratory depression, coma, and death. Primary care providers should try all available alternative treatments for pain or anxiety/insomnia before combining agents and limit dosage, duration, and frequently evaluate for opportunities to taper/discontinue and signs and symptoms of respiratory depression and sedation.

There are conflicting data about the teratogenicity of benzodiazepines. Most package inserts discourage or contraindicate use in pregnancy. Infants may experience withdrawal symptoms in the postnatal period. Breastfeeding infants whose mothers take benzodiazepines have been reported to experience sedation. Providers should exercise caution in prescribing benzodiazepines to women in pregnancy and consider using shorter acting benzodiazepines in women who are breastfeeding.

Nonbenzodiazepines
Eszopiclone, zolpidem, and zaleplon may cause respiratory depression when combined with other CNS depressants, disinhibition, emergent suicidal ideation, angioedema,

sleep driving and other complex behaviors, delirium in elderly patients, amnesia, and abnormal behaviors.

Ramelteon may cause respiratory depression or rare angioedema.

Suvorexant may cause worsening of depression, suicidal thinking, abnormal thinking, behavioral changes, daytime impairment, sleep driving and other complex behaviors, sleep paralysis, or cataplexy.

Suvorexant exerts its pharmacodynamics action by antagonizing orexin receptors. It is contraindicated in patients diagnosed with narcolepsy, as these patients have decreased or damaged orexin receptors. The authors advocate withholding its use in patients whose review of systems reveals the "narcoleptic triad" (excessive daytime sedation, cataplexy, and sleep paralysis); these patients should be referred for a sleep evaluation.

There are limited data on the safety of nonbenzodiazepine sedative–hypnotics in pregnancy, but use is discouraged. While the data are also limited for breastfeeding, the short half-life of the drugs reduces risk to the infant in breastfeeding. Low levels of eszopiclone have been found in the breast milk of nursing mothers.[22]

PRACTICAL RESOURCES

- Drugs.com: www.drugs.com/drug_interactions.html
  Drug interaction checker
- Quick Reference to Psychiatric Medication: www.psychceu.com/Quick_Reference_BW.pdf
  Psychotropic drug lists
- LactMed: https://toxnet.nlm.nih.gov/newtoxnet/lactmed.htm
  NIH website summarizing data about medications and breastfeeding

CASES AND QUESTIONS

CASE 1:

Mr. B is a 35-year-old man with HIV who presented to his primary care provider to be treated for systemic *Candida* infection, which has already failed two other antifungals. He is taking indinavir 800 mg q8 hours, emtricitabine 200 mg/tenofovir 300 mg daily, ritonavir 100 mg daily, sertraline 200 mg daily, trazodone 100 mg nightly, and buspirone 15 mg three times daily. Given his multiple failed treatments, you start ketoconazole 200 mg daily. He returns 4 days later with fever, chills, diarrhea, muscle aches, and confusion.

1. What is the most likely cause of his symptoms?
   A. Influenza
   B. Cryptococcal meningitis
   C. Serotonin syndrome
   D. Neuroleptic malignant syndrome
   E. HIV encephalopathy

Correct answer: C. *Although his symptoms could represent influenza, given the recent initiation of ketoconazole, a potent P450 3A4 inhibitor, it is more likely that he is suffering from a toxidrome brought on by decreased metabolism of his trazodone and buspirone, leading to increased levels of systemic serotonin in addition to the use of an SSRI, sertraline. Neuroleptic malignant syndrome does not usually cause diarrhea, although the other symptoms are similar, and the patient has not been started on a neuroleptic (antipsychotic) recently. HIV encephalopathy is a progressive neurocognitive disorder that would not present acutely or with the other physical symptoms described. Infectious causes of his symptoms are less likely but would need to be ruled out if supportive treatments do not resolve his symptoms.*

2. What other medications should be avoided in persons at risk for serotonin syndrome?
   A. Tramadol
   B. Sumatriptan
   C. Fentanyl
   D. Dextroamphetamine/amphetamine
   E. All of the above

Correct answer: E. *All of the medications listed increase serotonin levels. Tramadol and fentanyl (as well as other opioid analgesics) decrease serotonin reuptake. Amphetamines cause serotonin release and triptans are serotonin agonists at 5-HT1, which cause vasoconstriction.*

CASE 2:

Three months after hospitalization for exacerbation of schizophrenia, a 56-year-old woman follows up with her primary care provider. She admits that she hasn't been taking her olanzapine as prescribed because of a 16-pound weight gain. She has been hearing voices and feeling suspicious. She notes that another patient at the hospital was taking ziprasidone and was doing well and had lost weight, so she requests to switch to that medication.

1. Which baseline studies should the provider obtain if this switch is contemplated?
   A. Glucose or hemoglobin A1c
   B. ECG
   C. Lipid panel
   D. Weight
   E. All of the above

Correct answer: E. *A change in medication is warranted because the patient's psychosis is emerging and she was a nonadherent with olanzapine because of weight gain. Ziprasidone is a reasonable choice because it has a more favorable profile of metabolic side effects. Baseline monitoring of risk factors for the metabolic syndrome is recommended. Despite its favorable* *metabolic profile, ziprasidone has a larger effect on QTc, and this patient's gender and age put her at higher risk. Therefore, a baseline ECG is indicated.*

2. Which factors would argue against the use of ziprasidone?

A. QTc = 440 millisecond
B. AIMS = 0
C. Patient history of syncope, family history of sudden cardiac death of brother at age 42 years.
D. FBS = 121 mg/dL
E. Elevated fasting triglycerides and total cholesterol

Correct answer: C. *Syncopal episodes and family history of early, unexpected sudden death may indicate a genetic long QTc syndrome. It is prudent to use a different antipsychotic medication if a patient reports these risk factors. A baseline ECG with normal QTc would not rule out this possibility, and her age, gender, and family history would place her at increased risk for drug-induced QT prolongation.*

3. The patient is found to have no contraindications to ziprasidone, so she titrates slowly to 80 mg BID with food. Her psychiatric symptoms overall improve but she complains of feeling a sense of internal restlessness and anxiety. The most likely explanation for this experience is

_____.

A. agitation due to her psychosis
B. neuroleptic-induced tardive dyskinesia
C. parkinsonism
D. akathisia
E. generalized anxiety disorder

Correct answer: D. *The patient describes an internal, disturbing sensation of internal restlessness. It is imperative that this not be misdiagnosed as anxiety or agitation; there are reports of suicide by patients suffering akathisia. Parkinsonism is demonstrated with muscle stiffness, bradykinesia, or tremor. Akathisia can be distinguished from tremor by ability to suppress the movement and internal drive to continue to move. Akathisia can be treated with beta-blockers. Dyskinetic movements are involuntary, nonrhythmic, and without any sense of discomfort.*

CASE 3:

Ms. A is a 73-year-old married woman who has been in overall good physical and mental health with no psychiatric history. She takes lisinopril 5 mg daily for essential hypertension and amitriptyline 25 mg qhs for years for migraine prevention. She had complaints of urinary frequency, urge incontinence, and urinary leakage and was started on oxybutynin, which recently was titrated up to 5 mg four times daily. For the last several days, she had difficulty sleeping and was taking one to two tablets of acetaminophen 325 mg/diphenhydramine 25 mg at night.

Her husband brought her to the ER after she became confused, agitated, disoriented, complained of blurry vision and displayed fluctuating mental status.

1. The most likely diagnosis for the mental status change is _____.

A. schizophrenia
B. Alzheimer disease
C. encephalitis
D. delirium
E. psychosis

Correct answer: D. *Acute onset, disorientation, confusion, agitation, and autonomic signs are most consistent with delirium. Schizophrenia, Alzheimer disease, and psychosis do not present acutely and usually show a fluctuating course. There is no evidence to support encephalitis, although the presentation is consistent with encephalopathy.*

2. The prescribed medications with anticholinergic activity are _____.

A. diphenhydramine
B. amitriptyline
C. oxybutynin
D. lisinopril
E. A, B, and C

Correct answer: E. *Lisinopril is an ACE inhibitor, which lacks activity at cholinergic receptors. The anticholinergic activities of diphenhydramine, amitriptyline, and oxybutynin are well documented. The elderly are particularly susceptible to anticholinergic delirium, possibly secondary to age-related winnowing of cholinergic neurons.*

3. This syndrome demonstrates

_____.

A. pharmacokinetic drug interaction (CYP450)
B. pharmacodynamic drug interaction at the serotonin receptor
C. pharmacodynamic drug interaction at the muscarinic Ach receptor
D. pharmacokinetic drug interaction (protein binding)
E. pharmacodynamic drug interaction at the nicotinic Ach receptor

Correct answer: C. *The actions of these medications converge specifically on the muscarinic cholinergic receptor. Remember the mnemonic for anticholinergic delirium: "Blind as a bat (mydriasis), dry as a bone (decreased perspiration, urinary retention), hot as a desert (hyperpyrexia), mad as a hatter (mental status changes), red as a beet (flushing)." There are no pharmacokinetic interactions. Pharmacodynamic interactions occur at the site of action. The drugs in questions have no actions at other receptors listed, although amitriptyline has affinity for the serotonin transporter.*

REFERENCES

1. Anderson IM, McAllister-Williams RH, eds. *Fundamentals of Clinical Psychopharmacology*. 4th ed. Boca Raton: CBC Press; 2016.

2. The Flockhart Table ©2016 by The Trustees of Indiana University.

3. Stahl S, Muntner M. *Stahl's Essential Psychopharmacology*. 4th ed. Cambridge, UK: Cambridge University Press; 2013.

4. Stahl S. *Essential Psychopharmacology: The Prescriber's Guide*. 6th ed. Cambridge, UK: Cambridge University Press; 2017.

5. Nemeroff CB, Entusah R, Demitract M, et al. Comprehensive analysis of remission (COMPARE) with venlafaxine versus SSRIs. *Biol Psychiatry*. 2008;63: 424-434.

6. Papakostas GI, Thase ME, Fava M, et al. Are antidepressant drugs that combine serotonergic and noradrenergic mechanisms of action more effective than the selective serotonin reuptake inhibitors in treating major depressive disorder? A meta-analysis of studies of newer agents. *Biol Psychiatry*. 2007;62:1217-1227.

7. Bauer M, Bschor T, Phennig A, et al. World Federation of Societies of Biological Psychiatry (WFSBP) guidelines for biological treatment of unipolar depressive disorders in primary care. *World J Biol Psychiatry*. 2007;8(2):67-104.

8. Kennedy SH, Lam RW, McIntyre RS, et al. Canadian Network for Mood and Anxiety Treatments (CANMAT) 2016 clinical guidelines for the management of adults with major depressive disorder: section 3. Pharmacological treatments. *Can J Psychiatry*. 2016;61(9):540-560.

9. Lam RW, Kennedy SH, Grigoriadis S, et al. Canadian Network for Mood and Anxiety Treatments (CANMAT) clinical guidelines for the management of major depressive disorder in adults. III. Pharmacotherapy. *J Affect Disord*. 2009;117(suppl 1):S26-S43.

10. Pirraglia PA, Stafford RS, Singer DE, et al. Trends in prescribing of selective serotonin reuptake inhibitors and other newer antidepressant agents in adult primary care. *Prim Care Companion J Clin Psychiatry*. 2003;5(4): 153-157.

11. Huang H, Coleman S, Bridge JA, Yonkers K, Katon W. A meta-analysis of the relationship between antidepressant use in pregnancy and the risk of preterm birth and low birth weight. *Gen Hosp Psychiatry*. 2014;36(1):13-18.

12. Calabrese JR, Bowden CL, Sachs GS, et al. A double-blind placebo-controlled study of lamotrigine monotherapy in outpatients with bipolar I depression. *J Clin Psychiatry*. 1999;60:79-88.

13. Toxnet Toxicology Data Network. National Institutes of Health U.S. National Library of Medicine. https://toxnet.nlm.nih.gov.

14. Swartz MS, Stroup TS, McEvoy JP, et al. What CATIE found: results from the schizophrenia trial. *Psychiatr Serv*. 2008;59(5):500-506.

15. Cooper SJ, Reynolds GP, Barnes T, et al. BAP guidelines on the management of weight gain, metabolic disturbances and cardiovascular risk associated with psychosis and antipsychotic drug treatment. *J Psychopharmacol*. 2016;30(8):717-748.Fountoulakis KN, Grunze IH, Vieta E, et al. The International College of Neuro-Psychopharmacology (CINP) treatment guidelines for bipolar disorder in adults (CINP-BD-2017), part 3: the clinical guidelines. *Int J Neuropsychopharmacol*. 2017;20(2):180-195.

16. Riordan HJ, Antonini P, Murphy MF, et al. Atypical antipsychotics and metabolic syndrome in patients with schizophrenia: risk factors, monitoring, and healthcare implications. *Am Health Drug Benefits*. 2011;4(5):292-302.

17. New Zealand Medicines and Medical Devices Safety Authority. Drug-induced QT prolongation and Torsades de Pointes – the facts. *Prescriber Update*. 2010;31(4):27-29.

18. Vigod SN, Gomes T, Wilton AS, Taylor VH, Ray JG. Antipsychotic drug use in pregnancy: high dimensional, propensity matched, population based cohort study. *BMJ*. 2015;350:h2298.

19. Sirdifield C, Anthierens S, Creupelandt H, et al. General practitioners' experiences and perceptions of benzodiazepine prescribing: systematic review and meta-synthesis. *BMC Fam Pract*. 2013;14:191.

20. Sateia MJ, Buysse DJ, Krystal AD, et al. Clinical practice guideline for the pharmacologic treatment of chronic insomnia in adults: an American Academy of Sleep Medicine clinical practice guideline. *J Clin Sleep Med*. 2017;13(2):307-349.

21. Benca RM. Diagnosis and treatment of chronic insomnia: a review. *Psychiatr Serv*. 2005;56(3):332-343.

22. Gaillot J, Heusse D, Hougton GW, et al. Pharmacokinetics and metabolism of zopiclone. *Pharmacology*. 1983;27(suppl 2):76-91.

IV

SPECIAL CLINICAL TOPICS

20

GERIATRIC BEHAVIORAL HEALTH

Ana Hategan, MD, Calvin H. Hirsch, MD, and Glen L. Xiong, MD

CLINICAL HIGHLIGHTS

- Anxiety and depressive disorders are one of the most common psychiatric disorders among older adults.
- The most common anxiety disorders in old age are generalized anxiety disorder and specific phobia, with fear of falling.
- Late-life anxiety disorder is often comorbid with major depressive disorder.
- Comorbidity of major depressive disorder with generalized anxiety disorder in late life is associated with a poorer prognosis, longer duration to respond to treatment, and partial remission of illness.
- Older adults with late-onset depression are more likely to present with cognitive symptoms, which tend to resolve as the patient's depressive episode improves with treatment.
- Suicide occurs most frequently in depressive disorder; depressed patients aged 65 years or older have the highest suicide rate.
- Major depressive disorder is comorbid with multiple systemic medical conditions (e.g., arthritis, migraine and other pain syndromes, chronic pulmonary obstructive disease, hypertension).
- Two-thirds or more who commit suicide are seen by primary care physicians within a month of their deaths, and up to one-half within 1 week.
- The main types of dementia include the neurodegenerative forms (Alzheimer dementia, dementia with Lewy bodies, and frontotemporal dementia) and vascular dementia.
- Unless there is a competing cause for mortality, dementias usually progress to a state of complete functional dependence that may require institutional placement.

INTRODUCTION

Anxiety and major depressive disorders are common conditions in late life with a high rate of recurrence and chronicity, disability, and poor response to treatment. As with anxiety disorder, depressive disorder is one of the most common psychiatric disorders among older adults. Late-onset depression has distinct morphologic and clinical features, with a first onset occurring after age 60 or 65 years. Feeling sad as part of normal aging is a misconception that contributes to the underdiagnosis and undertreatment of depression in this population. The *Diagnostic and Statistical Manual of Mental Disorders*, 5th edition (*DSM-5*) changed the classification of depressive disorders, in which the broad category of mood disorders was removed and the depressive disorders have been separated from the bipolar disorders.

Cognitive impairment is commonly seen in late-life anxiety and depression and includes deficits in verbal and nonverbal learning, working and short-term memory, attention, visual and auditory processing, processing speed, and problem-solving. Differentiating anxiety- and depression-related cognitive impairment from cognitive symptoms of dementia is often challenging owing to age-associated clinical manifestation of anxiety and depression, polypharmacy, drug–drug interactions, predisposition to adverse drug events, and multiple comorbidities in older adults.

Confusion is a cognitive dysfunction, for which clinicians are frequently requested to see patients in a primary care setting. "Confusion" can be a symptom of mild cognitive impatient, dementia, delirium, major depressive disorder, or psychotic disorder. Differentiating among them can be challenging, especially when such psychiatric syndromes occur concurrently (e.g., delirium superimposed on dementia). Until another cause is identified, the confused older patient should be assumed to have delirium, which is often reversible with management of the underlying cause for delirium.

Furthermore, cognitive impairment of dementia is commonly accompanied, and even preceded, by neuropsychiatric symptoms (e.g., deterioration in emotional control, social behavior, or motivation), which can make the differential diagnosis rather complex. This chapter reviews the most common behavioral health problems (i.e., anxiety, depression, dementia) in the old age encountered in primary care.

LATE-LIFE ANXIETY DISORDERS

CLINICAL SIGNIFICANCE

Prevalence

The prevalence of late-life anxiety disorders (and clinically significant anxiety symptoms) ranges from 1.2% to 15% (15% to 52%) in community samples and from 1% to 28% (15% to 56%) in clinical settings.[1] Generalized anxiety disorder may be the most common late-life anxiety disorder and has a prevalence similar to that in younger adults, while panic disorder and obsessive-compulsive disorder are less common.[1] Generalized anxiety disorder and specific phobias account for 90% of presentations of late-life anxiety.[2] Moreover, studies show that between 50% and 97% of cases of late-life generalized anxiety disorder represent late-life exacerbations of an earlier-onset disorder, often undiagnosed.[3] Fear of falling is specific to older adults, with high rates and significant distress and functional impairment.[1]

Economics

Anxiety disorders tend to have an early onset and run a chronic but fluctuating course over a lifetime, with exacerbations or recurrent symptoms. Adults with anxiety disorders report an average duration of symptoms of 20 years or more.[1] They tend to be high life-long utilizers of health care, compared with adults with other psychiatric conditions, and they are more likely to seek care for their symptoms from a primary care physician rather than from a mental health professional, with the result that a medical cause for the symptoms often is sought.[4]

Clinical Burden; Medical Comorbidities

Anxiety disorders are highly impairing in late life. A clinical presentation of worry in generalized anxiety disorder predominates more so than a panic attack in old age, which is a reversal of anxiety presentation in earlier adulthood (see *Table 20-1*). This decrease in incidence of panic attacks in late life may be explained by age-related dampening of physiological autonomic responses.[1]

The clinical burden of anxiety disorders in older adults is associated with decreased independence, decreased life satisfaction, poor self-perception of health, poor adherence to treatment, increased loneliness, and increased risk for placement in a long-term care facility.[5-7] Late-life anxiety disorders may be associated with poor concentration and/or memory impairment and often accompany depressive and substance use disorders. When they occur as a behavioral complication of dementia, they can have multifarious presentations, ranging from excessive worry to agitation and aggression. Older patients suffering from an anxiety disorder have an increased risk of functional decline, development of disability, and premature mortality. Caring for an older patient with an anxiety disorder adds to caregiver burden and can lead to caregiver burnout. The nonspecific nature of many late-life anxiety symptoms, such as fatigue, abdominal pain, and headaches, can lead to unnecessary and costly diagnostic studies,[4] and these symptoms can be erroneously attributed to other comorbid conditions, delaying diagnosis and prolonging psychiatric morbidity. Moreover, the co-occurrence of major depressive disorder and generalized anxiety disorder in late life is associated with a worse prognosis than either disorder alone, as well as a longer duration to respond to treatment (at least 50% more time), and a greater likelihood of only achieving a partial remission of the depressive disorder.[1]

DIAGNOSIS

Diagnostic Considerations

Late-life anxiety disorders are often underdiagnosed and undertreated, especially because their clinical presentation differs from that seen in younger adults. Patients with late-life anxiety disorders tend to[1]:

- Report physical symptoms (e.g., dizziness, pain) rather than psychological distress
- Have comorbid medical conditions whose spectrum of potential symptoms can overlap with the anxiety-associated symptoms (e.g., complaints of fatigue in a patient with heart failure or hypothyroidism; "dizziness" in a patient with paroxysmal atrial fibrillation), which can result in the misattribution of the psychiatric symptoms
- Take multiple medications (polypharmacy), whose side effects may contribute to anxiety symptoms (e.g., beta-agonists, thyroid replacement therapy) or modify them (beta-blockers)

Older adults often seek treatment for anxiety symptoms from their primary care physician instead of a psychiatrist. Primary care physicians must remain alert to recognize and accurately attribute somatic symptoms to an anxiety disorder in older adults. Late-life anxiety disorder is often comorbid with major depressive disorder, which also requires recognition and treatment (see section on Late-life Depressive Disorders in this chapter). Anxiety symptoms can be the manifestation of a primary psychiatric disorder (e.g., generalized anxiety disorder), or can be secondary to another medical condition (e.g., dementia), or can be induced by substance/medication use (e.g., caffeine, levodopa, albuterol).

The multimorbidity, prevalent among older patients, compounds the diagnostic challenge because of symptom overlap with depressive disorders (e.g., insomnia, fatigue, concentration difficulties, psychomotor agitation) and/or systemic medical conditions (e.g., abdominal and chest complaints, headaches, shortness of breath). As discussed later in this chapter, a thorough history is key to making the diagnosis. *Table 20-2* shows

TABLE 20-1 Main Characteristics of Early-Onset versus Late-Onset Anxiety Disorders[8-13]

DISORDER TYPE	CHARACTERISTICS FOR EARLY ONSET	CHARACTERISTICS FOR LATE ONSET
Generalized anxiety disorder (GAD)	Worry topics: future, work Prevalence is 0.7%-9%	Worry topics: health, family, finances Frequent comorbidity with hypertension Poor health-related quality of life Nearly 50% with onset >age 50 years
Specific phobia	Prevalence is higher in early life	May underreport symptoms Fear of falling is common; 60% have a history of falling; 30% have no such history; more prevalent in women; increases with age
Social phobia (social anxiety disorder)	Presentation similar to that seen in older adults Life-time prevalence slightly decreases with age Prevalence is 5%	Common subtypes: eating food around strangers, being unable to urinate in public washrooms Stressful life events (e.g., death of spouse) are common; major depression, specific phobia, and personality disorder are common comorbidities
Agoraphobia	Most cases have early onset Can manifest within the context of panic attacks Prevalence is 0.6%	Can occur poststroke or another medical condition; can impact activities needed for rehabilitation Most do not have concurrent panic disorder More common in women, widowed/divorced, with comorbid chronic physical conditions and/or psychiatric disorders
Obsessive-compulsive disorder (OCD)	Common themes: contamination, symmetry, counting rituals	Common themes: handwashing, fear of having sinned Rarely begins in late life; most patients have symptoms for decades Late onset can occur in history of cerebral lesions (e.g., basal ganglia), suggesting neurodegenerative pathophysiology Prevalence decreases with age; up to 0.8% in age ≥60 years
Panic disorder	Symptoms are more severe than in older adults	Late onset in age >60 years is rare; panic attacks are commonly comorbid with systemic medical and psychiatric disorders; anxiety symptoms of shortness of breath, dizziness, or trembling can overlap with age-related medical conditions and may wax and wane Panic attack may present with more shortness of breath, but fewer physical symptoms overall
Posttraumatic stress disorder (PTSD)[a]	Commonly starts earlier in life.	Past trauma recollections can lead to new-onset PTSD Can present with more somatic symptoms of PTSD Alzheimer disease, vascular dementia, or alcohol-related dementia may worsen PTSD symptoms in patients whose symptoms were previously well controlled

[a]*No longer considered an anxiety disorder, but classified in* DSM-5 (Diagnostic and Statistical Manual of Mental Disorders, Fifth Edition) *in the category of trauma and related disorders.*

TABLE 20-2 Assessment and Management Tips in Late-Life Anxiety Disorders in Primary Care Setting[1]

ASSESSMENT ELEMENTS	MANAGEMENT TIPS
• Illness severity • Psychiatric comorbidity • Physical illness comorbidity • Prior treatments • Cognitive status • Medical workup	• Provide psychoeducation about diagnosis and treatment • Start one or more of the first-line options (e.g., SSRI, SNRI, CBT, bibliotherapy) • With medications: start low, go slow, but treat long to remission target • Avoid or discontinue harmful medications (e.g., anticholinergics, antihistaminergics, sedatives) • Avoid benzodiazepine prescription as possible • Provide sequent follow-up within the first month of treatment or dose change to encourage adherence • Measure treatment response • If poor response, consider augmentation treatment and refer to specialists if necessary • Provide maintenance treatment

the key assessment elements required in diagnosing late-life anxiety disorders.[1] Primary care practitioners must determine whether there is:

• A recurrence of a preexisting anxiety disorder versus a new-onset presentation (see *Table 20-1*)[8-13]
• A comorbid depressive disorder and/or another anxiety disorder
• Physiological effects of another medical condition
• Physiological effects of a substance or medication use

Figure 20-1 highlights the diagnostic criteria for the most common anxiety disorders in older adults: generalized anxiety disorder and specific phobia.[14] For a complete list of diagnostic criteria of the anxiety disorders, the reader is referred to the *DSM-5*.[14] Suggested screening questions to establish whether the worry is excessive are shown in Box 20-1.

BOX 20-1 COMMON QUESTIONS TO ESTABLISH WHETHER ANXIETY OR WORRY IS EXCESSIVE

Are you a worrier/nervous person?

How much of the time do you spend worrying or feeling anxious?

Do you worry more or are you more anxious than other people you know?

Do your family or friends believe that you worry too much or you are overly concerned about things?

Do you avoid doing certain things because of your worry/concern?

Generalized anxiety disorder is characterized by at least 6 months of excessive anxiety or worry about a number of daily life domains (e.g., health, relationships, finances), difficulty in controlling the worry, and associated physical symptoms (i.e., restlessness, fatigue, muscle tension, insomnia) that cause distress and impairment in important areas of functioning (see *Figure 20-1*). Specific phobia is characterized by persistent irrational fear of an object or situation and the desire to avoid the phobic object or situation (see *Figure 20-1*).

Agoraphobia can be a common phobia in old age[11] (see *Table 20-1*). Late-life agoraphobia may be precipitated by psychosocial stressors and interferes with life satisfaction. Unlike their younger counterparts, older adults do not always present with agoraphobia concurrent with panic disorder, but it can follow a traumatic event (e.g., fall). The fear of falling is much more common among older than younger adults and occurs in 60% of those who have previously fallen.[9] These patients become housebound and may have a poor postfall rehabilitation.[15]

Rating scales for anxiety disorder and its comorbidity: Anxiety disorders along with depressive disorders are among the most common psychiatric presentations in primary care and clinical specialty populations, regardless of age.[16] Identifying and managing both disorders is necessary. Scales such as Generalized Anxiety Disorder (GAD)-7 for anxiety and Patient Health Questionnaire (PHQ)-9 for depression are brief validated screening and rating tools.[16] The GAD-7 and GAD-2 (the abbreviated 2-item version) have good sensitivity and specificity in detecting generalized anxiety, panic, and social anxiety disorders. The optimal cutoff point is ≥10 on the parent scales (GAD-7 and PHQ-9) and ≥3 on the abbreviated versions (GAD-2 and PHQ-2). The PHQ-9 and its

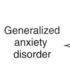

Generalized anxiety disorder
• Excessive anxiety/worry
• Plus ≥3: 1) restlessness; 2) fatigue; 3) concentration difficulty; 4) irritability; 5) muscle tension; 6) insomnia
• Distress/impairment in important areas of functioning
• Duration >6 months

Specific phobia
• Marked fear/anxiety about specific object/situation
• Phobic object/situation is actively avoided or endured with intense fear/anxiety, which is out of proportion to the actual danger
• Distress/impairment in important areas of functioning
• Duration >6 months

FIGURE 20-1 Key elements of the *DSM-5* (*Diagnostic and Statistical Manual of Mental Disorders*, Fifth Edition) diagnostic criteria for common anxiety disorders in older adults.[14]

abbreviated 8-item (PHQ-8) and 2-item (PHQ-2) versions have good sensitivity and specificity for detecting depressive disorders.[16] A short screening tool for posttraumatic stress disorder (PTSD) is the Primary Care PTSD Screen for *DSM-5* (PC-PTSD-5).[17]

Differential Diagnosis

Systemic medical illness is either commonly associated with or mimic anxiety disorder, which needs to be ruled out. In primary care, gastrointestinal symptoms may accompany anxiety and depression.[18] In one study, the prevalence of anxiety disorder was nearly fourfold in patients with gastrointestinal symptoms (stomach pain, constipation, loose stool or diarrhea, nausea, gas, or indigestion) compared with those without anxiety-related symptoms (19.4% vs. 5.6%; $P < .001$).[18] With each additional gastrointestinal symptom, the odds ratio (OR) for diagnosis of specific anxiety disorders increased significantly; in patients with generalized anxiety disorder and one gastrointestinal symptom, OR 3.7 (95% confidence interval [CI] 2.0-6.9), in patients with two gastrointestinal symptoms, OR 6.5 (95% CI 3.1-13.6), and in patients with three gastrointestinal symptoms, OR 7.2 (95% CI 2.7-18.8).

In patients with neuropsychiatric symptoms of dementia, anxiety symptoms can often manifest indirectly through physical signs or symptoms (e.g., restlessness, wringing hands, fidgeting, sleep disturbance, wandering), as well as through behavioral manifestations, such as agitation and irritability (as discussed in the section on Dementia in this chapter). Delusions or hallucinations can result in anxiety symptoms (e.g., a patient who sees a crying child in her bedroom as part of her psychotic experiences may become anxious about needing to protect it).

Differentiating primary from secondary anxiety disorder is important. *Table 20-3* shows some key elements to consider in determining whether the clinical presentation is due to a primary versus secondary anxiety disorder. Polypharmacy is common among older adults, and some medications and other substances (e.g., prescribed and illicit psychostimulants, steroids, beta-agonists, thyroxine, levodopa, albuterol, caffeine, alcohol) may cause or exacerbate anxiety disorders. A careful review of the medications (prescribed and over-the-counter) and substance use is important when considering the differential diagnosis of anxiety disorders.

BIOPSYCHOSOCIAL TREATMENT

Overview of Treatment

Less than 30% of patients with an anxiety disorder ever seek treatment.[4] Older adults with anxiety-related symptoms most often seek treatment from a primary care clinician.[19] Treatment of late-life anxiety disorder remains a challenge, given concerns about medication side effects, especially in frail, medically ill patients. The general principle for prescribing medications for older adults is to start low, go slow, and treat long to

TABLE 20-3 Red Flags for a Primary versus Secondary Cause of Anxiety in the Context of Physical Illness	
Supported elements for primary anxiety disorder	Anxiety symptoms occur before physical illness
	Depressive disorder occurs before physical illness
	No newly started prescribed and/or over-the-counter medications or natural products
	Presence of major life events or other risk factors for anxiety disorders
	History of increased anxiety when facing the feared object or situation
	History of avoidance behavior
Supported elements for secondary anxiety disorder	Anxiety symptoms occur postdiagnosis of physical illness
	Symptoms of a systemic medical condition are known to mimic those of anxiety (e.g., hyperthyroidism, respiratory illness, angina, arrhythmia)
	Anxiety symptoms are known side effects of newly started prescribed and/or over-the-counter medications or natural products
	Polypharmacy
	Absence of life events or other risk factors for anxiety disorders
	Absence of psychiatric history of anxiety disorders

remission target (see *Table 20-2* for management tips). Starting with one-quarter to one-half of the usual starting dose of an antidepressant, and increasing dose slowly, with regular follow-up and reassurance, is often necessary.

Psychopharmacology

Antidepressants are recommended but not always tolerated, whereas benzodiazepines are generally avoided because of serious side effects including cognitive impairment, rebound withdrawal symptoms, dependence, incontinence, falls, and fall-related trauma and mortality. Activating antidepressants (e.g., bupropion) and psychostimulants (e.g., methylphenidate) should be avoided because they may worsen anxiety symptoms. Tricyclic antidepressants, although potentially effective, are associated with anticholinergic and cardiac toxicity, rendering them potentially inappropriate medications for older patients. Trazodone can be used for anxiety-related insomnia but can add to the serotonin burden when simultaneously using a selective serotonin reuptake inhibitor (SSRI) or serotonin norepinephrine reuptake inhibitor (SNRI). *Table 20-4* shows common pharmacologic treatment options for late-life anxiety syndromes.[1,8,20-25]

Improvement in symptoms preferably should be assessed objectively through standardized questionnaires as well as by general report from the patient or

TABLE 20-4 Common Medications Used in Older Adults[1,8,20-25]

DRUG CLASS	MEDICATION (STARTING DOSE/DAY)[a]	SIDE EFFECTS/COMMENTS
Antidepressants	Citalopram (10 mg) Escitalopram (5 mg)	SIADH/hyponatremia, risk of bleeding, risk of falls, anorexia, akathisia, headache, agitation, GI complaints, constipation QTc prolongation warning by the US FDA and Health Canada: citalopram max 20 mg/day in patients over 60 years First-line treatment for depression, GAD, panic disorder, OCD, PTSD Citalopram has been used for agitation in Alzheimer dementia[25]
	Sertraline (25 mg)	SIADH/hyponatremia, risk of bleeding, risk of falls, anorexia, akathisia, headache, agitation, GI complaints, diarrhea, constipation First-line treatment for depression, GAD, panic disorder, OCD, PTSD
	Venlafaxine XR (37.5 mg)	Dose-related increase in BP, nausea, constipation, SIADH/hyponatremia, risk of bleeding, risk of falls First-line treatment for depression, GAD, panic disorder, OCD, PTSD; useful for neuropathic pain
	Duloxetine (30 mg)	Dry mouth, nausea, constipation, SIADH/hyponatremia, risk of bleeding First-line treatment for depression, GAD, panic disorder, OCD, PTSD; useful for neuropathic pain, fibromyalgia
	Mirtazapine (7.5-15 mg)	Sedation, weight gain, constipation, mild anticholinergic effects, decreased WBC More sedating when used at lowest doses (<15 mg) First-line treatment for depression and anxiety
	Bupropion XL (150 mg)	Dry mouth, agitation, constipation; can lower seizure threshold No data to support use in anxiety disorders First-line treatment for depression
Mood stabilizers	Lithium (150-300 mg QHS)	GI upset, tremor, benign leukocytosis, hypothyroidism, hyperparathyroidism, interstitial nephropathy, diabetes insipidus, neurotoxicity (with toxicity), cardiac conduction abnormalities Pretreatment workup and monitoring studies: CBC, TSH, calcium, eGFR, serum lithium level, ECG
	Valproate (125-250 mg QD-BID-TID)	Headache, tremor, dizziness, ataxia, nausea, vomiting, diarrhea, constipation, weight gain, somnolence, thrombocytopenia, hepatotoxicity, pancreatitis, hyponatremia, suicidal behavior/ideation, hyperammonemia Pretreatment workup and monitoring studies: CBC, liver enzymes, serum valproate level; check for serum hyperammonemia if altered mental status (consider urea cycle enzyme deficiency as cause of hyperammonemia)
	Lamotrigine (12.5-25 mg QD-BID)	Dizziness, ataxia, confusion, headaches, nausea, vomiting, diarrhea, blurred vision, Stevens–Johnson syndrome Increased risk of suicidal ideation/behavior
Anxiolytics/ sedatives/ hypnotics	Buspirone (5 mg BID)	Effective for GAD, but not for panic disorder; may take 2-4 weeks to take effect Second-line treatment for anxiety
	Lorazepam (0.25-0.5 mg QD-BID)	Older adults are prone to CNS depression; if used, start very low dose, depending on patient response, to avoid cognitive impairment and falls Paradoxical reactions: anxiety, agitation, excitation
	Trazodone (12.5-25 mg QHS-BID-TID)	Orthostasis, QTc prolongation, priapism Can be used in behavioral variant frontotemporal dementia, max daily dose 100-300 mg
	Doxepin (3-6 mg QHS)	Anticholinergic side effects in doses >6 mg/day Used for insomnia Contraindicated in patients with urinary retention
	Melatonin (1-3 mg QHS)	Drowsiness, headache, dizziness, nausea Used in jet lag, circadian rhythm sleep disorders, delayed phase sleep disorder

TABLE 20-4 Common Medications Used in Older Adults[1,8,20-25] (continued)

DRUG CLASS	MEDICATION (STARTING DOSE/DAY)[a]	SIDE EFFECTS/COMMENTS
Cognitive enhancers	Donepezil (5 mg)[b,c] Galantamine ER (8 mg) Rivastigmine (1.5 mg BID, 5 cm² transdermal) Memantine (5 mg QD-BID)[d]	Can improve anxiety/irritability among patients with Alzheimer dementia Cholinesterase inhibitors: all three approved for mild and moderate, and severe (donepezil only) Alzheimer dementia. Dose-dependent cholinergic side effects: nausea, vomiting, diarrhea, muscle cramps, dizziness, fatigue, anorexia. Transdermal formulation: three times less GI side effects Memantine: approved for moderate to severe Alzheimer dementia. Dose-limiting side effects: dizziness, headache, somnolence, confusion
Antipsychotics	Class-wide side effects: sedation, anticholinergic symptoms, orthostatic hypotension, EPS, QTc prolongation, metabolic side effects, cognitive decline, cerebrovascular adverse events, and death in patients with dementia. Prominent side effects for specific medications noted below; some are used as augmentation strategy to antidepressants	
	Haloperidol (0.25-0.5 mg BID)	Parkinsonism, akathisia, dyskinesia Avoid if QTc >500 ms Increased mortality
	Olanzapine (2.5-5 mg)	Anticholinergic, weight gain, hyperglycemia, hypertriglyceridemia Avoid in diabetes mellitus
	Risperidone (0.25-0.5 mg QD-BID)	EPS, hyperprolactinemia, pedal edema
	Quetiapine (12.5-25 mg QD-TID)	QTc prolongation, orthostatic hypotension, anticholinergic, weight gain, hyperglycemia, hypertriglyceridemia
	Aripiprazole (2 mg)	Akathisia, parkinsonism

[a]*Patients aged >75 years or those >60 years with frailty and multiple medication comorbidities require a lower dose.*
[b]*Dose of 10 mg daily is administered after a dose of 5 mg daily for 4-6 weeks; 23 mg daily is administered after a dose of 10 mg daily for at least 3 months.*
[c]*U.S. FDA approved a once-daily, sustained-release 23-mg tablet.*
[d]*If creatinine clearance ≤30 mL/minute, the maximum dose should not exceed 10 mg daily.*

EPS, extrapyramidal symptoms; GAD, generalized anxiety disorder; GI, gastrointestinal; OCD, obsessive-compulsive disorder; PTSD, posttraumatic stress disorder. BID, twice daily; QD, once daily; QHS, at bedtime; TID, thrice daily, SIADH, syndrome of inappropriate antidiuretic hormone; CBC, complete blood count; TSH, thyroid-stimulating hormone; ECG, electrocardiogram; CNS, central nervous system.

informant. An increase in the dose of the antidepressant should be considered at 2 weeks if there has been no subjective or objective improvement, or if the symptoms remain severe and disabling; otherwise, waiting a full 4 to 6 weeks before dose adjustment of the antidepressant is warranted.

Psychopharmacology Pearls

- Start low, go slow, and treat long to remission target for anxiety disorder.
- Start with one-quarter to one-half of the usual starting dose of a medication for anxiety, and increase dose slowly, with regular follow-up and reassurance.
- Antidepressants are recommended but not always tolerated.
- Benzodiazepines are generally avoided.

Psychosocial Approaches

Psychotherapy for anxiety disorders in older adults is often used in conjunction with pharmacotherapy. Psychotherapeutic approaches include cognitive behavioral therapy (CBT), exposure therapy, and bibliotherapy.[1,26,27] CBT in older adults with generalized anxiety disorder is associated with improvements in worry severity and comorbid depressive symptoms. Enhanced models of CBT, modified to better meet the needs of older adults by using large print and mnemonics to reinforce core concepts, have been shown to be more effective than standard CBT in both individual and group format.[20] CBT for anxiety disorder is based on behavioral exposure to anxiety-provoking objects or situations, cognitive restructuring, and modifying avoidance behaviors. *Table 20-5* lists common age-specific examples of maladaptive avoidance behaviors.[8,20]

Other Treatment Considerations

Both SNRIs and SSRIs can prolong the QTc and should be used cautiously with other serotonin agonists and drugs known to prolong the QTc. They also

TABLE 20-5 Common Age-Specific Examples of Maladaptive Avoidance Behaviors[8,20]

AVOIDANCE BEHAVIOR	FEAR OF OBJECT/SITUATION
Public transportation	Fear of falling
Driving	Fear of inability to see or react appropriately
Social events	Fear of inability to hear owing to loss of hearing
Aid to enhance functioning (e.g., cane, walker, hearing aid)	Fear of appearing old or frail
Seeking needed help	Fear of becoming a burden, losing independence/autonomy
Discarding unwanted items (hoarding)	Fear of needing the item sometime in the future

can stimulate inappropriate secretion of antidiuretic hormone, leading to hyponatremia. Consequently, older patients should have a baseline electrocardiogram (ECG) before starting an SSRI/SNRI and should have a serum sodium checked within approximately 2 weeks of starting the drug and after dose increases.

Benzodiazepine and GABA-benzodiazepine-receptor drugs for the treatment of the insomnia associated with anxiety disorders similarly increase the risk of cognitive impairment, delirium, impaired balance, falls, and fall-related fractures in older patients and should be avoided. Melatonin, melatonin-receptor agonists (e.g., ramelteon), and trazodone are safer alternatives, and the latter can work additively with serotonergic antidepressants.

Education, Prevention, Treatment Adherence Issues

In the primary care setting, lack of familiarity with antidepressant medication and concern about side effects often result in failure to optimize treatment doses, resulting in no or only partial remission. It is essential that the patient receive close follow-up, especially within the first month, ideally through office visits but at least by telephone or HIPAA-secure* electronic communication.

Because of the long-term nature of anxiety disorders, it is not uncommon for primary care clinicians to encounter an older patient who has been on long-term benzodiazepine therapy (≥6 months) for a history of chronic anxiety or PTSD. Despite their increased vulnerability to adverse

*Health Insurance Portability and Accountability Act: U.S. legislation aimed at ensuring the security and privacy of health-related information contained in medical records and electronic communication.

reactions from benzodiazepines, older adults have the highest prevalence of long-term use of benzodiazepines.[28,29] Alprazolam is associated with a particularly high rate of dependency and addiction, and withdrawal reactions can be severe, even when treated with another benzodiazepine.[30] Because of the difficulty weaning older patients off benzodiazepines (especially alprazolam), the benzodiazepine often continues to be renewed, especially when the drug appears to be controlling symptoms without apparent untoward side effects. Alprazolam can and should be tapered off, but, depending on the dose and frequency, the taper can sometimes take weeks to months. To prevent a recurrence of anxiety during the taper, initiation of an SSRI or SNRI should be considered.

WHEN TO REFER TO PSYCHIATRIC CLINIC?

- Severe anxiety symptoms
- Minimal improvement despite upward titration of medication and psychotherapeutic interventions
- Chronic anxiety symptoms interfering with function
- Medication review/reassessment of severe anxiety case previously seen in psychiatric clinic

LATE-LIFE DEPRESSIVE DISORDERS

CLINICAL SIGNIFICANCE

Prevalence

The lifetime prevalence of major depressive disorder in the general population is estimated at 15% to 17%.[31] The 1-year prevalence in those aged 65 years or older is 1% to 4%.[31] A significant number of older adults suffer from subthreshold symptoms of depression identified by fewer than five *DSM-5* criteria (formally diagnosed as other specified depressive disorder or unspecified depressive disorder). The prevalence of both major depressive disorder and clinically significant depressive symptoms vary by clinical setting, with the lowest rates observed in community settings and the highest rates in long-term care facilities (see *Figure 20-2*).[31] In younger adults, depression is more common in females than males (1.7-fold greater incidence in women).[31] However, at ages older than 65 years, both women and men show a decline in depression rates, and the prevalence becomes similar between them.[32]

Economics

In the 2013 Global Burden of Disease study, major depressive disorder was among the top 10 leading causes of years lived with disability in every country studied.[33] Depressive disorder is associated with a disease burden in health-adjusted life years greater than the combined burden for multiple cancers (breast, colorectal, lung, and prostate).[34,35]

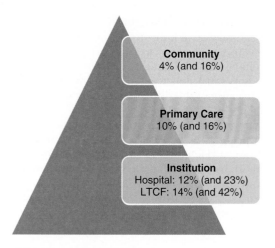

LTCF, long-term care facility

FIGURE 20-2 Prevalence rates of late-life major depressive disorder (and depressive symptoms) in various settings. LTCF, long-term care facility. Data derived from Glover J, Srinivasan S. Assessment of the person with late-life depression. *Psychiatr Clin North Am.* 2013;36:545-560.

Clinical Burden; Medical Comorbidities

As with late-life anxiety, the term "late-life depression" includes both older adults who are presenting with de novo (first-time) depressive disorders (referred as late-onset depressive disorders) and aging patients with a history of depressive disorders presenting earlier in life (referred as early-onset depressive disorders). *Table 20-6* summarizes the key characteristics between early-onset and late-onset depressive disorders.[31,36,37]

Older adults with major depressive disorder are more likely to present with cognitive symptoms such as impaired concentration and memory, decreased processing speed, and executive dysfunction, which may resemble symptoms similar to dementia, known as "pseudodementia."[36] Differentiating "pseudodementia" from dementia with neuropsychiatric symptoms of depression relies on history. The onset of cognitive symptoms before the emergence of depressive symptoms suggests a diagnosis of dementia. In those with poor insight and lack of collateral information from an informant, this differential diagnosis can be challenging. In cases where a diagnosis of underlying dementia

TABLE 20-6 Main Characteristics of Early-Onset versus Late-Onset Depressive Disorders[31,36,37]

CHARACTERISTIC	EARLY-ONSET DEPRESSION	LATE-ONSET DEPRESSION
Age of onset	Younger than 60-65 years	Older than 60-65 years
Psychiatric history	Usually present	Usually absent
Family psychiatric history	Usually present	Usually absent
Medical history	Usually low/normal for age	Usually higher
Neuroimaging abnormalities	Cortisol release → early damage to hippocampus; decreased BDNF → decreased neurogenesis	More structural brain changes: increased WMH, hippocampal atrophy, frontal–subcortical disruption
Clinical presentation	More expressed depressive symptoms (suicidal thoughts, thoughts of worthlessness); higher substance misuse comorbidity; poor social support At risk for suicide Mild cognitive impairments: reduced concentration, indecisiveness	Less expressed depressed mood, but more somatic complaints; more anhedonia and apathy; more irritability/social withdrawal/agitation symptoms, less guilt or sexual disinterest; higher medical comorbidity; better social support Somatic symptoms overlap with comorbid disease, medication side effects Higher risk for suicide More cognitive impairments: reduced selective attention, working memory/retrieval, new learning, processing speed, executive function More cardiovascular risk factors
Treatment response	Usually better	Usually worse
Course and prognosis	Episodic; more frequent episodes; longer duration; fewer residual symptoms; relapses at usual risk; usually full functional recovery	Usually chronic; fewer episodes; usually more residual symptoms; higher relapse risk, more rapid; usually less functional recovery; worse prognosis; increased morbidity/mortality

BDNF, brain-derived neurotrophic factor; WMH, white matter hyperintensities.

is unclear, clinicians can empirically start an antide-pressant and monitor whether there is any improvement in cognition after resolution of the depressive symptoms. Resolution of cognitive symptoms supports the diagnosis of pseudodementia. However, patients with mild cognitive impairment or early dementia and associated depression can experience improvement in cognitive performance as the depression improves but not a full return to normal cognitive function. Epidemiologic studies have linked late-life depression to an increased risk of dementia.[38] Thus, older patients treated for depression with apparent resolution of associated cognitive impairment are at increased risk for cognitive decline and should undergo annual neurocognitive screening as part of health maintenance.

Major depressive disorder may have a recurrent course. The recurrence rate of a major depressive episode was found to be 26.8% to 34.7% over a period of 3 years and 65% over a period of 23 years.[34,35] Suicide occurs most frequently in depressive disorder. The 12-month prevalence of suicide attempts in patients with major depressive disorder is more than 20-fold higher compared with those without major depressive disorder,[39] with as high as 15% of patients with major depressive disorder committing suicide.[40] Depressed patients aged 65 years or older have the highest suicide rate[41] (also see Box 20-2). Notably, these numbers may be lower for community dwelling adults, as most studies on depressive disorders and suicide were based on inpatient populations. As the cohort of baby boomers (persons born between 1946 and 1964) continues to age, it is estimated that suicide rates will increase, further highlighting the importance of adequate assessment and treatment of major depressive disorder in late life.

BOX 20-2   SUICIDE RISK FACTORS IN A MAJOR DEPRESSIVE EPISODE[14]

Age >65 years

Male sex

Presence of suicidal or homicidal ideation, intention, or plans

Access to means of suicide (i.e., firearms)

Previous suicide attempt or self-harm behavior

Family history of suicide

History of legal problems

Stressful life events

Presence of psychotic symptoms

Comorbid personality disorders

Comorbid anxiety symptoms

Comorbid alcohol or illicit substance use

Comorbid chronic physical illness

Major depressive disorder is comorbid with multiple systemic medical conditions (e.g., arthritis, migraine and other pain syndromes, chronic pulmonary obstructive disease, hypertension). In a study in primary care setting, the prevalence of major depressive disorder was nearly fivefold in patients with gastrointestinal symptoms compared with those without gastrointestinal symptoms (19.1% vs. 3.9%, $P < .001$).[18]

Major depressive disorder is also comorbid with generalized anxiety disorder (lifetime prevalence of this comorbidity is 39.2% in the Canadian Community Health Study), as well as alcohol and other substance use disorders. As noted, late-life depression has been associated with an increased risk of later developing mild cognitive impairment and dementia.[39,42,43] In a large community-based sample in the Netherlands that examined comorbidity of anxiety and depressive disorders in patients aged 55 to 85 years found that nearly 48% of older adults with major depressive disorder also had a comorbid anxiety disorder, whereas approximately 26% of those with anxiety disorders also had a major depressive disorder.[44] Preexisting anxiety disorders increases the risk of developing depressive disorders.[8] Comorbid major depressive disorder with generalized anxiety disorder or panic disorder in late life is associated with greater memory decline than depression alone, greater and prolonged symptom severity, substance dependence, poorer adherence and response to treatment, and worse overall prognosis than patients with either disorder alone, and a greater likelihood of suicidal ideation, especially in older men.[8]

Two-thirds or more who commit suicide are seen by a primary care physician within a month of their death, and up to one-half within 1 week.[45] Geriatric Depression Scale-Suicide Ideation (GDS-SI) includes 5 items drawn from the GDS (items no. 3, 7, 11, 12, and 14), assigning a response of "yes" or "no" to each item (see *Box 20-3*).[46] Both the 15-item GDS and 5-item GDS-SI appear to differentiate older primary care patients who expressed suicidal ideation from those who do not. This screen may effectively identify patients for whom a more in-depth suicide risk assessment would be warranted. The GDS-SI demonstrated sensitivity and specificity equivalent to that of the 15-item GDS in terms of identifying people at risk for suicide.

BOX 20-3   GERIATRIC DEPRESSION SCALE (GDS)-SUICIDE IDEATION SCREENING ITEMS[46]

Do you feel that your life is empty?

Do you feel happy most of the time?

Do you think it is wonderful to be alive?

Do you feel pretty worthless the way you are now?

Do you feel that your situation is hopeless?

Table 20-7 enlists common predisposing, precipitating, and protective factors for late-life depressive disorder,[31,34,47] while *Box 20-2* shows the suicide risk factors for a major depressive episode.[14] Studies suggest that a late-life major depressive disorder nearly doubles the risk of developing dementia.[42] Conversely, patients with dementia (particular Alzheimer disease or vascular dementia) are at increased risk of developing depression; up to 24% of patients with Alzheimer dementia meet criteria for major depressive disorder.[48] This bidirectional risk relationship between depressive disorder and dementia makes the diagnosis and management challenging in these patients.

DIAGNOSIS

Diagnostic Considerations

A major depressive episode presents with depressed mood, along with at least four other associated symptoms, which affect daily functioning (see *Figure 20-3*).[14] For a complete review of the *DSM-5* diagnostic criteria for depressive disorders, the reader is referred to the *DSM-5* manual.[14]

Acknowledgment of a depressed mood is common among depressed younger adults, but older adults with depression may present atypically, with behavioral changes and somatic complaints, and may even deny feeling depressed. Signs and symptoms of depression in the older adult include loss of interest in previous enjoyable activities, social withdrawal, irritability, loss of appetite and weight loss, loss of interest in appearance or hygiene, and (as in late-life anxiety disorders) nonspecific somatic complaints such as fatigue or complaints of worsening physical symptoms without corresponding physical changes, such as complaints of worsening knee pain in a patient with stable osteoarthritis. Depression has been associated with exacerbation of chronic pain.[49] Some clues to picking up the diagnosis of depressive disorder in the primary care are illustrated in *Box 20-4*. Behaviors to alert clinicians of potential suicide in older adults are listed in *Box 20-5*.

BOX 20-4   CLUES TO PICKING UP THE DIAGNOSIS OF DEPRESSIVE DISORDER IN PRIMARY CARE PATIENTS

Help-seeking behavior

Persistent complaints of "bad nerves," gastrointestinal symptoms, pain, headache, fatigue, weight loss, insomnia, multiple unspecific symptoms

Diurnal variation in symptoms (e.g., pain worse in the morning in depression, worse as day progresses in osteoarthritis)

Frequent calls and visits to primary care physician

High health care service utilization

BOX 20-5   BEHAVIORS TO ALERT CLINICIANS OF POTENTIAL SUICIDE

Preoccupation with death

Agitation

Increased alcohol use

Giving away personal belongings

Reviewing the will

Nonadherence to treatment

Purchasing a firearm

Figure 20-4 presents a summary of the assessment of late-life depression, which starts with determining the diagnostic criteria for a major depressive episode, followed by context assessment and differential diagnosis.

Rating scales for depressive disorder. A targeted screening in primary care is recommended for older adults at high risk of depression involving a number of situations as shown in *Table 20-8*. There are several standardized screening and rating scales for depression in late life. Case-finding and surveillance commonly include the 5-item, 15-item, and 30-item versions of the Geriatric Depression Scale (GDS), used for patients who are cognitively intact or have mild cognitive impairment and are able to provide a reliable history. The GDS was designed to omit somatic complaints whose prevalence in older adults can yield false-positive depression screening. The Cornell Scale for Depression in Dementia is an informant-based questionnaire that is used for patients with moderate to severe cognitive impairment but is also useful when language barriers prevent directly assessing the patient's mood. PHQ-9 items and its abbreviated 2-item version (PHQ-2) also downplay somatic complaints and have good performance characteristics in older patients. Hamilton Depression Rating Scale (HAM-D) and Beck Depression Inventory (BDI) both were developed for adults in general and thus represent second-line screening instruments for the older patients. The Center for Epidemiological Studies-Depression Scale (CES-D) has been used extensively in epidemiologic studies across wide age ranges, including older adults. The PHQ-2 contains two screening questions for depression: "Over the past 2 weeks, how often have you been bothered by the following problems: (1) Little interest or pleasure in doing things? (2) Feeling down, depressed, or hopeless?" A positive screening for depression is followed by a clinical interview.

Differential Diagnosis

If an older adult presents with first-onset depression, it would be important to rule out comorbid systemic medical conditions as the cause of the depressive symptoms (e.g., hypothyroidism, hyperparathyroidism,

TABLE 20-7 Risk Factors and Protective Factors for Late-Life Depressive Disorder[31,34,47]		
PREDISPOSING FACTORS	**PRECIPITATING FACTORS**	**PROTECTIVE FACTORS**
• Female sex • Widowed/divorced • Bereavement • Prior depression • Cerebrovascular changes • Disabling physical illness • Polypharmacy • Alcohol misuse • Low social support • Caregiver burnout • Personality structure (e.g., dependence/relationship problems)	• Recent bereavement • Recent residence move • Adverse life events • Social isolation • Persistent sleep difficulties	• Healthy physical status • Normal cognitive status • Optimal social support • Meaningful social activities

> • Symptoms are present during a 2-week period (symptom 1 or 2 must be present), ≥5 of: (1) depressed mood; (2) decreased interest/pleasure in activities; (3) appetite/weight change; (4) insomnia/hypersomnia; (5) psychomotor agitation/retardation; (6) fatigue/loss of energy; (7) feelings of worthlessness/inappropriate guilt; (8) poor concentration; (9) recurrent thoughts of death/suicidal ideation with/without a plan, or a suicide attempt.
> • Medical-/substance-induced conditions are excluded.

Major depressive episode

FIGURE 20-3 Highlights of the *DSM-5* (*Diagnostic and Statistical Manual of Mental Disorders*, Fifth Edition) diagnostic criteria for a major depressive episode.[14]

Cushing disease, Addison disease, Parkinson disease, pancreatic cancer, brain tumors, multiple sclerosis).[50]

Routine laboratory evaluation for depression includes a complete blood count, renal and hepatic function tests, thyroid function tests, and electrolytes. In addition, serum calcium, magnesium, phosphate, albumin, and vitamin B_{12} should be considered, especially if nutritional status is a concern. As indicated, hemoglobin A1c and lipid profile should be considered in someone with a history of diabetes mellitus and dyslipidemia, especially if second generation

antipsychotics are used. A urinalysis or chest X-ray may help to identify infection sources. An ECG is warranted in those with cardiac history, especially with the increased risk of depression in those with a recent myocardial infarction.[51] Notably, a baseline ECG is useful because pharmacologic treatment of depression may prolong QTc (e.g., SSRIs, tricyclic antidepressants, antipsychotics). Neuroimaging may be considered, especially if psychotic symptoms or cognitive deficits are present. Generally, a standard metabolic workup for depression as a screen for underlying medical disorders is not cost-effective. Preferably, the workup for an associated medical condition should be informed by epidemiology (incidence/prevalence of the condition) and begin with a thorough review of systems

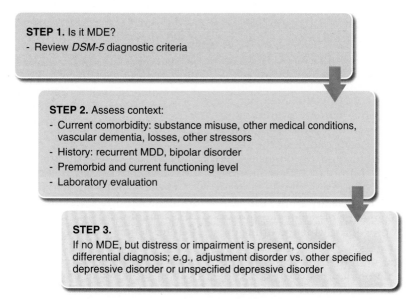

STEP 1. Is it MDE?
- Review *DSM-5* diagnostic criteria

STEP 2. Assess context:
- Current comorbidity: substance misuse, other medical conditions, vascular dementia, losses, other stressors
- History: recurrent MDD, bipolar disorder
- Premorbid and current functioning level
- Laboratory evaluation

STEP 3.
If no MDE, but distress or impairment is present, consider differential diagnosis; e.g., adjustment disorder vs. other specified depressive disorder or unspecified depressive disorder

DSM-5, Diagnostic and Statistical Manual of Mental Disorders, 5th edition; MDE, major depressive episode; MDD, major depressive disorder

FIGURE 20-4 Steps for the assessment of depression. *DSM-5, Diagnostic and Statistical Manual of Mental Disorders, Fifth Edition;* MDD, major depressive disorder; MDE, major depressive episode.

High-risk Situations for depression	Recently bereaved with unusual symptoms (e.g., active suicidal ideation, guilt not related to the deceased, psychomotor retardation, mood-congruent delusions, marked functional impairment, reaction that seems out of proportion to the loss)
	Socially isolated patient
	Persistent complaints of patchy memory difficulties
	Chronic disabling illness, and diagnosis of dementia, Parkinson disease, or stroke
	Recent major physical illness (e.g., within 3 months)
	Persistent sleep difficulties
	Significant somatic concerns
	Recent onset of anxiety disorder
	Refusal to eat or neglect of personal care

followed by a careful physical examination. The findings can then be used to select appropriate diagnostic studies. For example, in a patient with epigastric pain, weight loss, and depression, pancreatic cancer should enter the differential diagnosis. Complaints of constipation, new polyuria, and mild confusion should raise concern about hypercalcemia. In modern clinical laboratories, automated analyses usually include multiple laboratory tests (e.g., a comprehensive chemistry panel), which are more cost-effective than order the individual chemical analyses.

BIOPSYCHOSOCIAL TREATMENT

Overview of Treatment

A combination of biological and psychosocial interventions should be considered for the majority of patients who have depression. Patient preferences, past response to treatment, and service availability need to be considered in the elaboration of the treatment plan. Treatment is predicated on determining whether the patient has a unipolar versus bipolar depression. Because bipolar depression should benefit from referral to a psychiatric specialty clinic, this section focuses on the management of major depressive disorder (or unipolar depression), which is often the province of the primary care.

Treatment options are designed for the type and severity of depression. Major depressive disorder of mild or moderate intensity should be treated with antidepressants, or with psychotherapy, or with a combination of both.[48] Those with major depressive disorder of severe intensity without psychotic symptoms should be offered a combination of antidepressants and concurrent psychotherapy if services are available, and there

is no contraindication to either treatment. Although these patients should be referred to psychiatric services, electroconvulsive treatment (ECT) should be considered if antidepressant trials combined with psychotherapy have been ineffective.[48] Furthermore, patients with psychotic depression should receive a combination of antidepressant plus antipsychotic or ECT.

Psychopharmacology

Physicians should start the antidepressant at half of the recommended dose for younger adults. If the medication is tolerated, reaching an average dose within 1 month with weekly reassessments is recommended. Improvement in symptoms can be measured by using a validated scale (e.g., improvement is defined as 50% reduction on the HAM-D scores); however, targeting remission of depressive symptoms is the goal of therapy. If there is no evidence of improvement after at least 2 weeks on an average antidepressant dose, further dose optimization is recommended until there is some clinical improvement, there is limiting side effects, or the maximum recommended dose is reached.[48] An adequate trial must be ensured before considering a switch in antidepressants. Before commencing a new treatment strategy, it is important to reevaluate diagnosis and that pharmacotherapy is a suitable option. Switch should be made if there is *no improvement* in depressive symptoms after at least 4 weeks at the maximum tolerated or recommended dose, or there is *insufficient improvement* after 8 weeks at the maximum tolerated or recommended dose.[48] When *significant improvement* has occurred, but there is no full recovery after an adequate trial, physicians should consider the following:

- A further 4 weeks of treatment with or without augmentation with another antidepressant, lithium, aripiprazole, quetiapine, or specific psychotherapy (e.g., cognitive behavioral, interpersonal, problem-solving); augmentation strategies require supervision by experienced physicians.
- A switch to another antidepressant (same or another class) after reviewing with the patient the potential risk of losing any significant improvement made with the first choice of antidepressant.

Figure 20-5 shows the treatment algorithm for managing varying responses after a first-line antidepressant.

Table 20-9 lists some of the management considerations for clinicians when treating depressed older adults.[48,52,53] "Treatment-resistant" depression describes depression that has failed two or more trials of antidepressants. As a first step in managing a treatment-resistant depression, it is always advisable to review the working diagnosis, medication adherence, expand the differential diagnosis, and uncover comorbidities that may be complicating the course. Most studies on the efficacy of antidepressants and adjunctive strategies have been done in the general adult population, and evidence for older adult population is still lacking. *Table 20-4* shows common medications used to treat depression.[1,8,20-25]

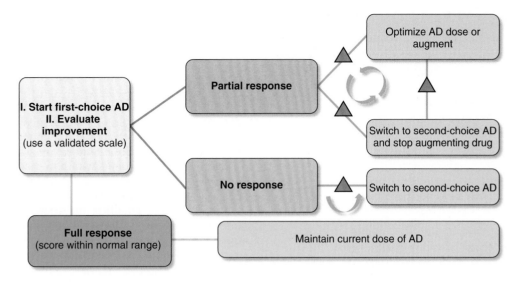

Reevaluate diagnosis; AD, antidepressant

FIGURE 20-5 Treatment algorithm for managing varying responses following a first-line antidepressant (AD). ▲ Reevaluate diagnosis.

Psychopharmacology Pearls

- Treatment options are designed for the type and severity of depression.
- The selection of an antidepressant is based on the side effect profile, potential drug–drug interactions, previous response to treatment, cost, and patient preference.
- Targeting remission of depressive symptoms should be the goal of therapy.

Psychological Approaches

CBT, interpersonal psychotherapy (IPT), and behavioral activation are recommended by the American Psychiatric Association (APA) 2010 guidelines as first-line psychotherapies in the acute treatment of major depressive disorder.[54] CBT remains the first-line psychological treatment for depressive disorder in both the acute and maintenance phase of treatment. Maintenance treatment should be considered for patients with recurrent major depressive disorder, chronic depressive disorder, or any risk factors for recurrence (e.g., ongoing residual symptoms, psychosocial stressors).[54] CBT and mindfulness-based cognitive therapy are first-line treatment options used in the maintenance phase of adults with depressive disorder.[55] In older adults with depressive disorder, CBT, behavioral activation, problem-solving therapy, brief dynamic therapy, and reminiscence therapy are considered effective interventions.[48] The psychosocial intervention called "managing cancer and living meaningfully" (CALM) addresses areas in patients with terminal or potentially terminal disease with the goals of decreasing death anxiety and depressive symptoms and improving attachments and spiritual

well-being.[56] Access to CBT and other nonpharmacologic treatments varies according to insurance coverage and the availability of trained physicians. In the United States, many outpatient mental health professionals do not accept the principal old age insurance, Medicare, because of low reimbursement rates.

Other Treatment Considerations

Adverse events can be minimized by careful selection of medications. Antidepressants should be used even in patients with multiple comorbidities who have shown to have similar efficacy rates compared with use in healthy seniors.[48] Comorbid anxiety disorders should be identified and treated, as they will adversely influence the outcome of depression. Use of fluoxetine as the first-line antidepressant is not recommended given its long half-life and risk of drug–drug interaction with many of the drugs prescribed in older adults. When switching medications, it is generally safe to reduce the current agent while starting low doses of the alternate agent. Specific drug interaction profiles need to be checked for both medications involved during this overlap, as antidepressants commonly interact with each other. Physicians should avoid the use of benzodiazepines for treatment of depressive symptoms in older adults.[48] When benzodiazepines must be used to prevent acute withdrawal, there should be a review and gradual discontinuation when feasible. Antidepressants, especially SSRIs, should not be abruptly discontinued but should be tapered off over a period of 7 to 10 days when possible.

Education, Prevention, Treatment Adherence Issues

The patient–clinician relationship is an important factor in achieving better treatment adherence. Clinicians should provide older depressed adults with education

TABLE 20-9 Management Considerations in the Selection and Monitoring of the Psychotropic Treatment of a Geriatric Depressed Patient[48,52,53]

Recommend	• Good AD options: sertraline, citalopram, escitalopram, venlafaxine, bupropion, mirtazapine • Select ADs with lowest risk of drug–drug interactions and anticholinergic effects • Consider augmentation with: lithium, antipsychotics • Consider urgent ECT referral for acutely suicidal patients, required rapid response to maintain safety, psychotic depression, AD intolerance, unstable medical conditions
Monitor	• Monitor for suicidal ideation and risk • Check sodium levels 1 month after starting SSRIs/SNRIs, before switching to another AD owing to poor response/tolerance, or when there are symptoms of hyponatremia (e.g., fatigue, malaise, delirium) • With citalopram: monitor for QTc, discontinue if persistent QTc >500 ms • With TCAs (nortriptyline, desipramine): monitor for postural hypotension, anticholinergic side effects, QTc prolongation, serum drug levels • With mood stabilizers: monitor over time for adverse events • When benzodiazepines must be used to prevent acute withdrawal, consider discontinuation as soon as feasible
Avoid	• Potential for CYP450 drug–drug interactions: fluoxetine, paroxetine, fluvoxamine • Personal/family history of QTc prolongation: citalopram • Active cerebral or other bleeds, history of SIADH/current hyponatremia: SSRIs, SNRIs • ECG conduction abnormalities and postural hypotension: TCAs • TCAs are not first-line treatment owing to side effect profiles (e.g., sedation, orthostatic hypotension, anticholinergic side effects, QTc prolongation, ventricular arrhythmias) • Cognitive and motor side effects: benzodiazepines

AD, antidepressant; CYP450, cytochrome P450; ECG, electrocardiogram; ECT, electro-convulsive treatment; SIADH, syndrome of inappropriate antidiuretic hormone; SNRIs, serotonin norepinephrine reuptake inhibitors; SSRIs, selective serotonin reuptake inhibitors; TCAs, tricyclic antidepressants.

regarding biological, psychological, and social aspects of depression; effective coping strategies; and lifestyle changes that will assist their recovery.

For patients with comorbid dementia and major depressive disorder, clinicians should select antidepressants that have low anticholinergic properties (e.g., citalopram, escitalopram, sertraline, venlafaxine, bupropion). For patients with comorbid dementia and psychotic depression, a combination of antidepressant and antipsychotic medication is usually the first choice.[48] Patients with strokes should be monitored closely for the onset of depression as a common complication of stroke even in those who do not endorse depressive symptoms.[48]

Clinicians should monitor older patients for recurrence of depression during the first 2 years after treatment. Older patients with a first depressive episode who achieve remission should be treated for a minimum of 1 year with their full therapeutic dose.[48] When discontinuing antidepressant treatment after remission of symptoms, a slow taper over months is recommended, with resuming the full therapeutic dose if there are signs of relapse or recurrence. Older patients who have had more than two depressive episodes, or required ECT, should continue to take antidepressant maintenance treatment indefinitely.[48] In long-term care facilities, the response to antidepressant treatment should be evaluated monthly after initial improvement, at quarterly care conferences, and at the annual assessment after remission of depressive symptoms.

WHEN TO REFER TO PSYCHIATRIC CLINIC?

Conditions that should benefit from referral:

• Depressive disorder with suicidal ideation or intent
• Psychotic depression
• Bipolar disorder

Conditions that may benefit from referral:

• Major depressive episode, severe
• Depressive disorder with comorbid substance abuse
• Depressive disorder with comorbid dementia

DEMENTIA
CLINICAL SIGNIFICANCE
Prevalence

The prevalence of the general population aged 60 years or older with all-cause dementia is 5% to 7% in most world regions.[57] The prevalence of dementia rises substantially with age and nearly doubles every 5 years, with approximately 1% to 4% at age 65 years.[58] However, a recent study looking at the participants in the Framingham Heart Study shows that the incidence of dementia has declined over the past three decades, although the factors contributing to this decline have not been fully elucidated.[58] The prevalence of mild cognitive impairment ranges from 2% to 10% at age 65 years[58]; up to 80% of patients with mild cognitive impairment will develop dementia within 6 years.[59] Alzheimer disease is the most common cause of dementia.[60] In clinic samples, vascular dementia is the second most common cause of dementia.[61] Age-adjusted rate of 14.6/1,000 per person-year for vascular dementia compares with 19.2/1,000 per person-year for Alzheimer disease.[62] Frontotemporal dementia represents between 2% and 10% of all patients diagnosed with dementia, depending on studies.[63,64] Its prevalence ranks after Alzheimer dementia and Lewy body dementia and is the leading cause of early-onset dementia in patients younger than 65 years. One study found that Lewy body dementia represented 20% of all cases of dementia, whereas vascular dementia represented 5.6%, respectively.[64]

Economics

It was estimated that in 2010, 35.6 million persons worldwide suffered from dementia, with projected numbers expected to almost double every 20 years, reaching 115.4 million by 2050.[57] Dementia is associated with a significant economic cost and is similar to the financial burden of heart disease and cancer.[65]

Clinical Burden; Medical Comorbidities

The term "dementia" is subsumed under the newly named entity referred to in the *DSM-5* as major neurocognitive disorder.[14] Mild neurocognitive disorder is a *DSM-5*-recognized term for the less severe level of cognitive impairment (also referred to as mild cognitive impairment), considered to be a potential prodrome of dementia.[14] This section reviews the diagnosis, typical clinical presentation, differential diagnosis, and treatment considerations in common types of dementia.

A decline in one or more cognitive domains, along with a concern about cognition on the part of the patient, a knowledgeable informant or the clinician, and performance on an objective cognitive assessment that falls below the expected level or that has been observed to decline over time, characterizes mild cognitive impairment. Core features of mild cognitive impairment and dementia exist on a spectrum of cognitive and functional impairment. Dementia is an acquired cognitive syndrome with an insidious onset, gradual progression, and impairment in two or more cognitive domains sufficient to cause decline in daily function.[14] The cognitive impairment in dementia affects domains of memory and learning, thinking, orientation, language, comprehension, calculation, and judgment, whereas consciousness is not affected. Functional impairment (or a decline in the ability to perform daily activities) is a required criterion for the diagnosis of all-cause dementia[14] (see *Table 20-10* for diagnostic criteria for all-cause dementia). Instrumental activities of daily living (IADLs) typically begin to decline at the stage of mild cognitive impairment and include household chores performance, meal

---

TABLE 20-10 Highlights of the *DSM-5* (*Diagnostic and Statistical Manual of Mental Disorders*, Fifth Edition) Diagnostic Criteria for All-Cause Dementia and the Main Types of Dementia[14]

All-Cause Dementia

- Substantial cognitive impairment in one or more cognitive domains
- Interference with independence in everyday activities
- Cognitive deficits do not occur exclusively in the context of delirium and are not better explained by a major psychiatric disorder
- *Specify:* with or without behavioral disturbance (e.g., psychotic symptoms, mood disturbance, agitation, apathy, other behavioral symptoms)

⇓

Alzheimer Dementia	Frontotemporal Dementia	Dementia with Lewy Bodies	Vascular Dementia

• Criteria for dementia are met
• Insidious onset and gradual progression of impairment in ≥2 cognitive domains
  ○ *Probable* if (1) or (2):
    1. Evidence of causative genetic mutation from family history or genetic testing
    2. All three are present: (1) clear evidence of decline in memory and learning and ≥1 other cognitive domain; (2) progressive, gradual cognitive decline, without extended plateaus; (3) no evidence of mixed etiology
  ○ *Possible* Alzheimer disease is diagnosed if above criteria are not met
	• Criteria for dementia are met
	• Either (1) or (2):
	  1. *Behavioral variant:*
	    a. ≥3 of:
	      • disinhibition
	      • apathy/inertia
	      • loss of sympathy/empathy
	      • perseverative/compulsive/ritualistic behavior
	      • hyperorality/dietary changes
	    b. Decline in social cognition and/or executive abilities
	  2. *Language variant:* decline in speech production, word finding, object naming, grammar, word comprehension
		• Criteria for dementia are met
		• Insidious onset and gradual progression
		  ○ *Core diagnostic features:* (1) fluctuating cognition/variations in attention and alertness; (2) recurrent visual hallucinations, well-formed and detailed; (3) spontaneous parkinsonism (onset after development of cognitive decline)
		  ○ *Suggestive diagnostic features:* (1) meets criteria for REM sleep behavior disorder; (2) severe antipsychotic sensitivity
		  ○ *Probable:* 2 core features, or 1 suggestive feature + ≥1 core features
		  ○ *Possible:* 1 core feature, or ≥1 suggestive features
			• Criteria for dementia are met
			• Probable or possible
			• ≥1 of the following for *probable*:
			  ○ neuroimaging evidence of vascular disease
			  ○ temporal relationship between vascular disease and dementia
			• *Code:* with/without behavioral disturbance
			• *Specify:* mild, moderate, severe

preparation, shopping, driving, using public transportation, and management of finances.[66] Basic activities of daily living (ADLs) are impaired in the moderate to severe stages of dementia and include dressing, grooming, toileting, bathing, ambulating, and eating.[66]

As previously discussed in the sections on Late-life Anxiety Disorders and Late-life Depressive Disorders in this chapter, the cognitive impairment is commonly accompanied, and even preceded, by neuropsychiatric symptoms, described as deterioration in emotional control, social behavior, or motivation. These neuropsychiatric symptoms can be prominent and disabling, affecting almost all patients with dementia in the course of the disease. These include agitation, depression, apathy, delusions, hallucinations, and sleep impairment, which are serious conditions that are increasingly becoming a focus of attention in primary care. These symptoms have serious adverse consequences for patients and caregivers, such as greater impairment in ADLs, cognitive decline, quality of life, caregiver depression, and earlier institutionalization.[67]

Mild cognitive impairment and dementia are on a clinical continuum and affect each patient differently, depending on the patient's premorbid personality. During the phase of mild cognitive impairment, the patient and family commonly notice mild changes in memory and other cognitive abilities that, by definition, have minimal or no impact on the patient's daily activities.[14] Mild cognitive impairment that primarily affects short-term memory is termed *amnestic* mild cognitive impairment and, when progressive, most commonly evolves into Alzheimer-type dementia; mild cognitive impairment involving multiple domains of cognition most commonly progresses to mixed or ischemic vascular dementia. Not all patients with the amnestic mild cognitive impairment progress to dementia, and a longitudinal follow-up is essential.[68] The differentiation of mild cognitive impairment and syndromal dementia is important because cognitive enhancers (see below) are

generally *not* indicated in the mild cognitive impairment phase and do not prevent progression to dementia. In California and Utah in the United States, there is mandatory reporting of dementia to the state, and California physicians can be subject to disciplinary action if they fail to report dementia to the Department of Motor Vehicles. In Canada, the requirement to report drivers who are deemed unfit to drive varies among the provinces. The criterion that the patient's ADLs be minimally affected in mild cognitive impairment can complicate the differentiation between mild cognitive impairment and early dementia, as the intellectual complexity of daily activities, including hobbies, varies from patient to patient. Thus, a chess player whose game deteriorates noticeably may be diagnosed earlier than a patient whose daily regimen consists largely of watching television.

Although the diagnosis of dementia can be straightforward in the moderate to severe stages, it is more difficult to diagnose in the earlier stages and (as noted previously) can be difficult to distinguish from mild cognitive impairment. Other cognitive domains than memory may be impaired first, or exclusively, depending on which parts of the brain are affected by the underlying disease process. According to the *DSM-5*, six cognitive domains can be affected in both mild cognitive impairment and dementia and include learning and memory, language, complex attention, perceptual motor function, executive function, and social cognition.[14]

Figure 20-6 shows the typical clinical characteristics of the four main types of dementia.[14] In typical Alzheimer dementia, the core clinical feature is impaired episodic memory (i.e., the collection of past personal experiences that occurred at a particular time and place) characterized by impaired free recall of recently acquired information that is not normalized by cueing. Amnestic mild cognitive impairment is generally viewed as the precursor stage to Alzheimer dementia.[14]

Alzheimer dementia
Progressive cognitive and functional decline
Amnestic and nonamnestic phenotypes
Early loss of insight
Probable diagnosis: cognitive changes and Alzheimer biomarker evidence required

Vascular dementia
Attentional deficits, slowed processing speed, retrieval difficulties, dysexecutive syndrome, and depression
Symptom overlap with Alzheimer dementia
Stepwise progression and focal neurologic signs
Mild motor signs in subcortical subtype

Types of dementia

Dementia with Lewy bodies
Cognitive changes, movement disorder, visual hallucinations, sleep disturbance, and autonomic changes
Alpha-synuclein deposits present in neurons

Frontotemporal dementia
Early personality and behavior, or language changes
Younger age at onset
Strong familial component
Focal atrophy of frontal/temporal lobes on structural neuroimaging

FIGURE 20-6 Clinical characteristics of the main types of dementia.[14]

Although a cognitive concern by the patient or family/caregiver is usually the main reason for assessment, it is important for clinicians to identify those at risk for vascular dementia. This may help in prevention of further cognitive decline, functional and behavioral changes by controlling vascular risk factors, and lifestyle modification. The presence of cognitive impairment in a patient with a history of stroke or stroke-like event (e.g., transient ischemic attack), affecting neurologic function, should raise suspicion of vascular dementia. Sudden-onset, step-wise decline (although not always present) should raise suspicion of vascular contribution to the cognitive impairment. Small-vessel disease in the periventricular white matter can produce a variant of ischemic vascular dementia that has an insidious onset and slowly progressive course and at times can be difficult to differentiate from Alzheimer disease.

Behavioral variant frontotemporal dementia has a subtle onset with progressive deterioration in behavior and function that generally precede memory impairment.[61] Frontal lobe–associated behavioral changes involve alterations in social conduct, personality, social cognition, and/or executive abilities[14] (see *Table 20-10* for the *DSM-5* diagnostic criteria). Patients may become disinhibited or become apathetic, fail to show appropriate emotional reactions (abulia), be inattentive to personal hygiene, have loss of sympathy and empathy, and engage in repetitive and stereotyped behavior, which may mimic obsessive-compulsive disorder. Hoarding, impaired persistence on tasks, and utilization behavior (i.e., the patients grab and play with objects in their visual field and within reach) can develop.[63] Dietary changes (e.g., ingestion of inedible food, carbohydrate and sweet cravings, binge behavior with food, tobacco, or alcohol) and hyperorality (i.e., excessive compulsions to place items in their mouth) are common. Deficits in executive tasks, such as planning and problem-solving, along with poor judgment and insight, are also common in the earlier stages of the frontotemporal dementia, helping to differentiate it from early Alzheimer or vascular dementia.[14]

The dementia with Lewy bodies is marked by complex and heterogeneous cognitive, other neuropsychiatric, motor, sleep, and autonomic symptoms. The early manifestation of dementia with Lewy bodies may involve a combination of cognitive and/or noncognitive symptoms.

The typical Alzheimer dementia progresses slowly, in which the clinical diagnosis is established approximately 3 years after symptom onset and shows a mean cognitive decline of approximately 3 to 4 Mini-Mental State Examination (MMSE) points per year in untreated patients.[69] The signs and symptoms linked to the phases of all-cause dementia can be understood in three stages, as outlined in *Table 20-11*.[14]

Neurodegenerative dementia is associated with increased mortality. In a study, the median survival of patients with Alzheimer dementia was 5.7 years from initial clinic presentation and 11.8 years since retrospectively determined symptom onset.[70] Frontotemporal dementia has a shorter median survival, which is 3 to 4 years from the time of diagnosis.[71]

TABLE 20-11 Clinical Stages of Dementia[14]

Early stage	Onset is gradual onset is gradual; signs and symptoms often overlooked Common symptoms: forgetfulness of recent events, lost in familiar places, word-finding difficulties, decision-making difficulties, lost interest in activities/hobbies, depression, apathy, unusual anger/aggression on occasion
Moderate stage	Signs and symptoms become clearer, more restricting Common symptoms: increased forgetfulness of recent events and names, lost in familiar places, difficulty with communication, increased assistance with living safely at home, increased assistance with personal care, wandering, repeated questioning, vocalizing, disturbed sleep, hallucinations, disinhibition, aggression
Severe stage	Near full dependence and inactivity Common symptoms: unawareness of time and place, unable to find way around, difficulty recognizing relatives, friends, and familiar objects, bladder/bowel incontinence, increasing need for assisted self-care, difficulty walking, confined to wheelchair/bed, aggression toward caregiver (kicking, hitting)

DIAGNOSIS

Diagnostic Considerations

The cognitively impaired patients may have comorbid psychiatric illness (e.g., depressive disorder). However, neuropsychiatric symptoms of dementia (e.g., depression, apathy) can also occur in all dementia types, but the relative timing of their onset can offer clues to the underlying diagnosis. For example, in frontotemporal dementia, behavioral manifestations of executive dysfunction usually precede memory impairment, and language impairment that exceeds short-term memory dysfunction may reflect a subcortical (vascular) or frontotemporal etiology. Because Alzheimer dementia is the most common type of dementia, it would seem reasonable to assume that cases of presumptive cognitive impairment are actually due to Alzheimer disease. However, this assumption is not always correct, and misdiagnosis can impact management. In advanced old age, a higher proportion of dementias are mixed, e.g., a combination of Alzheimer and vascular pathology. It is now recognized that chronic cerebral ischemia and even moderate closed head injury in older adults can stimulate the formation of neurofibrillary tangles and amyloid deposition that are considered the hallmark of Alzheimer disease.

Dementia can be diagnosed with different degrees of certainty based on the extent of the cognitive deficits and biomarker abnormalities. The diagnostic evaluation of dementia includes a detailed history provided by the patient and a knowledgeable informant, a thorough physical examination, including mental status examination, a standardized neuropsychological testing, or, in its absence, another quantified cognitive assessment.[14] For example, the typical cognitive deficits of Alzheimer dementia are insidious in onset, with early problems noted in episodic (short-term) memory. As the disease progresses, other cognitive domains become impaired (e.g., language, visuospatial, executive function). The diagnosis of dementia can be complex, especially when atypical presentations occur. Primary care physicians can refer patients with frontotemporal dementia, rapid cognitive decline, and atypical dementia presentations to a geriatric psychiatrist, geriatrician, or neurologist to identify or confirm the diagnosis and to assist in coordinating a plan of care for patients, their caregivers, and their primary care clinicians.

Clinical History

Patients with dementia may have reduced insight and underestimate the problem, which emphasizes the importance to obtain a history from a knowledgeable informant as well as the patient. Inconsistencies in the history obtained from the patient and the informant can provide useful clues. It is important to exclude whether medication (prescribed or over-the-counter) contributes to the patient's cognitive deficit. A family history of dementia, with the age of onset, should also be noted. Because family members may be reluctant to provide historical information that could upset the patient, it is helpful to interview the caregiver separately. One tactic is to ask the caregiver to leave the examination room so that a medical assistant can take full orthostatic vital signs, allowing 6 to 10 minutes alone with the caregiver. Extended history taking in service of care planning for a patient with cognitive impairment is reimbursed by the U.S. Centers for Medicare and Medicaid under the new CPT billing code, G0505, which can be used in conjunction with chronic care management CPT codes.[72] Because family caregivers of patients with dementia commonly experience considerable caregiver stress with high rates of depression, the time spent alone with the family member can be used to assess their overall coping with the caregiver role and can provide an opportunity to educate them regarding community-based services such as adult day health care and long-term care options suitable for the patient.

Physical Examination

Physical examination should address weight loss, nutritional status, dehydration, cardiovascular disease, cerebrovascular disease, and metabolic illness. Neurologic examination should include sensory function, gait assessment, frontal release signs, focal neurologic deficits, and movement disorders.[73] In early Alzheimer disease, the neurologic examination should be normal; if neurologic findings are present, the diagnosis of probable Alzheimer disease should be questioned. The exception is cranial nerve I, subserving olfaction. Patients with early Alzheimer disease, and often pre-Alzheimer patients still in the phase of mild cognitive impairment, may lose the ability to recognize familiar smells. To test olfactory sense, the patient, with eyes closed, can be asked to identify the smell of freshly ground coffee kept in a sealed container for that purpose.

Frontal physical signs (e.g., primitive reflexes—snout, suck, rooting, grasp; paratonia) are common in frontotemporal dementia. A visual field defect or parkinsonian features may suggest a vascular dementia or dementia with Lewy bodies. In those with severe cognitive impairment, cataract-related loss of visual acuity can increase visual hallucinations, which needs evaluation.[74] Optimizing hearing function may reduce sensory deprivation that may contribute to cognitive impairment.

Mental status examination should include a formal assessment of cognitive function. Depression rating scales are recommended to assist in differentiating major depressive disorder from dementia and in monitoring response to antidepressants. Suicide risk assessment (see the section on Late-life Depressive Disorders in this chapter) should be integrated in the clinical examination because suicide risk increases in the older adults.

Cognitive Assessment

Table 20-12 summarizes common brief screening cognitive tests utilized in primary practice. Many brief cognitive tests have been utilized in primary care, including GPCOG and Mini-Cog.[75,76] While the MMSE is probably the most popular cognitive screening tool widely used by clinicians, it does not evaluate executive function. The Montreal Cognitive Assessment (MoCA), available on the World Wide Web in multiple languages, screens all the cognitive domains and has been validated as a screening tool for mild cognitive disorder.[77] The Mini-Cog[78] is a brief screening instrument suitable for the outpatient setting that involves drawing a clock and recalling 3 items. When abnormal, it should be followed by a more in-depth assessment like the MoCA. Other brief cognitive tests include the verbal fluency test (e.g., semantic—animals or fruits; or phonemic—words that begin with letter F; and having the patient name as many items as possible in 1 minute); and the "go, no-go" test (e.g., the patient is instructed to tap once if the examiner taps once and to not tap if the examiner taps twice). Serial administrations of the cognitive test can quantify the progress of the disease.

A cooperative patient is required in these performance-based tests. However, the overall score is often less important than the pattern of scoring. Scoring perfectly on a cognitive screening test does not preclude the diagnosis of cognitive disorder, and a single test may not suffice, especially when an older adult has learning difficulties, a lower education level, or a language barrier. Highly educated patients with dementia may have normal scores but have deficiencies in insight, judgment, and other areas of cognitive function. Attention and motivation deficits due to anxiety and depressive disorders can influence cognitive test results. Collateral information from a knowledgeable informant thus is critical.

Investigations

There are no specific laboratory tests to diagnose dementia during life. Laboratory investigations are helpful to rule out other factors that may be contributing to the cognitive impairment, such as hypothyroidism and low vitamin B_{12}. As part of the workup for cognitive impairment, most

TABLE 20-12 Common Brief Screening Tests for Cognitive Impairment in the Primary Care Patients[75,76]

ABBREVIATION	TEST NAME	COMMENTS
CDT	Clock Drawing Test	Quick to administer; offers limited assessment; less influenced by education and culture than is MMSE/MoCA; detects moderate Alzheimer dementia in primary care
VFC	Verbal Fluency Categories	Measure of executive function, language, semantic memory; influenced by education
Mini-Cog	Mini-Cog	Combines three-term registration and recall with clock drawing
MIS	Memory Impairment Screen	Easily administered, even to illiterate patients
GPCOG	General Practitioner Assessment of Cognition	Includes informant questions
TMT	Trail Making Test	Measures cognitive abilities of speed and fluid intelligence
MoCA	Montreal Cognitive Assessment	Detects mild cognitive impairment; MMSE score of 24 is equivalent to MoCA of 18 to detect mild cognitive impairment.[76]
MMSE	Mini-Mental State Examination	Cutoff score 23/24; takes longer to administer; assesses patients presenting with memory deficits, but limited sensitivity to frontal and subcortical changes; influenced by age/education

guidelines recommend checking laboratory studies for thyroid-stimulating hormone (TSH), vitamin B$_{12}$, folate, and a rapid plasma reagin (RPR), if indicated. In recent years, the incidence of tertiary syphilis has risen, especially among men with HIV, making this screening test relevant once again. Other laboratory studies that may be additionally helpful include vitamin D, ammonia, and thiamine, depending on the medical comorbidities such as lack of sun exposure, cirrhosis, and malnutrition, respectively. Vitamin D receptors are found throughout the body including the brain, but the association with dementia remains controversial. For the diagnosis of Alzheimer dementia, biomarkers include characteristic patterns of hypometabolism seen on positron emission tomography and elevated levels of tau and decreased levels beta-amyloid in the cerebrospinal fluid. However, these tests remain largely experimental, and more work is needed to define how these results can be routinely applied to patients in the clinical setting. Neuroimaging (structural and functional) is used in clinical practice to rule out other causes of cognitive impairment, such as a brain tumor or vascular disease, and to identify characteristic changes that suggest Alzheimer dementia (e.g., hippocampal atrophy) or another cause of dementia. Magnetic resonance imaging (MRI) with gadolinium contrast is required for accurate hippocampal evaluation and to evaluate for small lacunar infarcts and the extent of periventricular white matter hyperintensities (reflecting small-vessel ischemia). In a patient with the triad of cognitive impairment, urinary incontinence, and a broad-based or "magnetic" gait (with or without a history of falls), either a computed tomography (CT) or MRI scan can be used to look for ventriculomegaly out of proportion to cortical atrophy, suggesting normal pressure hydrocephalus. The electroencephalogram (EEG) has little diagnostic value in Alzheimer dementia because of expected diffuse slowing, unless EEG is performed to rule in or out rare causes of dementia, such as the rapidly progressive prion disease,

Creutzfeldt–Jakob disease. Formal neuropsychological testing by a psychologist can establish the pattern and degree of cognitive impairment when diagnostic uncertainty remains, such as in patients who perform well on screening tests but whose family reports declines in performance in daily intellectual tasks such as handling finances.

Biomarkers (e.g., neuroimaging, cerebrospinal fluid proteins) have considerable overlap among Alzheimer dementia, other types of dementia, and cognitively normal older adults, and cannot serve as specific diagnostic features.[79] The most accurate and definite diagnosis is typically obtained from the biopsy-related histologic examination; however, biopsy is not indicated owing to a high risk/benefit ratio.[79] Brain autopsy serves as the "gold standard" for the definite diagnosis of dementia.[79]

For diagnosis of Alzheimer disease, neuropathologic findings of extracellular beta-amyloid plaques and intraneuronal tau-containing neurofibrillary tangles are the gold standard. The association of the age of onset, family history, and genetic makeup strengthens the diagnosis. The association of the apolipoprotein E e4 allele with Alzheimer dementia is significant; however, apolipoprotein E genotyping is neither fully specific nor sensitive to be used alone as a diagnostic test for Alzheimer dementia.[80]

Differential Diagnosis

Most causes of confusion in older adults can usually be determined based on the history, medication review, physical examination, including mental status examination, and laboratory evaluation. One of the most important diagnoses to rule out is delirium. Typical delirium has disturbances of attention and consciousness, with an acute onset and fluctuating course, which are hallmarks of delirium.[14] Delirium should be considered a medical emergency, regardless of whether the patient is agitated (hyperactive delirium) or calm and/or somnolent (hypoactive delirium); both can be a central nervous system manifestation of a potentially serious infection, metabolic derangement, or organ system injury and require urgent evaluation and management in the emergency department or acute care hospital. In this section, we have focused on the evaluation and management of dementia, which is one of the most important predisposing factors for delirium.[14]

Other differential diagnosis in dementia includes psychiatric disorders (e.g., anxiety, depressive, psychotic, and substance-related disorders), brain infection, thyroid disease, vitamin deficiencies (e.g., B_{12}, thiamine), metabolic disease, brain tumors, and cerebrovascular disease.[81] Developmental intellectual disability, although it may have features suggestive of Alzheimer disease, does not constitute a dementia. Frontotemporal dementia, Lewy body dementia, Parkinson disease dementia, normal pressure hydrocephalus, and Korsakoff syndrome may all be mistaken for Alzheimer dementia.[82] Patients with progressive supranuclear palsy often present with cognitive and behavioral changes in the later stages, which can resemble Alzheimer disease, although the neurologic symptoms (upward and lower gaze palsy and parkinsonism) provide distinguishing features.

BIOPSYCHOSOCIAL TREATMENT

Overview of Treatment

There is currently no cure for any type of dementia, although the progression of infection-associated dementia, such as caused by tertiary syphilis and HIV, can be arrested by appropriate antibiotic and antiretroviral treatment, respectively. For other dementias, treatment remains symptomatic, although novel treatments in various stages of clinical trials are being investigated. Because the pathologic processes seen in Alzheimer disease may develop as early as a decade before the development of clinical symptoms, currently approved treatments may be "too little, too late." As the dementia progresses, the loss of functional independence, first in instrumental activities of daily living (e.g., bill paying, shopping), then in basic activities of daily living (e.g., toileting, bathing), requires increasing amounts of caregiver time. An important part of the primary care of a dementing illness is monitoring changes in functional status and corresponding caregiver burden. Although many families want to keep their loved one at home until the end, caregiving, often performed by an elderly spouse, may exceed the caregiver's abilities and require that the patient be institutionalized. The primary care clinician therefore should be familiar with the family's network of primary and secondary caregivers (i.e., spouse, children, paid in-home support services) and the availability of resources to pay for long-term care. Either directly or through a referral to a social worker, the primary care clinician should educate the family about the spectrum of long-term care resources in the community, so that counseling with regard to placement can reflect

a balance between the patient's and family's wishes, what is needed, and what they can afford. Families should be counseled to investigate long-term care options *before* there is an emergent need. The thought of institutionalizing a family member often triggers guilt as well as anxiety about the quality of care, and institutionalization of a family member furthermore may be frowned upon from a cultural or social perspective. A physician's recommendation of institutionalization because of care or safety issues sometimes can assuage the family's sense of guilt.

Early diagnosis of dementia helps both the patient and family begin the process of planning for the future. An integral part of planning entails becoming educated in the natural history of the dementia. In North America, patients and families can be referred to the website of the U.S. Alzheimer's Association or the Alzheimer Society of Canada (or to a local branch) for information about the stages and what to expect.[83,84] Clinicians and family members should clarify the goals of care for the patient at each clinical stage; this includes discussing advance directives for end-of-life care.

A large part of the longitudinal care of dementia in the primary care setting entails screening for and managing behavioral complications of the neuropsychiatric symptoms, including agitation and its common forms of manifestation (see *Figure 20-7*), which affect up to 90% of demented patients during the course of their illness.[85] Behavioral issues add to the burden of caregiving, pose a risk factor for elder mistreatment, and constitute a major reason for institutionalization. *Figure 20-8* outlines a summary flowchart for the identification and management of distressing behaviors in dementia.

Psychopharmacology

Cholinergic and glutamatergic deficiencies are implicated in Alzheimer dementia, cholinergic deficits in Lewy body dementia, and serotonergic and dopaminergic deficiencies in frontotemporal dementia, although the exact biochemical basis of these dementias is not well understood. All currently approved treatment is classified as a "cognitive enhancer"; none have been shown to arrest or slow progression, and the effects tend to be small. However, even when the slope of decline is not affected, optimizing the patient's cognitive and functional status has the potential for delaying loss of cognitive and self-care skills that affect the patient's quality of life and the amount of caregiving needed.[86] Cholinergic neurotransmission plays an important role in learning and memory; treatment with cholinesterase inhibitors (donepezil, rivastigmine, and galantamine) has shown modest effects in clinical trials.[24] Glutamate is also required for memory and learning. Memantine has a low-affinity antagonism to N-methyl-D-aspartate (NMDA)-type receptors, which may prevent excitatory amino acid neurotoxicity. Evidence is minimal for a benefit of memantine in mild to moderate stages of Alzheimer dementia.[87] In a study of combining memantine treatment to patients with moderate to severe Alzheimer dementia already receiving donepezil,

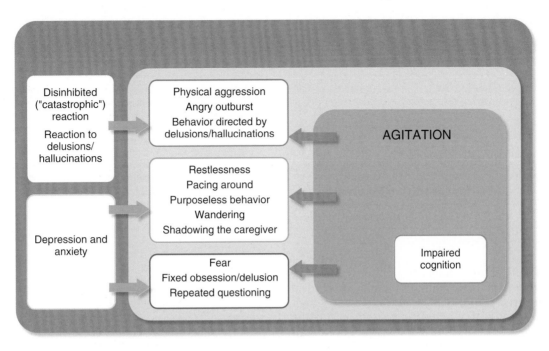

FIGURE 20-7 Common clinical manifestations of agitation in dementia.

there were statistically significant additional benefits on measures of cognition, ADLs, and global outcome and behavior, and it was well tolerated.[88]

No cognitive enhancers have been approved for treatment of mild cognitive impairment. The three cholinesterase inhibitors are approved by the U.S. Food and Drug Administration (FDA) as monotherapy for the symptomatic treatment of patients with mild to moderate Alzheimer dementia, and donepezil for the severe stage of illness, in particular. Rivastigmine is FDA approved for the treatment of mild to moderate Parkinson disease dementia. Memantine is approved by the U.S. FDA for the treatment of patients with moderate to severe Alzheimer dementia. Galantamine has been used for

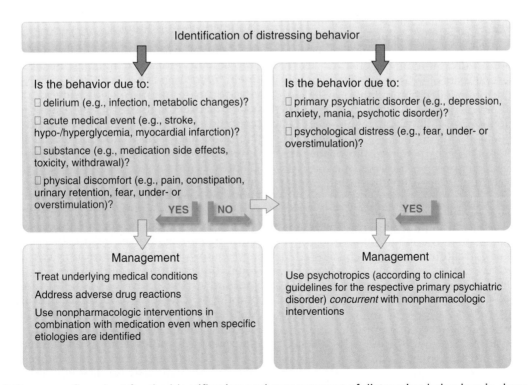

FIGURE 20-8 Summary flowchart for the identification and management of distressing behaviors in dementia.

TABLE 20-13	Common Medication Classes for Treatment of Dementia				
	First Line			**Second Line**	
Medications	Antipsychotic (preferable second generation)	Antidepressant (preferably SSRI)	Cholinesterase inhibitor and/or memantine	Mood stabilizer (divalproex, carbamazepine)	Centrally acting beta-blocker
			⇓		
Indications	Reactions to delusions Depression and anxiety	Depression and anxiety Disinhibited ("catastrophic") reaction	Impaired cognition	Disinhibited ("catastrophic") reaction	Depression and anxiety

SSRI, selective serotonin reuptake inhibitor.

the treatment of vascular dementia, while rivastigmine for the treatment of Lewy body dementia. In clinical practice, the three cholinesterase inhibitors are generally used interchangeably based on tolerance and the convenience of administration. For example, donepezil can be administered once daily; rivastigmine is available in a patch for patients unwilling or unable to take by mouth. Many clinicians will prescribe memantine in early Alzheimer disease when a cholinesterase inhibitor cannot be used. *This textbook does not endorse off-label use of any cognitive enhancer.*

Because of their cholinergic properties, all cholinesterase inhibitors can slow heart rate. Therefore, cholinesterase inhibitors should be used cautiously in patients with bradycardia (heart rate <65 beats/minute), concomitant use of a beta-blocker, or a history of syncope.

There are four main domains that clinicians need to discuss with the patient or substitute decision-maker when prescribing cognitive enhancers for dementia: set realistic treatment expectations, address possible side effects, consider when to switch, and consider when to discontinue medications. Switching agents for loss of response after several years of treatment with a cognitive enhancer is not recommended because this usually indicates the natural progression of the disease stage rather than loss of response. Addition of memantine, rather than switching to a second cholinesterase inhibitor, is a more reasonable option. The patient or his or her substitute decision-maker must be informed of the risks and benefits of continuation versus discontinuation of treatment. When a medication is discontinued because of a perceived lack of effectiveness, the dose should be tapered and stopped, with monitoring over the following 1 to 3 months. If there is evidence of an observable decline, reinstating treatment may be considered if feasible.[89]

Table 20-13 shows common first-line and second-line medication classes utilized in the treatment of dementia. Additionally, *Table 20-4* presents some characteristics of the cognitive enhancers for cognitive symptoms and psychotropic medications for neuropsychiatric symptoms of dementia in patients who fail to respond to nonpharmacologic interventions.[1,8,20-25]

Psychopharmacology Pearls

- Cholinesterase inhibitors should be used cautiously in patients with bradycardia, concomitant use of a beta-blocker, or a history of syncope.
- Switching agents for loss of response after several years of treatment with a cognitive enhancer is not recommended because this usually indicates the natural progression of the disease stage rather than loss of response.
- Many clinicians will prescribe memantine in early Alzheimer disease when a cholinesterase inhibitor cannot be used.

Behavioral Approaches

In primary care setting, family and caregivers are key collaborators and need to be involved in treatment planning. The first line of treatment should always be to identify and address the underlying cause or precipitant of the distressing behavior whenever possible (e.g., pain, constipation, infection). Nonpharmacologic treatment should be the primary intervention for patients with dementia and neuropsychiatric symptoms (e.g., agitation, depression, anxiety, apathy, delusions, hallucinations, sleep impairment), and clinicians and caregivers must be knowledgeable about and respond promptly and appropriately to address the patient's needs while searching for the most likely trigger (see *Figure 20-8* on identification and management of behaviors). The nonpharmacologic interventions should always be considered first, tailored to the individual patient, and their impact should be carefully monitored through the use of standardized behavioral assessment tools such as the Cohen-Mansfield Agitation Inventory.[90] The nonpharmacologic interventions are summarized in *Table 20-14* and, although used in randomized clinical trials, they are not exhaustive and should only be considered

TABLE 20-14 Summary of the Nonpharmacologic Interventions for Neuropsychiatric Symptoms of Dementia, by Category[91]

CATEGORY	INTERVENTION
Structured activities	Recreational activities Physical activities Outdoor walks
Sensory stimulation/ relaxation	Massage and touch Individualized music Controlled multisensory stimulation Art therapy Aromatherapy
Social contact (real or simulated)	Individualized social contact Pet therapy Simulated interactions/family videos
Behavioral therapy	Differential reinforcement Stimulus control
Environmental modifications	Remove clutter and unnecessary objects Use labeling or other visual cues Reduced stimulation Light therapy
Training and development	Training programs for family caregivers Staff education Staff support

once thorough assessment has been completed.[91] The nonpharmacologic interventions should be utilized in combination with medication, even when specific etiologies are identified. The clinician must educate the patient and family caregiver that a particular strategy may be effective for one patient but not for another. This is because any specific strategy may not have been evaluated for effectiveness in all dementia patients with the same presenting behavior problem.[91]

Other Treatment Considerations

Legal issues should be addressed early in the disease course and include discussion for completion of durable power of attorney and advance directives.[92] The patient's decisional capacity must be assessed each time a medical decision is needed. Addressing the patient's driving ability is paramount; driving evaluations may be repeated at least every 6 months. A road competency test may be needed if there is unclear clinical assessment. Clinicians need to comply with the local disclosure laws to motor vehicle departments regarding notification of patients with impaired driving due to cognitive impairment.[89] Working with family is crucial because the car keys or the automobile may need to be removed. The patient may ultimately progress into disease when full supervision at home to preserve safety is necessary. Placement to a skilled nursing facility that specializes in the care of patients with dementia usually follows.

Education, Prevention, Treatment Adherence Issues

Early education about diagnosis and treatment, with regular follow-ups scheduled at least every 3 months, is necessary. Every visit should include assessment of whether the patient can still safely live at home. Monitoring response to nonpharmacologic strategies may require more frequent visits. Events that trigger problematic behaviors should be identified and minimized.[89] Psychiatric admission can be considered for severely agitated, aggressive, psychotic, or suicidal patients, but the availability of inpatient psychiatry for dementia-related psychiatric disorders varies, based on health insurance and the number of psychiatric beds in the community. In the United States, Medicare does not cover psychiatric hospitalization for dementia-related psychiatric disorders, with the result that patients may require admission to an acute care hospital with psychiatric consultation. Primary caregivers have an increased risk of burnout and depression, which requires screening for and strategies to prevent depression by facilitating respite care opportunities (e.g., employing an in-home caregiver, attending an adult senior center).

WHEN TO REFER TO PSYCHIATRIC CLINIC?

- Rapidly progressive Alzheimer dementia (>4 MMSE points/6 months) where the diagnosis is uncertain
- Rapid clinical decline in known Alzheimer patients who should be reassessed for comorbid conditions
- Atypical presentations (early onset, nonamnestic presentations, early motor signs, seizures, apathy, and psychotic symptoms)
- Presence of neuropsychiatric symptoms that cannot be explained by the typical course of the underlying dementia

CASES AND QUESTIONS

CASE 1: The Anxious Mrs. A

Mrs. A is a 78-year-old retired teacher who lives alone in an apartment since her spouse died 2 years ago. She complains to you, her primary care physician, about extreme fatigue and sleep difficulties. Six months ago she fell and sustained a left intertrochanteric hip fracture after tripping over the doormat while walking outside the building. She underwent open reduction and internal fixation followed by 4 weeks of rehabilitation and is now able to walk but she has developed multiple fears associated with falling. She is afraid she will lose her balance and fall again, and that she may "faint" (although she does not feel dizzy) when alone, and consequently she no longer goes out by herself. She now insists that one of her children accompany her on the rare occasion when she goes out shopping. She describes herself as always being nervous, which has worsened since the death of her spouse. She does not use illicit substances or alcohol. She takes chlorthalidone for hypertension and acetaminophen (paracetamol) as needed for pain related to her osteoarthritis. She worries about the future and her health and has difficulty initiating sleep because of her concerns. In addition, she feels impatient with her children and grandchildren, easily irritable, tense, and on edge when they come to visit her.

1. What are the working diagnoses?
   A. Generalized anxiety disorder, agoraphobia, and specific phobia (fear of falling)
   B. Generalized anxiety disorder, panic disorder, and bereavement
   C. Major depressive disorder, panic disorder, and agoraphobia
   D. Specific phobia, major depressive disorder, chronic pain
   E. Agoraphobia, panic disorder, specific phobia (fear of falling)

   Correct answer: A. *Generalized anxiety disorder and specific phobias are common in older adults. Fear of falling is specific to older adults, with high rates and significant distress and functional impairment. As in this case, her fear of falling and its impact on her daily function would be similar in presentation to agoraphobia in the more severe manifestation. As in this case, agoraphobia can follow a traumatic event such as a fall. The fear of falling is much more common among older than younger adults (e.g., 60% of those who have previously fallen). Therefore, her diagnoses are generalized anxiety disorder, agoraphobia, and specific phobia (fear of falling).*

2. Mrs. A is adamant that she would not wish to initiate an antidepressant trial. What is the next step?
   A. She is willing to start CBT.
   B. She is only interested in short visits with her primary care physician to check her physical status.
   C. She requests information about naturopath remedies for anxiety.
   D. She demands that she receives alprazolam, as her friend told her to take.
   E. She believes eating healthy and regular exercising is the treatment.

   Correct answer: A. *CBT in older adults with generalized anxiety disorder is associated with improvements in worry severity. CBT for anxiety disorder is based on behavioral exposure to anxiety-provoking objects or situations, cognitive restructuring, and modifying avoidance behaviors.*

3. If Mrs. A is interested in medications, which of the following is relatively contraindicated?
   A. Buspirone
   B. Sertraline
   C. Bupropion
   D. Venlafaxine
   E. Escitalopram

   Correct answer: C. *Of the choices, bupropion does not have regulatory approval for anxiety disorders and is relatively contraindicated, as bupropion use is associated with increase in anxiety. SSRIs, SNRIs, and buspirone are reasonable to initiate as treatment options.*

CASE 2: The Depressed Mr. D

Mr. D is an 84-year-old man, recently diagnosed with stage D prostate cancer with several metastases to his thoracic and lumbar vertebrae. He has been started on androgen deprivation therapy, with a marked reduction in his serum prostate-specific androgen from 34 to 2.4 ng/mL (μg/L). He confides in you, his new primary care physicians, of his wish to die. He reports that he no longer enjoys anything in his life, he wakes up at 4:00 am and is unable to return to sleep, feels fatigued, has poor appetite, with a 35-lb weight loss, and has difficulty concentrating and making decisions. He is living alone at home, has a limited social network, and no formal supports. Mr. D has one daughter living nearby who is supportive. His back pain has slightly improved with a recently started opioid analgesic, but his insomnia and fatigue persist as does his poor appetite. He has not shaved in over 2 weeks.

Upon your examination, he appears disheveled and describes his mood as "alright." He particularly denies feeling depressed and attributes his insomnia to bone pain and the rest of his symptoms to his cancer. When asked to elaborate about his death wish, he replies that he has felt lonely since the death of his wife 3 months previously, is tired of living, and is ready to die. His affect is blunted. He becomes tearful when discussing his late wife. There is no evidence of psychotic symptoms. He is alert and oriented to the four spheres (person, space, time, and circumstances). He scores 27 out of 30 on the Montreal Cognitive Assessment (MoCA); he lost a point each on the Trails Making Test Part B, attention, and delayed recall. He refuses to complete the clock drawing test. His PHQ-9 score is 20 (consistent with severe depression). A physical examination shows mild temporalis muscle wasting and decreased strength but no focal motor abnormalities concerning for spinal cord compression. His laboratory investigations are remarkable for mild anemia (hemoglobin, 11.5 g/dL [115 g/L]) and an albumin of 2.8 g/dL (28 g/L). Electrocardiogram shows normal sinus rhythm. There are no other medical disorders or medication problems that could have contributed to his presentation.

1. What is the diagnosis?

    A. Anxiety disorder
    B. Mild neurocognitive disorder
    C. Posttraumatic stress disorder
    D. Persistent complex bereavement disorder
    E. Major depressive disorder

    Correct answer: E. *Mr. D's diagnosis is major depressive disorder.*

2. Although initially reluctant, Mr. D agrees to start an antidepressant. Which antidepressant is proposed?

    A. Bupropion
    B. Citalopram
    C. Mirtazapine
    D. Amitriptyline
    E. Trazodone

    Correct answer: C. *Activating antidepressants (e.g., bupropion) should be avoided because they may worsen anxiety symptoms. Tricyclic antidepressant (amitriptyline), although potentially effective, is associated with anticholinergic and cardiac toxicity, and is generally avoided in order patients. Trazodone can be used for anxiety-related insomnia but can add to the serotonin burden in patients simultaneously using drugs with serotonergic effects (e.g., the analgesic tramadol, or an SSRI or SNRI). Citalopram is a reasonable first-choice antidepressant, but it may interfere with the QTc and serum sodium. Because of his history of insomnia, anorexia, and weight loss, mirtazapine is most appropriate course of action.*

3. Mr. D is being seen in follow-up every 1 to 2 weeks to ensure treatment adherence, address any adverse effects, and complete serial depression scales to document response to treatment. After 8 weeks of antidepressant therapy, on a repeated MoCA, he scores 30 out of 30 and his PHQ-9 score is 3 (full remission of depression). He now understands that he has the potential for sustained remission from his prostate cancer and wants to enjoy whatever time he has remaining but still worries about dying alone. What is the best course of psychotherapy in his case?

    A. Managing cancer and living meaningfully (CALM)
    B. Cognitive behavioral therapy (CBT)
    C. Supportive therapy
    D. Interpersonal psychotherapy (IPT)
    E. Problem-solving therapy

    Correct answer: A. *Although CBT and other nonpharmacologic treatment options are suitable choices for this patient, access to these varies according to insurance coverage and the availability of trained physicians. However, the psychotherapeutic intervention called "managing cancer and living meaningfully" (CALM) addresses areas in patients with terminal or potentially terminal disease with the goals of decreasing death anxiety and depressive symptoms and improving spiritual well-being; therefore, the most suitable option is A.*

CASE 3: The Confused Mr. C

Mrs. C asked you for an urgent house call to see her husband, a 79-year-old man with mild cognitive impairment (with an MMSE of 27 out of 30, and a clock drawing test with visuospatial and constructional deficits, both done 1 year previously). He has developed parkinsonism and had repeated falls over the past 6 months. During the previous night, Mr. C became suddenly more confused, agitated, and attempted to leave the house. He endorsed vivid visual hallucinations of children running into his room whom he believed were lost and Mr. C was attempting to find their parents. There was no previous history of depressive or psychotic disorder. A medication review indicated that Mr. C did not take any antiparkinsonian medication, but he recently started to take over-the-counter dimenhydrinate for insomnia. Upon your current assessment, MMSE is now 0, and Mr. C is mostly uncooperative with the examination. You are unable to perform a physical examination owing to his agitation.

1. What is the working diagnosis?

    A. An acute worsening of his cognitive impairment, perceptual disturbances, and psychomotor agitation, in keeping with a diagnosis of delirium
    B. Alzheimer dementia
    C. Parkinson disease dementia
    D. Recurrent major depressive disorder, with psychotic symptoms
    E. Psychotic disorder

    Correct answer: A. *A delirium superimposed on a mild cognitive impairment or dementia with Lewy bodies would be plausible; however, Parkinson disease dementia is improbable because of his cognitive impairment (visuospatial and constructional deficits) predating the parkinsonism. Early parkinsonism excludes a diagnosis of Alzheimer dementia. He has no history of depressive or psychotic episodes, which make these diagnoses unlikely. Mr. C is likely suffering from a delirium caused by the anticholinergic medication (dimenhydrinate).*

2. You send Mr. C to the local hospital for further evaluation. Physical and laboratory workups prove negative. Although there is some improvement with the discontinuation of dimenhydrinate (an anticholinergic medication that has triggered delirium), his agitation remains uncontrolled the following day. What is the next course of action?

    A. Quetiapine 12.5 mg at bedtime
    B. Lorazepam 1 mg twice daily
    C. Haloperidol 1 mg at bedtime
    D. Chlorpromazine 25 mg at bedtime
    E. Trazodone 25 mg twice daily

    Correct answer: A. *Chlorpromazine has anticholinergic properties, and therefore it is contraindicated in delirium. Lorazepam is also*

continued

contraindicated in delirium, except for alcohol and benzodiazepine withdrawal syndromes and delirium due to neuroleptic malignant syndrome. Haloperidol is considered gold-standard symptomatic treatment for delirium; however, the geriatric dose is lower than in option C and generally not tolerated in cases of parkinsonism. Although trazodone may help with general agitation, it is not the traditional medication for delirium. Owing to the patient's parkinsonism, a low-dose quetiapine (12.5 to 25 mg QD or BID) can be considered in view of symptomatic treatment of agitation owing to delirium triggered by an anticholinergic medication.

3. His confusion and agitation slowly improve over the next week, and his visual hallucinations become less frequent and troubling to him. His MMSE score is now 23 out of 30, although the clock drawing test remains abnormal. On examination, his affect is euthymic, and his parkinsonism remains unchanged. What is the probable diagnosis?

   A. Dementia with Lewy bodies
   B. Alzheimer dementia
   C. Mild cognitive impairment
   D. Major depressive disorder
   E. Frontotemporal dementia

   Correct answer: A *Based on the history provided, there is no indication of personality or behavioral changes to suggest frontotemporal dementia, neither a depressed mood to suggest major depressive disorder. The presence of early parkinsonism excludes Alzheimer disease. The current MMSE score of 23 out of 30 excludes a mild cognitive impairment. Because of the presence of cognitive impairment (visuospatial deficits), persistent visual hallucinations, and parkinsonism, the probable diagnosis is dementia with Lewy bodies.*

PRACTICAL RESOURCES

- **The Well**: https://thewellhealth.ca
  A tool to support primary care physicians in reducing harm in patients who exhibit signs, symptoms, or behaviors suggestive of a psychiatric disorder. Considerations and resources are included in the tool to aid in decision-making. For example, this article on keeping patients safe: https://thewell-health.ca/wp-content/uploads/2017/03/CEP_MHA_V1.pdf and this discussion aid for assessing functional impairments: https://thewellhealth.ca/wp-content/uploads/2017/01/Assessing-Functional-Impairments-Discussion-Aid.pdf
- **National Institute on Aging**: https://www.nia.nih.gov/
  Provides an initiative on aging well and offers strategic directions for research on aging

- **Canadian Coalition for Seniors' Mental Health**: http://ccsmh.ca/projects/depression/
  Provides tools for health care professionals for the assessment and treatment of depression in older adults
- **Alzheimer's Association**: https://www.alz.org
  The Alzheimer's Association is the U.S. leading health organization in Alzheimer's care, support, and research
- **Alzheimer Society**: http://www.alzheimer.ca/en
  The Alzheimer Society is working nationwide to improve the quality of life for Canadians affected by Alzheimer disease and other dementias and advance the search for the cause and effective treatment

REFERENCES

1. Lenze EJ, Wetherell JL. A lifespan view of anxiety disorders. *Dialogues Clin Neurosci.* 2011;13(4):381-399.
2. Krasucki C, Howard R, Mann A. Anxiety and its treatment in the elderly. *Int Psychogeriatr.* 1999;11:25-45.
3. McCurry SM, Gibbons LE, Logsdon RG, et al. Anxiety and nighttime behavioural disturbances. Awakenings in patients with Alzheimer's disease. *J Gerontol Nurs.* 2004;30:12-20.
4. Lépine JP. The epidemiology of anxiety disorders: prevalence and societal costs. *J Clin Psychiatry.* 2002;63(suppl 14):4-8.
5. DeBours E, Beekman A, Geerlings S, et al. On becoming depressed or anxious in late life: similar vulnerability factors but different effects of stressful life events. *Br J Psychiatry.* 2001;179:426-431.
6. Lenze EJ, Karp JF, Mulsant BH, et al. Somatic symptoms in late-life anxiety: treatment issues. *J Geriatr Psychiatry Neurol.* 2005;18:89-96.
7. Gibbons LE, Teri L, Logsdon R, et al. Anxiety symptoms as predictors of nursing home placement in patients with Alzheimer's disease. *J Clin Geropsychol.* 2002;4:335-342.
8. Bassil N, Ghandour A, Grossberg GT. How anxiety presents differently in older adults. *Current Psychiatry.* 2011;10(3):65-72.
9. Alcalde Tirado P. Fear of falling. *Rev Esp Geriatr Gerontol.* 2010;45(1):38-44.
10. Cairney J, McCabe L, Veldhuizen S, et al. Epidemiology of social phobia in later life. *Am J Geriatr Psychiatry.* 2007;15(3):224-233.
11. McCabe L, Cairney J, Veldhuizen S, et al. Prevalence and correlates of agoraphobia in older adults. *Am J Geriatr Psychiatry.* 2006;14(6):515-522.
12. Chacko RC, Corbin MA, Harper RG. Acquired obsessive-compulsive disorder associated with basal ganglia lesions. *J Neuropsychiatry Clin Neurosci.* 2000;12:269-272.
13. Mittal D, Torres R, Abashidze A, et al. Worsening of post-traumatic stress disorder symptoms with cognitive decline: case series. *J Geriatr Psychiatry Neurol.* 2001;14(1):17-20.

14. American Psychiatric Association. *Diagnostic and Statistical Manual of Mental Disorders.* 5th ed. Arlington, VA: American Psychiatric Publishing; 2013.

15. Kressig R, Wolf SL, Sattin RW, et al. Associations of demographic, functional, and behavioral characteristics with activity-related fear of falling among older adults transitioning to frailty. *Age Ageing.* 2001:1456-1462.

16. Kroenke K, Spitzer RL, Williams JB, Löwe B. The patient health questionnaire somatic, anxiety, and depressive symptom scales: a systematic review. *Gen Hosp Psychiatry.* 2010;32(4):345-359.

17. Prins A, Bovin MJ, Smolenski DJ, et al. The Primary Care PTSD Screen for DSM-5 (PC-PTSD-5): development and evaluation within a veteran primary care sample. *J Gen Intern Med.* 2016;31(10):1206-1211.

18. Mussell M, Kroenke K, Spitzer RL, Williams JB, Herzog W, Löwe B. Gastrointestinal symptoms in primary care: prevalence and association with depression and anxiety. *J Psychosom Res.* 2008;64(6):605-612.

19. Mohlman J, Bryant C, Lenze EJ, et al. Improving recognition of late life anxiety disorders in Diagnostic and Statistical Manual of Mental Disorders, Fifth Edition: observations and recommendations of the Advisory Committee to the Lifespan Disorders Work Group. *Int J Geriatr Psychiatry.* 2012;27(6):549-556.

20. Cassidy KL, Rector NA. The silent geriatric giant: anxiety disorders in late life. *Geriatrics and Aging.* 2008;11(3):150-156.

21. Katzman MA, Bleau P, Blier P, et al. Canadian clinical practice guidelines for the management of anxiety, posttraumatic stress and obsessive-compulsive disorders. *BMC Psychiatry.* 2014;14(1):S1.

22. Crone CC, Gabriel GM, DiMartini A. An overview of psychiatric issues in liver disease for the consultation-liaison psychiatrist. *Psychosomatics.* 2006;47(3):188-205.

23. McIntyre RS, Baghdady NT, Banik S, Swartz SA. The use of psychotropic drugs in patients with impaired renal function. *Prim Psychiatr.* 2008;15(1):73-88.

24. Massoud F, Leger G. Pharmacological treatment of Alzheimer disease. *Can J Psychiatry.* 2011;56(10):579-588.

25. Porsteinsson AP, Drye LT, Pollock BG. Effect of citalopram on agitation in Alzheimer disease: the CitAD randomized clinical trial. *J Am Med Assoc.* 2014;311(7):682-691.

26. Calleo JS, Bush AL, Cully JA, et al. Treating late-life GAD in primary care: an effectiveness pilot study. *J Nerv Ment Dis.* 2013;201(5):414-420.

27. Brenes GA, Danhauer SC, Lyles MF, Hogan PE, Miller ME. Telephone-delivered cognitive behavioral therapy and telephone-delivered nondirective supportive therapy for rural older adults with generalized anxiety disorder: a randomized clinical trial. *JAMA Psychiatry.* 2015;72(10):1012-1020.

28. Airagnes G, Pelissolo A, Lavallee M, Flament M, Limosin F. Benzodiazepine misuse in the elderly: risk factors, consequences, and management. *Curr Psychiatry Rep.* 2016;18(10):89. doi:10.1007/s11920-016-0727-9.

29. Kurko TA, Saastamoinen LK, Tahkapaa S, et al. Long-term use of benzodiazepines: definitions, prevalence and usage patterns - a systematic review of register-based studies. *Eur Psychiatry.* 2015;30(8):1037-1047.

30. Sachdev G, Gesin G, Christmas AB, Sing RF. Failure of lorazepam to treat alprazolam withdrawal in a critically ill patient. *World J Crit Care Med.* 2014;3(1):42-44.

31. Glover J, Srinivasan S. Assessment of the person with late-life depression. *Psychiatr Clin North Am.* 2013;36:545-560.

32. Albert PR. Why is depression more prevalent in women? *J Psychiatry Neurosci.* 2015;40(4):219-221.

33. Global Burden of Disease Study 2013 Collaborators. Global, regional, and national incidence, prevalence, and years lived with disability for 301 acute and chronic diseases and injuries in 188 countries, 1990-2013: a systematic analysis for the Global Burden of Disease Study 2013. *Lancet.* 2015;386(9995):743-800.

34. Knöchel C, Alves G, Friedrichs B, et al. Treatment-resistant late-life depression: challenges and perspectives. *Curr Neuropharmacol.* 2015;13:577-591.

35. Lam RW, McIntosh D, Wang JL, et al. Canadian Network for Mood and Anxiety Treatments (CANMAT) 2016 clinical guidelines for the management of adults with major depressive disorder: section 1. Disease burden and principles of care. *Can J Psychiatry.* 2016;61(9):510-523.

36. Valiengo L, Stella F, Forlenza OV. Mood disorders in the elderly: prevalence, functional impact, and management challenges. *Neuropsychiatr Dis Treat.* 2016;12:2105-2114.

37. Fountoulakis KN, O'Hara R, Iacovides A, et al. Unipolar late-onset depression: a comprehensive review. *Ann Gen Hosp Psychiatry.* 2003;2(1):11.

38. Mirza SS, Wolters FJ, Swanson SA, et al. 10-year trajectories of depressive symptoms and risk of dementia: a population-based study. *Lancet Psychiatry.* 2016;3(7):628-635.

39. Patten SB, Williams JVA, Lavorato DH, et al. Descriptive epidemiology of major depressive disorder in Canada in 2012. *Can J Psychiatry.* 2015;60(1):23-30.

40. Angst J, Angst F, Stassen HH. Suicide risk in patients with major depressive disorder. *J Clin Psychiatry.* 1999;60(2):57-62.

41. Dines P, Hu W, Sajatovic M. Depression in later-life: an overview of assessment and management. *Psychiatr Danub.* 2014;26(1):78-84.

42. Byers AL, Yaffe K. Depression and risk of developing dementia. *Nat Rev Neurology.* 2011;7(6):323-331.

43. Saczynski JS, Beiser A, Seshadri S, et al. Depressive symptoms and risk of dementia. *Neurology.* 2010;75(1):35-41.

44. Beekman AT, de Beurs E, van Balkom AJ, et al. Anxiety and depression in later life: co-occurrence and communality of risk factors. *Am J Psychiatry.* 2000;157(1):89-95.

45. Unützer J, Tang L, Oishi S, et al. Reducing suicidal ideation in depressed older primary care patients. *J Am Geriatr Soc.* 2006;54:1550-1556.

46. Heisel MJ. Screening for suicide ideation among older primary care patients. *J Am Board Fam Med.* 2010;23(2):260-269.

47. Cole MG, Dendukuri N. Risk factors for depression among elderly community subjects: a systematic review and meta-analysis. *Am J Psychiatry.* 2003;160:1147-1156.

48. Buchanan D, Tourigny-Rivard MF, Cappeliez P, et al. National guidelines for seniors' mental health: the assessment and treatment of depression. *Can J Geriatr.* 2006;9(suppl 2):S52-S58.

49. Velly AM, Mohit S. Epidemiology of pain and relation to psychiatric disorders. *Prog Neuropsychopharmacol Biol Psychiatry.* 2017; pii: S0278-5846(17)30194-X.

50. Cosci F, Fava GA, Sonino N. Mood and anxiety disorders as early manifestations of medical illness: a systematic review. *Psychother Psychosom.* 2015;84(1):22-29.

51. Choi NG, Kim J, Marti CN, et al. Late-life depression and cardiovascular disease burden: examination of reciprocal relationship. *Am J Geriatr Psychiatry.* 2014;22(12):1522-1529.

52. FDA Drug Safety Communication: Revised recommendations for Celexa (citalopram hydrobromide) related to a potential risk of abnormal heart rhythms with high doses. March 28, 2012. http://www.fda.gov/Drugs/DrugSafety/ucm297391.htm. Accessed April 26, 2017.

53. Menza MA, Liberatore BL. Psychiatry in the geriatric neurology practice. *Neurol Clin.* 1998;16(3):611-633.

54. Gelenberg AJ, Freeman MP, Markowitz JC, et al. *Practice Guideline for the Treatment of Patients with Major Depressive Disorder.* 3rd ed. American Psychiatric Association; 2010. https://psychiatryonline.org/pb/assets/raw/sitewide/practice_guidelines/guidelines/mdd.pdf. Accessed April 26, 2017.

55. Parikh SV, Quilty LC, Ravitz P, et al. Canadian Network for Mood and Anxiety Treatments (CANMAT) 2016 clinical guidelines for the management of adults with major depressive disorder: section 2. Psychological treatments. *Can J Psychiatry.* 2016;61(9):524-539.

56. Nissen R, Freeman E, Lo C, et al. Managing Cancer and Living Meaningfully (CALM): a qualitative study of a brief individual psychotherapy for individuals with cancer. *Palliat Med.* 2011;26(5):713-721.

57. Prince M, Bryce R, Albanese E, Wimo A, Ribeiro W, Ferri CP. The global prevalence of dementia: a systematic review and metaanalysis. *Alzheimers Dement.* 2013;9(1):63-75.e2.

58. Satizabal CL, Beiser AS, Chouraki V, Chêne G, Dufouil C, Seshadri. Incidence of dementia over three decades in the Framingham heart study. *N Engl J Med.* 2016;374:523-532.

59. Molin P, Rockwood K. The new criteria for Alzheimer's disease - implications for geriatricians. *Can Geriatr J.* 2016;19(2):66-73.

60. Blennow K, de Leon MJ, Zetterberg H. Alzheimer's disease. *Lancet.* 2006;368(9533):387-403.

61. Hebert R, Brayne C. Epidemiology of vascular dementia. *Neuroepidemiology.* 1995;14(5):240-257.

62. Kalaria RN, Maestre GE, Arizaga R, et al. Alzheimer's disease and vascular dementia in developing countries: prevalence, management, and risk factors. *Lancet Neurol.* 2008;7(9):812-826.

63. Kirshner HS. Frontotemporal dementia and primary progressive aphasia, a review. *Neuropsychiatr Dis Treat.* 2014;10:1045-1055.

64. Aarsland D, Rongve A, Nore SP, et al. Frequency and case identification of dementia with Lewy bodies using the revised consensus criteria. *Dement Geriatr Cogn Disord.* 2008;26(5):445-452.

65. Hurd MD, Martorell P, Delavande A, Mullen KJ, Langa KM. Monetary costs of dementia in the United States. *N Engl J Med.* 2013;368(14):1326-1334.

66. Marshall GA, Amariglio RE, Sperling RA, Rentz DM. Activities of daily living: where do they fit in the diagnosis of Alzheimer's disease? *Neurodegener Dis Manag.* 2012;2(5):483-491.

67. Lyketsos CG. Neuropsychiatric symptoms in dementia: overview and measurement challenges. *J Prev Alzheimers Dis.* 2015;2(3):155-156.

68. Petersen RC, Smith GE, Waing SC, et al. Mild cognitive impairment: clinical characterization and outcome. *Arch Neurol.* 1999;56(3):303-308.

69. Schmidt C, Wolff M, Weitz M, Bartlau T, Korth C, Zerr I. Rapidly progressive alzheimer disease. *Arch Neurol.* 2011;68(9):1124-1130.

70. Jalbert JJ, Daiellio LA, Lapane KL. Dementia of the alzheimer type. *Epidemiol Rev.* 2008;30:15-34.

71. Knopman DS, Roberts RO. Estimating the number of persons with frontotemporal lobar degeneration in the US population. *J Mol Neurosci.* 2011;45:330-335.

72. Medicare's Cognitive Impairment Assessment and Care Planning Code: Alzheimer's Association Expert Task Force Recommendations and Tools for Implementation. http://www.alz.org/careplanning/downloads/cms-consensus.pdf. Accessed June 16, 2017.

73. Doraiswamy PM, Steffens DC, Pitchumoni S, Tabrizi S. Early recognition of Alzheimer's disease: what is consensual? What is controversial? What is practical? *J Clin Psychiatry.* 1998;59(suppl 13):6-18.

74. Knopman DS, DeKosky ST, Cummings JL, et al. Practice parameter: diagnosis of dementia (an evidence-based review). Report of the Quality Standards Subcommittee of the American Academy of Neurology. *Neurology.* 2001;56(9):1143-1153.

75. Brown J. The use and misuse of short cognitive tests in the diagnosis of dementia. *J Neurol Neurosurg Psychiatry.* 2015;86:680-685.

76. Trzepacz PT, Hochstetler H, Wang S, Walker B, Saykin AJ, Alzheimer's Disease Neuroimaging Initiative. Relationship between the Montreal Cognitive Assessment and Mini-mental State Examination for assessment of mild cognitive impairment in older adults. *BMC Geriatr.* 2015;15:107. doi:10.1186/s12877-015-0103-3.

77. Montreal Cognitive Assessment. http://www.mocatest.org. Accessed June 16, 2017.

78. Mini-Cog™. http://mini-cog.com. Accessed June 16, 2017.

79. Beach TG, Monsell SE, Phillips LE, Kukull W. Accuracy of the clinical diagnosis of Alzheimer disease at National Institute on Aging Alzheimer's Disease Centers, 2005–2010. *J Neuropathol Exp Neurol.* 2012;71(4):266-273.

80. Mayeux R, Saunders AM, Shea S, et al. Utility of the apolipoprotein E genotype in the diagnosis of Alzheimer's disease. Alzheimer's Disease Centers Consortium on Apolipoprotein E and Alzheimer's Disease. *N Engl J Med.* 1998;338:506-511.

81. Schott JM, Warren JD. Alzheimer's disease: mimics and chameleons. *Pract Neurol.* 2012;12(6):358-366.

82. Rogan S, Lippa CF. Alzheimer's disease and other dementias: a review. *Am J Alzheimers Dis Other Demen.* 2002;17:11-17.

83. Alzheimer's Association. https://www.alz.org. Accessed June 16, 2017.

84. Alzheimer Society of Canada. http://www.alzheimer.ca/en. Accessed June 16, 2017.

85. Kazui H, Yoshiyama K, Kanemoto H, et al. Differences of behavioral and psychological symptoms of dementia in disease severity in four major dementias. *PLoS One.* 2016;11(8):e0161092.

86. Feldman H, Gauthier S, Hecker J, et al. Efficacy of donepezil on maintenance of activities of daily living in patients with moderate to severe Alzheimer's disease and the effect on caregiver burden. *J Am Geriatr Soc.* 2003;51(6):737-744.

87. Schneider LS, Dagerman KS, Higgins JP, McShane R. Lack of evidence for the efficacy of memantine in mild Alzheimer disease. *Arch Neurol.* 2011;68(8):991-998.

88. Tariot PN, Farlow MR, Grossberg GT, et al. Memantine treatment in patients with moderate to severe Alzheimer disease already receiving donepezil: a randomized controlled trial. *J Am Med Assoc.* 2004;291(3):317-324.

89. Gauthier S, Patterson C, Chertkow H, et al. Recommendations of the 4th Canadian Consensus Conference on the Diagnosis and Treatment of Dementia (CCCDTD4). *Can Geriatr J*. 2012;15(4):120-126.

90. Cohen-Mansfield Agitation Inventory (CMAI). https://www.pdx.edu/ioa/sites/www.pdx.edu.ioa/files/CMAI_Manual%20%281%29.pdf. Accessed June 16, 2017.

91. Gitlin LN, Kales HC, Lyketsos CG. Managing behavioral symptoms in dementia using nonpharmacologic approaches: an overview. *J Am Med Assoc*. 2012;308(19):2020-2029.

92. Grossberg GT, Lake JT. The role of the psychiatrist in Alzheimer's disease. *J Clin Psychiatry*. 1998;59(suppl 9):3-6.

21

CHILD AND ADOLESCENT BEHAVIORAL HEALTH

Myo Thwin Myint, MD, Rohail Kumar, MD, Kimberly Kavanagh, MD, and
Mary Margaret Gleason, MD

INTRODUCTION

As many as one in five children and youth will experience a psychiatric problem before age 21 years.[1] Pediatric primary care providers (PCPs) have long-standing relationships with children and their families and are often the first-line providers in pediatric mental health care. In this chapter, we will review the major presentations of attention deficit hyperactivity disorder (ADHD), autism spectrum disorder (ASD), disruptive behavior patterns, anxiety, and depressive disorders, which are conditions for which first-line management can often begin in the primary care setting. A number of other disorders can present in pediatric populations, including gender dysphoria, reactive attachment disorder, disruptive mood dysregulation disorder, bipolar disorder, substance use disorders, and psychotic illnesses, but assessment and management of these disorders are generally not within the scope of primary care and should be managed by or in collaboration with a mental health provider.

Although the diagnostic criteria for pediatric disorder are, for the most part, similar to those in adulthood, some adaptations to clinical care are warranted. Children's cognitive, behavioral, and emotional development occurs in the complex interactions between genetics, epigenetics, and environments, which may offer protection or risk for psychiatric disorders and are considered in the assessment. The child's family and caregiving environment is the most prominent context and can both influence and be influenced by a child's symptoms. Rapid developmental changes also affect the presentation of psychiatric problems as well as the assessment and treatment plans.

Only a quarter of children with mental health problems are identified in primary care and most do not receive any treatment.[2] This unmet need causes suffering to the child and family. Financially, the costs of mental health problems are equivalent to costs of physical health problems, approximately $247 billion annually in the United States with implications for child, the family, the educational, justice, and medical systems, among others.[3,4] Costs to children include exclusion from social, family, and educational experiences that could provide a foundation for future development and learning. Parents may lose workdays for clinical and school appointments and often experience substantial emotional strain and sleep deprivation. Educational costs, such as special education services, represent the second highest category of expenditure after health care costs for children with mental health problems.[3] Involvement with the juvenile justice system, related to symptoms of severe disruptive behavior patterns, developmental delays, and substance use disorders, creates additional societal costs. Children with physical health conditions and family or social adversities are at higher risk for mental health problems, compounding the impact on them, their families, and society.

CONSIDERATIONS FOR SCREENING AND ASSESSMENT IN CHILDREN

Child mental health problems should be considered in any child who presents with a chief complaint related to school or home functioning problems, atypical pain, somatic symptoms, or adherence concerns related to other medical treatment. The American Academy of Pediatrics' (AAP) periodicity schedule requires a "psychosocial/behavioral assessment" at every well-child visit, with specific screening for ASDs at 18 and 24 months, and formal screening for substance use and depression in adolescence.[5]

Interviewing the parents and the child, separately and together, offers the richest source of information related to mental health concerns. Supplementary information from teachers, guidance counselors, therapists, and foster care workers, among others, contribute essential data.

Validated parent, teacher, and youth report measures can facilitate efficient review of treatment effects in multiple contexts (*Table 21-1*). For school-age

TABLE 21-1 Assessment

Domain		What to look for	To identify	ASD	DISRUPTIVE BEHAVIOR	ADHD	MOOD	ANXIETY
				Considerations specific to the disorder				
Physical examination	Dysmorphology	Dysmorphic facial features	Evidence of genetic syndromes or teratogen exposure	Especially Fragile X, fetal alcohol syndrome		Especially Fragile X, fetal alcohol syndrome		Consider Williams syndrome, Prader–Willi
	Size for age and growth curve		Evidence of genetic/endocrine syndromes or teratogen exposure; nutritional insufficiency (genetics, food insecurity, deprivation, eating disorder)	Macrocephaly?	Obesity associated with DBD in young children		Weight gain or loss may be associated with depression	
	Vital signs	Heart rate, blood pressure	Indicators of thyroid dysfunction, substance use	Safety for medications	Safety for medications	Safety for medications	Hypothyroidism can present as depression	Hyperthyroidism can be associated with anxiety
	Skin and hair	Full skin examination	Scars/bruising or signs of self-injurious behaviors, substance use, non-accidental injuries	Signs of neurocutaneous syndromes		Signs of physical abuse may be associated with disruptive behavior patterns	Signs of self injurious behaviors (scars) are not uncommon	Alopecia, evidence of skin picking
	HEENT			Otitis media with effusion if language delays			Thyromegaly	Thyromegaly

(continued)

TABLE 21-1 Assessment (continued)

			ASD	DISRUPTIVE BEHAVIOR	ADHD	MOOD	ANXIETY
Neuro	General assessment of neurologic functioning, targeted examination as indicated	Evidence of other CNS process	Macrocephaly, hypertonia (toe walking), stereotypies				
Mental Status examination							
Appearance/behavior	Clothing appropriate for context and season	Reflects caregiving environment (young children) or thought process (adolescents)					
Behavior	Cooperativeness with PCP and parent, activity level, physical movement		May have limited eye contact and cooperativeness with PCP, may have difficulty with social reciprocity, may have high levels of activity (consider ADHD)	May show range of cooperativeness. If high activity, consider ADHD	Level of activity may be age-appropriate or very high. Do not need to see high level of activity if hyperactivity established in two settings or if inattentive ADHD	May show low eye contact, limited engagement. May show typical or low activity/movement	May show low eye contact, limited engagement with PCP, and more interaction with parent
Mood	What the child says he or she feels	Can child comment on feelings that match the history presented?		Check for mood component of presentation		To confirm diagnosis	To confirm diagnosis, Comorbid mood symptoms are common
Affect	What feeling you see on his or her face	Sometimes affect belies assurances that the child "feels fine"; Does affect match the context (looks sad talking about sad topics)?	Affect may be disconnected from content of discussion	Generally not affected	May appear angry but often shows neutral/euthymic affect	Generally flat or sad appearing	May show limited feelings, may look nervous, or may seem irritable

Speech	Rate, volume, rhythm	Delayed or absent verbal communication, may have flat intonation, volume may not be appropriate for context	Generally typical; but assess for delays	May interrupt frequently, more rapid speech	Generally normal or slow speech. Rapid, non-interruptable speech would suggest possibility of mania	May be very quiet, slow rate, or typical
Thought process	How organized is the child's thinking?	Cognitive process — May show unexpected connection in thinking or highly perseverative ("stuck") thinking	Generally age-typical	May be scattered because of distractibility	Generally organized; if seems highly disorganized, assess for signs of psychosis, hallucination	Generally organized
Thought content	What is on the child's mind?	May show highly restricted and limited interests	Generally age-typical but may have perseverations on aggression or shame/guilt	Generally age-typical	Assess for suicidality, homicidality, ability to think about the future	Assess for what fears, suicidality, homicidality, ability to think about the future. If fears are not reality based (delusional), explore signs of psychosis
Hallucinations	Any perceptual changes?	Assessing for signs of psychosis. Para-omnic events are generally not related to psychosis				May be present with severe depression

(continued)

TABLE 21-1 Assessment (continued)

	ASD	DISRUPTIVE BEHAVIOR	ADHD	MOOD	ANXIETY
Cognition	Developmental status, orientation to time, memory, and ability to problem solve	Comorbid developmental delays common	Concentration likely impaired	Memory and problem solving may be impaired	Concentration, memory may be impaired
		Rule out developmental delays and learning problems			
Insight	Ability to understand how symptoms are influencing functioning in age-appropriate way	Problems in thinking, appreciating importance of the problem, ability to participate in treatment			
Judgment	Ability to make thoughtful decisions in age-appropriate way	Concerns about safety and ability to participate in treatment			
Screening tool	Efficient way to track symptoms — M-CHAT 18-33 months	General measure such as PSC, PSC-17	Vanderbilt ADHD Rating Scale (teacher and parent)	PHQ-9 (12-18), general measure like PSC for younger children	SCARED (8-18 years)

ADHD, attention deficit hyperactivity disorder; ASD, autism spectrum disorder; DBD, disruptive behavior disorder; HEENT, Head, Eye, Ear, Nose, and Throat Examination; M-CHAT, modified checklist for autism in toddlers; PCP, primary care provider; PHQ, Patient Health Questionnaire; PSC, Pediatric Symptom Checklist; SCARED, Screen for Child Anxiety and Related Emotional Disorders.

children and adolescents, the Pediatric Symptom Checklist (PSC) and the shorter PSC-17 are well-established, nonproprietary measures that track both mood and behavioral patterns. Nearly half of all children in the United States have experienced at least one adverse childhood event and these must be considered and asked about.[6] Using a tool such as the Safe Environment for Every Kid (SEEK) or Adverse Childhood Experiences (ACES) Screening Tool to assess the child's environmental risks may be a useful supplement to the social history.[7-9] More than one appointment may be necessary to obtain sufficient information for diagnosis.

Assessment of children includes attention to the child's functioning in multiple settings and the contribution of those environments to the symptoms or resilience. Specific components of the history include the following:

Symptoms: Review frequency, intensity, duration, progression and context of the primary symptoms and review of disruptive behavior patterns, signs of ADHD, anxiety, mood, social reciprocity, development and learning, and substance use.
Impairment: How do the symptoms affect the child and family's functioning and ability to participate in activities typical for development and culture?
Risk factors: What might contribute to the problem? Consider medical conditions, family history, social factors, especially quality of caregiving at home and at school, exposure to violence, unpredictable experiences, problems with basic needs (food, housing, and safety), bullying, and child-specific risk factors such as developmental delays, gender, and age.
Strengths: What are the protective factors including relationships with stable adults, ability to interact with peers, access to social and/or financial resources, intelligence, motivation for treatment, and the lack of risk factors described above?
Development: Review the child's past and current developmental status. Evaluate the timing of developmental milestones. What are the child's grades? Has there been any retention in a grade?

INFANT OR PRESCHOOL CHILD

Parent–child relationships are the foundation for all ages, but especially for this age group, who cannot describe their experiences verbally and who depend on caregivers to shape their emotional and physical worlds. Observations of parent–child interactions offer a view into parental sensitivity, responsiveness, and mutual enjoyment of the relationship. A clinician can assess the child's developmental level, relational capacity, and joy potential by playing brief games such as peek-a-boo. The validity of diagnostic criteria for many disorders has been established in young children, and these disorders cause significant impairment and deserve treatment, although assessment generally requires partnering with a specialist.[10]

ADOLESCENT

Recognizing the adolescent's need for confidentiality and autonomy guides the assessment process. Both the parent and child should be aware of the bounds and limits of confidentiality. In addition to the other aspects of the history, adolescent assessment examines substance use and sexual development including identity and activity.

PHYSICAL EXAMINATION AND MENTAL STATUS OBSERVATIONS

The summary of the components of the physical examination in a child with concerns of mental health problems is provided in *Table 21-1.* For all children, vital signs, growth trajectories, skin, and neurological examinations may be helpful in ruling out other conditions or identifying safety risks such as self-injurious behaviors. The pediatric mental status examination includes the same components as for adults but often requires interactions and developmentally specific approaches. In the primary care setting, PCPs should use every opportunity to observe the patient's interaction with others, especially during elements of the examination that provide opportunities to observe the child and child's responses to stressors such as separation or immunizations.

Observations of the child's mental status add important information to the assessment and must be developmentally grounded to avoid pathologizing typical behaviors. Noting how the parent and child interact in the room and whether the child's patterns of behavior are different with the parent compared with the PCP is valuable. For example, a child may follow all directions from the provider but swears at the parent, which may suggest specific challenges in the caregiving relationship. Most of the components of the mental status examination are completed observationally while taking the history and the physical examination. Only mood, thought process, and perceptions require specific questions. Cognition, when it is a concern, may require additional interview questions as well.

All children over 3 to 4 years of age should be asked to report about his or her own mood, consequences to misbehaviors, and exposure to major life events ("have any scary or big things happened to you?"). As with adults, asking about suicidality does not cause suicidality, so assessing for suicidal thoughts or plans is an important component of a mental status examination for children with depression, irritability, and/or anxiety for children who are older than 6 years. Questions such as *"Do you ever wish you weren't alive? Wished you were dead? How close have you come to hurting yourself?"* can be understood by most school-age children and older. Preoccupations with death, aggression, or sexualized activities may be evident in play or during an interview. Hopefulness and future orientation may also be assessed by asking a child what he or she wants to be when he or she grows up or for three wishes of what they wish would happen to them. Perceptual changes or hallucinations are commonly sleep-related and rarely associated with a psychiatric problem in preschool- and young school-age children, although would if present should prompt an assessment for intoxication or central nervous system (CNS) problem.

TREATMENT OF CHILDREN

Treatment for child psychiatric problems almost invariably requires multimodal approaches. Psychosocial, family-focused approaches including psychoeducation and support are fundamental. Research for treatments has some limitations, especially related to medications in preschoolers and school-age children[10] (*Table 21-2*). All treatments should be monitored closely for expected or atypical adverse effects. Treatment failures warrant reassessment of the diagnosis and consideration of additional services as well as alternative treatments.

- Start low, go slow... but be aware that because of differences in absorption, distribution, metabolism, and excretion, children may require relatively higher doses to achieve the same plasma level.
- When starting a medication, have a plan for duration of the treatment trial if effective.
- Establish effective communication with mental health providers treating the child.

Psychoeducation for families and the patient can increase engagement and adherence, and decrease stigma and stress. Resources that provide a range of useful and accessible information for families include the AAP's healthychildren.org and American Academy of Child and Adolescent's (AACAP) Facts for Families and Resource Guides (aacap.org). For younger children, zerotothree.org has a range of useful handouts. Additional disorder-specific resources will be described in each of the following sections.

TABLE 21-2 Commonly Used Medications in Primary Care

NAME	FORMULATION: BRAND NAME	THERAPEUTIC DOSES (TOTAL mg/d) SCHOOL AGE AND ADOLESCENT[b]	COMMON SIDE EFFECTS	SERIOUS SIDE EFFECTS
ADHD—stimulants				
Dextroamphetamine (d-amp)	IR TAB: d-amp, Dexedrine, Zenzedi IR SOL: ProCentra ER CAP: d-amp	2.5-40 (IR) 5-40	Decreased appetite Initial insomnia Abdominal pain Headaches Mood changes Small increases in BP and HR	Misuse Divergence Cardiac arrhythmias in susceptible individuals
Lisdexamfetamine	CAP: Vyvanse CHEW: Vyvanse	30-70		
Mixed amphetamine salts (MAS)	IR TAB: MAS, Adderall ER: MAS, Adderall XR ER TAB: Evekeo ER ODT: Adzenys ER SUSP: Dyanavel XR	2.5-40 5-40 2.5-40 6.3-18.8 2.5-20		
Methylphenidate (mph)	IR TAB: mph, Ritalin IR CHEW: mph IR SOL: mph, Methylin ER TAB: mph, Metadate ER ER CAP: mph, Metadate CD, Ritalin LA, Aptensio XR ER CHEW: Quillichew ER ER SUSP: Quillivant XR OROS: mph, Concerta Transdermal patch: Daytrana (9 hours)	All IR forms: 5-60 20-60 10-60 20-60 18-72 10-30 10-unspecified		
Dexmethylphenidate (d-mph)	IR TAB: d-mph, Focalin ER CAP: d-mph, Focalin XR	5-20 (IR)/30 (ER)		

TABLE 21-2 Commonly Used Medications in Primary Care   (continued)

NAME	FORMULATION: BRAND NAME	THERAPEUTIC DOSES (TOTAL mg/d) SCHOOL AGE AND ADOLESCENT[b]	COMMON SIDE EFFECTS	SERIOUS SIDE EFFECTS
ADHD—alpha agonists				
Clonidine	IR TAB: clonidine, Catapres[a] ER TAB: clonidine ER, Kapvay Transdermal patch: Catapres TTS[a] (wkly)	0.1-0.4	Somnolence Hypotension Fatigue Bradycardia	Death (with overdose)
Guanfacine	IR TAB: guanfacine[a] ER TAB: guanfacine ER, Intuniv	1-4		
ADHD—SNRI				
Atomoxetine	CAP: Strattera	Start 0.5 mg/kg/d titrated to 1.2/mg/kg/d (maximum 80)	GI symptoms Somnolence Irritability	Hepatic failure
Depression/anxiety—SSRI				
Citalopram	TAB: citalopram, Celexa[a] SOL: citalopram[a]	20-40	GI symptoms Headaches Changes in sleep Activation Sexual side effects	Suicidal behaviors Mania Serotonin syndrome
Escitalopram	TAB: escitalopram, Lexapro SOL: escitalopram, Lexapro	10-20		
Fluoxetine	TAB: Fluoxetine, Prozac, Rapiflux, Sarafem, Selfemra CAP: fluoxetine, Prozac SOL: fluoxetine	10-60		
Sertraline	TAB: sertraline, Zoloft SOL: sertraline, Zoloft	25-200		
Irritability in ASD—atypical antipsychotic				
Aripiprazole	TAB: aripiprazole, Abilify ODT: Abilify Discmelt SOL: Abilify	2-30	Sedation/Fatigue GI problems Increased appetite Drooling	Metabolic syndrome Hyperprolactinemia, Extrapyramidal effects Neuroleptic malignant syndrome
Risperidone	TAB: Risperdal ODT: Risperdal M-Tab Sol: Risperdal	0.5-6		

[a] Not FDA approved, but supported by empirical data or professional treatment guidelines.
[b] Except for d-amphetamine and mixed amphetamine salts, no medications have FDA psychiatric indications for use in children younger than 5 years.
Key: ADHD, attention deficit hyperactivity disorder; ASD, autiam apectrum disorder; BP, blood pressure; CAP, capsule; CHEW, chewable; DR, delayed release; ER, extended release; HR, heart rate; INJ, injection; IR, immediate release; ODT, orally dissolving tablet; OROS, osmotic release oral system; SNRI, serotonin–norepinephrine reuptake inhibitors; SOL, solution; SSRI, selective serotonin reuptake inhibitor; SUSP, suspension; Tab, tablet.

ATTENTION DEFICIT AND HYPERACTIVITY DISORDER

CLINICAL SIGNIFICANCE

ADHD is the most commonly treated mental health problem in pediatric primary care. Pediatric prevalence is approximately 5% to 8%, with 4% persisting into adulthood.[11] The core symptoms are extreme hyperactivity/impulsivity, and/or inattention in more than one setting, causing functional impairment. ADHD costs the United States $21 to 44 billion annually in health care and $15 to 25 billion in education.[12] Clinically, ADHD is associated with educational difficulties, relationship difficulties, and safety concerns (motor vehicle accidents, substance use, and high-risk sexual behavior).[13] Importantly, ADHD is both overdiagnosed and underdiagnosed in the United States.[11] Thus, a structured approach is warranted to ensure accurate identification of those with symptoms of ADHD, accurate diagnosis, and appropriate treatment.

DIAGNOSIS

ADHD diagnosis requires systematic assessment of the diagnostic criteria (*Box 21-1*). The history should specifically confirm the presence of symptoms in more than one setting, onset before age 12 years (although children may be diagnosed after that age if symptoms were present earlier), and impairment (including school difficulties, interpersonal problems, or safety risks). Validated tools such as the Vanderbilt ADHD Rating Scales for children 6 years and above can increase assessment efficiency but does not replace reviewing the history from the child and family.[13]

BOX 21-1 ATTENTION DEFICIT HYPERACTIVITY DISORDER

- Pervasive and impairing inattention and/or hyperactivity and impulsivity
- Six or more symptoms (five or more symptoms for 17+-year-olds) in each or both domains
- Symptoms
  - Evident before 12-year-olds
  - Present in two or more settings
  - Persist at least 6 months
  - Cause impairment
- **Inattention:**
  1. Makes careless mistakes
  2. Trouble maintaining focusing
  3. Seems not to be listen
  4. Does not follow through on tasks
  5. Has trouble organizing
  6. Avoid tasks requiring mental effort
  7. Loses things
  8. Gets distracted
  9. Forgets simple things
- **Hyperactivity and impulsivity:**
  1. Moves a lot (fidget)
  2. Gets out of seat
  3. Runs or (adolescents) feels restless
  4. Is loud/trouble being quiet
  5. Is always on the go
  6. Talk too much
  7. Answers before question is finished
  8. Trouble waiting for turn
  9. Frequently interrupts

The differential diagnosis of ADHD is broad and developmentally specific. A thorough assessment should examine the patterns of impulsivity and hyperactivity, the timing, and context of the symptoms and review anxiety, mood, disruptive behavior patterns, exposure to trauma, developmental status, and social skills, all of which may present as impulsive or disorganized behaviors, especially in young children. Assessment of very young children requires time to observe them in multiple settings as well as obtain history from multiple reporters, ideally by a specialist in early childhood development or mental health. In older children, the same differential diagnosis should be considered, but in most cases can be adequately assessed in one or more PCP visits. Hyperactivity is often not seen in the office, which should not preclude the diagnosis if symptoms occur in two other settings.

Assessment includes review of sleep patterns, especially signs of obstructive sleep apnea, and consideration of genetic syndromes that present with ADHD, such as Fragile X, hearing problems, absence seizures, or other CNS disorders.[13] In children with pica or children younger than 6 years, the assessment should also consider lead toxicity. In adolescents, the history should examine substance use, depression, and anxiety, especially in the inattentive presentation. In preparation for possible stimulant treatment, clinicians should review cardiac risk factors including personal and family history of syncope, chest pain, and family history of sudden death or pediatric cardiac disease, with cardiac workup before starting a stimulant medication only if the screening identifies specific risk factors.[14]

BIOPSYCHOSOCIAL TREATMENT

ADHD requires a chronic care model approach. Successful treatment of ADHD relies on effective education about the disorder, course, and treatment as well as a developmentally specific treatment plan that will include behavioral and/or pharmacologic approaches (*Figure 21-1*). Regular follow-up with reporters from both school and home is an integral part of the treatment plan. In all cases, providing information about behavioral ADHD management strategies is valuable.

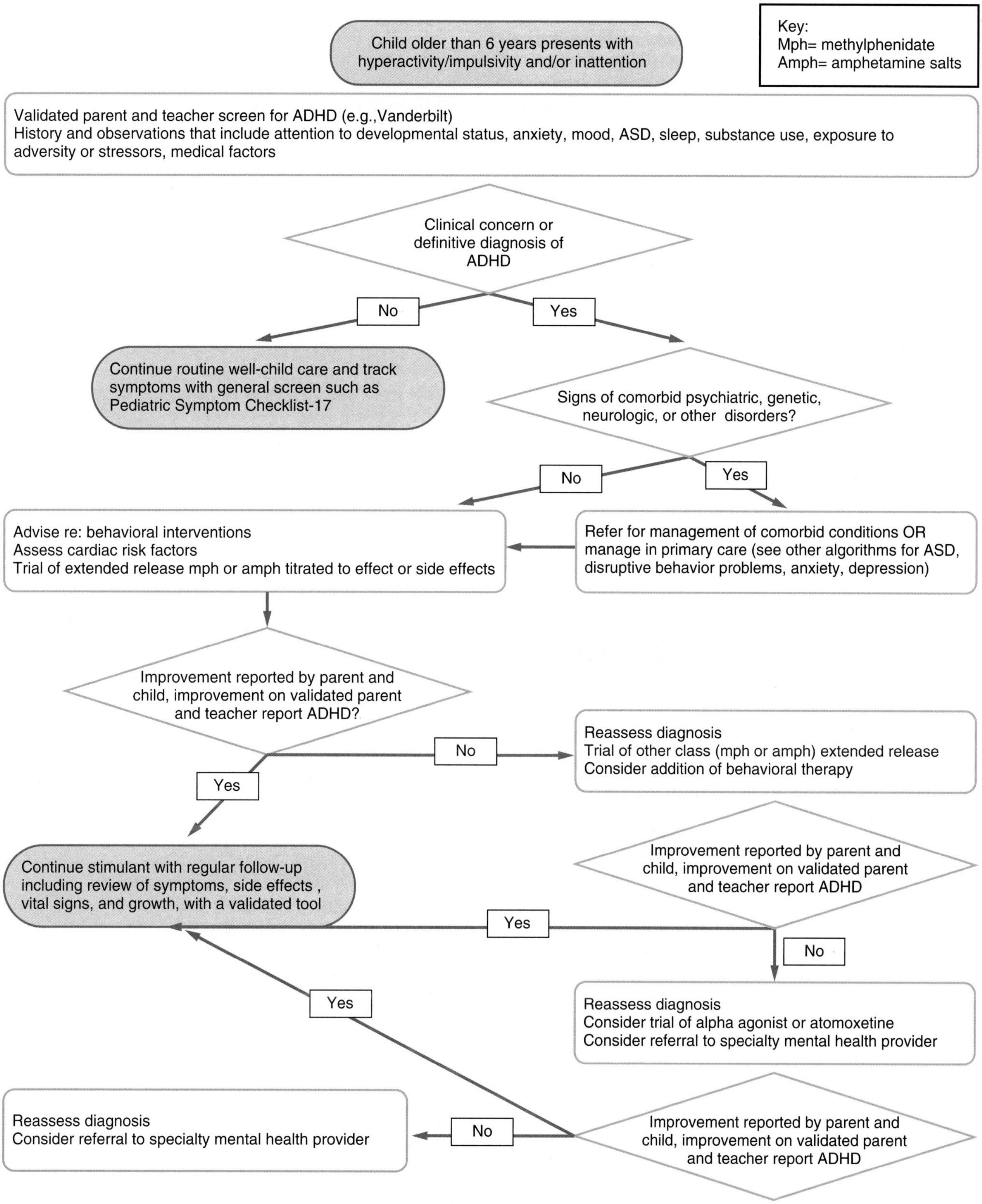

Key:
Mph= methylphenidate
Amph= amphetamine salts

Child older than 6 years presents with hyperactivity/impulsivity and/or inattention

Validated parent and teacher screen for ADHD (e.g.,Vanderbilt)
History and observations that include attention to developmental status, anxiety, mood, ASD, sleep, substance use, exposure to adversity or stressors, medical factors

Clinical concern or definitive diagnosis of ADHD

No

Yes

Continue routine well-child care and track symptoms with general screen such as Pediatric Symptom Checklist-17

Signs of comorbid psychiatric, genetic, neurologic, or other disorders?

No

Yes

Advise re: behavioral interventions
Assess cardiac risk factors
Trial of extended release mph or amph titrated to effect or side effects

Refer for management of comorbid conditions OR manage in primary care (see other algorithms for ASD, disruptive behavior problems, anxiety, depression)

Improvement reported by parent and child, improvement on validated parent and teacher report ADHD?

No

Reassess diagnosis
Trial of other class (mph or amph) extended release
Consider addition of behavioral therapy

Yes

Continue stimulant with regular follow-up including review of symptoms, side effects, vital signs, and growth, with a validated tool

Improvement reported by parent and child, improvement on validated parent and teacher report ADHD

Yes

No

Reassess diagnosis
Consider trial of alpha agonist or atomoxetine
Consider referral to specialty mental health provider

Yes

Reassess diagnosis
Consider referral to specialty mental health provider

No

Improvement reported by parent and child, improvement on validated parent and teacher report ADHD

FIGURE 21-1 Pathway for attention deficit and hyperactivity disorder (ADHD).

Pharmacotherapy is the mainstay of ADHD treatment for children older than 6 years.[13] *Table 21-2* reviews the details of the many formulations of medications for ADHD. Both methylphenidate and amphetamine formulations are equally effective as first-line agents, and PCPs may select a treatment based on family history, formulation, and the PCP's comfort. The medications are generally well-tolerated, with the most common adverse effects of sleep and appetite disturbances and mood changes.[13] School-age children should receive extended-release formulations given in the morning to cover the school day. Rapid (weekly) dose titration to an effective dose without adverse effects can be accomplished if good communication is established with family. To avoid undertreatment, monthly monitoring with PCP is recommended when changing doses. Treatment effects can be monitored using the Vanderbilt ADHD Rating Scale completed by teachers and parents. Sleep, appetite, mood, vital signs (weight, height, blood pressure, and pulse), and growth parameters should be checked at each visit as well. If a first trial is ineffective, reconfirming the diagnosis is the first step, followed by switching to the other stimulant class. With accurate diagnosis, three-quarters of children will respond after two trials.[15] If both trials fail with adequate dosing, reassessment of diagnosis, adherence, and adequate evaluation and treatment of comorbid conditions is warranted. Second- and third-line approaches may include alpha agonists or atomoxetine, and consideration of consultation with a child psychiatrist or developmental-behavioral pediatrician. In all adolescents and families with histories of substance use, monitoring for diversion or misuse of medication is recommended by testing for both presence of the prescribed drug and absence of other drugs and alcohol. Medications with lower risk of misuse, such as atomoxetine, alpha agonists, or lisdexamfetamine may be considered in youth with substance use disorders, although stimulants are not fully contraindicated. Stimulants are less effective in preschoolers than in older children and have higher rates of adverse effects, so should only be used in this age group if therapy has failed or if significant safety risks require rapid response.[16] Drug "holidays" are not recommended as standard care but may be considered for children whose symptoms are not impairing outside of the school setting and a child has medication-related weight loss or slowed growth trajectory secondary to the stimulant.

- Stimulants are first-line treatment for ADHD in children older than 6 years.
- Once a stimulant is started, avoid undertreatment by adequate monitoring of treatment effects.
- Success rates of treatment are high with accurate diagnosis; reconsider diagnosis with any treatment failure.

Nonpharmacologic approaches should be considered for all children with ADHD. Behavioral therapies can reduce symptoms of ADHD in children older than 6 years, although they are less effective than stimulants.[17] Concurrent therapy with medication is more effective than medication alone for children with comorbid anxiety, developmental delays, and public insurance.[18] For preschool-aged children, evidenced-based behavior therapy is recommended as first-line treatment.[10] These approaches are based on similar models as those described in Disruptive Behavior Problems section.

- For young children, family-focused behavioral therapy is first-line treatment.
- Structured behavioral strategies that recognize children's positive behaviors and using concrete tokens (stickers, stars) and a safe strategy, effective for discipline (timeout), can reduce symptoms of ADHD.
- Teachers should be offered information to support children with ADHD.

Education about ADHD is critical for engagement and adherence. Specifically, families should know that ADHD is a chronic condition, develop adaptations to ADHD, and support the child in developing self-management skills. Family-focused resources abound, including Parents Med Guide (parentsmedguide.org), Healthychildren. org, the National Institute of Child Health Quality tool kit (nichq.org), and Children and Adults with Attention-Deficit/Hyperactivity Disorder (CHADD.org).

Indications for referrals:

- Preschooler with suspected ADHD
- Two or more ineffective or intolerable trials of ADHD medications
- Multiple comorbid conditions or uncertain diagnosis

AUTISM SPECTRUM DISORDERS
CLINICAL SIGNIFICANCE

ASDs are characterized by atypical social interaction and communication, and stereotyped behaviors or restricted interests. Autism occurs in 1 in 86 children in the United States.[19] Early intervention is the best approach for ASDs, but in current practice, treatment too often starts years after a parent has voiced concerns.[20] ASDs affect the entire family, with implications for direct medical and developmental costs and lost work productivity for parents involved in intense therapies, but the most significant costs are incurred in the educational setting.[21] ASDs are commonly associated with genetic syndromes, seizure disorders, eating and nutritional problems, sensory and motor abnormalities, and gastrointestinal concerns, among many others.[22]

DIAGNOSIS

The AAP recommends universal use of a measure such as the Modified Checklist for Autism in Toddlers, Revised (MCHAT-R) at 18 and 24 months to screen for ASD.[22] Screening is also recommended at other visits if a parent or provider is concerned, especially if both are concerned or the child has a sibling with ASD.

ASD often presents with communication difficulties manifested by regression, delay, or atypical development, typically in the second year of life. Problems with communication may include verbal communication as well as problems with eye contact, gestural communication (pointing), and the typical reciprocity of conversations (*Box 21-2*). The repetitive and restrictive behaviors include extremely rigid routines, repetitive movements ("stereotypies") such as hand flapping, or an intense preoccupation with parts of an object (e.g., spinning wheels on a toy car). Sensory hyper- or hyposensitivity manifests as distress with exposure to the sensation and may interfere with eating, wearing clothing, and socially normative behaviors.

BOX 21-2 AUTISM SPECTRUM DISORDER

- Lack of appropriate communicating and interaction in socially expected manner consistent with these examples
  1. Difficulty with back-and-forth of social exchange
  2. Limited nonverbal communication (e.g., atypical eye contact)
  3. Trouble with starting and sustaining relationships
- Highly focused, recurrent, constricted, behavior and interests (two or more)
  1. Highly scripted, repetitive language, activities, or speech
  2. Requires unchanging routines/distress with transitions
  3. Intense fixation on circumscribed interests
  4. Excessively high or low sensitivity to sensory input

Table 21-1 summarizes the elements of the physical examination important to assess in children with concerns for ASD. Of particular importance is the child's capacity for social reciprocity, attempts to engage eye contact, reciprocal conversation in older children, and any moments of joint attention in which the PCP and child are looking at the same object together and communicating with each other through eye contact or verbally. This reciprocal interaction is a core deficit in ASDs.

Evaluations by audiology, speech and language, occupational and physical therapy, and early intervention programs (available in all US states under the Individuals with Disabilities Education Act for children under 36 months) or special education (over 36 months to 21 years enrolled in school) should be part of an assessment for children with suspected ASD. The diagnosis of ASD is a clinical diagnosis, and formal testing is not required if the diagnosis is clear. However, formal autism evaluation that includes the Autism Diagnostic Observational Schedule can aid in less clear presentations and for all children can support a parent's advocacy for services. Specialty clinics for ASD can offer more extensive education to families as well as local and Web-based resources.[22]

Children diagnosed with ASD should have testing for Fragile X syndrome, chromosomal microarray, and Woods lamp examination to identify neurocutaneous disorders. Other testing, including other genetic or metabolic testing, neuroimaging, lead levels, electroencephalography, can be selected based on the history or physical examination.[22]

The differential diagnosis for ASD generally includes global developmental delays, specific speech or language disorders, hearing impairment, selective mutism, and (in older children) obsessive–compulsive disorder or psychosis. Extreme neglect in families or in institutional care can cause quasi-autism, which is indistinguishable from ASD at presentation but resolves after placement in a safe environment.[23]

In addition to the differential, it is important for clinicians to actively assess for the common conditions that may co-occur with ASD, most commonly ADHD, anxiety disorders, affective disorders, and oppositional defiant disorder (ODD), as well as intellectual disabilities. The assessment should consider these diagnoses using developmentally specific approaches.

BIOPSYCHOSOCIAL TREATMENT

Treatment for ASD requires a multidisciplinary approach that may include developmental, behavioral, educational, family interventions tailored to the needs of the child (*Figure 21-2*). Family education, support, and family-driven care are key components to the treatment plan. Families may derive support through the child's treaters, parent groups, and/or clinical care.

No medications are proven effective in treating the core symptoms of ASD. However, the U.S. Food and Drug Administration (FDA) has approved indications for risperidone and aripiprazole to treat irritability in autism in children as young as 5 years and 6 years, respectively. Comorbid conditions in children with ASD may be treated with medications as well. Because children with ASDs may experience higher rates of adverse effects or atypical adverse effects, low starting doses may be helpful and treatment should be monitored closely clinically and with recommended laboratory testing (*Table 21-2*). A number of pseudomedical approaches have no evidence to support their use and may be dangerous, including chelation (except for documented lead toxicity), hyperbaric oxygen, secretin injections, and stem cell treatment.[24]

- Treating comorbid conditions is the first-line pharmacotherapy approach in children with ASD.
- Medications should be used in conjunction with developmental and behavioral interventions.
- Children with ASD may have higher rates of adverse effects than neurotypical children.

Nonpharmacologic interventions are the main interventions to treat the core symptoms of ASD. Treatment should be tailored to the child's specific needs but may include behavioral therapy, medical management of comorbid conditions, educational interventions, speech therapy, and occupational therapy. Treatment for comorbid physical and mental health problems is

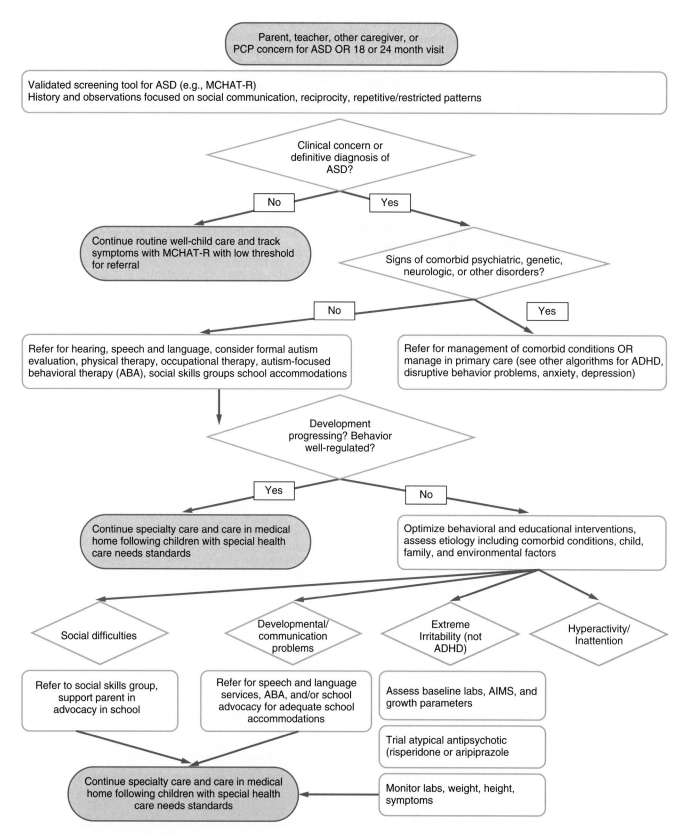

FIGURE 21-2 Pathway for autism spectrum disorders (ASDs). ADHD, attention deficit and hyperactivity disorder; MCHAT-R, Modified Checklist for Autism in Toddlers, Revised; PCP, primary care provider.

critical. Among the behavioral interventions, applied behavior analysis (ABA) has the most extensive empiric support for its effect on cognitive and language outcomes.[25] ABA breaks down complex tasks into smaller components and supports children's motivation for adaptive behaviors. Other effective interventions including parent management training, cognitive behavioral therapy, and social skills training can address clinical concerns related to ASD.

- Interventions focused on core symptoms of ASD include speech and language therapy, ABA, and social skills training.
- Many evidence-based therapies for comorbid conditions can be adapted to treat those conditions in children with ASD.
- Family support is a critical component of intervention.

Ensuring that families have access to accurate information is especially important in ASDs, as the Internet is rife with inaccurate and sometimes dangerous information. In addition to the AAP, AACAP, and Zero to Three, AutismSpeaks.org has an extensive library of resources, including an invaluable resource called the "first 100 days kit" for families immediately after diagnosis, and provides tips for behavioral support.[26] AACAP's Autism Medication Resource Guide also provides excellent information related to treatment.[24]

Indications for referral:

- All children with ASD (to speech and language therapists, ±occupational therapy, and physical therapy)
- Children whose diagnosis is not clear or with significant comorbidity or with significant level of parent concerns or questions (to ASD specialists or multidisciplinary specialty teams if available)
- Young children with significant social interaction problems and/or disruptive behaviors (to ABA and/or developmental-behavioral pediatrics or mental health evaluation)
- Children with comorbid psychiatric conditions for whom medication is considered and/or when first-line treatments are ineffective

DISRUPTIVE BEHAVIOR PROBLEMS
CLINICAL SIGNIFICANCE

Disruptive behavior problems, including explosive moods, aggression, and noncompliance, are among the most common presenting concerns of parents in pediatric primary care. Disruptive behaviors may represent a wide range of specific disorders, but the term traditionally encompasses ODD and conduct disorder (CD) (*Boxes 21-3 and 21-4*). Many other disorders, including anxiety, mood, neurodevelopmental, sleep, trauma-related, and psychotic disorders may present with patterns of disruptive behaviors and must be distinguished from these two disorders. Worldwide, 113 million youth experience a disruptive behavior disorder (DBD).[27] Although substantial variation occurs, approximately 4% to 8% of youth are affected by a disruptive behavior problem.[27]

BOX 21-3 OPPOSITIONAL DEFIANT DISORDER

- Four or more symptoms for at least 6 months
- Often:
  1. Loses temper
  2. Gets annoyed easily
  3. Seems resentful
  4. Argues with adults
  5. Defies rules
  6. Annoys others purposely
  7. Blames others
  8. Seems vindictive

BOX 21-4 CONDUCT DISORDER

- Recurrent severe rule-breaking behaviors three or more symptoms in the last 12 months with at least one in the last 6 months
- Harms others
  1. Bullies others
  2. Starts physical fights
  3. Uses weapon that can seriously injure
  4. Intentionally harms others
  5. Intentionally harms animals
  6. Steals in face–face confrontations
  7. Forces sexual activity
- Harms property
  1. Sets fires
  2. Destroying property (other ways)
- Stealing and lying
  1. Entered building/vehicle to steal
  2. Deceives to get things
  3. Steals nontrivial items without face–face confrontation
- Serious rule breaking
  1. Stays out past curfew (before age 13 years)
  2. Runs away overnight (at least twice)
  3. Skipped school (before age 13 years)

The costs of disruptive behavior patterns are substantial in the school system. ODD predominantly affects the school system, costing approximately $3,000 (US)/youth/year. CD is associated with $15,000 per year in costs to health care, education, and juvenile justice services.[28] Disruptive behavior problems commonly co-occur with other psychiatric disorders, especially anxiety, depression, learning problems, and substance use disorders.[29]

DIAGNOSIS

The diagnostic process for children presenting with a disruptive behavior problem requires careful attention to the differential diagnosis in the primary care setting. As noted above, almost every psychiatric disorder in childhood can present with disruptive behavior problems, so careful consideration of the differential diagnosis is important, with an appreciation that the symptoms cannot occur exclusively in the context of psychosis, mood disorder, or substance use disorder. It should be noted that ODD occurs in higher rates in youth with ADHD and may co-occur with mood, anxiety, and learning problems as well. An effective treatment plan requires identification of the underlying process and comorbid conditions.

The history related to the disruptive behavior patterns can be seen as analogous to the history for pain. It should include when it started, what it looks like/characteristics of this child's patterns, time course for each event, what makes it better, what makes it worse, and what has been tried to reduce it.

The history taking for children with disruptive patterns requires some specific components. Safety, including access to weapons and guns, is a critical part of the history. Risk factors for disruptive behavior problems include prenatal substance exposure, especially tobacco, developmental delays/learning problems, exposure to adversities including violence in the home, bullying/peer problems, parental conflict or divorce or caregiving separations, school failure, and stressful family financial status. Disruptive behavior patterns are seen in higher rates among children with a family history of mood problems, CD, and substance use disorders, reflecting genetic and/or environmental associations.

Specific signs of ODD and CD are presented in *Boxes 21-3 and 21-4*. Using a broad screening tool such as the PSC-17 for children may help to identify emotional patterns that might co-occur with or underlie the disruptive patterns.[30] The SEEK or an ACES Screening Tool screen may be helpful, but no screen takes the place of taking a history that reviews the stressors that may be associated with an individual child's disruptive behavior patterns.

Observations can inform the diagnostic process (*Table 21-1*). For disruptive behavior patterns, the child's mental status and the tone of parent–child interactions are critical observations. Specific observations include a child's inability to separate from a parent (suggesting anxiety), or harsh parenting tone or threats of later punishment (which may contribute to disruptive behaviors), or overly protective or inconsistent parent behaviors (suggestive of difficulty with limit setting).

Laboratory studies rarely assist with the diagnosis, but testing for lead toxicity, thyroid dysfunction or other endocrinopathies, pregnancy, or substance use may be clinically indicated.

BIOPSYCHOSOCIAL TREATMENT

Treatment for DBDs is predominantly psychosocial, focused on reducing exacerbating factors, enhancing a child's motivation for compliance, and supporting the family in adjusting communication and discipline strategies (*Figure 21-3*).

- Medications have been studied for treatment of signs of DBDs, such as aggression, but not for specific disorders. Pharmacotherapy of comorbid conditions is recommended before pharmacotherapy focused on DBDs. Stimulants and atypical antipsychotic agents, and to a lesser extent alpha agonists, have been shown to be effective in reducing aggression.[31] Of these, stimulants have the safest profile for use in primary care settings and would be recommended as first line if behavioral interventions have not been effective. Atypical antipsychotic agents may be considered in conjunction with behavioral strategies for severe aggression with close monitoring of growth and metabolic adverse effects.
- There is no medication to produce "good behavior."
- Treatment of comorbid conditions that have evidence-based support for use of pharmacologic interventions is recommended.
- Stimulants are the safest medications for PCPs to use for DBD when behavioral interventions have failed.

In preschoolers and school-age children, all effective therapies focus on supporting parents to apply fundamental behavioral principles described in the following list.[32] In older children, evidence-based treatments not only include these approaches, but also explicitly address family communication strategies, learning to regulate strong emotions, and provide the child with individual coping strategies. Educational advocacy is often a component.[31,33] PCPs can begin to introduce behavioral principles by encouraging parents to motivate their child to engage in positive behaviors by praising them for appropriate, but not for inappropriate behaviors.

Principles of behavioral intervention:

- Positive parenting approach:
  - Pair positive reinforcement (e.g., praise) with positive behaviors (use liberally)
  - Withdraw attention from (e.g., "ignore") mid-level provocative or annoying, but safe, child behaviors (selective use)
  - Implement safe, consistent consequences (e.g., time out) for unsafe or unacceptable behaviors (use sparingly)

PCPs are first-line providers for addressing typical and clinical disruptive behavior patterns. Handouts from trusted resources such as the American Academy of Pediatrics' HealthyChildren.org or zerotothree.org can be helpful. Early referral to empirically supported treatment approach is recommended, as early treatment is associated with persistent changes in behavior.[32]

Indications for referral:

- Unsafe aggression toward other children
- Symptoms meeting the level of a psychiatric disorder persistent more than 3 months
- High level of parental stress or concern
- Lack of response to handouts and primary care guidance
- Diagnostic uncertainty

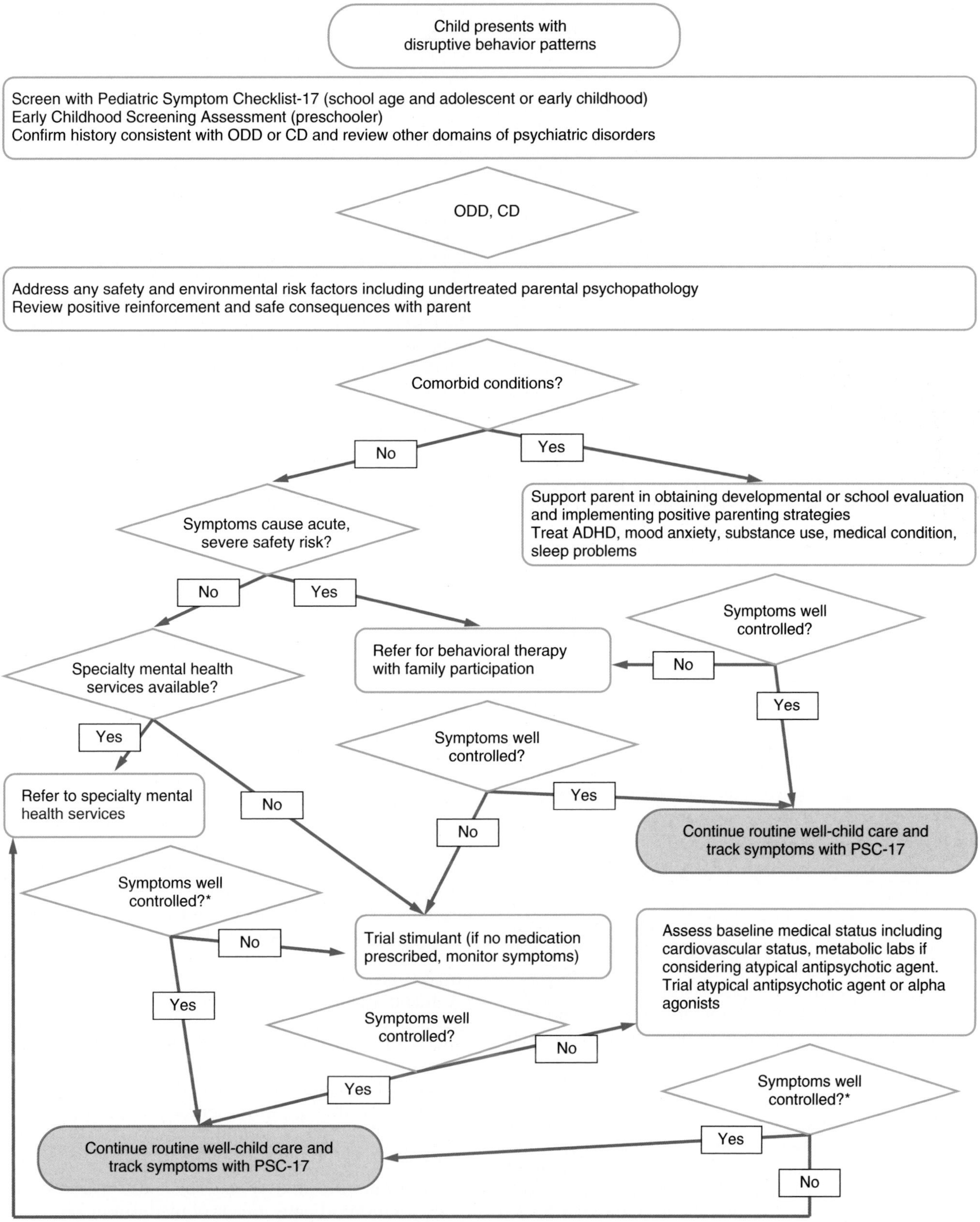

FIGURE 21-3 Pathway for disruptive behavior problems. ADHD, attention deficit and hyperactivity disorder; ASD, autism spectrum disorder; CD, conduct disorder; ODD, oppositional defiant disorder.

ANXIETY DISORDERS

CLINICAL SIGNIFICANCE

Developmentally normative fears, such as preschoolers' fear of the dark, school-age children's fear of separation and strangers, and adolescents' concerns about peer and school issues are commonly discussed with PCPs in health maintenance visits.[34] Pathologic fears are distinguishable because they prevent the child from participating in developmentally and culturally typical activities or cause substantial family reactions/accommodations to the fears.

Anxiety affects 117 million children worldwide, with a prevalence rate of approximately 6.5%.[27] Anxiety disorders cause distress and interfere with educational, familial, and peer activities. Separation anxiety disorders may interfere with a parent's employment when a child cannot attend school or childcare. Pediatric anxiety disorders contribute to physical health costs because of frequent somatic complaints such as headaches or abdominal pain without corresponding physical findings.[35] Strikingly, only a third of youth who meet criteria for an anxiety disorder receive treatment.[1]

All anxiety disorders, including separation anxiety disorder, social phobia, selective mutism, generalized anxiety disorder, and panic disorder can occur in the pediatric population.[35] Selective mutism and separation anxiety disorder often present more in preschool- and school-age children, whereas panic disorder tends to have an adolescent onset.[36] Generalized anxiety disorder shows an increased incidence in adolescent girls but can be present in all ages. Obsessive–compulsive disorder and posttraumatic stress disorder (PTSD) (see Chapters 6 and 7), formerly classified as anxiety disorders, but which have distinct trajectories and treatment responsiveness, also present in children beginning in the preschool ages.

DIAGNOSIS

Anxiety should be considered in any clinical presentation because children with anxiety may range from overly inhibited behavioral patterns to showing dysregulated behaviors that mimic disruptive patterns. Signs of specific anxiety disorders in children are similar to those in adults (see Chapter 5), although developmental differences may influence how these diagnostic criteria present as well as the relative prevalence of specific disorders.

A full history should review the onset of the pattern overall, as well as the environmental context triggers for anxiety, factors that perpetuate the anxiety, factors that help the anxiety resolve, and how caregivers respond to anxiety. It is important to assess for individual as well as family avoidance of triggers and accommodation to the patterns, as families may not be aware of how they have adjusted to avoid anxiety triggers, especially if it is long-standing. Comorbidity is common among children with anxiety disorders, with many children having more than one anxiety disorder, but also commonly concurrent DBDs, ADHD, and/or mood disorders.[35]

When anxiety is suspected, the Screen for Children's Anxiety and Related Emotional Disorders (SCARED) can be helpful in clarifying different types and relative intensity of anxiety.[37] Family history of anxiety may contribute to the development of anxiety genetically and through the caregiving environment, as can other stressors, which should be reviewed thoroughly.

For children with OCD presentations and/or tics, especially abrupt onset, consideration of pediatric autoimmune neuropsychiatric disorder associated with strep (PANDAS) is warranted, although will not influence immediate treatment. For children with signs of PTSD, assessment of safety and risks is the first step. Subsequently, each symptom should be reviewed with the parent and child to ensure identification of children with symptoms as many PTSD symptoms are or represent internal experiences that may not be readily identified by caregivers independently.

Differential diagnosis of pediatric anxiety disorders includes typical development, parental anxiety, medication side effects (e.g., steroids, beta agonists), cardiac arrhythmias (rare), mood disorders, and adaptive response to frightening events including maltreatment or bullying.

BIOPSYCHOSOCIAL TREATMENT

Treatment for pediatric anxiety is multimodal and includes psychoeducation for the child, family, and school as appropriate, in addition to psychotherapy and consideration of psychopharmacologic approaches. In adolescents, combination of psychotherapy and a selective serotonin reuptake inhibitor (SSRI) results in a faster treatment effect than psychotherapy alone and lower safety risk than medication alone[38] (*Figure 21-4*).

Psychopharmacologic treatment is recommended for children older than 6 years with moderate–severe anxiety or children with mild anxiety for whom behavioral approaches have not been effective. SSRIs have the strongest efficacy data in treating non-PTSD pediatric anxiety disorders, with a moderate effect size.[39,40] Fluoxetine, escitalopram, and sertraline have substantial safety and efficacy data and FDA indications in adolescents, so they are recommended for treatment of pediatric anxiety in primary care.[41] No medications have been shown to be effective in treating pediatric PTSD, although comorbid symptoms and conditions including sleep, comorbid anxiety, ADHD may be managed pharmacologically.[42] Combination therapy with medication and psychotherapy shows the most rapid and strongest effects for pediatric anxiety in the short term and up to 3 years later.[43]

- Children with anxiety may be more aware of and report more somatic effects of medication.
- Concurrent psychotherapy and pharmacotherapy is likely to yield most rapid onset and most durable effect.
- FDA black box should be reviewed, although large studies have not demonstrated significant increase in suicidality in anxious youth.

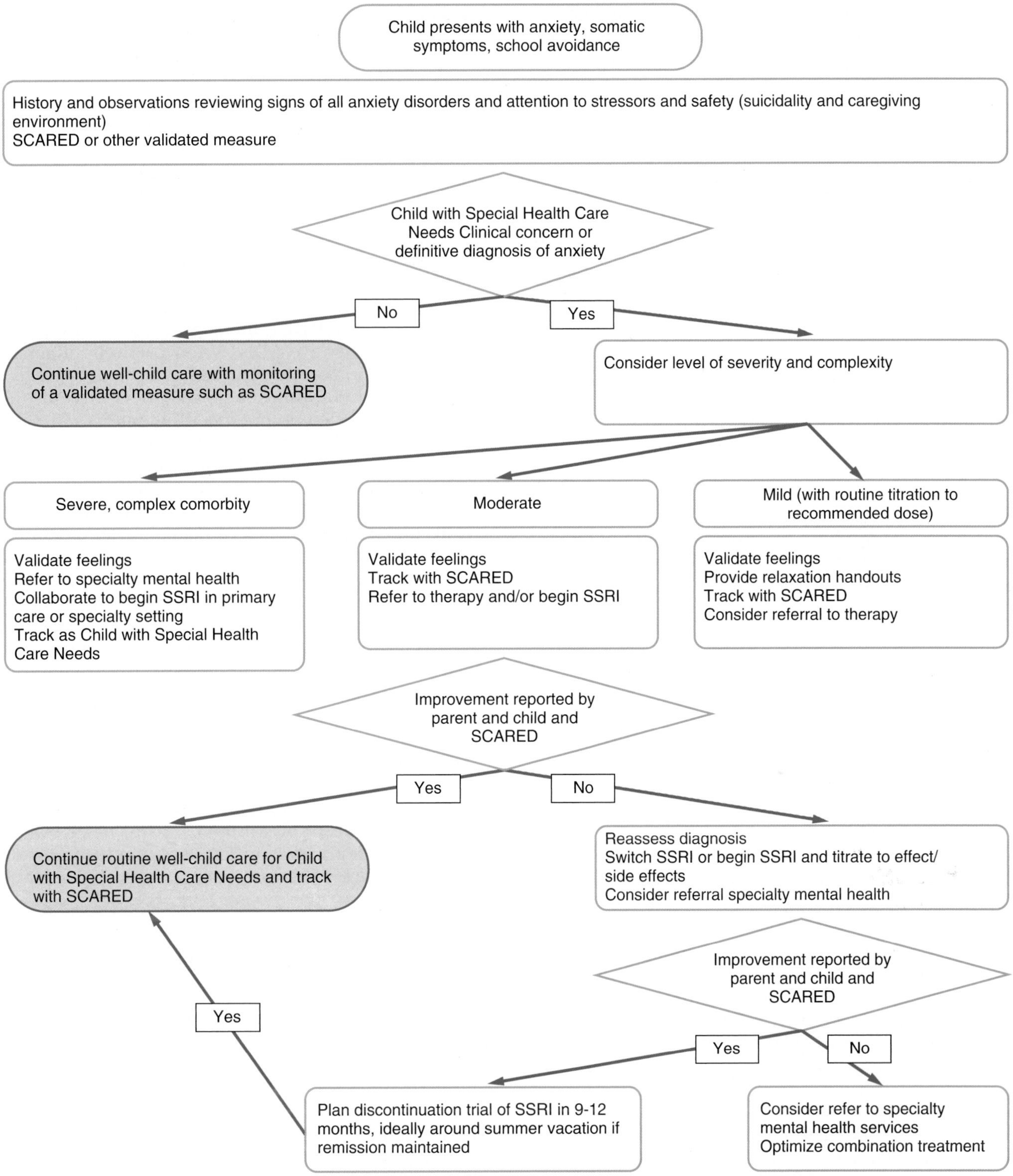

FIGURE 21-4 Pathway for anxiety disorders.

Psychotherapy, especially cognitive behavioral therapy, offers effective and durable treatment for pediatric anxiety (CBT).[44] A form of CBT, exposure and response prevention (ERP), involves a cycle of rating distress, learning relaxation strategies, and practicing exposure to anxiety triggers, followed by rating of distress, use of strategies, and rerating of distress.[44] Strategies for younger children tend to rely on more behavioral coping strategies (relaxation) and for older children include both behavioral and cognitive strategies such as analyzing automatic and maladaptive thoughts.

PCPs can offer children and families training in relaxation strategies including breathing and/or muscle relaxation and can educate families about the foundations of CBT. Families can praise and positively reinforce developing "brave" behaviors and stop avoiding the anxiety triggers themselves. Behavioral strategies originally developed for disruptive behavior problems, such as parent training to increase positive reinforcement for "brave" behaviors, can effectively reduce anxiety symptoms in preschoolers.[45] Relaxation strategies abound on the Internet with apps and handouts and are reviewed on the American Association of Depression and Anxiety (aada.org) Web page.[46] Books by anxiety experts including John March, Tamar Chansky, and Phillip Kendall can be useful in supporting families.[47-49]

PCP's can track symptoms, using a measure such as the SCARED, at least every 6 months if the child is receiving treatment outside the medical home. The PCP may be involved with providing information to the school about needed accommodations including in-school counseling, academic expectation adjustments, and helping educate the school to not to perpetuate avoidance behaviors, such as sending a child home from school for complaints of abdominal pain that has already been assessed and found to be associated with anxiety.

Indications for referral:

- Impairing anxiety in preschool child, for whom therapy is first line
- Any child with anxiety whose family is interested in therapy
- No improvement with psychopharmacologic monotherapy
- Comorbid conditions make clear diagnosis and/or treatment plan difficult to develop

DEPRESSIVE DISORDERS
CLINICAL SIGNIFICANCE

Depression affects 1% to 2% of preschool- and school-age children and 5% to 8% of adolescents, with higher rates among teen girls.[50] Depression presents with depressed mood, neurovegetative signs, cognitive changes, guilt, and suicidal ideation or actions. It is among the leading correlates of suicide and predicts adult anxiety, substance use, suicidality, and physical health problems. Emotional disorders such as depression are more costly than other mental health problems in children, in large part owing to hospitalization costs.[3] Depression is associated with individual suffering, peer relationship problems, family functioning, academic functioning problems, and costs to parents' employment.[51] More than half of adolescents with depression have at least one comorbid condition and many have more.[50] Depression is also associated with physical health problems, especially asthma, pain syndromes, chronic fatigue, epilepsy, and headaches and should be differentiated from thyroid dysfunction.[52]

DIAGNOSIS

The diagnostic criteria for pediatric depression are the same for children and adolescents compared with adults and only slightly modified for preschoolers.[53,54] The most important step in diagnosis of depression in pediatrics is to identify it. The AAP recommends universal screening for adolescent depression with depression-specific measures such as the Patient Health Questionnaire-2.[55]

The differential diagnosis for depressive symptoms is broad and includes any physical health conditions that may cause similar low energy, changes in appetite, and decreased hope as well as psychiatric illnesses including dysthymia, adjustment disorder, disruptive mood dysregulated disorder (DMDD), bipolar disorder, anxiety, substance use, inattentive ADHD, and psychotic illnesses. Dysthymia is a chronic, but less symptomatic/severe depressive disorder. Adjustment disorders present with mood symptoms that do not meet full criteria for major depressive disorder (MDD) in response to a stressor. DMDD is a newly described diagnosis of chronic irritability and excessive emotional reactivity without the cycles of bipolar disorder. Bipolar disorder includes distinct periods greater than a week of mania, meaning euphoria or intense irritability with decreased need for sleep, intense focused activities, rapid speech and thoughts, and extreme risk-taking behaviors.[53] It should be noted that subthreshold depressive symptoms are a risk factor for MDD and other adverse outcomes and warrant tracking in primary care. Severe depression may present with hallucinations and/or delusions, which must be distinguished from other psychotic illnesses and should trigger referral.

Diagnosis depends on a careful history with the patient and parent individually. History includes the criteria for depression with attention to the timing and context of the onset of symptoms, patterns of exacerbation and relief, and associated symptoms of anxiety, ADHD, disruptive behavior patterns, substance use, and hallucinations.

BIOPSYCHOSOCIAL TREATMENT

Treatment recommendations for pediatric depression depend on age and severity, but always include substantial psychoeducation, addressing life stressors, and parental psychopathology. Recommendations for adolescents tend to be more widely agreed on in the United States, whereas the limits of the literature make recommendations in younger children more challenging (*Figure 21-5*).

Fluoxetine has been shown to be effective in treating pediatric depression and is the SSRI with a positive safety:efficacy ratio in children younger than 12 years.[41] Escitalopram and sertraline have been shown to be more effective than placebo in treating adolescent depression.[56] Other medications have very little support and are not recommended for use in primary care. Based on existing evidence, unless a child has high risk of adverse effects or strong preference, fluoxetine is a reasonable first-line treatment. Common side effects are reviewed in

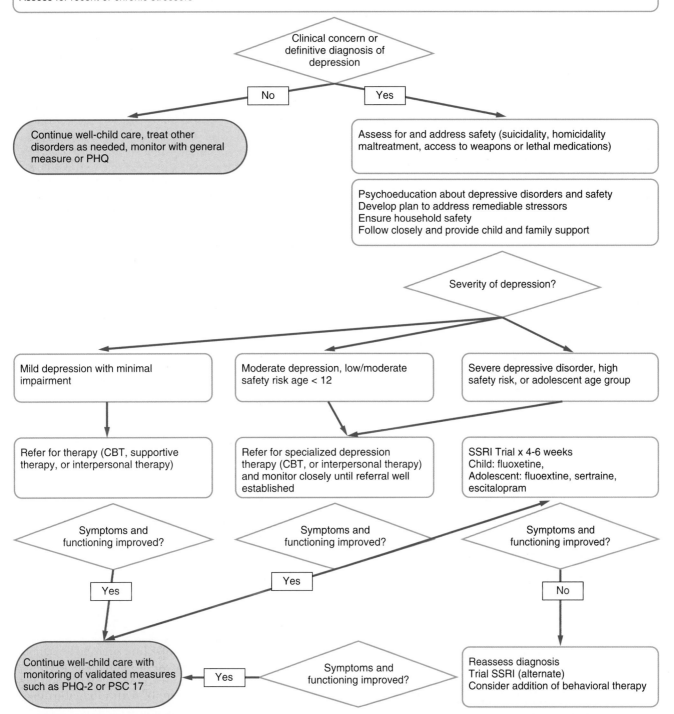

FIGURE 21-5 Pathway for depressive disorders. PHQ, Patient Health Questionnaire; PSC, Pediatric Symptom Checklist; SCARED, Screen for Children's Anxiety and Related Emotional Disorders; SSRI, selective serotonin reuptake inhibitor.

Table 21-2. The highest-risk side effects of mania and suicidal ideation occur rarely, 5% and 2%, respectively, but constitute emergencies requiring immediate attention. Development of a safety plan is a critical part of treatment planning. Clinically, it may be helpful to have the child confirm the plan directly with the provider and the parent in the office. The FDA recommends follow-up weekly in the first month after initiation or dose change of an antidepressant and biweekly in the second month for individuals younger than 25 years. If a first SSRI is not effective, reassessment of the diagnosis and comorbid diagnosis is warranted and an alternate SSRI may be tried. When they are effective, SSRIs should be continued 9 to 12 months after remission of symptoms in the first episode of depression.

- Careful review of signs of mania is necessary before starting an SSRI because of the higher risk of triggering mania in children with bipolar disorder.
- Informed consent should include the black box warning about suicidality and also the risks associated with untreated depression including completed suicide.
- The lowest rate of relapse with treatment discontinuation is in the summertime.

For mild depression, supportive therapy or other proven treatments may be the primary treatment. For moderate or severe depression, an evidence-based treatment such as CBT or interpersonal therapy (IPT) is recommended, although the research supporting these treatments for depression in children is less than that for adults or for pediatric anxiety disorders.[50] CBT focuses on developing skills to address maladaptive thought or behavior processes. IPT is less available in the United States compared with other countries.

- Supportive therapy can be helpful for mild depression, with family involvement especially for young children.
- Evidence-based treatments for depression provide psychoeducation about the course and treatability of depression and addressing misconceptions and stigma about the cause of impairment.
- Recommendations of healthy lifestyle such as sleep hygiene, exercise, and reducing modifiable stressors (school stress, bullying) may be helpful.
- Referrals to therapy commonly fail, so PCPs should continue to see children with depression regularly until therapy is established.

In addition to the common resources, the Anxiety and Depression Association of America offers valuable handouts and podcasts for youth and parents. GLAD-PC.org offers a primary care tool kit. Parentsmedguide.org offers guidance about psychopharmacologic treatment.

Indications for referral:

- Children younger than 12 years with depression not responding to supportive approaches
- Adolescents with comorbid psychiatric conditions, including psychosis or substance use
- Adolescents not responding to first- or second-line SSRI monotherapy
- Symptomatic parents of children with depression

PRACTICAL RESOURCES

- Child Psychiatry: AACAP.org
- Child well-being Healthychildren.org
- Young children: zerotothree.org
- ADHD: CHADD.org

CASES AND QUESTIONS

CASE 1:

Max is an 18-month-old-immigrant boy who presents for a well-child visit. He does not make eye contact or point. He has about two spontaneous words and can imitate and repeat others. He does not play at all with his older brother. He has significant temper tantrums multiple times a week, often when his favorite toy is taken away from him and is very difficult to comfort.

1. What is the most likely diagnosis?
   A. ASD
   B. Normal development
   C. Bipolar disorder
   D. Intermittent explosive disorder
   E. Oppositional defiant disorder

   Correct answer: A. *Max has deficits in social communication and social interactions. Although his symptoms are disruptive, they are not consistent with intermittent explosive disorder or ODD. None of the history is suggestive of mania/hypomania to make the diagnosis of bipolar.*

2. What screen for social development does the American Academy of Pediatric recommend at 18-month visit?
   A. PSC-17
   B. Autism-specific screening tool such as the M-CHAT-R/F only
   C. Informal developmental surveillance
   D. A and B
   E. B and C
   F. None

   Correct answer: B. *The AAP recommends formal screening for autism at 18 and 24 months as well as developmental screening. The PSC-17 is used in older children and developmental surveillance is insufficient to identify autism in a timely manner.*

3. Which aspect of the history is most concerning for his age?
   A. Repeating words
   B. Lack of joint attention skills (pointing)
   C. Having a favorite toy
   D. Having an attachment to his favorite toy
   E. Having temper tantrum

Correct answer: B. *Joint attention skill is important component of social development and typically present earlier than 18 months. Having a favorite toy, being attached to it, and having a temper tantrum when taken away can all be typical behavior for this age. Cooperative play tends to develop at an older age.*

4. What workups, labs, and referrals should be ordered?

   A. Wood lamp examination to identify tuberous sclerosis
   B. Chromosome microarray analysis
   C. Lead test
   D. Hearing evaluation
   E. E.All of the above

   Correct answer: E. *Anyone with suspected ASD should be evaluated for neurocutaneous disorders and other genetic disorders because of high comorbidities. Lead toxicity and hearing impairment can also present with similar symptoms.*

CASE 2:

Amy is an 11-year-old transgender girl who presents with behavior concerns. She will not sit still and is always running/skipping around. She talks excessively. She has trouble concentrating except playing video games. She interrupts family members and fidgets. She gets into trouble for not following directions, not completing homework, and not listening. The examination, including neuro examination, is unremarkable except for hyperactivity.

1. What additional steps should be done to diagnose?

   A. Obtain both parent and teacher assessments using a validated tool such as Vanderbilt Scale
   B. Full diet journal to assess sugar intake
   C. TSH and Free T4
   D. Neuroimaging and EEG
   E. Lead level

   Correct answer: A. *It is important to assess the symptoms present in at least two settings and causing impairment. One of the ways to accomplish is to utilize validated tools. Although the dietary sugar intake contributing to ADHD symptom is not established, a diet journal would not help in making diagnosis. Without other signs and symptoms, additional labs, imagining, or workup is unnecessary.*

2. Which medication should be chosen first?

   A. Atomoxetine or other SNRIs
   B. Bupropion or other antidepressants
   C. Clonidine or other alpha agonists
   D. Dextroamphetamine or other stimulants
   E. Escitalopram or other SSRIs

   Correct answer: D. *Stimulants are the first-line treatment for ADHD in school-age children and older. Although other medication such as*

atomoxetine and clonidine can be used to treat ADHD, they are not considered first line. There is no FDA indication for bupropion or escitalopram to treat ADHD.

3. If Amy has been 4 years old, what would have been the first-line treatment?

   A. Guanfacine because it is less sedating
   B. Behavioral therapy because the evidences show high effect
   C. Fluoxetine because it has the most coverage for other comorbidities
   D. Dextroamphetamine because it has FDA approval for children as young as 3 years old
   E. Aripiprazole because it will manage disruptive behaviors the most

   Correct answer: B. *Behavioral therapy is first-line treatment for preschool-age children with ADHD. If adequate therapy fails and there is a high risk, medication can be considered. There is no indication to use atypical antipsychotics such as aripiprazole for this patient.*

CASE 3:

Ben is a 16-year-old brought in by parents for low mood and energy after death of his friend 6 months ago. He has not been sleeping well. He has been eating more and gained significant weight. He stopped his favorite activities, failed several examinations recently. He is irritable and defensive.

1. What is the least likely diagnosis?

   A. Major Depressive Disorder
   B. Substance use disorder
   C. Persistent depressive disorder
   D. Binge eating disorder
   E. Bereavement

   Correct answer: A. *Any youth presenting with these symptoms should be assessed for MDD, persistent depressive disorder, bereavement, and substance use disorder. Increased appetite is likely related to his mood or substance use (e.g., cannabis) rather than binge eating disorder.*

2. Should suicidal thinking be assessed?

   A. Yes, he is at higher risk but he should be assessed in private.
   B. Yes, he is at higher risk but his parents can answer accurately.
   C. Yes, he is at higher risk but gaining weight is a future oriented protective factor.
   D. No, he is at lower risk because of his family involvement.
   E. No, because assessing suicidal thinking will make him start to think about suicide.

continued

Correct answer: A. *Despite having concerned family, he is at risk for suicide because of depression. Comprehensive risk assessment including suicide should be done alone with him after explaining the scope and limit of confidentiality. Assessing for thoughts of suicide does not lead to development of suicidal thinking.*

3. If depression has been diagnosed, what treatment option should be recommended?

   A. SSRIs such as fluoxetine and escitalopram
   B. Psychotherapy such as cognitive behavioral therapy and interpersonal therapy
   C. Both SSRI and psychotherapy
   D. Any of the above
   E. None of the above—watchful waiting

   Correct answer: D. *When depression has been diagnosed, treatment should be recommended. However, the choice between psychotherapy, medication, or combination treatment will depend on the severity of symptoms, availability of evidence-based therapy provider, and patient and family's preference and ability to receive treatment.*

ACKNOWLEDGMENTS

With thanks to Lauren Kaczka-Weiss and Kathryn Sigalow for their contributions to the effort.

REFERENCES

1. Merikangas KR, He JP, Brody D, Fisher PW, Bourdon K, Koretz DS. Prevalence and treatment of mental disorders among US children in the 2001-2004 NHANES. *Pediatrics.* 2010;125(1):75-81.

2. Kelleher KJ, Campo JV, Gardner WP. Management of pediatric mental disorders in primary care: where are we now and where are we going? *Curr Opin Pediatr.* 2006;18(6):649-653.

3. Guevara JP, Mandell DS, Rostain AL, Zhao H, Hadley TR. National estimates of health services expenditures for children with behavioral disorders: an analysis of the medical expenditure panel survey. *Pediatrics.* 2003;112(6):e440-e446.

4. Perou R, Bitsko RH, Blumberg SJ, et al. Mental health surveillance among children—United States, 2005-2011. *MMWR Surveill Summ.* 2013;62(suppl 2):1-35.

5. AAP. *Bright Futures Periodicity Schedule.* 2107. Available at https://www.aap.org/en-us/documents/periodicity_schedule.pdf. Cited July 12, 2017.

6. National Survey of Children's Health NSCH 2011/12. *Data query from the Child and Adolescent Health Measurement Initiative, Data Resource Center for Child and Adolescent Health website.* 2011. Available at www.childhealthdata.org. Cited July 21, 2017.

7. Dubowitz H, Lane WG, Semiatin JN, Magder LS, Venepally M, Jans M. The safe environment for every Kid model: impact on pediatric primary care professionals. *Pediatrics.* 2011;127(4):e962-e970.

8. Marie-Mitchell A, O'Connor TG. Adverse childhood experiences: translating knowledge into identification of children at risk for poor outcomes. *Acad Pediatr.* 2013;13(1):14-19.

9. Purewal SK, Harris NB. Screening for adverse childhood experiences (ACEs) in an integrated pediatric care model. *Zero to Three J.* 2016;36(3):10-17.

10. Gleason MM, Goldson E, Yogman MW, et al. Addressing early childhood emotional and behavioral problems: technical report. *Pediatrics.* 2016;138(6):e20163025.

11. Thomas R, Sanders S, Doust J, Beller E, Glasziou P. Prevalence of attention-deficit/hyperactivity disorder: a systematic review and meta-analysis. *Pediatrics.* 2015;135(4):e994-e1001.

12. Doshi JA, Hodgkins P, Kahle J, et al. Economic impact of childhood and adult attention-deficit/hyperactivity disorder in the United States. *J Am Acad Child Adolesc Psychiatry.* 2012;51(10):990-1002.e2.

13. AAP. ADHD: clinical practice guideline for the diagnosis, evaluation, and treatment of attention-deficit/hyperactivity disorder in children and adolescents. *Pediatrics.* 2011;128(5):2654.

14. Southammakosane C, Schmitz K. Pediatric psychopharmacology for treatment of ADHD, depression, and anxiety. *Pediatrics.* 2015;136(2):351-359.

15. Faraone SV, Buitelaar J. Comparing the efficacy of stimulants for ADHD in children and adolescents using meta-analysis. *Eur Child Adolesc Psychiatry.* 2010;19(4):353-364.

16. Gleason MM, Egger HL, Emslie GJ, et al. Psychopharmacological treatment for very young children: contexts and guidelines. *J Am Acad Child Adolesc Psychiatry.* 2007;46(12):1532-1572.

17. Fabiano GA, Pelham WE Jr, Coles EK, et al. A meta-analysis of behavioral treatments for attention-deficit/hyperactivity disorder. *Clin Psychol Rev.* 2009;29(2):129-140.

18. Hinshaw SP. Moderators and mediators of treatment outcome for youth with ADHD: understanding for whom and how interventions work. *Ambul Pediatr.* 2007;7(1):91-100.

19. Developmental Disabilities Monitoring Network Surveillance Year. Prevalence of autism spectrum disorder among children aged 8 years-autism and developmental disabilities monitoring network. *MMWR Morb Mortal Wkly Rep.* 2014;63(2):1.

20. Zuckerman KE, Lindly OJ, Sinche BK. Parental concerns, provider response, and timeliness of autism spectrum disorder diagnosis. *J Pediatr.* 2015;166(6):1431-1439.e1.

21. Lavelle TA, Weinstein MC, Newhouse JP, Munir K, Kuhlthau KA, Prosser LA. Economic burden of childhood autism spectrum disorders. *Pediatrics.* 2014;133(3):e520-e529.

22. Myers SM, Chris Plauché Johnson the Council on Children with Disabilities. The Council on children with, management of children with autism spectrum disorders. *Pediatrics.* 2007;120(5):1162-1182.

23. Rutter M, Kreppner J, Croft C, et al. Early adolescent outcomes of institutionally deprived and non-deprived adoptees. III. Quasi-autism. *JCPP (J Child Psychol Psychiatry).* 2007;48(12):1200-1207.

24. AACAP. *Autism Spectrum Disorders Parents Medication Guide.* Washington, DC; 2016.

25. Siu AL, US Preventive Services Task Force (USPSTF), Bibbins-Domingo K. screening for autism spectrum disorder in young children US preventive task force recommendation statement. *J Am Med Assoc.* 2016;315(7):691-696.

26. AutismSpeaks. *First Hundred Days Kit.* Available at https://www.autismspeaks.org/family-services/tool-kits/100-day-kit. Cited July 14, 2017.

27. Polanczyk GV, et al. Annual Research Review: a meta-analysis of the worldwide prevalence of mental disorders in children and adolescents. *J Child Psychol Psychiatry.* 2015;56(3):345-365.

28. Foster EM, Jones DE. The conduct problems prevention research group, the high costs of aggression: public expenditures resulting from conduct disorder. *Am J Public Health.* 2005;95(10):1767-1772.

29. Costello EJ, Mustillo S, Erkanli A, Keeler G, Angold A. Prevalence and development of psychiatric disorders in childhood and adolescence. *Arch Gen Psychiatry.* 2003;60(8):837-844.

30. Gardner W, Murphy M, Childs G, et al. The PSC-17. *Ambul Child Health.* 1999;5(3):225-236.

31. Scotto Rosato N, Correll CU, Pappadopulos E, et al. Treatment of maladaptive aggression in youth: CERT guidelines, II: treatments and ongoing management. *Pediatrics.* 2012;129(6):e1577-e1586.

32. Eyberg SM, Nelson MM, Boggs SR. Evidence-based psychosocial treatments for children and adolescents with disruptive behavior. *J Clin Child Adolesc Psychol.* 2008;37(1):215.

33. Pliszka S, AACAP Work Group on Quality Issues. Issues, Practice parameter for the assessment and treatment of children and adolescents with attention-deficit/hyperactivity disorder. *J Am Acad Child Adolesc Psychiatry.* 2007;46(7):894-921.

34. Weems CF, Costa NM. Developmental differences in the expression of childhood anxiety symptoms and fears. *J Am Acad Child Adolesc Psychiatry.* 2005;44(7):656-663.

35. Connolly SD, Bernstein GA. Practice parameter for the assessment and treatment of children and adolescents with anxiety disorders. *J Am Acad Child Adolesc Psychiatry.* 2007;46(2):267-283.

36. Beesdo K, Knappe S, Pine DS. Anxiety and anxiety disorders in children and adolescents: developmental issues and implications for DSM-V. *Psychiatr Clin North Am.* 2009;32(3):483-524.

37. Connor DF, Carlson GA, Chang KD, et al. Juvenile maladaptive aggression: a review of prevention, treatment, and service configuration and a proposed research agenda. *J Clin Psychiatry.* 2006;67(5):808-820.

38. March JS, Silva S, Petrycki S, et al. The Treatment for Adolescents with Depression Study (TADS): long-term effectiveness and safety outcomes. *Arch Gen Psychiatry.* 2007;64(10):1132-1143.

39. Strawn JR, Welge JA, Wehry AM, Keeshin B, Rynn MA. Efficacy and tolerability of antidepressants in pediatric anxiety disorders: a systematic review and meta-analysis. *Depress Anxiety.* 2015;32(3):149-157.

40. Pediatric OCD Treatment Study (POTS) Team. Cognitive-behavior therapy, sertraline, and their combination for children and adolescents with obsessive-compulsive disorder: the Pediatric OCD Treatment Study (POTS) randomized controlled trial. *J Am Med Assoc.* 2004;292(16):1969-1976.

41. Bridge JA, Iyengar S, Salary CB, et al. Clinical response and risk for reported suicidal ideation and suicide attempts in pediatric antidepressant treatment: a meta-analysis of randomized controlled trials. *J Am Med Assoc.* 2007;297(15):1683-1696.

42. Cohen JA, Mannarino AP, Perel JM, Staron V. A pilot randomized controlled trial of combined trauma-focused CBT and sertraline for childhood PTSD symptoms. *J Am Acad Child Adolesc Psychiatry.* 2007;46(7):811-819.

43. Piacentini J, Bennett S, Compton SN, et al. 24- and 36-week outcomes for the child/adolescent anxiety multimodal study (CAMS). *J Am Acad Child Adolesc Psychiatry.* 2014;53(3):297-310.

44. AACAP. Practice parameter for the assessment and treatment of children and adolescents with anxiety disorders. *J Am Acad Child Adolesc Psychiatry.* 2007;46(2):267-273.

45. Carpenter AL, Puliafico AC, Kurtz SM, Pincus DB, Comer JS. Extending parent-child interaction therapy for early childhood internalizing problems: new advances for an overlooked population. *Clin Child Fam Psychol Rev.* 2014;17(4):340.

46. ADAA. *Mental Health APps.* 2015 . Available at https://www.adaa.org/finding-help/mobile-apps. Cited July 3, 2017.

47. March JS, Benton C. *Talking Back to OCD.* NY: Guilford Press; 2007.

48. Chansky T. *Freeing Your Child from Anxiety.* 2nd ed. NY: Harmony Books; 2014.

49. Kendall PC, Podell JL, Gosch E. *The Coping Cat Parent Companion.* Ardmore, PA: Workbook Publishing; 2010.

50. Thapar A, Collishaw S, Pine DS, Thapar AK, et al. Depression in adolescence. *Lancet.* 2012;379(9820):1056-1067.

51. Jaycox LH, Stein BD, Paddock S, et al. Impact of teen depression on academic, social, and physical functioning. *Pediatrics.* 2009;124(4):e596-e605.

52. Pinquart M, Shen Y. Depressive symptoms in children and adolescents with chronic physical illness: an updated meta-analysis. *J Pediatr Psychol.* 2010;36(4):375-384.

53. APA. *Diagnostic and Statistical Manual-5.* Washington, DC: APA Press; 2013.

54. Gleason MM, Goldson E, Yogman MW, Council on Early Childhood, Committee on Psychosocial Aspects of Child and Family Health, Section on Developmental and Behavioral Pediatrics. Addressing early childhood emotional and behavioral problems (Policy Statement). *Pediatrics.* 2016;138(6):e20163025.

55. AAP. *Bright Futures Periodicity Schedule.* 2016. https://www.aap.org/en-us/documents/periodicity_schedule.pdf.

56. AACAP. Practice parameter for the assessment and treatment of children and adolescents with depressive disorders. *J Am Acad Child Adolesc Psychiatry.* 2007;46(11):1504-1526.

22

SUICIDE AND VIOLENCE RISK ASSESSMENT

Amy Barnhorst, MD and Cameron Quanbeck, MD

INTRODUCTION

Primary care physicians will evaluate and treat patients at risk for both suicide and violence in the course of their practice. Patients at risk for suicide are more likely to be in treatment with a primary care physician than with a psychiatrist, so it is important for primary care doctors to be able to identify patients at risk and intervene appropriately. Violence in primary care patients most often happens in the clinic itself, and proper prevention and management of violence risk can be crucial for staff and patient safety.

CLINICAL HIGHLIGHTS

Assessment and Management of Suicide Risk

- Screening at-risk patients for suicidal thinking in the primary care setting can prevent suicides.
- A number of studies in primary care settings indicate that providers often do not ask patients with depression if they have suicidal thoughts.
- Patients who commit suicide are more likely to have seen a primary care doctor than a mental health professional in the month before their death. Therefore, primary care physicians may be uniquely poised to intervene with suicidal patients.
- Patients who commit suicide within a month of seeing a primary care provider are predominately older males with chronic physical illnesses who live alone.
- Suicide risk assessment involves balancing nonmodifiable and modifiable risk factors for suicide against factors that protect against suicide. One key modifiable risk factor for suicide in the primary care setting is psychiatric illness, particularly depression coupled with severe anxiety.
- Screening at-risk patients for suicidal thinking is important in assessing suicide risk and will not cause a patient to start thinking about suicide.

- Research has shown that most patients who commit suicide tell family and friends of their wish to die. Therefore, obtaining collateral information from relatives or friends can be an invaluable strategy for detecting patients at high suicide risk.
- Seventy-five percent of patients reported having planned their suicide attempt for less than an hour before acting, and nearly a quarter of them planned it for less than 5 minutes. Care should be taken to mitigate impulsivity when possible (e.g., decreasing alcohol use) and to restrict access to high-lethality suicide methods (e.g., firearms and lethal medications).
- If clinicians determine that a patient is at significant acute risk of suicide, they should have a "plan of action" in place that ensures the patient is quickly referred to a mental health professional.

Assessment and Management of Violence Risk

- Most primary care providers report experiencing violent behavior from their patients and these experiences can have a negative impact on work performance.
- Patients with a history of violence and substance abuse are most likely to behave aggressively in the primary care setting; the emergency department is the setting where violence is most common.
- A common precipitant to an assault on a primary care provider is after a patient is told "no."
- Effective strategies to diffuse potential violence include early recognition, avoiding arguments or taking an authoritarian stance, empathizing with the patient's frustration, and providing choices for the patient.

ASSESSMENT AND MANAGEMENT OF SUICIDE RISK

CLINICAL SIGNIFICANCE

One in ten patients seen in primary care settings meets criteria for major depressive disorder. Depression is particularly common in patients presenting for treatment of a chronic medical condition, with a prevalence of about 30% to 40%. Primary care providers see depressed patients routinely and most are managing these patients with antidepressant pharmacotherapy. Suicidal thinking is a feature of depression and suicide is a potential outcome. One in five patients will report suicidal thoughts during a course of treatment for depression, particularly those with more severe symptoms.[1] Clinicians should therefore be familiar with assessing and managing suicide risk.

However, although depression is common in primary care settings, it is not the only condition strongly associated with suicide, and patients presenting without depressive symptoms may still be at an elevated risk. Schizophrenia, borderline personality disorder, and bipolar disorder carry lifetime risks of suicide of more than 10 times that of the general population.[2] Alcohol use is also strongly associated with suicide, and one study showed that 33% percent of people who completed suicide had alcohol in their system when they did so. Alcohol may also predispose people to making attempts with a higher expectation of death; people who used firearms as a suicide method were more likely to be intoxicated than people who overdosed.[3]

Alcohol's disinhibiting qualities may partially explain its relationship to suicide, as there is evidence to show that the majority of serious suicide attempts are impulsive. One study examined people who had survived a serious suicide attempt that would have likely resulted in their death if not for an emergent medical or surgical intervention. Investigators questioned them about the time leading up to their attempt. Seventy-five percent reported having planned their suicide attempt for less than an hour before acting, and nearly a quarter of them planned it for less than 5 minutes. This is one reason that restricting people's access to suicide methods with high lethality has been proven to be an effective method in reducing suicides[4]—they often use what is available to them in the short time-frame in which they are suicidal before acting.

Despite the fact that most patients are not planning their suicide attempt far in advance, primary care clinicians may be better positioned than mental health professionals to identify patients at risk of suicide, planned or impulsive. This is because clinical contact of depressed patients with primary care providers in the period preceding a suicide is more common than contact with mental health professions. Nearly half of these patients have contact with their primary care physician in the month before their death, particularly older adults.[5] In contrast, only 20% of those who die by suicide see a mental health professional in the month before their death.[6] Although it is not known whether or not these suicides were preventable, this suggests the clinical encounter immediately before suicide can be an opportunity to identify suicide risk and plan appropriate interventions. In patients who are at risk but not currently suicidal at the time of the visit, this may include addressing untreated psychiatric symptoms, reducing alcohol use, and counseling them and their support systems about access to lethal means.

Studies suggest that primary care providers could do a better job at identifying patients at risk for suicide. A recent study examined whether or not suicidal thinking was explored in a group of patients who made an unannounced visit to a primary care clinic complaining of depressive symptoms and requesting an antidepressant. Fewer than half (42%) of patients were asked about suicidal ideations.[7] Another study examined whether or not suicidal thinking was explored by primary care physicians in the last visit before suicide in a group of patients who committed suicide within a month of contact. Sixty-two percent of these patients were not asked about suicidal thinking, and in half of these cases, the provider had little knowledge of the patient's life circumstances.[8]

SUICIDE RISK ASSESSMENT IN THE PRIMARY CARE SETTING

The finding that many of those who commit suicide have seen a primary care provider shortly before their death has led to investigations that attempt to profile the type of patient at risk. One study compared differences between older adults who committed suicide within 30 days of visiting a primary care provider with older primary patients who did not commit suicide. Those who committed suicide had more depressive illness, greater physical illness burden, and functional limitations and were more likely to be prescribed antidepressants, antianxiety agents, and opiate analgesics.[9] A similar study investigated the differences between older men and women who committed suicide shortly after a primary care visit. Male suicides outnumbered female by a ratio of 3:1. Men were more likely to be single or widowed than women. Men were more likely to use hanging as a primary suicide method, whereas women tended to overdose on medications, which suggests care should be exercised in prescribing medications that can be lethal in overdose. In both men and women, the primary complaint involved physical, not psychiatric, symptoms.[10] Another study found that older adults were more likely to complain of physical symptoms before suicide, whereas younger adults were more likely to seek help for psychiatric symptoms.[11] These data lead to the conclusion that older, nonpartnered men with physical symptoms, especially pain and functional limitations, are at an elevated risk of suicide in a primary care setting. Although many individuals in this large demographic may not be at risk, it may be worth focusing suicide risk screening questions on these types of patients.

The assessment of suicide risk is not as simple as asking a patient, "Have you been having suicidal thoughts?" Inquiring about suicidal thinking is important, but is only one piece of performing a suicide risk assessment. The assessment also involves an examination of risk factors for suicide balanced against factors protective against suicide. The more suicide risk factors and fewer protective factors, the greater the risk. There is no specific set of risk factors that have been shown to predict whether or not a patient will commit suicide; because suicide is a very rare event, it is nearly impossible to design and carry out a study with that goal. If primary care providers are aware of key risk and protective factors, however, they can use sound clinical judgment to identify at-risk patients and take steps to reduce the likelihood a suicide will occur.

TABLE 22-1 Risk Factors for Suicide

Key nonmodifiable risk factors for suicide

- A past suicide attempt, particularly a serious attempt
- Male gender
- Advanced age (>65 years)
- Caucasian or Native American ethnicity
- Divorced, separated, or widowed
- Unemployment (particularly recent loss of job in those <45 years)
- Alcohol dependence (particularly when facing losses)
- Childhood sexual and physical abuse
- Chronic neurologic illness
- A family history of suicide

Key modifiable risk factors for suicide

- Major depressive episode, especially with prominent anxiety symptoms causing insomnia, psychomotor agitation, decreased concentration, and an inability to experience pleasure
- Alcohol abuse
- Hopelessness
- Suicidal ideation and plan (although some patients intent on suicide may deny these thoughts to health care providers)
- Access to lethal means (e.g., firearms, certain medications, etc.)

Nonmodifiable Risk Factors

Certain risk factors are static and cannot be changed with clinical intervention. They include demographic factors (e.g., age, gender, and ethnicity) and certain features of a patient's clinical history. They are important to recognize because they will indicate which type of patient is at highest risk (*Table 22-1*).

Demographic Risk Factors

Older males are statistically the most likely to die by suicide; elderly men (85 years or older) are at greatest risk with an annual prevalence of 60 suicides per 100,000.[12] Although women attempt suicide three times more often than men, men are four times more likely to die by suicide.[13] There are several reasons for the increased risk in men: (1) substance misuse (e.g., alcoholism) is more prevalent among men; (2) men are less willing than women to seek help; (3) men attempt suicide using more lethal methods (e.g., firearms) than women; and (4) females tend to be more socially embedded than men.[13] Nevertheless, a significant number of women commit suicide and their risk cannot be discounted. Women with a history of depression and suicide attempts are likely to have poor outcomes postpartum and have increased suicide risk, especially within the first month of delivery.[13]

Caucasians and Native Americans are the ethnic groups at highest risk. Their risk of suicide is twice that of African-Americans, Hispanics, and Pacific Islanders.[13] When examining ethnicity as a risk factor, it is important to also consider age. Suicide rates in all ethnic groups rise sharply from ages 10 to 24, but then plateau into adulthood. Among Caucasian Americans, there is a marked increase in suicide rate in older age, which is not observed in African-Americans.[12] Thus, African-American men commit suicide earlier in life than do Caucasian men (mean ages 34 and 44, respectively).[14] African-American females have a remarkably low suicide rate. They are nine times less likely to commit suicide than are Caucasian women. This low suicide rate has been attributed to protective factors of religion and extended kin networks.

Clinical History

The most robust nonmodifiable risk factor for suicide is a previous attempt, particularly a past serious attempt.[12] A previous attempt dramatically increases the risk of eventual death by suicide. Previous attempters are 38 times more likely to complete suicide than are nonattempters. Serious attempts can be distinguished from less serious attempts if the previous attempt (1) involved a high degree of intent (e.g., when asked, the patient tells you that, before the attempt, he or she fully expected to die and was surprised when he or she did not); (2) involved a degree of planning, including measures to avoid discovery; and (3) involved lethal or violent methods that resulted in physical injuries.[13]

Other Factors

Other important nonmodifiable risk factors include being divorced, separated, or widowed; a family history of suicide; a history of childhood abuse (sexual or physical); unemployment (recent job loss is a common precipitant to suicide in males under the age of 45 years); and having a chronic physical illness, particularly a neurologic illness (epilepsy, multiple sclerosis, Huntington disease, and brain and spinal cord injuries). Certain nonneurologic illnesses associated with increased suicide risk include human immunodeficiency virus (HIV)/acquired immunodeficiency syndrome (AIDS) and chronic heart, lung, kidney, and prostate diseases.[13] In a recent study, older primary care patients (≥65 years) were asked if they were having thoughts they wished they were dead. Those with chronic medical conditions, especially a recent myocardial infarction, were the most likely to report having death wishes.[15]

Modifiable Risk Factors

Patients with a psychiatric disorder are at increased risk for committing suicide. The condition that carries the greatest risk is depression in the form of either major depressive disorder or bipolar disorder. Patients with these disorders are 20 times more likely to commit suicide than those without a mental disorder.[13] Substance misuse, particularly alcoholism, also increases suicide risk. Those with heavy alcohol use are particularly likely to commit suicide when faced with life stressors caused by their misuse: (1) loss or disruption of a close personal relationship (e.g., divorce), (2) job loss, and (3) legal and financial difficulties.[13]

Psychological autopsies (a focused evaluation of the deceased's life and emotional state before death) conducted on suicide victims have found that 90% meet criteria for one or more psychiatric disorders, predominately a major depressive episode.[12] A study involving a large sample of patients with recurrent depression found that the presence of certain symptoms was predictive of suicide within the ensuing year. These symptoms were (1) global insomnia (e.g., disruption of all phases of sleep), (2) psychomotor agitation (e.g., restlessness, pacing), (3) severe anxiety, (4) panic attacks, (5) difficulty concentrating, (6) severe anhedonia (e.g., an inability to experience pleasure), and (7) alcohol abuse.[16] Depressed patients who are also anxious are more likely to act on suicidal impulses than those with psychomotor slowing.[12]

The strong association between anxiety and suicide has been found in other settings. In a retrospective study of psychiatric inpatients who committed suicide, the vast majority (80%) exhibited signs of anxiety and agitation in the week before death.[12] Primary care patients with anxiety disorders have an increased risk of suicidal ideations and attempts in both the short and long term. Patients with anxiety symptoms coupled with depression have a significantly greater suicide risk than those with depression alone.[17] Other key modifiable risk factors for suicide are strong feelings of hopelessness[18]; a wish to destroy the lives of survivors (revenge suicide); extreme feelings of worthlessness, shame, or guilt; and polarized thinking (e.g., rigid thinking in which a patient is unable to consider options other than suicide).[13]

Access to lethal means is another modifiable risk factor for suicide. The presence of a firearm in the home is associated with a nearly fivefold increase in risk for suicide.[19] The risk of suicide in those who have recently purchased a handgun is nearly 60 times greater than that of the general population.[12] Medications with high lethality in overdose, such as lithium or fentanyl, are also potentially dangerous to the suicidal patient. If a patient has even low-level or passive suicidal ideation, steps should be taken to ensure that if their suicidality escalates or they make an impulsive attempt, they do not have access to methods with low survival rates. Research has shown that the removal of access to lethal means reduces not only suicide by that method, but also overall suicide in the study population, and does not result in a substitution of another suicide method.[4]

In cases of concern, medications with high overdose potential can be bubble packed or prescribed in small quantities at a time. Patients and family members should be counseled to make firearms less accessible by giving them to someone else for storage, or separating the ammunition from the weapon and keeping both locked. Some states have laws where guns can be temporarily relocated by law enforcement in times of crisis, and clinicians should familiarize themselves with what options are available in their state.

Protective Factors

Having strong reasons for living is inversely correlated with hopelessness, suicidal ideations, and depression.[13] Those reasons for living include having family and other social support, responsibility for children, and an expectation that current emotional pain is temporary and a hope that things will improve in future.[12] Patients with strong religious beliefs are also at a decreased risk of suicide, particularly those who practice Catholicism and Judaism.[13] The belief that killing oneself is morally wrong and sinful and results in eternal damnation is a strong deterrent to suicide. A cultural sanction against suicide (the view that suicide is shameful) is another protective factor.[12] Other protective factors include rewarding work, a good therapeutic alliance, and healthy and well-developed coping skills[13] (*Box 22-1*). Older primary care patients (≥65 years) who display a positive affect are less likely than those who do not to report suicidal thinking.[20]

BOX 22-1 PROTECTIVE FACTORS FROM SUICIDE: REASONS TO LIVE

- Strong religious (eternal damnation) or cultural beliefs (shame) against suicide
- A strong social network
- Responsibility for children
- Hope for the future
- Good therapeutic alliance
- A positive affect

Eliciting Suicidal Ideations

Any patient presenting with a primary complaint of depression, anxiety, or substance misuse should be screened for suicidal ideation, as they are at elevated risk for self-harm.[21] Additionally, patients in other categories of elevated risk should also be screened, for example, older unpartnered males with chronic medical conditions. Questions about suicidal ideation should be asked later in a clinical encounter, after rapport with a patient has been established. For example, as part of screening for depression, thoughts of death and suicide should be asked after screening for the other eight depressive symptoms. *Figure 22-1* illustrates a line of questioning designed to elicit suicidal ideations in at-risk patients. It is also very important to recognize that asking about suicidal thinking does not "plant" suicidal ideas in a patient's mind.[22] It is common for primary care providers to hold this view. One in five primary care providers believed

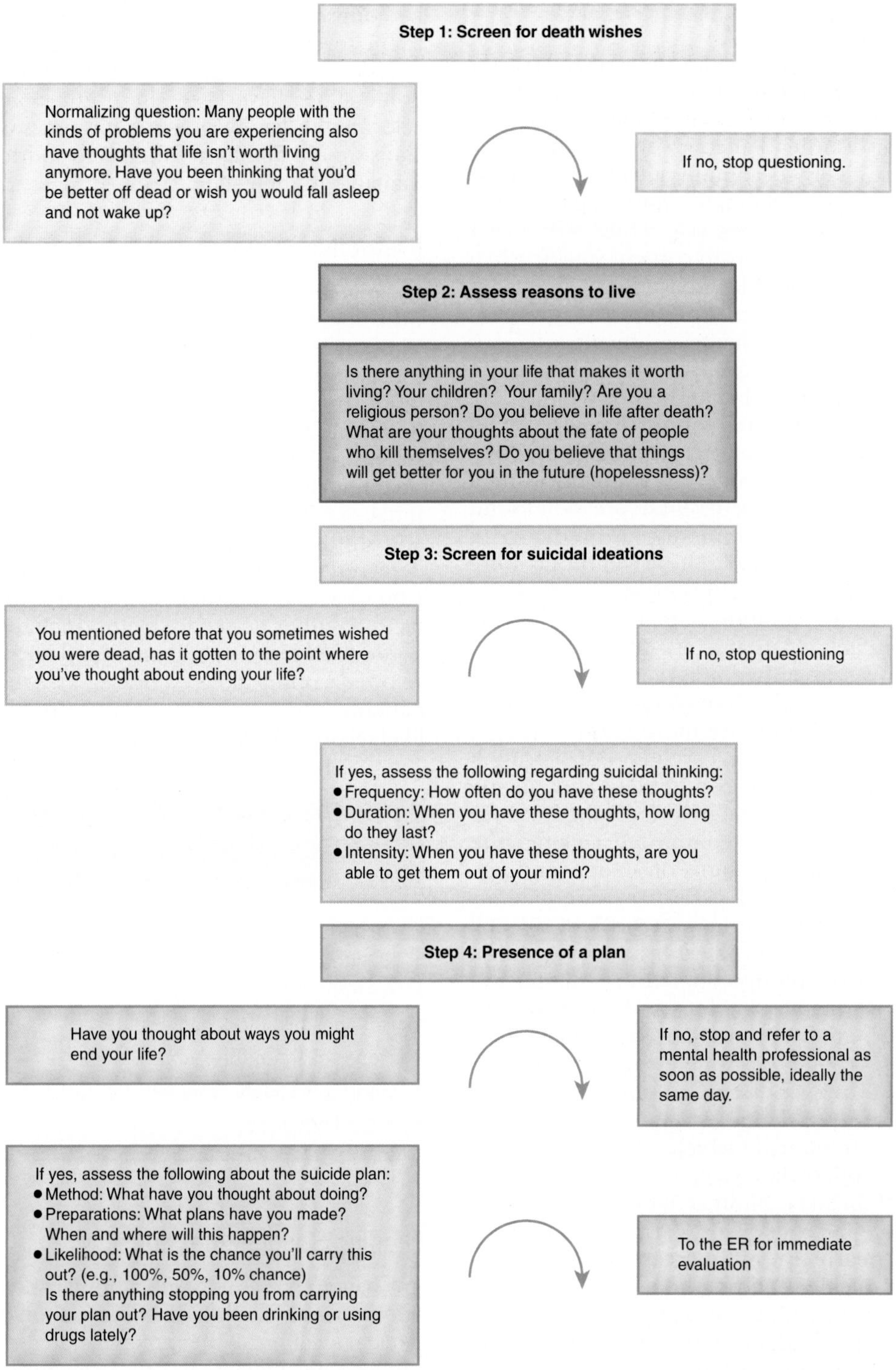

Step 1: Screen for death wishes

Normalizing question: Many people with the kinds of problems you are experiencing also have thoughts that life isn't worth living anymore. Have you been thinking that you'd be better off dead or wish you would fall asleep and not wake up?

If no, stop questioning.

Step 2: Assess reasons to live

Is there anything in your life that makes it worth living? Your children? Your family? Are you a religious person? Do you believe in life after death? What are your thoughts about the fate of people who kill themselves? Do you believe that things will get better for you in the future (hopelessness)?

Step 3: Screen for suicidal ideations

You mentioned before that you sometimes wished you were dead, has it gotten to the point where you've thought about ending your life?

If no, stop questioning

If yes, assess the following regarding suicidal thinking:
● Frequency: How often do you have these thoughts?
● Duration: When you have these thoughts, how long do they last?
● Intensity: When you have these thoughts, are you able to get them out of your mind?

Step 4: Presence of a plan

Have you thought about ways you might end your life?

If no, stop and refer to a mental health professional as soon as possible, ideally the same day.

If yes, assess the following about the suicide plan:
● Method: What have you thought about doing?
● Preparations: What plans have you made? When and where will this happen?
● Likelihood: What is the chance you'll carry this out? (e.g., 100%, 50%, 10% chance) Is there anything stopping you from carrying your plan out? Have you been drinking or using drugs lately?

To the ER for immediate evaluation

FIGURE 22-1 Eliciting suicidal thinking in at-risk patients. ER, emergency room.

that asking depressed patients about suicidal thinking will cause a patient to begin thinking about it. There is no evidence this is true and, on the contrary, many patients report feeling relieved when they are asked.[21]

The intensity and duration of suicidal ideations are predictive of eventual suicide.[13] More ominous is the development of a suicide plan. Thirty-four percent of those with suicidal ideations go on to devise a suicide plan. Up to 70% of patients who develop a plan go on to make a suicide attempt, usually within the year after the onset of suicidal thinking.[12] A suicide plan dramatically increases risk, especially when the plan (1) is detailed and specific, (2) is formulated to escape detection, and (3) involves a violent and irreversible method (e.g., jumping off a bridge, shooting oneself, or carbon monoxide poisoning). Certain behaviors, such as writing a suicide note and giving away personal possessions, indicate an intensification of suicidal thinking and a strong subjective desire to die.[13]

Past research has shown that in the last clinical contact before a suicide, most patients will give providers no indication they are about to end their lives.[24] A study of psychiatric inpatients who committed suicide in the hospital or immediately after discharge found that the vast majority (77%) denied suicidal thoughts at their last clinical contact.[24] This finding extends to primary care settings as well. In only 19% to 54% of primary care encounters did suicidal patients explicitly inform primary care providers of life-ending thoughts and plans.[6] Elderly patients, commonly seen in primary care settings, are much less likely than younger patients to endorse having suicidal ideations.[12]

Although the reasons why many of those who commit suicide did not communicate their intentions to health care professionals can never be known, there are several possible reasons. Patients who are intent on committing suicide may hide their intentions from providers because they don't want to be stopped. Patients who are considering suicide but ambivalent about it may not feel comfortable disclosing these deeply personal thoughts in the absence of a strong empathic connection with their provider. And evidence suggests that the majority of patients who commit suicide likely fall into the category of those who make serious attempts impulsively with little planning. In contrast to those who are actively considering suicide at the time of the encounter, this group may honestly deny suicidal ideation at their visit. However, they are likely to have other risk factors, including depression, social stressors, and a history of impulsive behaviors, that put them at risk for a future, unplanned attempt.

It is very important to be aware that many patients who commit suicide, however, do communicate the desire to end their lives to the people they are closest to. In one study of suicide completers, only 18% told a health care provider of their suicidal ideas, but 60% told a spouse and 50% told a relative of the wish to end their lives.[24] It is also critical to recognize that a brief encounter in the office offers a limited view of what is occurring in a patient's life. To get a broader perspective you need to speak with someone who knows the patient well and sees him or her on a regular basis. If you screen an at-risk patient for suicidal thinking and he or she denies suicidal thinking but you are concerned about his or her risk, a call to a family member or friend can be invaluable in preventing a suicide. A patient's recent behaviors and communications outside the office can be important when making an accurate assessment of suicide risk. In practice, it is always ideal to have the patient's permission to contact collateral sources and to protect patient confidentially unless explicitly stated. However, there is an emergency exception to confidentiality. In dangerous situations (e.g., risk of suicide, impending assault, medical emergency), confidentiality can be breached.

BIOPSYCHOSOCIAL TREATMENT
Disposition and Referral of Suicidal Patients

As shown in *Figure 22-1*, screening for suicidal thinking can result in four possible clinical situations: (1) no desire to die or thoughts of death, (2) death wishes but no thoughts of harming self, (3) suicidal ideations without a plan, and (4) suicidal ideations with a plan. In general, patients in categories 1 and 2 can effectively be managed in primary care settings. Providers should engage their social support systems as sources of collateral information as well as collaborators in care. They should discuss the importance of avoiding alcohol and substances and restricting access to lethal medication and firearms. Close follow-up should be provided with both the patient and their close supports. Patients in the higher-risk categories should be referred to mental health specialists for further assessment, treatment, and monitoring.

Patients who have been having active suicidal ideations without a specific plan should be seen as soon as possible by a mental health professional, ideally the same day, for further evaluation and triage. In cases where there is suspicion for a risk of suicide, family or friends may be able to provide important collateral. Patients with active suicidal ideation and a specific plan in mind should be sent to the emergency room for immediate evaluation. If an actively suicidal patient is unwilling to go to the emergency room and attempts to leave the clinicians office, a call to the local police department for involuntary detainment may be indicated. Clinicians should familiarize themselves with clinic policies and state laws regarding involuntary commitment and have a low threshold to secure an involuntary hold in those who are at moderate or high acute risk for suicide and unwilling to get immediate mental health treatment.

Medicolegal Issues

Primary care providers who assume the responsibility for treating a patient with a mental illness will generally be held to the same liability standard as mental health professionals. Consequently, primary care providers who have a patient commit suicide while under their care may be named in malpractice litigation. Asking the patient or family members to get rid of guns in the home can be an important issue in malpractice litigations. Most importantly, if a patient under your care commits suicide and a malpractice suit is brought against you, whether or not you assessed and documented suicide risk will be crucial in determining if the care you provided was negligent.[23]

Another emerging issue in suicide malpractice cases is the use of antidepressant therapy. There is a twofold increase in nonfatal suicide attempts during the first 9 days of treatment with selective serotonin reuptake inhibitors (SSRIs), particularly in adolescent and young adults. This is likely due to the propensity of these agents in some patients to initially increase levels of anxiety and agitation. Patients should be closely monitored for the development of suicidal ideations in the first 2 weeks after therapy is initiated. Prescribing practices should be tailored to prevent the possibility of an overdose, particularly avoiding antidepressants that are highly lethal like tricyclics. Although there may be a short-term risk of emergent suicidality with antidepressant treatment and overdose risk must be considered, it is also important to detect and treat depression effectively. Studies on primary care patients who attempted suicide found that those on antidepressants were not dosed adequately. Physicians should document that they considered the risks and benefits of starting antidepressant therapy and discussed the potential risks with their patient.[23]

ASSESSMENT AND MANAGEMENT OF VIOLENCE RISK

CLINICAL SIGNIFICANCE

Violence in primary care settings is common.[25] In a survey of general practitioners, two-thirds reported experiencing aggressive behavior (verbal abuse, threats to commit violence, or physical assault) from patients in the previous year. Primary care providers who experience work-related violence report that it impairs their job performance because it leads to anxiety and difficulty concentrating in the work environment.[26] Primary care providers who are less experienced, work in lower socioeconomic and socially disadvantaged areas, and treat patient populations with a high prevalence of substance misuse and mental health disorders are at increased risk for workplace violence.[25]

VIOLENCE RISK ASSESSMENT IN THE PRIMARY CARE SETTING

Certain risk factors increase the likelihood a patient will behave aggressively. Past behavior is the best predictor of future behavior. A history of violence is the most powerful long-term predictor of future violence.[27] Primary care providers are most often assaulted by patients who misuse substances.[28] An important short-term risk factor for violence is recent verbal or physical aggression.[29] Symptoms that indicate a patient is at imminent risk for becoming assaultive include (1) psychomotor agitation, (2) a hostile or angry affect, (3) verbal threats to harm others, (4) attacks on objects, (5) intense staring, and (6) a poor therapeutic alliance or resistance to treatment.[29,30]

Past research has identified specific environments, situations, and patient interactions in the health care setting that most frequently trigger a patient assault.[31-33] The health care environment with the highest number of assaults is the emergency department (ED). Evening and early morning hours are the highest-risk times, as these are when patients are most likely to be intoxicated. Patients frustrated by long waiting times in the clinic or ED can become angered to the point they resort to violence as a response. Enforcement of hospital rules can precipitate patient violence. Patients who disagree with their physicians or feel dissatisfied with their treatment (including the health care system in general) can become upset and aggressive.

BIOPSYCHOSOCIAL TREATMENT

Awareness of common precipitants to patient assault is a key component in efforts to prevent violence (*Box 22-2*). Clinicians regarded as experts in de-escalating potentially explosive situations stress the importance of early intervention in the emotional process that can culminate in a physical assault. Early recognition of pre-escalation, as evidenced by pacing, staring, yelling, demanding, and psychomotor agitation, is paramount. An empathic stance also has the potential to diffuse the situation early. *Box 22-3* summarizes proactive steps that can be taken in this case to help diffuse the situation and decrease the risk for violent behavior. If a patient becomes aggressive without an identifiable external trigger, the motivation for the violence is often related to psychotic symptoms. A psychiatry consultation should be obtained for further evaluation and treatment of a possible cognitive (e.g., delirium) or psychotic disorder (e.g., schizophrenia).

BOX 22-2 SITUATIONS AND INTERACTIONS WITHIN THE HEALTH CARE SYSTEM ASSOCIATED WITH VIOLENCE

- Long waiting times in the emergency department of clinic
- Disagreement with the physician's treatment plan
- Dissatisfaction with treatment or the health care system in general
- Enforcement of hospital and clinic policies and rules
- Providing care in acute care settings during evening and early morning hours
- Providing care to patients experiencing psychotic symptoms
  - Paranoid delusions are most associated with violence
  - Seen in patients with delirium and major psychotic disorders

---

BOX 22-3 CLINICAL INTERVENTIONS THAT CAN BE TAKEN TO DE-ESCALATE A PATIENT AND PREVENT A PHYSICAL ASSAULT (BASED ON PRACTICE POINTERS CLINICAL CASE)

- *Step 1: Recognize patients who are escalating emotionally*
  - Verbal abuse, psychomotor agitation, hostility, and staring indicate a patient is escalating
  - Appropriate intervention at this stage may avert physical aggression
- *Step 2: Read the situation and the meaning of the behavior*
  - A frustrated patient may be upset and arriving for the appointment on time and having to wait over an hour
  - Patients may become angry about their time being wasted, their needs not being unmet or feeling disrespected
- *Step 3: Connect with the patient*
  - Approach the patient maintaining an adequate distance
    - Agitated patients need increased interpersonal space
  - Speak in a calm voice
  - Instill in patient a sense of control
    - For example: "May I speak with you? You seem very upset right now—can we talk about it?"

continued

- *Step 4: Empathize with the patient and validate emotions*
  - For example: "Sir, I'm really sorry about the long wait. I can imagine it is really frustrating to show up on time and have to wait this long to be seen. I know your time is very important...."
- *Step 5: Depersonalize the situation*
  - Anger can create cognitive distortions that lead to mistaking the intentions of others; for example: "This doctor is putting me off.... He doesn't care about me!"
  - Communicate openly and honestly
    - For example: "You know, the reason I'm so far behind is that I had to deal with an emergency situation earlier this afternoon and send a patient to the hospital. Sometimes these things happen; I hope you understand. I'm doing my best to catch up and get to you."
- *Step 6: Give the patient choices*
  - Asking an escalating patient to make a decision diverts focus from the inciting stimulus and helps in regaining emotional control
  - For example: "Is there anything I can do for you that will make waiting here easier for you? You could take a walk around the building and I could call you when I'm ready to see you, or I could offer you some different magazines and a glass of water...."

CASES AND QUESTIONS

CASE 1: Suicide Risk Assessment

A 76-year-old Caucasian male with COPD, type 2 diabetes, peripheral neuropathy, and osteoarthritis presents with complaints of "horrible insomnia." His wife of 40 years passed away 2 years ago and he is currently living alone. His daughter lives in a nearby town and visits him on a weekly basis. One year prior, his daughter noticed he was having trouble getting around the house to attend to household duties, so she hired a home health aide 4 hours a day to assist him. She is concerned because he is depressed and has little energy to participate in pleasurable activities.

He endorses feeling depressed most days, has lost interest in things he used to enjoy, and has had some trouble focusing enough to read the daily paper. On chart review, you note he has lost 10 pounds since he was last seen in the clinic 3 months ago. When you ask him if he has recently thought that life isn't worth living or if he wished he were dead, he breaks eye contact with you and lowers his head. He responds, "No," then pauses and softly says "No" a second time. You provide him with education on depression and he agrees, somewhat reluctantly, to take an antidepressant. Something about his response to your question about death wishes keeps bothering you.

After obtaining the permission from the patient, you call his daughter and ask if she's noticed anything

different or concerning about him lately. She tells you she has noticed he doesn't watch football anymore, which is something he used to love to do, and that she has to remind him to eat, as he doesn't seem interested in food. She is also worried about his drinking, having recently found a bunch of empty bottles of vodka in his garage. His neighbor told her he seems to be up late at night, pacing the rooms of his house.

1. Which of the following interventions is *most* likely to decrease this patient's risk of suicide in the immediate future?
   A. Initiation of an SSRI
   B. Motivational interviewing for alcohol cessation
   C. Referral for psychodynamic psychotherapy
   D. Removal of firearms and lethal medications from the home
   E. Contacting more family members for further collateral information

   Correct answer: D. *Since firearms are the most lethal form of suicide method, removing firearms and lethal medications from the home is most commonly recommended in clinical practice.*

2. Which of the following is a protective factor for suicide in this patient?
   A. His age
   B. His gender
   C. His relationship with his daughter
   D. His medical history
   E. His current mood

   Correct answer: C. *A strong supportive family or social support is often seen as a protective factor. Lack of social support is often seen as a risk factor for suicide.*

3. Treatment of which of the following is *least* likely to have an impact on this patient's risk of suicide in the future?
   A. His alcohol use
   B. His depressive symptoms
   C. His insomnia
   D. His COPD
   E. His anxiety

   Correct answer: D. *The other more immediate psychiatric symptoms are more likely to impact the patient's suicide risk, compared with COPD. Chronic medical conditions are often considered "static" (nonmodifiable) risk factor for suicide, assuming that the condition is not acute and no amenable to any immediate medical interventions.*

4. Which of the following is *true* about asking patients questions about suicide?
   A. Discussing suicide with depressed patients can put the idea in their head and lead to attempts.

continued

B. In cases where the provider believes the danger of self-harm is an imminent threat, he or she can disclose information to parties in a position to help (i.e., family members, law enforcement) without a release of information.

C. Suicidal patients will usually spontaneously offer up their thoughts about suicide to a provider.

D. If patients say they have had any suicidal thoughts in the last year, they should be immediately sent to the ED for further evaluation.

E. Asking about suicidal thoughts in primary care settings is generally ineffective, as suicidal patients rarely present to primary care.

Correct answer: B. *This patient has multiple risk factors for suicide including depressed mood, advanced age, loss of his wife, chronic medical illness, possible preparation for suicide, and likely alcohol abuse. Even though the patient reported "no" to wanting to end his life, there is valid justification for concern given the way he answered the question. Referring this patient to the emergency room for a suicide assessment if clinically indicated could prove to be life-saving.*

This patient likely has major depressive disorder and should be treated with both psychotherapy and an antidepressant. While on medication for his depression, he should be monitored by both a mental health professional and his primary care provider on a frequent basis for the first 6 months of therapy. Additionally, his daughter and other sources of social support should be involved in his care to what extent possible and cautioned of his potential risk of suicide. His anxiety, insomnia, alcohol abuse, and depression should all be treated to minimize his future risk. Care should be taken to minimize his access to large amounts of potentially lethal medications, and firearms and ammunition should be removed from the home when possible.

CASE 2: Looking for Pre-escalation

Mr. Green is a 56-year-old patient with type 2 diabetes and hypertension who was recently transferred to your care by a primary physician who recently retired. He has been scheduled to see you for a routine follow-up. Earlier in the afternoon, you encountered and dealt with an emergent situation with one of your patients and are subsequently running behind schedule. Mr. Green arrived to his appointment on time and has been wait-ing for over an hour to see you. The clinic receptionist rushes back to see you between patients and expresses concern about his behavior. She tells you, "At first he seemed all right with having to wait, but he just started yelling at me and demanding to be seen immediately. I keep on telling him that you'll see him soon and ask him to sit down but that just seems to make him angrier. Now he's pacing around the room and staring at me. What should I do?"

1. Which of the following is likely the underlying cause of this patient's behavioral escalation?

A. Unmet personal needs and dissatisfaction with his treatment

B. An undiagnosed psychotic disorder

C. Suboptimal treatment for major depressive disorder

D. Traumatic brain injury

E. Substance intoxication

Correct answer: A. *This is the most common cause of violence in medical settings.*

2. What would be an appropriate intervention for the receptionist at this time?

A. Confront the patient about his behavior, matching his angry affect.

B. Do nothing; his anger will probably subside.

C. Call an emergency psychiatric consultation.

D. Tell the patient if he keeps this up, he will not be seen in clinic today at all.

E. Call for other staff to be present for safety; try to address his concerns in a calm and rational manner.

Correct answer: E. *Staying calm and approaching the patient in a nonconfrontation manner while having another staff serving as a backup is the most rational approach.*

3. All of the following are physical warning signs of potential impending violence *except*:

A. Pacing

B. Staring

C. Posturing

D. Punching objects

E. Crying

Correct answer: E. *This patient displays many of the physical signs of impending violence, including posturing, staring and angry speech. In situations where a patient begins to escalate and there is concern for violence, it is crucial to intervene early and try to meet his or her needs while maintaining the safety of the staff. For instance, the receptionist (after making sure she is not alone with the patient) might briefly explain the emergent nature of why the doctor is late and say, "I understand your time is important and that this is frustrating for you." This patient can also be offered alternatives to a longer wait time. For example, he can be given the option of making another appointment or provided an accurate time frame for which he will be waiting. Empathic connection and early de-escalation are key in these situations.*

CASE 3: Maintenance of Safety Is Paramount

You are working a weekend shift in an urgent care clinic. A nurse approaches you and hands you a patient's chart. She tells you, "This patient, Mr. Johnson, is a big-time drug seeker. He is always coming in here with these bogus pain complaints and demanding OxyContin and other narcotics. You aren't gonna give him any, are you?"

The first thing Mr. Johnson tells you is, "Hey, doctor, I got the worst migraine headache ever. The only thing that will take care of it is a shot of Demerol. Just give me that shot and I'll be out of here." You begin to question Mr. Johnson in detail about the onset, duration, and location of his pain. His answers are vague, nondescript, and contradictory. As the interview progresses, he gets increasingly hostile and eventually blurts out, "What's with all the stupid questions? I already told you what I need! Do your goddamn job and give me the shot or I'll sue you!" You exit the room and review Mr. Johnson's medical records. They chronicle numerous urgent care visits for various pain complaints, which are unsubstantiated by objective findings. He demands opiates at each visit and often receives a prescription for a small supply of opiates with instructions to follow up with his primary care physician. He has a history of heroin dependence and has been arrested in the past for assault. After consulting with a colleague, you determine that he is likely seeking abusable medication and prepare to speak with him about the issue.

1. Which of the following precautions should be taken when going into the examination room to speak with this patient?

   A. Going in alone to maintain patient privacy
   B. Confronting him with documented proof of his past heroin use
   C. Leaving the door of the room open and standing near it
   D. Dictating the course of care in an authoritative fashion
   E. Ensuring the room is well-stocked with sharp objects or potential projectiles

   Correct answer: C. *Ensuring a mode of exit is paramount to ensuring safety in highly assaultive scenarios.*

2. Which of the following is *not* risk factor for violence in this patient?

   A. His history of assault
   B. His illicit drug use
   C. His loud manner of speech
   D. His gender
   E. His frequent visits to the clinic

   Correct answer: E. *Frequent visits to the clinic is the least likely risk factor for violence.*

3. Which of the following symptoms should prompt a referral to psychiatry in a patient who appears at risk for violence?

   A. Loud, angry speech
   B. Demanding increasing doses of opiod medications
   C. Responding to auditory hallucinations
   D. A family history of suicide
   E. A diagnosis of malingering

Correct answer: C. *Primary care providers should take precautions when preparing to deny a patient's request. Although necessary at times, telling a patient "no" is a common precipitant to assaults on medical staff.[29] In this case, giving the patient the narcotics he is demanding may facilitate him leaving the clinic, but will be counterproductive in the long term because the behavior will be reinforced. Box 22-4 details how to approach and manage a patient in this situation in a manner that protects your safety and will not escalate the situation further. Rarely is violence caused by an underlying severe mental illness, and in such cases, the patient should be referred to a mental health care provider.*

TELLING A PATIENT "NO": TIPS FOR PROTECTING YOUR SAFETY AND PREVENTING FURTHER ESCALATION OF THE SITUATION

- *Never* enter a room with a potentially violent patient and situate yourself in a position where you can be cornered without a route of escape
- *Always* notify your colleagues about your concerns for possible violence so that they are aware and can help if needed
  - Ask another staff member to accompany you if you don't feel safe
  - In some instances, notifying hospital security to stand by is appropriate
- *Avoid* taking an authoritarian stance with a patient; becoming argumentative only serves to fuel the escalating process
  - Agitated and angry patients don't respect your authority; don't think that being a physician protects you from violence
- When denying a request, explain your reasoning to the patient and how you are acting in his or her best interest
  - For example: "Sir, your records indicate that you have a history of heroin use. Giving you narcotic medication for your headache will place you at risk for relapse. I want to do what's best for you. I can offer you some nonnarcotic pain medications instead. What do you think?"

PRACTICAL RESOURCES

- National Suicide Prevention Lifeline: Sponsored by the U.S. Department of Health and Human Services: The Substance Abuse and Mental Health Administration: www.suicidepreventionlifeline.org; 1-800-SUICIDE or 1-800-273-TALK (8255)
- American Psychiatric Association Guidelines for Suicide Prevention: http://www.psychiatryonline.com/pracGuide/pracGuideTopic_14.aspx

REFERENCES

1. Vannoy SD, Duberstein P, Cukrowicz K, et al. The relationship between suicide ideation and late-life depression. *Am J Geriatr Psychiatry.* 2007;15:1024-1033.

2. Chesney E, Goodwin GM, Fazel S Risks of all-cause and suicide mortality in mental disorders: a meta-review. *World Psychiatry.* 2014;13(2):153-160.

3. Kaplan MS, McFarland BH, Huguet N, et al. Acute alcohol intoxication and suicide: a gender-stratified analysis of the National Violent Death Reporting System. *Inj Prev.* 2013;19(1):38-43.

4. Barber CW, Miller MJ. Reducing a suicidal person's access to lethal means of suicide a research agenda. *Am J Prev Med.* 2014;47:264-272.

5. Luoma JB, Martin CE, Pearson JL. Contact with mental health and primary care providers before suicide: a review of the evidence. *Am J Psychiatry.* 2002;159:909-916.

6. Blashki G, Pirkis J, Epid A, et al. Managing depression and suicide risk in men presenting to primary care physicians. *Prim Care Clin Office Pract.* 2006;33:211-221.

7. Feldman MD, Franks P, Duberstein PR, et al. Let's not talk about it: suicide inquiry in primary care. *Ann Fam Med.* 2007;5:412-418.

8. Milton J, Ferguson B, Mills T. Risk assessment and suicide prevention in primary care. *Crisis.* 1999;20(4):171-177. Conwell Y, Lyness JM, Duberstein P, et al. Completed suicide among older patients in primary care practices: a controlled study. *J Am Geriatr Soc.* 2000;48(1):23-29.

9. Harwood DM, Hawton K, Hope T, et al. Suicide in older people: mode of death, demographic factors, and medical contact before death. *Int J Geriatr Psychiatry.* 2000;15:736-743.

10. Salib E, Tadros G. Elderly suicide in primary care. *Int J Geriatr Psychiatry.* 2007;22:750-756.

11. Simon RI. *Suicide risk: assessing the unpredictable.* In: *Textbook of Suicide Assessment and Management.* Washington, DC: American Psychiatric Publishing; 2006:1-32.

12. American Psychiatric Association. Practice guidelines for the assessment and treatment of patients with suicidal behaviors. *Am J Psychiatry.* 2003;160(suppl):1-60.

13. Garlow SJ, Purselle D, Heninger M. Ethnic differences in patterns of suicide across the life cycle. *Am J Psychiatry.* 2005;162:319-323.

14. Kim YA, Bogner HR, Brown GK, et al. Chronic medical conditions and wishes to die among older primary care patients. *Int J Psychiatry Med.* 2006;36(2):183-198.

15. Fawcett J, Scheftner WA, Fogg L, et al. Time-related predictors of suicide in major affective disorder. *Am J Psychiatry.* 1990;147(9):1189-1194.

16. Sareen J, Cox BJ, Afifi TO, et al. Anxiety disorders and risk for suicidal ideation and suicide attempts. *Arch Gen Psychiatry.* 2005;62:1249-1257.

17. Beck AT, Brown G, Berchick RJ, et al. Relationship between hopelessness and ultimate suicide: a replication with psychiatric outpatients. *Am J Psychiatry.* 1990;147(2):190-195.

18. Kellermann AL, Rivara FP, Somes G, et al. Suicide in the home in relation to gun ownership. *N Engl J Med.* 1992;327:467-472.

19. Hirsch JK, Duberstein PR, Chapman B, et al. Positive affect and suicide ideations in older adult primary care patients. *Psychol Aging.* 2007;22(2):380-385.

20. Raue PJ, Brown EL, Meyers BS, et al. Does every allusion to possible suicide require the same response? *J Fam Pract.* 2006;55(7):605-612.

21. Schulberg HC, Hyg MS, Bruce ML, et al. Preventing suicide in primary care patients: the primary care physician's role. *Gen Hosp Psychiatry.* 2004;26:337-345.

22. Simon RI, Sadoff RL. *Malpractice law: an introduction.* In: *Psychiatric Malpractice: Cases and Comments for Clinicians.* Washington, DC: American Psychiatric Press; 1992:23-55.

23. Mays D. Structured assessment methods may improve suicide prevention. *Psychiatric Ann.* 2004;34:367-372.

24. Magin PJ, Adams J, Sibbritt DW, et al. Experiences of occupational violence in Australian urban general practice: a cross-sectional study of GPs. *Med J Aust.* 2005;183:352-356.

25. Coles J, Koritsas S, Boyle M, et al. GPs, violence and work performance—'just part of the job?' *Aust Fam Physician.* 2007;36:189-191.

26. Quanbeck CD. Forensic psychiatric aspects of inpatient violence. *Psychiatry Clin North Am.* 2006;29:743-760.

27. Tolhurst H, Baker L, Murray G, et al. Rural general practitioner experience of work-related violence in Australia. *Aust J Rural Health.* 2003;11:231-236.

28. Quanbeck C, McDermott B. *Inpatient settings.* In: *Textbook of Violence Assessment and Management.* Washington, DC: American Psychiatric Publishing; 2008:295-318.

29. Lanza ML, Zeiss RA, Rierdan J. Non-physical violence: a risk factor for physical violence in health care settings. *AAOHN J.* 2006;54:397-402.

30. Carmi-Iluz T, Peleg R, Freud T, et al. Verbal and physical violence towards hospital- and community-based providers in the Negev: an observational study. *BMC Health Serv Res.* 2005;5:54.

31. Gates DM, Ross CS, McQueen L. Violence against emergency department workers. *J Emerg Med.* 2006;31:331-337.

32. May DD, Grubbs LM. The extent, nature, and precipitating factors of nurse assault among three groups of registered nurses in a regional medical center. *J Emerg Nurs.* 2002;28:11-17.

23

SOMATIC SYMPTOM AND RELATED DISORDERS

Matthew Reed, MD, MSPH, Bharat R. Sampathi, BA,
Robert M. McCarron, DO, DFAPA, and Glen L. Xiong, MD

A 32-year-old man with no medical history presents to an urgent care clinic complaining of "gas in the stomach," shortness of breath, and squeezing back pain that prevents him from working. Other symptoms include a "jumping sensation in the legs" and "poor circulation in the hands and feet." He is unsure about what condition he might have. He is so concerned about his health that he has been sleeping in his car near the hospital for the past few days. He has seen numerous doctors over the past 6 months and, after an extensive medical workup, has been told there are no obvious medical problems.

CLINICAL HIGHLIGHTS

- Somatization is commonly encountered in the outpatient setting and often requires a long-term treatment plan.

- Psychiatric disorders, such as depression and anxiety, frequently coexist with somatic symptom and related disorders. We suggest using the AMPS (Anxiety, Mood, Psychotic, Substance) screening tool, see Chapter 2) when assessing the psychiatric review of systems. The prognosis of someone with a somatic symptom disorder will usually improve when comorbid psychiatric illness is promptly identified and treated.

- Although most patients with a somatic symptom and related disorder may benefit from psychiatric consultation, they often initially refuse to see a psychiatrist. Therefore, primary care practitioners play a key role in the treatment of these disorders.

- **The CARE MD treatment plan (*Table 23-3*) may be a useful approach for patients who have somatic symptom and related disorders.**

CLINICAL SIGNIFICANCE

Primary care practitioners encounter unexplained and perplexing somatic complaints in up to 40% of their patients.[1,2] However, medical explanations for common physical complaints such as malaise, fatigue, abdominal discomfort, and dizziness are found only 15% to 20% of the time.[3] Patients and primary care practitioners alike can become frustrated when symptoms persist without a clear etiology or when symptoms seem out of proportion for any of the patient's known medical conditions. Frustration is compounded when treatments targeting the symptoms are only partially effective. Abnormal thoughts, feelings, and behaviors may develop in response to somatic symptoms and can significantly disrupt daily life. This process of developing abnormal thoughts, feelings, and behaviors in relation to bothersome somatic symptoms is loosely termed somatization. Although it is difficult to reliably determine the prevalence of somatization due to changing definitions, most studies estimate a prevalence of 16% to 20% in primary care settings.[4]

The common occurrence of somatization carries a large financial burden. A retrospective review of over 13,000 psychiatric consultations found that somatization resulted in more disability and unemployment than any other psychiatric illness.[5] Moreover, patients with somatization in the primary care setting have more than twice the outpatient utilization and overall medical care costs when compared with patients without somatization. The direct costs related to the management of unexplained physical symptoms approach 10% of medical expenditures or over $100 billion annually in the United States.[6]

DIAGNOSIS

Disorders involving somatization are defined in the *Diagnostic and Statistical Manual of Mental Disorders, Fifth Edition (DSM-5)* under the category of "somatic symptom and related disorders." There are five key dis-orders from this category including somatic symptom disorder, illness anxiety disorder, conversion disorder (functional neurologic symptom disorder), psycho-logical factors affecting other medical conditions, and factitious disorder. Prior editions of the *DSM* included a requirement that general medical conditions be excluded before diagnosing a somatic symptom disor-der. With the release of *DSM-5*, this requirement has been eliminated.

To meet criteria for any of these disorders, one must have distressing somatic symptoms in addi-tion to abnormal thoughts, feelings, and behaviors in response to the symptoms. These symptoms must also result in a significant disruption of daily life (*Table 23-1*).

PATIENT ASSESSMENT

Other than completing a thorough history and phys-ical examination with indicated laboratory or radio-graphic tests, there are no specific diagnostic protocols for patients who have a somatic symptom disorder. It is important to review collateral history from other health care providers and family to help confirm the diagnosis and reduce redundant and unnecessary medical evalua-tions or interventions.

DIFFERENTIAL DIAGNOSIS

The differential diagnosis for unexplained physical symptoms seen in the primary care setting is extensive. *Table 23-2* lists some of the common *DSM-5* diagno-ses and the crosswalk to ICD-10 diagnostic codes. It is important to keep in mind that "unexplained" somatic symptoms may be due to (1) a medical condition that has not yet been diagnosed; (2) a medical condition that is present but not yet known to the medical com-munity at large; (3) a psychiatric condition such as malingering, factitious disorder, or one of the somatic symptom and related disorders; or (4) both a general medical condition and one of the abovementioned psy-chiatric conditions. Somatic symptom disorder is no longer a "diagnosis of exclusion" but is instead based on the presence of distressing somatic symptoms plus abnormal thoughts, feelings, and behaviors in response to those symptoms. A patient may have a chronic med-ical condition with somatic symptoms, but their abnor-mal thoughts, feelings, and behaviors related to those symptoms may qualify them for an additional diagnosis of somatic symptom disorder.

Before establishing the diagnosis of a somatic symp-tom disorder, one should attempt to rule out the inten-tional production of physical or psychological symptoms. A patient with malingering is focused on feigning illness to gain external incentives such as financial compen-sation, controlled substances, shelter, or escape from occupational duty or criminal prosecution. Factitious dis-order involves the purposeful and sometimes elaborate

TABLE 23-1 Somatic Symptom and Related Disorders[7]

DISORDER	DEFINITION
Somatic symptom disorder	• Distressing somatic symptoms that result in significant disruption of daily life • Abnormal thoughts, feelings, or behaviors related to the somatic symptoms
Illness anxiety disorder (formerly hypochondriasis)	• Preoccupation with having or acquiring a serious illness • High level of anxiety about health disproportional to the real threat to health • Excessive health-related behaviors or maladaptive avoidance
Conversion disorder (also known as functional neurologic symptom disorder)	• Altered voluntary motor or sensory function • Symptoms are not due to a recognized neurologic or medical condition
Psychological factors affecting other medical conditions	• Psychological or behavioral factors adversely influence the course, treatment, or underlying pathophysiology of an existing medical condition
Factitious disorder	• Falsification of physical or psychological signs or symptoms (or induction of injury or disease) • There is no obvious external reward for the deception
Other specified somatic symptom and related disorder	• Diagnosis is used when full criteria for one of the abovementioned disorders is not met. • Reason for not meeting full criteria is added as a specifier • Pseudocyesis (false belief in being pregnant with signs/symptoms of pregnancy) is one specifier for this diagnosis
Unspecified somatic symptom and related disorder	• Diagnosis is used when full criteria for one of the abovementioned disorders is not met *and* the reason for not meeting the diagnosis is not specified

The abovementioned disorders (1) cause clinically significant distress or impairment in social or occupational functioning and (2) are not due to other general medical or psychi-atric conditions.

self-report of somatic complaints with the objective of assuming the "sick role." People with factitious disorder have no obvious external secondary gain. When treat-ing either condition, it is important to obtain collateral history (particularly from other area hospitals and pro-viders), conduct a focused physical examination, and consider both as diagnoses of exclusion. People who are malingering are not usually "antisocial." Instead, they

TABLE 23-2 Differential Diagnosis: *DSM-5* to ICD-10 Crosswalk

DSM-5 DIAGNOSIS	ICD-10 CODE
Somatic symptom disorder	F45.1
• With predominate pain	F45.42
Illness anxiety disorder	F45.21
Conversion disorder	
• With weakness or paralysis	F44.4
• With abnormal movement	F44.4
• With swallowing symptoms	F44.4
• With speech symptoms	F44.4
• With attacks or seizures	F44.5
• With anesthesia or sensory loss	F44.6
• With special sensory symptom (e.g., visual, olfactory, or hearing disturbance)	F44.6
• With mixed symptoms	F44.7
Psychological factors affecting other medical conditions	F54
Factitious disorder	F68.10
Other specified somatic symptom and related disorder	F45.8
Unspecified somatic symptom and related disorder	F45.9

TABLE 23-3 CARE MD—Treatment Guidelines for Somatic Symptom and Related Disorders

CBT/ Consultation	• Follow the CBT (cognitive behavioral therapy) treatment plan developed by the therapist and patient
Assess	• Address potential general medical causes for the somatic complaints • Treat comorbid psychiatric disorders
Regular visits	• Short frequent visits with focused examinations • Discuss recent stressors and healthy coping strategies • Over time, the patient should agree to stop overutilization of medical care (e.g. frequent emergency room visits or excessive calls and pages to the primary care provider)
Empathy	• "Become the patient" for a brief time • During visits, spend more time listening to the patient rather than jumping to a diagnostic test • Acknowledge the patient's reported discomfort
Medical– psychiatric interface	• Help the patient self-discover the connection between physical complaints and emotional stressors ("the mind–body" connection) • Avoid comments such as "your symptoms are all psychological" or "there is nothing wrong with you medically"
Do no harm	• Avoid unnecessary diagnostic procedures • When possible, minimize unnecessary requests for consultation to medical specialists

Modified from McCarron R. Somatization in the primary care setting. Psychiatr Times. 2006;23(6):32-34. Reprinted by permission of UBM Medica. Copyrighted 2016. UBM. 278723:0818DD.

are often emotionally troubled and under so much psychological stress that they engage in maladaptive and deceitful coping strategies, with resultant isolation from family, friends, and medical providers. Once a diagnosis of malingering is established, one should attempt to confront the patient in a supportive and reassuring way while trying to problem-solve using a multidisciplinary team approach. Assisting malingerers with urgent stressors and attempting to find appropriate ways to meet their needs can be effective, and a psychiatric referral is not normally indicated. However, if a diagnosis of factitious disorder is made, psychiatric consultation is strongly advised because this disorder can be difficult to treat and carries a poor long-term prognosis.

BIOPSYCHOSOCIAL TREATMENT

The treatment approach to somatic symptom and related disorders exemplifies the "art of medicine." Because these disorders occur on a wide-ranging diagnostic continuum, with elusive etiologies, it is difficult to apply a strict, evidence-based approach to treatment.[8,9] We propose a simplified treatment plan that is described by the acronym CARE MD (*Table 23-3*).[10] This approach encourages patients to be active participants in their care and serves as a guide to help primary care practitioners effectively work with people who have somatoform disorders.

COGNITIVE BEHAVIORAL THERAPY/ CONSULTATION

Consultation with mental health professionals and use of cognitive behavioral therapy (CBT) have been

NOT TO BE MISSED

- General medical condition(s)
- Depression
- Anxiety disorders
- Alcohol or substance-induced disorders
- Malingering

Emotions	Automatic Thoughts	Rational Reponse	Outcome
Specify feeling Rate 1–10 (10 rated as mo st intense)	"What is running through your head" (not an emotion or feeling)?	Why is the automatic thought inaccurate (be specific)?	Rerate feeling using 1–10 scale
"Sad" 8/10	"My pain will *never* go away."	"Not true—I am working hard with my doctor so my pain will get better over time." "Never is a strong word to use."	"Sad" 5/10
"Angry" 9/10	"*Everyone* thinks I'm faking my pain."	"My doctor listens to me and everyone is a lot of people!" "I know my family is trying to understand my pain and depression."	"Angry" 3/10
"Anxious" 9/10	"*Nobody* will ever figure out what is wrong with me and there is no reason to go on living."	"I know I have somatic symptom disorder and doing my CBT homework will only help me." Sometimes I feel like dying but I know I want to live."	"Anxious" 4/10

FIGURE 23-1 Sample dysfunctional thought record. CBT, cognitive behavioral therapy.

shown to decrease the severity and frequency of somatic preoccupations.[11,12] Kroenke and Swindle, in 2000, reviewed 31 controlled studies and concluded that CBT is an effective treatment for patients with somatization. Group therapy using CBT with an emphasis on education has also been found to be beneficial.[13] CBT generally consists of 10 to 20, 1-hour psychotherapy sessions with the goal of teaching patients how to take an active role in their treatment and developing skills that last a lifetime. This type of psychotherapy is based on the premise that negative, automatic, or "dysfunctional thoughts" are predominant in patients with somatic symptom and related disorders. Examples of such thoughts are "I will always be sick and never get better," "No one understands or believes my pain," and "Everyone thinks it's all in my head." Through a variety of mechanisms, patients learn to recognize and reconstruct dysfunctional thought patterns with resultant decreased somatic complaints. Patients should be encouraged to use a daily dysfunctional thought record (DTR) to self-monitor depressive or anxious emotions and associated negative thoughts. In collaboration with the therapist, primary care providers can learn to use brief cognitive behavioral techniques and quickly review a DTR during office visits. Additionally, we recommend that patients with somatic symptom, depressive, or anxiety disorders, as well as treating mental health and primary care practitioners, learn the basics of CBT. One of many practical resources includes the book *Feeling Good: The New Mood Therapy* by Davis Burns, MD.[14] The first 80 pages of this book are practical and teach the patient how to recognize dysfunctional thought patterns and complete "homework" that will reverse cognitive distortions, decrease somatization, and improve mood (*Figure 23-1*).

ASSESS MEDICAL AND PSYCHIATRIC COMORBIDITIES

Assessing patients on each visit for general medical problems that might explain troublesome physical complaints is essential. This is particularly important for patients who have a long history of somatic preoccupation and present with a new complaint or a worsening of existing symptoms. Up to 25% to 50% of patients with conversion disorder eventually have an identifiable, nonpsychiatric disease that explains their symptoms.[15] It is also important to screen for other common psychiatric diagnoses. Up to 50% of patients with somatic symptom and related disorders have concurrent anxiety or depressive disorders.[16,17] The number of unexplained somatic symptoms is highly predictive of comorbid mood and anxiety disorders as well as functional disability. Primary care clinicians can address frequently co-occurring depression by using the Patient Health Questionnaire (PHQ-9), a patient self-report tool that reliably screens for depression in the primary care setting (see Chapter 2). All patients with a score greater than 5 should be assessed for a possible major depressive disorder.

REGULAR VISITS

Regular visits with a single clinician are critical to the management of somatic symptom and related disorders. Short, frequent appointments or telephone encounters have been shown to decrease outpatient medical costs while maintaining patient satisfaction.[18] These encounters should include a brief but focused history and physical examination followed by open-ended questions such as "How are things at home?" "What is your number one, biggest problem?" or, if the patient is exposed to CBT, "Tell me about your most frequent negative thoughts since your last visit." Over time, patients can replace excessive emergency room visits or frequent calls to the clinic with this supportive, caring patient–provider interaction. Longer, less frequent visits can be reserved for assessment and treatment of other general medical disorders and health care maintenance. In sum, spending most of the time during the shorter, frequent visits on worrisome psychosocial stressors will provide an outlet for patients to better cope with somatic preoccupation.

EMPATHY

Empathy or briefly "becoming the patient" is important for developing a strong therapeutic alliance between the patient and the health care provider. The use of empathy can also minimize negative feelings or countertransference from providers. True empathic remarks such as "This must be difficult for you" or "It must be very hard to cope with what you are experiencing" are often therapeutic. Modeling empathic communication when frustrated family and friends are present may also help improve patient–family interactions outside of the clinic. Although there are clear benefits associated with an empathic communication style, it can at times be emotionally taxing for medical providers. To mitigate potential frustration or even burnout, we recommend the utilization of Balint groups or regularly scheduled, candid, and confidential discussions about challenging patient encounters with colleagues who experience similar clinical situations.

MEDICAL–PSYCHIATRIC INTERFACE

Patients diagnosed with a somatic symptom disorder should be educated about how emotions and stressors have a direct effect on their body. Understandably, many patients will not accept explanations for their unexplained physical symptoms with statements (or indirect communications) such as "It's all in your head," "There is nothing medically wrong with you," or "A psychiatrist will have to take care of your complaints." Instead, primary care practitioners should provide a diagnosis and, if necessary, arrange for a psychiatric consultation while remaining the primary point of contact for all medical issues. During short but frequent office visits, patients should be asked if their unexplained symptoms worsen as a primary stressor intensifies or if the symptoms improve as a primary stressor lessens. If the answer is affirmative

to both questions, allow the patient to gradually make the connection by asking an open-ended question such as "Do you have any thoughts on why this might be?" Essentially, it is best to help the patient self-discover the connection between the unresolved conflict or emotional stress and the somatic symptoms.

DO NO HARM

Doing no harm by avoiding unnecessary procedures or consultations is the most important part of treating patients with somatic symptom and related disorders. Providers should not deviate from clinical best practices to appease a patient or minimize their own frustration. While unnecessary invasive procedures should be avoided, routine health care maintenance should be emphasized and offered when indicated. These routine studies may be offered over time, rather than completing every test in one visit. Doing so will help keep to the principle of "short and frequent" visits. After taking reasonable steps to rule out general medical cause for the symptoms make the appropriate somatic symptom disorder diagnosis and treat accordingly.

PHARMACOTHERAPY

Antidepressants may be considered for the treatment of somatic symptom disorders, but we generally do not recommend starting such medications, especially on the first encounter. In our clinical experience, offering psychotropic medications for a somatic symptom disorder too quickly may reinforce the idea that the symptoms are exclusively psychiatric in nature and may impair the development of a trusting therapeutic relationship. On the other hand, antidepressants should be considered when comorbid depressive or anxiety disorders are discovered, and treatment is accepted by the patient. Even with a receptive patient, a significant amount of effort is typically required to educate about the potential psychiatric contribution to their unexplained physical ailment. The provider should only start psychotropic medications after establishing full collaboration with the patient.

WHEN TO REFER

- Patients with significant social or occupational dysfunction directly related to a somatic symptom and related disorder should be referred to a psychiatrist.
- Patients with comorbid psychopathology such as psychosis or suicidal ideation should receive an urgent psychiatric referral.
- In cases where a psychiatric referral is placed for somatization, the primary care provider should receive input from the psychiatrist but remain the primary care provider.

CASES AND QUESTIONS

CASE 1:

A 32-year-old man with no medical history presents to an urgent care clinic complaining of "gas in the stomach," shortness of breath, and squeezing back pain that prevents him from working. Other symptoms include a "jumping sensation in the legs" and "poor circulation in the hands and feet." He is unsure about what condition he might have. He is so concerned about his health that he has been sleeping in his car near the hospital for the past few days. He has seen numerous doctors over the past 6 months and, after an extensive medical workup, has been told there are no obvious medical problems. He does not take any medications. He smokes occasionally and denies illicit drug use. He is currently unemployed. Both parents are healthy with no family history of heart disease or cancer. The physical examination reveals an anxious and somewhat dramatic man who uses frequent hand gestures. He repeatedly states, "There is something wrong with my heart." The laboratory studies including complete blood count, basic chemistry panel, and thyroid studies are normal. Two weeks later, the patient returns to inquire about his laboratory tests. During this visit, he reports vague physical complaints and recalls that a neurologist had suggested that he might have problems in his spine. He admits to a history of depression more than 3 years ago, which improved on its own. He denies current depressed mood and states, "There is nothing wrong with my head." In fact, he becomes quite upset when the physician suggests that his symptoms could be related to depression or anxiety. He does concede that things have been stressful for him over the last few months and that he noticed a temporal correlation between the stress and the symptoms. He is motivated to get better and has no desire to collect disability. His physical examination was normal.

1. Which of the following is the most appropriate diagnosis for this patient?

   A. Somatoform disorder
   B. Illness anxiety disorder
   C. Somatic symptom disorder
   D. Malingering

   Correct answer: C. *This patient exhibits several symptoms that are vague, are seemingly disconnected, and do not suggest any obvious general medical etiology. This patient describes numerous somatic symptoms that are distressing and debilitating. His behavior is excessive as evidenced by repeated doctor visits and sleeping in his car near the hospital. He demonstrates a persistently high level of anxiety about his symptoms and has devoted excessive time and energy to doctor visits and medical workups. His symptoms have persisted for at least 6 months. He meets criteria for somatic symptom disorder. There is no reason to think he is intentionally feigning the*

symptoms for either external (e.g., financial) or internal (e.g., assuming the "sick role") gain, and therefore, he does not meet criteria for malingering or factitious disorder. He is not preoccupied with a specific illness or diagnosis so does not have illness anxiety disorder. Treatment should begin with the development of a supportive, nonjudgmental, and collaborative relationship. It is important that the provider spend sufficient time to understand the patient's symptoms and consequent suffering. The provider may explain to the patient that although the current symptoms may not point to a clear medical condition, continued monitoring is indicated. It is important to point out the dangers of unnecessary diagnostic tests and procedures, as they can lead to false-positive results and increased morbidity. We recommend close attention to health care maintenance and general counseling about diet, exercise, and smoking cessation. After a therapeutic alliance has been established, psychoeducation regarding unexplained physical symptoms could be introduced. Subsequent exploration of possible psychosocial precipitants of the distressing physical symptoms should be attempted. Assessment of concurrent psychiatric conditions using the AMPS screening tool should be ongoing. Referral to a mental health professional may also be considered. CBT is a well-studied first-line intervention for somatic symptom and related disorders. It is advisable for medical providers to become familiar with CBT principles and the use of a DTR, as this is an evidence-based approach studied in primary care settings.

CASE 2:

A 22-year-old woman with a history of insomnia, progressive fatigue, and poor concentration is brought to the emergency department by her family for the third time in 7 days to see the "on-call neurologist" for "seizures." The patient recently lost her job and reluctantly reports feeling severely depressed without suicidal ideation. When asked to recall what happens during a seizure, she states, "I feel confused and try to talk to people around me, but just keep shaking." There is no loss of consciousness, tongue biting, injuries, bowel or bladder incontinence, or postictal disorientation. She is unable to recall any emotional trigger before these episodes. When asked about any history of abuse, she pauses for some time but eventually denies any abuse. She has no other pertinent medical history and denies any illicit drug or alcohol use. Owing to financial difficulties, she recently moved in with her family. Her mother reports that this is very uncharacteristic of her daughter.

1. Which of the following is the most appropriate diagnosis for this patient?

   A. Epilepsy
   B. Conversion disorder

C. Somatic symptom disorder
D. Malingering

Correct answer: B. *Given her description of the seizures, it is unlikely she has a true seizure disorder. This young woman underwent a recent stressor (job loss) followed by the development of a nonintentional motor abnormality most consistent with psychogenic nonepileptic seizures, a conversion disorder. It is often challenging to differentiate psychogenic nonepileptic seizures from epileptic seizures without the use of video electroencephalography. Also consider that up to 30% of patients with psychogenic nonepileptic seizures have concomitant documented epilepsy, underscoring the importance of thorough evaluation and consultation with specialists. Further evaluation and potential treatment of her depressive symptoms with an antidepressant and/or CBT is indicated. There is generally a stressful event that precedes the development of conversion disorders. Identifying and addressing the emotional event may be helpful. In this case, further exploration of physical, sexual, or emotional abuse should be attempted in a private and safe environment without the presence of family members. It is not helpful to challenge the patient with statements such as, "your problem is strictly psychiatric" or "you do not have a medical problem." It is helpful to direct the patient toward functional recovery through the development of coping techniques and better anxiety management strategies. CBT is an evidence-based intervention that may help reduce the number of episodes and improve psychosocial function.*

CASE 3:

A 44-year-old man with no medical history is seen in an emergency room with complaint of "I cannot feel my face... I think I'm having a stroke." He can talk on the phone and eat solid and liquid foods without difficulty. He does not give permission to obtain collateral history from his family or friends. A nurse overhears him on the phone say, "It's cold out there and you better let me back in the house." When confronted, he admits his wife separated from him recently and that he is homeless. He also laments, "My face is paralyzed, and I need to be hospitalized." A neurologic examination and brain imaging are both normal. All laboratory values, including blood alcohol and toxicology screens, are also normal. The patient's response to reassurance from the emergency department physician is, "You better admit me...at least for tonight."

1. Which of the following is the most appropriate diagnosis for this patient?

   A. Factitious disorder
   B. Conversion disorder
   C. Somatic symptom disorder
   D. Malingering

Correct answer: D. *In this case, a thorough diagnostic workup was done, and it is likely that the patient is malingering to obtain shelter (external, secondary gain). Unlike those who have a somatic symptom disorder, patients who malinger intentionally report inaccurate information to realize a predetermined goal. Although it is often challenging, practitioners should try to empathize with patients who are malingering and focus on a solution to the actual problem. In this case, a discussion about housing options that do not include the hospital should be addressed with the patient in an assertive and nonpunitive manner. Collaboration with social workers and knowledge about local resources is important. The clinician can point out that admitting the patient to the hospital will not solve his housing problem or financial problems. Lastly, malingering should always be a diagnosis of exclusion and made only after a thorough history and physical examination have been completed. Factitious disorder should also be considered in this case. This diagnosis would apply if the patient was intentionally feigning symptoms to assume the "sick role" and gain medical attention from various health care practitioners. Patients with factious disorder are often resistant to participate in psychiatric evaluations and psychotherapy. The most important part of treatment is to recognize the disorder and do no harm by avoiding unnecessary procedures and consultations. These patients should be fully assessed for general medical, neurologic, and highly comorbid psychiatric disorders. It is important to note that, unlike malingering, somatic symptom and related disorders often originate from unconscious and unhealthy coping mechanisms to life stressors.*

PRACTICAL RESOURCES

- Merck Manual Online. Somatic Symptom and Related Disorders. http://www.merckmanuals.com/professional/psychiatric-disorders/somatic-symptom-and-related-disorders/overview-of-somatization
- Medscape. Somatic Symptom and Related Disorders. https://emedicine.medscape.com/article/294908-overview

REFERENCES

1. Katon W, Ries RK, Kleinman A. The prevalence of somatization in primary care. *Compr Psychiatry.* 1984;25(2):208-215.
2. Kroenke K. Symptoms in medical patients: an untended field. *Am J Med.* 1992;92(1A):3S-6S.
3. Kroenke K, Mangelsdorff AD. Common symptoms in ambulatory care: incidence, evaluation, therapy, and outcome. *Am J Med.* 1989;86(3):262-266.

4. de Waal MW, Arnold IA, Eekhof JA, et al. Somatoform disorders in general practice: prevalence, functional impairment and comorbidity with anxiety and depressive disorders. *Br J Psychiatry.* 2004;184:470-476.

5. Thomassen R, van Hemert AM, Huyse FJ, et al. Somatoform disorders in consultation–liaison psychiatry: a comparison with other mental disorders. *Gen Hosp Psychiatry.* 2003;25:8-13.

6. Neimark G, Caroff S, Stinnett J. Medically unexplained physical symptoms. *Psychiatry Ann.* 2005;35(4):298-305.

7. American Psychiatric Association. *Diagnostic and Statistical Manual of Mental Disorders.* 5th ed. Washington, DC: American Psychiatric Association; 2013.

8. Simon GE, Gureje O. Stability of somatization disorder and somatization symptoms among primary care patients. *Arch Gen Psychiatry.* 1999;56:90-95.

9. Allen LA, Escobar JI, Lehrer PM, et al. Psychosocial treatments for multiple unexplained physical symptoms: a review of the literature. *Psychosom Med.* 2002;64: 939-950.

10. McCarron R. Somatization in the primary care setting. *Psychiatr Times.* 2006;23(6):32-34.

11. Speckens AE, van Hemert AM, Spinhoven P, et al. Cognitive behavioural therapy for medically unexplained physical symptoms: a randomised controlled trial. *BMJ.* 1995;311:1328-1332.

12. Warwick HM, Clark DM, Cobb AM, et al. A controlled trial of cognitive behavioural treatment of hypochondriasis. *Br J Psychiatry.* 1996;169:189-195.

13. Kroenke K, Swindle R. Cognitive-behavioral therapy for somatization and symptom syndromes: a critical review of controlled clinical trials. *Psychother Psychosom.* 2000;9:205-215.

14. Burns D. *Feeling Good: The New Mood Therapy.* 2nd ed. New York: Avon Books; 1999.

15. Sadock BJ, Sadock VA. *Synopsis of Psychiatry.* Philadelphia: Lippincott Williams & Wilkins; 2015.

16. Allen L, Gara M, Escobar J. Somatization: a debilitating syndrome in primary care. *Psychosomatics.* 2001;42(1).

17. Kroenke K, Spitzer R, Williams J, et al. Predictors of psychiatric disorders and functional impairment. *Arch Fam Med.* 1994;3:774-779.

18. Smith C, Monson R, Ray D. Psychiatric consultation in somatization disorder. *Engl J Med.* 1986;14:1407-1413.

24

INSOMNIA

Scott G. Williams, MD, FACP, FAPA, FAASM and Vincent F. Capaldi, II, ScM, MD

- Chronic insomnia affects more than 10% of the population, and transient insomnia affects at least 30% to 35% of the general population.
- Evaluation of a sleep complaint should include a complete assessment of general medical and psychiatric comorbidities, as well as evaluation of legal and illicit substances.
- Insomnia should be treated as a separate clinical entity even if it occurs as part of an underlying medical, psychiatric, or substance-related problem.
- Current clinical guidelines recommend behavioral treatments (cognitive behavioral treatment of insomnia) as the first-line approach.
- Although short-term use of benzodiazepine receptor agonists can be useful, there are very few data showing effectiveness of pharmacologic treatments in patients with chronic insomnia.
- Always evaluate for driving safety, and understand that all sedative-hypnotic medications carry a risk for next-day effects. Benzodiazepines and anticholinergic agents should be used cautiously in elderly patients.

INTRODUCTION

According to the Institute of Medicine, an estimated 50 to 70 million Americans are affected by disorders of sleep and wakefulness. Sleep disorders are often divided into categories including sleep-related breathing disorders (obstructive sleep apnea), insomnia, restless legs syndrome, parasomnias, circadian rhythm disorders, and hypersomnia conditions. *Table 24-1* lists the ICD-10 coding for these associated disorders. Of these categories, arguably the most common sleep disorder is insomnia, which affects up to one-third of the general population.

CLINICAL SIGNIFICANCE

Although most with insomnia have transient symptoms, chronic insomnia can affect up to 10% of the population. Direct and indirect costs of insomnia approach $100 billion per year; however, sleep disorders in general go largely undertreated because of a combination of a lack of recognition and a lack of experienced clinicians. Although there has been some recent progress, medical school curricula still largely ignore sleep disorders, and the majority of clinical learning occurs during graduate medical education or as a staff physician. The pattern of sleep disturbances associated with various sleep disorders is presented in *Table 24-2*.

The majority of patients with insomnia suffer from comorbid conditions. Medical conditions most likely to cause insomnia include chronic pain and cardiopulmonary disease with resultant nocturnal dyspnea. Psychiatric conditions associated with insomnia include anxiety, depression, and psychosis. *Table 24-3* lists the specific patterns of sleep disruption associated with psychiatric conditions. Many substances can cause or contribute to insomnia. The most common over-the-counter substance implicated in chronic insomnia is caffeine, particularly when ingested within a few hours of sleep. Prescription medications such as beta agonists, stimulants, theophylline, certain antibiotics, and even lipid-lowering agents have been associated with sleep fragmentation or insomnia. Illicit drugs such as cocaine or methamphetamine can cause profound hyperarousal. Withdrawal from certain substances such as alcohol can also cause an insomnia syndrome. *Table 24-4* provides a more comprehensive list of medications associated with insomnia.

Because of the substantial comorbidity, insomnia has typically been thought to be solely secondary to these underlying conditions and is not treated as a separate entity; however, current thinking is that insomnia should be considered an independent condition warranting specific treatment in parallel with any other diagnosis. Untreated insomnia can worsen cardiovascular outcomes. Multiple studies have shown that focusing specifically on insomnia can improve other health-related outcomes, particularly for psychiatric disorders.

TABLE 24-1 ICD-10 Codes	
Breathing-related sleep disorder	G47.9
Circadian rhythm sleep disorder	G47.29
Dyssomnia not otherwise specified	G47.8
Hypersomnia due to [general medical condition]	G47.1
Insomnia due to [general medical condition]	G47.01
Narcolepsy	G47.41
Primary insomnia	F51.01
Sleep terror disorder	F51.4
Sleepwalking disorder	F51.3

DIAGNOSIS

The International Classification of Sleep Disorders, Third Edition, and the Diagnostic and Statistical Manual of Mental Disorders, Fifth Edition, are now aligned almost completely regarding the criteria for the diagnosis of chronic insomnia. Diagnostic criteria for insomnia are listed in *Box 24-1*. There has been a philosophical shift over the past few years to streamline the insomnia taxonomy. Previously, there were numerous insomnia subtypes such as psychophysiologic insomnia, paradoxical insomnia, inadequate sleep hygiene, and idiopathic insomnia. In part because patients cannot always easily be separated into discrete subtypes, and because the management is often similar, that current approach is to simply separate acute from chronic insomnia and not focus as much on whether it is a "primary" or a "secondary" condition.

TABLE 24-2 Predisposing Factors, Clinical Features, and Treatment of Common Primary Sleep Disorders

SLEEP DISORDER	PREDISPOSING FACTORS	CLINICAL FEATURES	TREATMENT
Obstructive sleep apnea-hypopnea (OSAH)	Nasopharyngeal abnormalities, craniofacial abnormalities, obesity, >40 years old, men > women (2:1), neurologic disorder (e.g., recent stroke)	Repetitive episodes of upper airway obstruction that occur during sleep, usually associated with oxygen desaturation. Episodes include loud snoring or gasps that last 20-30 seconds. Associated with morning headaches and increased daytime sedation	• Nasal continuous positive airway pressure (CPAP) • Behavioral therapies: avoid alcohol, tobacco, and sedative-hypnotics at night; weight loss if overweight; sleep on side, not back • Dental appliances: reposition lower jaw and tongue • Surgical interventions: resection of tonsils, uvula, or part of soft palate
Periodic limb movement disorder (PLMD)	OSAH, RLS, narcolepsy, increased age, chronic uremia, TCAs or MAOIs, withdrawal from sedating agents, incidence same in men and women	Periodic episodes of repetitive and stereotyped limb movements during non-REM sleep: extension of the big toe with partial flexion of the ankles, knees, or hips. Muscle contractions last 0.5-5 seconds, with 20- to 40-second interepisode intervals	• Treat underlying problem • Improve sleep hygiene • Relaxation therapy • Consider carbidopa, levodopa, pramipexole, FDA-approved sleep agent
Restless legs syndrome (RLS)	Pregnancy (>20 weeks gestation), uremia, iron deficiency anemia, rheumatoid arthritis, renal disease, alcoholism. Peak onset is middle age	Uncomfortable sensations in the legs or arms just prior to sleep onset. Described as "achy," "crawling," "pulling," "prickling," or "tingling." Those who suffer from RLS can have very severe insomnia	• Treat the underlying cause • Correct nutritional deficiency (vitamin B_{12}, folic acid, or iron) • Stop or decrease dose of offending medications • Consider: carbidopa or levodopa, pergolide, pramipexole, bromocriptine mesylate, ropinirole

Adapted with permission from International Classification of Sleep Disorders. 3rd ed. Darien, IL: American Academy of Sleep Medicine; 2014. Copyright © 2014 American Academy of Sleep Medicine.
FDA, Food and Drug Administration; MAOIs, monoamine oxidase inhibitors; REM, rapid eye movement; TCAs, tricyclic antidepressants.

TABLE 24-3 Characteristics of Sleep in Various Psychiatric Diagnoses

DSM-5 DIAGNOSIS	COMMON SLEEP COMPLAINTS AND SYMPTOMS
Major depressive disorder	• Difficulty falling asleep (early insomnia) • Frequent awakenings (middle insomnia) • Uncharacteristic early-morning awakening (terminal insomnia) • Hypersomnia ("I sleep all day long so I don't have to face my depression")
Manic episode	• Decreased need for sleep lasting days or weeks • Lack of fatigue despite lack of sleep • Extra work accomplished during usual sleep times ("I stayed up all night and cleaned the whole house")
Posttraumatic stress disorder	• Difficulty falling asleep, which is often associated with anxiety about being abused or traumatized • Physiologic hyperarousal • Very light sleep, with exquisite sensitivity to sounds and other stimuli • Hyperstartled response if awakened by external stimuli • Frequent awakenings • Nightmares
Generalized anxiety disorder	• Prone to *psychophysiologic insomnia* • Difficulty falling asleep due to preoccupation and excessive worry about several stressors
Psychotic disorders	• Hallucinations (e.g., "The voices laugh and scream at me at night, so I can't sleep") • Paranoid thoughts
Attention deficit hyperactivity disorder	• Difficulty falling asleep due to physical hyperactivity • Activating effects of stimulants

BOX 24-1   GENERAL CRITERIA FOR THE DIAGNOSIS OF INSOMNIA

1. Difficulty initiating or maintaining sleep, awakening too early, nonrestorative or poor quality of sleep
2. Sleep difficulty occurs despite adequate opportunity and circumstances for sleep
3. At least one of the following forms of daytime impairment related to the nighttime sleep difficulty occurs:
   - Fatigue or malaise
   - Attention, concentration, or memory impairment
   - Social or vocational dysfunction or poor school performance
   - Mood disturbance or irritability
   - Daytime somnolence
   - Motivation, energy, or initiative reduction
   - Prone to errors or accidents at work or while operating a car or other machinery
   - Muscle tension, headaches, or gastrointestinal symptoms
   - Preoccupation with sleep or lack of sleep

Adapted from: International Classification of Sleep Disorders. 3rd ed. Darien, IL: American Academy of Sleep Medicine; 2014.

BIOPSYCHOSOCIAL TREATMENT

Treatment of insomnia includes a variety of interventions including behavioral, psychological, and sometimes pharmacologic. The underlying causes of sleep complaints are varied. Adequately treating insomnia patients starts with an accurate diagnosis and addressing the underlying etiology. A clinician must first identify and address modifiable factors such as sleep hygiene, medical illnesses, psychosocial stressors, and underlying psychiatric conditions before initiating treatment with a sedative-hypnotic medication. A sleep aid may be initiated earlier if the patient has time-limited adjustment insomnia. Medications should also be considered if symptoms persist despite addressing acute stressors.

PHARMACOLOGIC TREATMENTS FOR INSOMNIA

The ideal sleep aid should promote sleep onset and sleep maintenance without next-day side effects such as grogginess, headaches, and fatigue. The FDA has approved three classes of medications for the treatment of insomnia (*Table 24-5*): benzodiazepine gamma-aminobutyric acid A (GABAA) receptor agonists (BZDs), nonbenzodiazepine GABAA receptor agonists (BzRAs), and melatonin receptor agonists. Common BZD side effects include daytime

TABLE 24-4 Medications Known to Cause Insomnia

CLASS	MEDICATION
Antiepileptics	Lamotrigine
Antidepressants	Bupropion
	Fluoxetine
	Venlafaxine
	Phenelzine
	Protriptyline
Beta-blockers	Propranolol
	Pindolol
	Metoprolol
Bronchodilators	Theophylline
	Levalbuterol
	Albuterol
	Formoterol
	Salmeterol
Decongestants	Pseudoephedrine
	Phenylpropanolamine
Steroids	Prednisone
Stimulants	Dextroamphetamine
	Methamphetamine
	Methylphenidate
	Modafinil
	Pemoline
	Armodafinil

sedation, transient amnesia, cognitive impairment, motor incoordination, dependence, tolerance, and rebound insomnia. In general, BZDs should be limited to healthy patients and used cautiously in the elderly and those with multiple medical problems. Although not FDA approved specifically for insomnia, other medications with sedative properties have been useful in treating some patients with insomnia. BzRA may have a decreased side effect profile when compared with BZDs. BzRAs include eszopiclone, zaleplon, zolpidem, and zolpidem extended release. The melatonin receptor agonist ramelteon (Rozerem) also reduces time to fall asleep without next-day psychomotor and memory effects. Ramelteon (and melatonin) is associated with less concern for dependence, perhaps owing to its less immediate effects on sleep. Limited data exist on the efficacy of non–FDA-approved medications for insomnia such as antidepressants, second-generation antipsychotics, and antihistamines. *Table 24-6* summarizes sedating

medications that may be useful for patients with insomnia, although selection should be based on the underlying psychiatric conditions. Of the FDA-approved medications, only eszopiclone and zolpidem continuous release (CR) have been approved for use without a specified time limit. The other medications have approved use limited to 35 days or less. Finally, most of the FDA-approved medications for insomnia also carry an FDA black box warning for complex sleep-related behaviors, which may include sleep driving, making phone calls, and preparing and eating food while asleep. Although dangerous outcomes from these behaviors are rare, primary care practitioners should discuss and document the potential for these behaviors with patients who suffer from insomnia.

PSYCHOLOGICAL APPROACHES

Because pharmacotherapy is not intended for long-term use, nonpharmacologic interventions should be considered before or concurrently with sedative-hypnotic medications. Primary care patients who have insomnia often take sedative-hypnotic agents well beyond the recommended time frame. Discontinuing these medications can lead to increased anxiety and irritability as well as rebound insomnia. The inclusion of a psychosocial treatment approach for insomnia is safe and can be used indefinitely.

Sleep Hygiene Education

Extrinsic factors often cause, worsen, or perpetuate poor sleep. Therefore, it is important to educate patients about the impact of lifestyle and behavioral factors on sleep, and to give specific suggestions to improve sleep hygiene (*Table 24-7*).

Sleep Restriction

This therapy is based on the premise that those with insomnia can increase their sleep time and sleep efficiency by inducing temporary sleep deprivation through voluntarily reducing their time in bed. For example, people who try to sleep at night and suffer from insomnia should be encouraged to restrict daytime or early evening naps.

Stimulus Control

Stimulus control may be helpful when insomnia is caused by a "bedtime environment" that is conducive to staying awake rather than sleeping. A patient's report that he can "never" sleep in his own bed, but sleeps very well in unfamiliar environments, is a clue that he has developed a maladaptive response to his sleep environment. This is a common phenomenon of psychophysiologic insomnia. For example, this occurs when wake-promoting activities such as watching TV, studying, and paying bills are done in the bedroom (or on the bed). The treatment focuses on breaking these associations by teaching patients to avoid activities that promote wakefulness in the bedroom (or sleep environment) and to only use the bedroom for sleeping. If sleep is not possible, the patient is encouraged to leave the bedroom until a definitive urge to sleep is present.

TABLE 24-5 Food and Drug Administration (FDA)-Approved Drugs for Insomnia

DRUGS	ADULT DOSE (mg)	HALF-LIFE (hours)	ONSET (minutes)	PEAK EFFECT (hours)	MAJOR EFFECTS/CLINICAL COMMENTS
Benzodiazepines (BZDs)					***Caution*** *in elderly patients.* Tolerance to BZDs develops to the sedative, hypnotic, and anticonvulsant effects. High doses can cause respiratory depression. Avoid in patients with obstructive sleep apnea-hypopnea
Estazolam (ProSom)	1-2	10-24	60	½-1½	Short-term (7-10 days) treatment for frequent arousals and early-morning awakening. Not as useful for initial insomnia. **Caution** in those with liver disease
Flurazepam (Dalmane)	15-30	47-100	15-20	3-6	Short-term (7-10 days) treatment for middle and terminal insomnia. Increased daytime sedation over time
Temazepam (Restoril)	15-30	6-16		2-3	Short-term (7-10 days) treatment for sleep onset and maintenance. Doses ≥30 mg/day: morning grogginess, nausea, headaches, and vivid dreaming
Benzodiazepine receptor agonists (BzRAs)					
Eszopiclone (Lunesta)	2-3	6-9	Rapid	1	In elderly start with 1-2 mg. Rapid onset; should be in bed when taking medication. For faster sleep onset, do not ingest with high-fat foods. No tolerance after 6 months
Zaleplon (Sonata)	5-20	1	Rapid	1	Short-term (7-10 days) treatment for initial insomnia
Zolpidem (Ambien, Ambien CR)	5-20	1.4-4.5	30	2-4	Short-term (7-10 days) treatment for initial and middle insomnia (generic form is available). Rapid onset; should be in bed when taking medication. For faster sleep onset, do not ingest with food
Zolpidem CR (Ambien CR)	12.5	1.4-4.5	30	2-4	Short-term (7-10 days) treatment for initial and middle insomnia (generic form is available). Rapid onset; should be in bed when taking medication. For faster sleep onset, do not ingest with food
	6.25-12.5	1.4-4.5	30	2-4	Used for sleep induction and sleep maintenance
Melatonin agonist					
Ramelteon (Rozerem)	8	1-2	30	1-1½	Used for initial and middle insomnia. For faster sleep onset, do not ingest with high-fat foods. No tolerance or potential for addiction. **Contraindicated** with fluvoxamine. Should not be used concurrently with melatonin

All sedative-hypnotics should be used with caution and at a lower starting dose when given to the elderly. All sedative-hypnotics should be taken only if the patient plans to go to bed immediately after taking the medication.

Adapted with permission from International Classification of Sleep Disorders. 3rd ed. Darien, IL: American Academy of Sleep Medicine; 2014. Copyright © 2014 American Academy of Sleep Medicine.

Cognitive Behavioral Therapy

Cognitive behavioral therapy (CBT) presumes that cognitive distortions lead to negative emotions and behavior, which may cause or worsen insomnia. This therapy includes identifying, challenging, and replacing cognitive distortions and beliefs regarding sleep and loss of sleep with realistic thoughts and beliefs. For example, a college student may catastrophize inability to fall asleep with failing an examination. However, when this belief is examined in detail, the inability to sleep may not necessarily cause her to fail the examination. Previous evidence of such an event may be used to refute this distorted cognition.

Progressive Relaxation Technique

Insomnia is associated with hyperarousal. With this technique, patients are taught how to recognize and control muscular tension through the use of exercises (sometimes using music or audio instructions) to reduce the anxiety and hyperarousal associated with insomnia.

TABLE 24-6 Drugs Commonly Used "Off-label" for Insomnia

DRUG	PERTINENT SIDE EFFECTS	COMMENTS
Antidepressants		
Mirtazapine (Remeron)	Somnolence and increased appetite	May be beneficial if patient has comorbid depression and insomnia. Mirtazapine's sedating effect is inversely dose dependent. As the dose increases, the noradrenergic activity counteracts the sleep-inducing H_1 antihistaminic effect of mirtazapine
Trazodone (Desyrel)	Residual daytime sedation, headache, orthostatic hypotension, priapism, cardiac arrhythmias	One of the most commonly prescribed agents for the treatment of insomnia. May be beneficial if patient has comorbid depression and insomnia. May be an acceptable alternative for patients for whom BzRAs are contraindicated (severe hypercapnea or hypoxemia, or history of substance abuse or dependence). Usually dosed much lower (50-100 mg) than when used for depression
Tricyclic antidepressants (TCAs)	Delirium, decreased cognition and seizure threshold, orthostatic hypotension, tachycardia, ECG abnormalities	**Avoid** in hospitalized patients because of their anticholinergic, antihistaminic, and cardiovascular side effects. Not recommended as a treatment for insomnia or other sleep problems unless comorbid depression is present. As with other antidepressants, TCAs are usually used at significantly lower doses than for depression
Antihistamines		
Diphenhydramine (Benadryl)	Residual daytime sedation, weight gain, delirium, orthostatic hypotension, blurred vision, urinary retention	Antihistamines are one of the most commonly used over-the-counter agents for chronic insomnia. If possible, avoid in patients >60 years old
Hydroxyzine (Vistaril)	Residual daytime sedation, weight gain, delirium, orthostatic hypotension, blurred vision, urinary retention	Efficacy as an anxiolytic has not been established. Not FDA approved for insomnia. **Avoid** in patients >60 years old and those with closed-angle glaucoma, prostatic hypertrophy, severe asthma, and COPD
Antipsychotics		
Quetiapine (Seroquel)	Sedation, orthostatic hypotension, metabolic derangements (e.g., weight gain, dyslipidemia, and glucose dysregulation)	The most sedating of the atypical antipsychotics; it is frequently used as a sleep aid. Not recommended for insomnia or other sleep problems unless there is comorbid psychotic or bipolar disorder. Is dosed much lower (25-100 mg) when used for insomnia. Other less expensive sedative-hypnotic agents should be used first

BzRAs, benzodiazepine receptor agonists; COPD, chronic obstructive pulmonary disease; ECG, electrocardiogram; FDA, Food and Drug Administration; TCAs, tricyclic antidepressants (doxepin, amitriptyline, imipramine, nortriptyline, desipramine).

TABLE 24-7 Principles and Tips for Good Sleep Hygiene

Sleep diary	• Monitor the amount of sleep during day and night
Regular sleep–wake schedule	• Go to bed at the same time each night • Wake up at same time each morning • Avoid naps during the day
Sleep-promoting nightly ritual	• Plan a relaxing, soothing routine for your last hour of wakefulness (e.g., if the time for "lights out" is 9:45 PM, start winding down by 8:45 PM) • Your last hour could include the following: dimming the lights; screening phone calls for urgent calls; showering, bathing, and doing other usual hygiene routines; changing into your bed clothes; reading relaxing or nonstimulating material; limiting yourself to read only up to your "lights out" time; listening to soothing music or other "white noise"
Avoid stressful or other mentally stimulating activities before bedtime	• Address tomorrow's activities, concerns, or distractions earlier in the day • Unless absolutely necessary, postpone anxiety-provoking conversations that require you to make important decisions, or may cause more conflicts, to a time when you are more alert, rested, and much more likely to make a sound decision

TABLE 24-7 Principles and Tips for Good Sleep Hygiene   (continued)

Do not lie in bed "wide awake"	• Trying to will yourself to sleep when you're not sleepy will make you more frustrated, not sleepier • Instead, get out of bed, and engage in mentally and physically nonstimulating activities that will relax, soothe, and, perhaps, even bore you • Do not frequently check the clock
Avoid stimulants, alcohol, and heavy meals at bedtime	• Have your last caffeine- and alcohol-containing food or drink at least 4 hours before you go to bed • Do not smoke within an hour of bedtime, and refrain from smoking if you wake up in the middle of the night • Do not eat a heavy meal within 2 hours of going to bed
Exercise	• Light, aerobic exercise for even 20-30 minutes earlier in the day promotes deep sleep • Avoid exercising within 2 hours of bedtime because it could actually be activating and interfere with sleep
Comfortable environment	• Sleep is promoted by darkness, quiet or soothing noises, and a relatively cool temperature (<68°F)

WHEN TO REFER

• Refractory insomnia
• Insomnia with a concurrent mood, anxiety, or psychotic disorder
• Suicidal ideation in the context of insomnia
• Need for supportive or cognitive behavioral psychotherapy

CASES AND QUESTIONS

CASE 1:

A 48-year-old man who has been sober for 6 weeks comes to the ambulatory care clinic saying he hasn't "slept a wink" since entering a residential treatment program 4 weeks ago. He stopped drinking alcohol "cold turkey" after his wife of 20 years and two daughters left him because of the patient's refusal to quit drinking. For the past 20 years, he drank up to one 12 pack of beer nightly and could not fall asleep unless he drank at least two beers before bedtime.

During the first week of sobriety, he had moderate cravings for alcohol and mild tremors that quickly resolved. His sleep was characterized by taking up to an hour to fall asleep and waking up feeling tired and groggy. By the end of his second week of sobriety, he fell asleep soon after going to bed and started to sleep through the night, especially after his wife allowed him to speak to his daughters.

Since the third week of sobriety, he has been living in a house with 23 other people who are in treatment for alcohol or substance dependence. The house has a strict "lights out" time of 10 PM. He shares a room with three other men and sleeps on the lower bunk of a bunk bed. During the first week in the program, his main problems were "falling asleep and staying asleep." Recently, he started getting out of bed to smoke a cigarette on the porch because he felt so restless and

anxious about not being able to fall asleep. During the day, he struggles to stay awake during group meetings. He wonders if he's "bipolar" because minor annoyances that never bothered him before, such as a housemate slurping his soup, make him extremely irritable. He also reports a mildly depressed mood that is directly related to his stressors and related insomnia.

1. What is the first-line treatment for this patient's insomnia symptoms?

   A. Eszopiclone
   B. Suvorexant
   C. CBT for insomnia
   D. Sleep hygiene

   Correct answer: C. *For this patient, treatment includes psychoeducation about the effects of psychosocial stressors, alcohol withdrawal, nicotine dependence, environmental factors (new temporary home), and being anxious about not being able to sleep (psychophysiologic insomnia). It would be important to reassure the patient that multiple significant, but modifiable, factors have converged to disrupt his sleep. First, several nonpharmacologic approaches should be tried: sleep hygiene (refraining from cigarette use before or during bedtime), environmental triggers (e.g., asking roommates to refrain from discussing the day's events, wearing earplugs, or dimming the alarm clock lights), and behavioral interventions (e.g., refraining from checking the time constantly). The use of CBT may be useful as it would address his depressed mood and related insomnia.*

2. Which of the following medications should be avoided in this patient?

   A. Mirtazapine
   B. Eszopiclone
   C. Suvorexant
   D. Trazodone

continued

Correct answer: B. *In this case, BZD and BzRA medication should be avoided, as these may trigger alcohol relapse. However, a brief course of one of the non–FDA-approved agents, such as diphenhydramine 25 mg, can be considered. The other listed options are also reasonable options.*

3. This type of insomnia is characterized by a preoccupation and anxiety about sleep:
   - **A.** Primary insomnia
   - **B.** Acute insomnia
   - **C.** Chronic insomnia
   - **D.** Psychophysiologic insomnia

   Correct answer: D. *Sleep disruption is very common during the first several months after the discontinuation of alcohol and other substances. During the first 2 weeks of sobriety, his differential diagnoses included insomnia due to alcohol withdrawal and adjustment (acute) insomnia. He started having symptoms of adjustment (acute) insomnia again with increased sleep latency and frequent awakenings (middle insomnia)—immediately after he started facing the new stressors of moving into a residential treatment facility and sleeping in a new, uncomfortable environment. He is also psychologically hyperaroused as he frequently thinks about the separation from his family.*

He also has symptoms of psychophysiologic insomnia, including preoccupation and anxiety about sleep, nodding off unintentionally during the day, and the sense that he needs cigarettes to relax his mind and body. Unfortunately, cigarettes are compounding the problem because nicotine is a central nervous system stimulant.

CASE 2:

A 53-year-old African-American woman who weighed 232 pounds and was 5′3″ tall presented to the ambulatory care clinic complaining of "really bad snoring" and frequent nighttime awakenings, some lasting 30 minutes or more. The patient usually goes to bed feeling "exhausted" and does not have problems falling asleep; however, she awakens 2 to 3 hours later because of a "rumbling" feeling in her stomach, and often feels nauseated. She usually gets up to urinate at this time but is unsure whether the need to urinate or the gastrointestinal (GI) symptoms wake her up at night. Sometimes her "allergies" act up at that time and she starts coughing. She hasn't had an asthma attack since childhood, but sometimes feels like she's about to have one. However, she calms herself by using deep breathing techniques that she learned at an employee wellness class and falls asleep again shortly thereafter. She usually awakens feeling fatigued and sleepy several hours later.

She can function relatively well in her job as a bookkeeper in the morning, especially after drinking a cup of regular coffee. By the early afternoon, she can barely keep her eyes open unless she has at least two shots of espresso. The patient often awakens with a pounding headache that is only slightly relieved with ibuprofen. On examination, you note that the patient has a large posterior pharynx and an enlarged neck. Medical history includes moderate hypertension that seems to be well controlled with an angiotensin-converting enzyme inhibitor. At this time, she is opposed to getting a sleep study or using an oral appliance or "any breathing device."

1. What is this patient's most likely diagnosis?
   - **A.** Obstructive sleep apnea—hypopnea
   - **B.** Willis–Ekbom disease
   - **C.** Central apnea syndrome
   - **D.** Periodic limb movement disorder

   Correct answer: A. *This patient presented with evidence of obstructive sleep apnea-hypopnea (OSAH): snoring, morbid obesity, daytime somnolence, awakening with a headache, a history of hypertension, and a large posterior oropharynx.*

2. Which of the following diagnoses are exacerbated by this underlying disorder?
   - **A.** Hypertension
   - **B.** Gastroesophageal reflux disorder (GERD)
   - **C.** Obesity
   - **D.** All of the above

   Correct answer: D. *Her GI symptoms that awaken her from sleep are suggestive of nocturnal gastroesophageal reflux, which is frequently associated with OSAH. Rather than her "allergies" acting up, she's probably coughing because of the reflux, which has gradually worsened after she gained 50 pounds over the past year. The morning headaches may be due to unrecognized apneic episodes and associated blood pressure spikes throughout the night.*

3. Which of the following labs are recommended for this patient?
   - **A.** Comprehensive metabolic panel
   - **B.** Thyroid-stimulating hormone
   - **C.** Complete blood count
   - **D.** All of the above

   Correct answer: D. *All of the options are reasonable initial workup labs.*

4. Which if the following is not a good initial treatment approach?
   - **A.** Recommend weight loss
   - **B.** Continuous positive airway pressure
   - **C.** Hypnotic medication
   - **D.** H2-blocker
   - **E.** Nutrition counseling

   Correct answer: C. *Hypnotic medication is relatively contraindicated as it could worsen sleep* *apnea by relaxing respiratory muscles further and may also reduce respiratory drive. Help the patient identify a few sleep hygiene problems, and assist her in developing a plan to address them. To prevent nocturnal GERD symptoms, advise the patient not to eat or drink anything within at least 2 hours of bedtime. Consider prescribing a bedtime dose of an antireflux agent. Encourage the patient to continue sitting up in bed and using deep breathing techniques if she continues to wake up with the above GI symptoms. In this case, weight loss is paramount. She should be given a referral for nutrition counseling and a weight management program. If symptoms persist after these interventions, consider revisiting the sleep study referral to rule out OSAH and possible treatment with continuous positive airway pressure.*

PRACTICAL RESOURCES

- The American Academy of Sleep Medicine (guidelines, practice parameters): http://www.aasmnet.org/
- The Insomnia Severity Index: https://biolincc.nhlbi.nih.gov/static/studies/masm/Insomnia%20Severity%20Index.pdf
- Insomnia smartphone application: http://t2health.dcoe.mil/apps/CBT-i

REFERENCES

1. American Academy of Sleep Medicine. *International Classification of Sleep Disorders*. 3rd ed. Darien, IL: American Academy of Sleep Medicine; 2014.
2. American Psychiatric Association. *Diagnostic and Statistical Manual of Mental Disorders*. 5th ed. Arlington, VA: American Psychiatric Association; 2013.
3. Bonnet M, Arand D. Hyperarousal and insomnia: state of the science. *Sleep Med Rev.* 2010;14:9-15.
4. Morganthaler T, Owens J, Alessi C, et al. Practice parameters for the behavioral treatment of bedtime problems and night wakings in infants and young children. *Sleep.* 2006;29:1277-1281.
5. Morgenthaler T, Kramer M, Alessi C, et al. Practice parameters for the psychological and behavioral treatment of insomnia: an update. *Sleep.* 2006;29:1415-1419.
6. National Institute of Health. NIH state-of-the-science conference statement on manifestations and management of chronic insomnia in adults. *NIH Consens Stat Sci Statements.* 2005;22:1-30.
7. Ohayon MM. Epidemiology of insomnia: what we know and what we still need to learn. *Sleep Med Rev.* 2002;6:97-111.
8. Riemann D, Spiegelhalder K, Feige B, et al. The hyperarousal model of insomnia: a review of the concept and its evidence. *Sleep Med Rev.* 2010;14:19-31.
9. Sateia M, Buysse D, Krystal A, Neubauer D, Heald J. Clinical practice guideline for the pharmacologic treatment of chronic insomnia in adults: an American Academy of sleep medicine clinical practice guideline. *J Clin Sleep Med.* 2017;13:307-349.
10. Schutte-Rodin S, Broch L, Buysse D, Dorsey C, Sateia M. Clinical guideline for the evaluation and management of chronic insomnia in adults. *J Clin Sleep Med.* 2008;4:487-504.
11. World Health Organization. *International Classification of Diseases.* 10th revision. Geneva, Switzerland: World Health Organization; 2007.

25

SEXUAL DYSFUNCTION

Mary Elizabeth Alvarez, MD, MPH

CLINICAL SIGNIFICANCE

Second only to pain, sexual dysfunction is probably the most commonly treated problem in the primary care clinic with entirely overlapping medical and psychiatric causes. Sexual dysfunction is a silent but common phenomenon in the primary care clinic, and clinician discomfort or lack of knowledge is the main barrier to patients' access to recovery.

The process that leads to a satisfying sexual encounter is complex but can be distilled to the process shown in *Figure 25-1.*

Both physiological and psychological glitches can occur anywhere in this process. Good history-taking and an appropriate physical examination with a directed workup can help make the diagnosis in most cases. In addition, treatments can often be provided without referral. In this chapter, I'll review the most common sexual dysfunctions and how they are treated.

When taking a history, all patients should be asked:

1. Do you have sex with men, women, or both?
2. Do you have any sexual concerns today?

Follow-up questions should address health behaviors that affect sexual function and are included in any social history. Exercise, diet, weight fluctuations, alcohol intake, drug use, and smoking all heavily influence sexual functioning and should be specifically addressed. Of course, you will ask about contraception and desire for pregnancy to both men who have sex with women and female patients. Important—but harder to ask about—are relationship histories including open-ended questions about masturbation, number of partners in the last year, and variations in sexual function between solo and partnered sexual episodes. Understanding there is no "normal" in the frequency and the wide variations of sexual expression, it's illuminating to ask how often the patient has sex and how often it is oral, vaginal, or anal. It is also important to gauge the level of distress and whether the patient identifies it as a problem or whether their partner is showing concern or distress.

Female sexual dysfunction is a significant public health problem that affects 41% of premenopausal women around the globe. About 12% of women in the United States report distressing sexual health concerns, although as many as 40% report sexual concerns overall.[1] While studies demonstrate varying results depending on sampling and methods, the prevalence of erectile dysfunction (ED) of men ranges between 6% in their 40s to 35% in their 60s. Know this: If you rarely address sexual dysfunction in your primary care visits, it's because of your own barriers to treat this group of disorders, not because of its rarity.

While each individual patient follows his or her own path, sexual appetite can change dramatically from youth and young adulthood through aging and

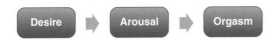

FIGURE 25-1 Sexual function.

pregnancy; menopause can have a dramatic effect on a woman's sexual functioning and the multifactorial effects of aging markedly affects a man's risk of ED. That said, it is realistic to expect healthy sexual appetites and functioning throughout the lifecycle and to not immediately attribute low sexual functioning to aging.

Chronic illness and pain have a direct effect on libido as well as arousal and orgasm; diabetes and atherosclerosis are responsible for the large part of sexual dysfunction among the primary care population who are seeking care for chronic diseases. Aging men with prostate disease also must cope with ED and difficulty with orgasm that can come with the disease or its treatments. Neurologic compromise and endocrine disorders are also commonly found in the primary care clinic and need to be ruled out before a sexual dysfunction can be diagnosed.

Although chronic disease often drives sexual dysfunction, the low-hanging fruit of treating it is the medications we prescribe for chronic conditions. Be careful to examine the medication list of your patients reporting sexual dysfunction and find alternatives for those commonly involved before launching a large workup for underlying causes (*Box 25-1*). It is often difficult to discern whether it is the disease or the treatment causing the sexual problem, so holding the medication or switching to another class is the first step.

BOX 25-1 COMMON MEDICATIONS THAT CAUSE PROBLEMS WITH SEXUAL DYSFUNCTION

Beta-blockers

5 alpha-reductase inhibitors

Alpha-blockers

Selective serotonin reuptake inhibitor (SSRI)

Androgen deprivation

Spironolactone

Anticholinergics

Benzodiazepines

Phenytoin

Antipsychotics

Hormonal contraception

DIAGNOSIS OF SEXUAL DYSFUNCTION

Sexual dysfunction diagnoses can be grouped according to the phase of the encounter it affects most. *hypoactive*

sexual desire is more common in women than men and can be primary (lifelong) or secondary. Of note, this is different from individuals who identify as asexual, or without any interest in sex. Arousal disorders are sorted by gender, with *female arousal disorder* being the counterpart to *male ED*. Orgasmic disorders vary widely in their ability to produce personal distress or interpersonal conflict. About half of women who do not consistently reach orgasm during sexual activity do not report distress. *Premature* or *delayed ejaculation* in men can vary in their time course and have both medical and behavioral treatments. Lastly, sexual pain disorders such as *vaginismus* and *vulvodynia/vestibulodynia* disproportionally affect women and have wide differential diagnoses for underlying causes and may often require specialty care. Fortunately, there are many effective treatments—both physical and psychological—and the primary care physician plays a key role in identifying the problem and validating the patient to receive care.

The differential diagnosis for the causes of sexual disorders is vast and screening for symptoms and history is the first step in deciding the next steps (*Table 25-1*).

When deciding on laboratory tests to order to assess dysfunction, understand that ordering a testosterone level is key to moving through the differential diagnosis for ED in men, but the situation is more complex for women. Decreased vaginal lubrication and dyspareunia are associated with low estradiol levels; however, the association between low sexual desire and lower estradiol levels has been inconsistent. Testosterone levels do not correlate with female sexual function or overall well-being, possibly because of the difficulty in accurately measuring free and total testosterone levels at the lower end of the female range. Although androgens are positively associated with improvements in all aspects of sexual functioning (e.g., subjective arousal, vaginal blood flow, sexual desire, orgasm), there is no lower level of testosterone that predicts sexual dysfunction, and androgen levels are not used to define an androgen deficiency syndrome in women. Laboratory testing is usually not needed to identify causes of female sexual dysfunction.[1]

FEMALE SEXUAL INTEREST/AROUSAL DISORDER

Known by many names, low libido, hypoactive sexual desire disorder (HSDD), and now female sexual interest/arousal disorder (FSIAD), FSIAD has always been used to describe distress or suffering caused by a patient's lack of desire for sexual contact. This is NOT used to describe a lifelong lack of interest in sex that causes no conflict, distress, or suffering. This is seen as a sexual orientation called asexuality, which does not cause distress. The shift in the definition from just low desire for sex to include problems with arousal is controversial, but the new name encompasses input from urologists to include inability to become aroused with sexual stimulation.

The epidemiology of low libido in women varies by how fully the sampled population is questioned on their

TABLE 25-1 Factors Contributing to Sexual Dysfunction

SOMATIC FACTORS	PSYCHOGENIC FACTORS	INTERPERSONAL FACTORS	PSYCHOSEXUAL FACTORS
Illness	Depression	Poor communication	Intimacy avoidance
Pregnancy	Anxiety	Relationship conflict	Religious conflict
Medications	Pregnancy fear	Abuse	Performance anxiety
Endocrine disorders	Contamination fear	Infidelity	Prior sexual trauma
Surgical sequelae	Hypochondriasis	Fear of intimacy	Intellectual defenses
Dermatoses/infections	Addiction	Poor models	Naiveté
Trauma/nerve damage	Paraphilia	Family system disruption	Unrealistic expectations

distress level. In a study of nearly 2000 women between ages 30 and 70 years in a stable relationship, the prevalence of low sexual desire was 36.2%, and the prevalence of distressing low sexual desire consistent with a diagnosis of HSDD was 8.3%, which shows a large difference between the presence of low libido and those women who feel its impact. Although the prevalence of low sexual desire increases with age, distress about low sexual desire decreases with age; thus, the prevalence of distressing low sexual desire stays relatively constant with increasing age. Interestingly, rates are about double in US women compared with women sampled in Europe.[2]

The pathophysiology of hypoactive sexual desire is multifactorial and highlights the interaction between the central nervous system (CNS) and peripheral nerve function. The pelvic organs are innervated by the sacral parasympathetic motor neurons, which are controlled by a specific group of neurons in the pontine brain stem, the pelvic organ stimulating center (POSC). Through long descending pathways, this POSC controls micturition, defecation, and sexual activities by stimulating different groups of sacral parasympathetic motor neurons. The pontine POSC is driven by the periaqueductal gray (PAG), which receives sensory information on the status of all pelvic organs. In addition, the PAG receives instructions from amygdala, hypothalamus, and other cortical structures. In humans, the PAG is controlled primarily by the medial orbitofrontal cortex, which is deactivated in women with desire and arousal disorder. In women with HSDD, deactivation of their medial orbitofrontal cortex produces a decrease in PAG–POSC activation, causing absence of vaginal vasocongestion and lubrication and decreased sexual behavior in general.[3]

DIAGNOSIS

As with other disorders in the *Diagnostic and Statistical Manual of Mental Disorders* (*DSM*), the symptoms of FSIAD cannot be entirely explained or caused by another medical, psychiatric disorder or psychosocial context. For example, the diagnosis is excluded if it is in the context of a sexual trauma, major depressive disorder, or relationship conflict. Be careful of diagnosing FSIAD when a patient is on a medication such as antidepressants or aromatase inhibitors, which is known to have a deleterious effect on sexual functioning across the spectrum. Also, be sure again to screen patients for substance use disorders, all of which alter sexual desire and responsiveness. As with any report of sexual difficulty, it is important to gather a social history to see if social stressors or relationship conflict underlies a recent change in libido or if the lack of desire is specific to the patient's long-term partner. It is a common sequela of betrayal and infidelity to experience a defensive decrease in sexual desire and is not FSIAD in this context. Severity is graded as mild, moderate, and severe; and symptoms must be present for at least 6 months during more than 75% of encounters. It may be useful to classify their respective disorders as lifelong or acquired and generalized (all partners, activities, forms of sexual expression) or situational (certain partners, practices). Women who begin sexual activity without a subjective experience of sexual desire but experience responsive desire during arousal phase and *are satisfied* with their sexual experiences and *not distressed* by the absence of subjective desire do not have FSIAD.[4]

To assess a woman for FSIAD, start with open-ended questions that focus on whether the lack of interest or arousal is bothersome or distressing in the relationship.

1. Do you feel like you have recently or always have had less desire for sex than your partners or peers?
2. Is it difficult for you to respond sexually to your partner's attempt to initiate sex?

Female Sexual Function Index (FSFI) is a 19-item instrument that has been used in clinical trials to measure overall sexual function, although the FDA is unaware of data that adequately establish the validity of the instrument. Although it is copyrighted, it can be downloaded for free at www.fsfiquestionnaire.com. Developed specifically for hypoactive sexual desire, the Decreased Sexual Desire Screener (DSDS) was designed for use in general practice by internists, family physicians, and gynecologists without expertise in sexual medicine (*Box 25-2*). In the validation study, the DSDS used by physicians without special expertise had a sensitivity of 0.84, specificity of 0.88, and overall diagnostic accuracy of 85.2% in the study sample, which had a 54% prevalence of HSD.[5]

BOX 25-2 DECREASED SEXUAL DESIRE SCREENER (DSDS)

The patient qualifies for the diagnosis of generalized, acquired hypoactive sexual desire disorder (HSDD) if she answers "YES" to all of questions 1 to 4, and your review confirms "NO" to all of the factors in question 5. The patient MAY qualify for the diagnosis of generalized, acquired HSDD if she answers "YES" to all of questions 1 to 4 and "YES" to any of the factors in question 5; clinical judgment is required to determine if the answers to question 5 indicate a primary diagnosis other than generalized, acquired HSDD. Comorbid conditions such as arousal or orgasmic disorder do not rule out a concurrent diagnosis of HSDD. The patient does NOT qualify for the diagnosis of generalized, acquired HSDD if she answers "NO" to any of the questions 1 to 4.[7]

1. In the past, was your level of sexual desire or interest good and satisfying to you?   YES   NO

2. Has there been a decrease in your level of sexual desire or interest?   YES   NO

3. Are you bothered by your decreased level of sexual desire or interest?   YES   NO

4. Would you like your level of sexual desire or interest to increase?   YES   NO

5. Please circle all the factors that you feel may be contributing to your current decrease in sexual desire or interest:

   A. An operation, depression, injuries, or other medical condition

   B. Medications, drugs, or alcohol you are currently taking

   C. Pregnancy, recent childbirth, menopausal symptoms

   D. Other sexual issues you may be having (pain, decreased arousal or orgasm)

   E. Your partner's sexual problems

   F. Dissatisfaction with your relationship or partner

   G. Stress or fatigue

Men can suffer with hypoactive sexual desire and should undergo a workup for low testosterone, but studies conflict about the threshold level of testosterone that would be considered causative if other symptoms of hypogonadism are absent. If the level is below 12 nmol/L in a man with low libido, it is reasonable to replace testosterone. If the symptoms also include ED, the treatment effect is likely to be greater. Ruling out pituitary tumor with prolactin (PL) level and assessing for adrenal insufficiency with serum cortisol if accompanied by other symptoms are important. It is also key to address sexual trauma, religious constraints, and interpersonal conflict in a man with hypoactive desire, particularly when erectile function is unaffected.

BIOPSYCHOSOCIAL TREATMENT

The first step to address problems with desire and arousal is to create a safe space to discuss it. Even a brief conversation can validate the suffering it causes—if any—and assess the patient's readiness to take steps to manage it. If the reduced desire is recent and in the context of interpersonal conflict, addressing the problems in the relationship is the first step to restore a healthy sexual relationship. Often by having the patients address conflict either on their own, with clergy, or with a couples counselor can remove barriers to sexual intimacy. It is often an enormous relief for the patient to have a nonjudgmental audience to discuss their evolving perceptions of sex. Those barriers to intimacy can be numerous, including problems with body image, past sexual trauma, a partner's criticism, or religious prohibitions. Behavioral activation where the patient names sexual activity that they are interested in engaging in, such as erotic touch, massages, grooming by her partner without the expectation of progressing to intercourse, can be a great next step. Referral to a therapist who specializes in sensate therapy may be useful to direct this intervention if the patient has difficulty conceptualizing or implementing this change in her relationship.

There are new horizons for pharmacologic treatment of hypoactive sexual desire in both sexes, which may encourage patients to seek treatment, but their use is fraught and not yet mainstream. Flibanserin and transdermal testosterone (off-label) are novel therapies for women with low sexual desire. Reviews show no increase in cancers, but concern for hirsutism and acne limits use. Double-blind studies have also shown that androgens profoundly influence sexual behavior in women, and they have been used to treat women with inadequate sexual desire. The benefit of using androgens in women, however, must be weighed against their virilizing side effects. Oral doses of 2.5 mg daily or 5.0 mg Monday through Friday of methyltestosterone or fluoxymesterone or parenteral doses of 50 to 100 mg of testosterone have been used.

Flibanserin, a centrally acting postsynaptic 5-HT1A (serotonin) receptor agonist and a 5-HT2A antagonist, has won FDA approval in premenopausal women. It works by downregulating suppressive serotonin and potentiating excitatory norepinephrine and dopamine in the networks that regulate sexual desire. Flibanserin appears to improve the number of "sexually satisfying events" on self-rating scales, although the clinical validity of the improvement has been called into question. It appears to be well tolerated without significant side effects with only 4% to 13% discontinuing because of side effects compared with 3% to 10% of placebo. The initial placebo-controlled trial was replicated twice in premenopausal women and showed the same efficacy in postmenopausal women but was not FDA approved for this age group. Because of an alcohol interaction study that showed a significantly increased risk of hypotension with syncope in men who consumed four drinks along with taking flibanserin, a Risk Evaluation and Management Strategy program was put in place for the drug, marketed as Addyi for pharmacists and prescribers. Bupropion has been used off-label to treat low libido in the setting of depression or to combat the libido limiting effects of SSRI treatment; it may work in the same way.

Of course, systemic hormones affect sexual desire both positively and negatively, and estrogen supplementation is a reasonable approach when the patient has other bothersome symptoms of premature ovarian failure, surgical menopause, or natural menopause. Localized treatment with estrogen or vaginal lubricants is helpful for pain and dryness as well as decreased sexual response but will not have a significant effect on desire. Although there are multiple randomized trials that support testosterone use for low desire in women, many trials have been stopped early and the FDA has never approved testosterone by any route for women. Testosterone supplementation is not recommended because of the inability to establish population-based norms for serum levels in women or correlate serum levels with symptoms. The unwanted effects of virilization also limit the routine use of testosterone in women. Consider referral to a specialist in sexual medicine or an endocrinologist, as 2014 Endocrine Society Guidelines on androgen therapy in women supports the short-term use of high physiological doses of testosterone in postmenopausal women with low desire. The guidelines note that endogenous testosterone levels do not predict response to this therapy; however, women should be monitored for signs of androgen excess.[4]

Oral contraceptives (OCs), while may decrease fear of pregnancy and therefore increase sexual interest and frequency, are an overlooked cause of female sexual dysfunction. The estimated prevalence of OC-induced sexual dysfunction ranges from 5% to 20% worldwide. Robust randomized controlled trials comparing various forms of contraceptives and measuring effect on sexual desire are lacking, but reports of sexual side effects are most often low desire. OCs such as drospirenone 3 mg/ethinyl estradiol (EE) 30 mg (Yasmin) and gestodene 75 mg/EE 20 mg (Meliane) should be the preferred choice because FSD symptoms are less likely to occur while patients are on these two OCs. Shortening the hormone-free interval (continuous dosing and 24-day hormone treatment with 4-day placebo vs. 21-day hormone/7-day placebo) also seems to have a beneficial effect on libido.[6]

TABLE 25-2 Prevalence of ED with Age

AGE (years)	MEDIAN PREVALENCE	RANGE
40-49	6%	1%-29%
50-59	16%	3%-50%
60-69	32%	7%-74%
70-79	44%	26%-76%

ERECTILE DYSFUNCTION

CLINICAL SIGNIFICANCE

Erectile dysfunction (ED) is a symptom and not a disease in and of itself. It is defined as the consistent or recurrent inability of a man to attain or maintain an erection sufficient for sexual intercourse. The duration of the problem should be at least 3 months, and there is a range of pathophysiology that can lead to ED. In a review of quality epidemiologic studies, the prevalence of ED reliably increased with age (*Table 25-2*).

In those studies that reported the severity of the ED, most men had either mild or moderate ED, while only a few of them had severe or complete ED. In one study, two-thirds of men (67.3%) with ED were bothered by it, which translated into only 10.4% of men receiving treatment. These studies suggest that treatment-seeking behavior is associated with greater severity of the ED and is affected by a man's relationship status, his attitudes and beliefs about the therapies available, and the people who he had discussed his ED with before seeking consultation.

Of course, heart and cerebrovascular disease and its risk factors are associated with ED because of their common vasculopathic pathway. While studies differ on obesity's effect on erectile function, the rise in obesity correlates with increased rates of ED over time. Both hypertension and its treatments are risk factors, and ED occurs 10 to 15 years earlier in diabetic men than in nondiabetic men. Lifestyle factors such as obesity, smoking, and activity level all affect erectile function and improve symptoms when reversed.

When taking a history, be sure to ask about onset and associations. ED with a sudden onset, intermittent course, or short duration also suggests psychogenic factors. Conversely, ED with a gradual onset, progressive course, or long duration suggests a predominantly organic cause.[7] Major life disruptions (new job, pregnancy, financial stress) can present with sexual fears and performance anxiety, so special attention to psychosocial factors is paramount to an adequate workup. Physical examination should include a survey for secondary sex characteristics, pulses, and sensations scars from previous surgery or trauma and a genital examination looking for fibrosis, hypospadias, and testicular size and consistency.[8]

TABLE 25-3 Drugs Commonly Associated with Erectile Dysfunction

DRUGS OF ABUSE	CARDIOVASCULAR	PSYCHIATRIC	OTHER
Cannabis	Thiazides	Serotonin reuptake inhibitors	Ketoconazole
Cocaine	Beta-blockers	Tricyclic antidepressants	H2 blockers
Opiates	Calcium channel blockers	Phenothiazines	Anti-gonadotropins
Nicotine	Spironolactone	Atypical antipsychotics	Statins (controversial)
Alcohol	Digoxin/amiodarone		Cyclophosphamide

DIAGNOSIS

As with other sexual disorders, the first place to look in a man's history to find the cause of ED is the medication list (*Table 25-3*). Any medication can influence a man's erections, but the most common agents are those that treat hypertension, although it can be difficult to discern whether it is the medication or the disease itself. In early studies from the 1970s and 1980s, the incidence of ED was 7% in normotensive men, 17% to 23% in hypertensive men, and 25% to 41% of men with treated hypertension. This is not true of high cholesterol, where statins appear to have no effect, and particularly low HDL correlates with ED symptoms in older men. Know that ED symptoms can appear as late as 6 months into treatment.[9] All patients reporting ED should be screened for drug and alcohol use, as this is a common reversible cause.

Disruption in any system (hepatic, renal, cardiac, pulmonary, and CNS) can lead to ED, so these should be ruled out with a thorough review of systems, focusing specifically on ruling out heart disease and depression. When signs and symptoms of endocrine disease are suspected, a serum testosterone level is obtained, and if the level is low, the PL levels and serum gonadotropin levels (FSH, LH) are evaluated. Marginally high PL is unlikely to be responsible for ED, but in subjects with significantly high levels (735 mU/L or 35 ng/mL), decreased libido was almost universally present (84.2%), whereas only fewer than 1% of patients consulting for sexual dysfunction had significantly high PL. Simply put, elevated PL is rare in patients reporting ED, but ED is common in patients with pituitary dysregulation. All patients with high PL levels should receive an MRI of the brain to rule out pituitary tumor.[5]

BIOPSYCHOSOCIAL TREATMENT

Testosterone supplementation does not benefit men with normal serum testosterone levels. In fact, in impotent men with normal serum levels, testosterone can compound the problem by increasing sexual desire without increasing performance. The Food and Drug Administration (FDA) uses a cutoff value of 300 ng/dL to define hypogonadism for clinical trial development and enrollment. Meanwhile, a consensus statement of multiple professional societies state that levels above 350 ng/dL

do not require treatment, and levels below 230 ng/dL (with symptoms) may require testosterone supplementation. The American Urological Association guidelines recommend that men with levels below 200 ng/dL be treated as hypogonadal, those with levels above 400 ng/dL be considered normal and between 200 and 400 ng/dL be treated if symptomatic.[10]

The mainstay of treatment when psychosocial stressors have been ruled out by the absence of morning erections is phosphodiesterase (PDE) inhibitors. Because ED can be a precursor to cardiovascular disease, risk stratification for heart disease with an adequate review of systems should be performed and further workup for moderate and high-risk patients (i.e., unstable angina) should be performed before reopening the door to sexual activity with a PDE inhibitor. Lifestyle modification and treating underlying heart disease and diabetes can often resolve the issue without intervention. Patients can expect a significant and rapid improvement in erectile function upon smoking cessation if they have smoked over 30 pack-years.[11] Negotiating medications for smoking cessation first before prescribing PDE inhibitors can be an effective contingency for lifestyle modification.

Consider the opposite of ED: priapism in men and persistent clitoral engorgement in women. Priapism can be ischemic (venous outflow obstruction, which is emergent), nonischemic (with intact venous outflow), or stuttering, which is intermittent, but can progress to ischemic if the erection lasts more than 4 hours. This is a common complication for men with sickle cell disease. Painful, rigid erections are likely ischemic and require emergent specialist intervention for detumescence. Nonpainful erections often come from trauma, could be delayed, but will likely detumesce on their own. Most priapism is secondary to intracavernosal injections of vasoactive drugs to treat ED or to hemoglobinopathies. Medications such as anticoagulants and trazodone can also cause it, but it can be idiopathic in 50% of cases. Pelvic solid organ malignancy or lymphoma should always be ruled out as causes of ischemic priapism. Ischemic priapism has to be treated emergently, but all priapism merits specialty attention. There is evidence for continuous dosing of PDE inhibitors for stuttering priapism to regulate penile vasculature, but that is beyond the scope of the primary care physician. There is no analogue of ischemic clitoral engorgement, so all cases can be treated by searching for the cause, which is often medications and stopping the offending agent. Search the medication list for agents that cause alpha-blockade including quetiapine and trazodone.

There is also persistent genital arousal disorder (PGAD) in women, which is more poorly understood. It can be related to spinal or pelvic nerve damage or psychological conflict about sexual activity, but it is defined as persistent arousal lasting for hours, days, or weeks, unrelated to sexual desire, not relieved by orgasm, and causing distress. It can be related to bladder dysfunction and restless legs and can be caused by medications such as trazodone. Because interventions can involve epidural nerve blocks or nerve stimulators, it should be evaluated by a specialist, as all treatments should be combined with psychosocial interventions.[12]

OTHER DISORDER OF SEXUAL DYSFUNCTION

EJACULATORY DISORDERS

Premature ejaculation (PE) can be classified as either lifelong or acquired and general or situational. It is controversial over whether the diagnostic criteria should focus on timing (before, during, or immediately after penetration) or on the man's inability to control it. Depending on the population and definition, PE has been diagnosed in 15% to 46% of presenting complaints in a sexual medicine clinic and in 29% of a healthy population sample. Acquired PE is often comorbid with ED, especially in older men.[13]

PE treatment for years has involved cognitive behavioral therapy (CBT) or other sexual therapies to improve the man's tolerance for sexual touch and prolong sexual activity before ejaculation, shifting the goals of sex away from penetration and orgasm toward mutual and coordinated pleasure. Improved communication about stimulation and how to control it are key to treating both acquired and lifelong PE. Now, there are effective pharmacologic augmentation strategies, and an FDA-approved drug, dapoxetine. SSRIs are often used off-label and on-demand, although PE can return when medication is stopped. Alpha-blockers can be effective and are used when men are dealing with urinary symptoms of BPH but can cause dizziness so can't be recommended. Local anesthetics such as topical lidocaine applied to the glans before sex have also been shown to be effective. PDE inhibitors can used when comorbid with ED. New modalities such as oxytocin receptor blockers and botulinum toxin injections are on the horizon but not yet proven safe in all populations.[14]

Delayed ejaculation (DE) is less prevalent of the two ejaculatory disorders, estimated at 1% to 4%. It involves a persistent delay or absence orgasm after normal arousal and excitement. It is difficult, but clinicians are asked to evaluate if the stimulation has been adequate for the age of the patient. The pathophysiology of DE is related to disruptions in ejaculatory apparatus, nerve damage, hormonal or neurochemical ejaculatory dysregulation, or psychosocial factors.

As with other sexual disorders, the evaluation of DE requires a focused history, which includes a detailed sexual history, and physical examination of the genitalia and open discussion of dynamics with his partner. Special focus should be spent on the context (partnered or self-stimulation), onset, and any related emotional conflicts. Laboratory tests for recent-onset DE should look for abnormal blood count, glucose level, hormone levels, or kidney function. If a correctable etiology is discovered, treatment is directed toward the reversal of this condition. In some cases, the DE may be a lifelong problem. Moreover, in some cases, the etiology of the DE may be irreversible, such as in the case of age-related sensation loss or diabetes-related neuropathy. In these instances, treatment may require a combination of behavioral modification, sexual therapy, or perhaps pharmaceutical drugs. Participation of the partner in therapy may sometimes be necessary.

Different psychosexual therapy strategies have been described for DE but with limited data to describe efficacy. There is no medication for DE approved by the U.S. FDA. The quality of evidence supporting the off-label use of medications for DE is low. However, there are numerous medications reported in the literature suggested to treat the condition. Cabergoline and bupropion are the two most commonly used. In addition, penile vibratory stimulation has been described as an adjunct treatment option for DE.[15]

GENITO-PELVIC PAIN/PENETRATION DISORDER: DYSPAREUNIA, VULVODYNIA, VESTIBULODYNIA, AND VAGINISMUS

Genito-pelvic pain/penetration disorder (GPPPD) is a cluster of different diagnoses involving distress and discomfort surrounding vaginal penetrative sex. Vulvodynia and vestibulodynia are cutting, searing, or burning pain with or without applied pressure to the area (unprovoked vs. provoked). Dyspareunia describes pain with vaginal penetration, and vaginismus is the painful contraction of vaginal muscles to prevent penetration. It can be lifelong or acquired after trauma, illness, or surgery. The differential diagnosis includes endometriosis, pelvic adhesions, ovarian or adnexal masses, hernias, and bowel or rectal disease. Although a pelvic examination is often difficult or intolerable, a nonpenetrating genital examination must be performed to rule out vulvar dermatoses and vaginal infections.

Good estimates find 16% of women have vulvodynia and 12% have provoked vestibulodynia. You should expect to find one in three women have primary or lifelong vestibulodynia and two in three women, acquired. It was previously believed that lifelong symptoms involved more organic factors and a poorer prognosis, but that appears on further study to be incorrect.[16]

Systematic desensitization techniques taught and practiced in the setting of sex therapy, or pelvic floor physical therapy is helpful both alone or in conjunction with other modalities such as relaxation training. Systematic desensitization has also been used successfully to treat PE in men but is helpful for women with inhibited orgasm, inhibited excitement, hypoactive sexual desire, comorbid with sexual aversions such as dyspareunia. Experimentally validated psychotherapeutic treatments include sensate focus, CBT, and guided imagery/hypnosis. Group therapy can be especially helpful when comorbid with paraphilias, compulsions, gender identity, and attraction dysphorias to normalize the social stigmas surrounding these disorders. Total remission may not be expected, but improvement in symptoms is a realistic goal.

When dyspareunia is related to surgical and medical menopause, ospemifene (Osphena) is a selective estrogen receptor modulator that has been shown to improve the vaginal maturation index, vaginal pH, and symptoms of vaginal dryness. The U.S. FDA has approved it for treatment of moderate to severe dyspareunia. The route of administration of estrogen can impact sexual function. Oral estrogens increase sex hormone–binding globulin, which reduces available free testosterone and may thereby adversely affect sexual function, whereas transdermal estrogens have no such effect. Topical estrogen applied vaginally has the lowest rate of side effects and highest rate of remission of systems, but women may find it difficult to administer.[17] There is a new agent that is FDA approved for dyspareunia related to menopause. It is prasterone (Intrarosa), an intravaginal application of dehydroepiandrosterone (DHEA). It is more extensively studied than the widely available over-the-counter DHEA supplements. It has been proven safe and effective for regular use when vulvovaginal atrophy due to ovarian failure is the cause of painful sex. The most common side effect is increased vaginal discharge.[18]

CASES AND QUESTIONS

CASE 1:

A 45-year-old G2P2 woman with hypothyroidism comes to have her levels checked because she's noticed a general sense of fatigue, low appetite, and excessive sleep. Her weight is stable, and her periods are regular but becoming heavy. Her social history is notable for being nonsmoking and drinking rarely but notes stress both at work and at home. She admits that her lack of interest in sex is causing difficulty in her marriage and she wonders if her hypothyroidism is to blame.

1. In addition to checking a thyroid stimulating hormone, what is your next step?
   A. Prescribe paroxetine 20 mg because she meets criteria for depression.
   B. Check her serum testosterone, FSH, and LH to assess for gonadal failure.

C. Refer for marital counseling.
D. Order MRI of the head and serum PL.
E. After reviewing risks and benefits, you put her on flibanserin for FSIAD.

Correct answer: B. *Medical causes should be ruled out before diagnosing either depression or a sexual disorder. While marital problems could be fueling her lack of sexual desire, she sees the causal relationship differently and may be struggled to engage in marital therapy. An MRI and PL level should be performed to work up a pituitary disorder if there are signs and symptoms such as headache, galactorrhea, visual disturbances, or amenorrhea.*

2. On follow-up where you review her laboratory results, she tells you that her mood has been poor for the last year with crying, low energy, excessive sleep and appetite, and poor concentration leading to conflict at work. You diagnose depression. Which antidepressant is least likely to cause sexual dysfunction??
   A. Paroxetine
   B. Duloxetine
   C. Bupropion
   D. Vortioxetine

   Correct answer: C. *Of the SSRIs, paroxetine is most likely to cause sexual side effects owing to nitric oxide synthase inhibition. All serotonergic drugs can cause sexual side effects, but bupropion can actually be prescribed to address sexual dysfunction with antidepressants.*

3. After her depression improves, she reports that she still has a low libido but has a physical response when her partner engages with sex and is able to orgasm sometimes with her partner, although not consistently. What is your next step?
   A. Prescribe flibanserin for female sexual interest/arousal disorder (FSIAD).
   B. Refer to a psychiatrist specializing in sexual disorders.
   C. Refer to a marital therapist.
   D. Briefly discuss conflicts in the relationships and share simple techniques to improve communication during sex.
   E. Reassure the patient and schedule follow-up for depression.

   Correct answer: D. *Most patients respond well to brief interventions in the primary care environment and prefer that to seeking specialty care, but if the problem persists or intensifies to an inability to become aroused, she may qualify for further treatment for FSIAD.*

CASE 2: ED Associated with Metabolic Syndrome Versus Performance Anxiety

A 39-year-old man presents in clinic due to difficulty getting erections, which has become more common over the last year, starting occasionally, now becoming more the norm. He can sometimes get an erection, but he has difficulty sustaining it. He notes that he has gained about 15 lbs in the 6 months, which he relates to getting a promotion at work that has him working at a desk now, whereas his former job was more active. His review of systems is relevant for increased dyspnea on exertion, and he becomes winded when playing football with his nephew. He inquires if medication such as sildenafil is right for him. One examination:

Weight 240 lbs, Height 70 inches
BP 145/89, P 94

Physical examination is significant for normal heart sounds, regular rate and rhythm, clear lungs, obese abdomen with striae, but normal genitalia.

1. What is your next step?

   A. Prescribe 50 mg sildenafil prn #10 tablets.
   B. Check am cortisol.
   C. Check testosterone and A1c before considering PDE inhibitor.
   D. Check ECG before considering PDE inhibitor.

   Correct answer: C. *A medical workup should be performed to rule out secondary causes of ED. Treatment of diabetes and hypertension can improve ED, which is much more common than Addison disease, and rapid weight gain is a much more common cause of striae than Cushing disease.*

2. His blood pressure does not improve with 10 lbs weight loss and following dietary approaches to stop hypertension diet. Which blood pressure medicine is least likely to cause ED?

   A. Hydrochlorothiazide
   B. Metoprolol
   C. Prazosin
   D. Amlodipine
   E. Lisinopril

   Correct answer: E. *Angiotensin converting enzyme inhibitors and angiotensin receptor blockers should be the first line in treating hypertension in the setting of ED.*

3. Even after he reaches his weight loss goals and his BP is controlled, he still notes difficulty sustaining erections. Which of the following causes of ED is epidemiologically most common and yet to be ruled out?

   A. Childhood sexual trauma
   B. Fetish
   C. Depression
   D. Excessive alcohol intake
   E. Specific phobia

Correct answer: D. *Alcohol and substance use disorders account for the remainder of secondary causes of ED after metabolic, vascular, endocrine, and neurologic disorders have been ruled out.*

CASE 3: Vaginismus versus Vestibulodynia

A 22-year-old woman presents for a consultation regarding contraception. She denies being sexually active but heard from a friend that oral contraceptive pills can control her heavy, symptomatic periods. She has painful cramps that is helped only somewhat by non-steroidal anti-inflammatory drugs and heating pad applications. She was 13 years at the age of menarche and has regular periods that last 7 to 8 days and soaks 5 to 6 pads on heavy days. On review of systems she admits to chronic constipation. She denies dysuria or vaginal discharge, but she says she never feels "clean down there." Her medical history is significant for a laparoscopic appendectomy in her teens. She had sex with one partner in high school but denies any sexual activity in the last year. On physical examination, her hymen is not intact, but she is unable to tolerate the introduction of a speculum due to pain and emotional distress. You suspect vaginismus. What are key items to the history that you need to know before taking the next step?

NONE

   A. Does she have sex with men, women, or both?
   B. Does she have anal, vaginal, or oral sex or a combination?
   C. Has she ever felt coerced or forced into sex without her consent?
   D. Has she ever had a sexually transmitted infection?
   E. All of the above

   Correct answer: E. *A full sexual history and screening for sexual trauma and past infections are important to assess for causes of vaginismus and therefore direct treatment.*

PRACTICAL RESOURCES

- Sexual Medicine Specialists referral network: International Society for the Study of Women's Sexual Health: www.isswsh.org
- Counselors and Therapists for sex therapy referral resources: American Association of Sexuality Educators: www.aasect.org

REFERENCES

1. Faubion SS, Rullo JE. Sexual dysfunction in women: a practical approach. *Am Fam Physician.* 2015;92(4):281-288.

2. West SL, D'Aloisio AA, Agans RP, et al. Prevalence of low sexual desire and hypoactive sexual desire disorder in a nationally representative sample of US women. *Arch Intern Med.* 2008;168:1441.

3. Holstege G. How the emotional motor system controls the pelvic organs. *Sex Med Rev.* 2016;4:303-328.

4. Parish SJ, Hahn SR. Hypoactive sexual desire disorder: a review of epidemiology, biopsychology, diagnosis, and treatment. *Sex Med Rev.* 2016;4:103-120.

5. Corona GC, Isidori AM, Aversa A, et al. Endocrinologic control of Men's sexual desire and arousal/erection. *J Sex Med.* 2016;13:317-337.

6. Lee JJML, Low LL, Ang SB. Oral contraception and female sexual dysfunction in reproductive women. *Sex Med Rev.* 2017;5:31-44.

7. Montorsi F, Adaikan G, Becher E, et al. Summary of the recommendations on sexual dysfunctions in men. *J Sex Med.* 2010;7:3572-3588.

8. Shamloul R, Ghanem H. Erectile dysfunction. *Lancet.* 2013;381(9861):153-165.

9. Crenshaw TL, Goldberg JP. *Sexual Pharmacology: Drugs that Affect Sexual Function.* New York: W.W. Norton & Company, Inc.; 1996.

10. Paduch DA, Brannigan RE, Fuchs EF, et al. *Laboratory Diagnosis of Testosterone Deficiency.* American Urological Association; 2013.

11. Mannino DM, Klevens RM, Flanders WD. Cigarette smoking: an independent risk factor for impotence? *Am J Epidemiol.* 1994;140:1003-1008.

12. Yafi FA, April D, Powers MK, et al. Penile priapism, clitoral priapism, and persistent genital arousal disorder: a contemporary review. *Sex Med Rev.* 2015;3(3):145-159.

13. Maurice WL. *Sexual Medicine in Primary Care.* Mosby, Inc.; 1999:192-195.

14. McMahon CG. Current and emerging treatments for premature ejaculation. *Sex Med Rev.* 2015;3:183-202.

15. Sadowski D, Butcher MJ, Köhler TS. A review of pathophysiology and Management options for delayed ejaculation. *Sex Med Rev.* 2016;4:167-176.

16. Pukall CF. Primary and secondary provoked vestibulodynia: a review of overlapping and distinct factors. *Sex Med Rev.* 2016;4:36-44.

17. Buster JE. Managing female sexual dysfunction. *Fertil Steril.* 2013;100(4):905-915.

18. Prasterone (Intrarosa) for dyspareunia. *Med Lett Drugs Ther.* 2017;59(1529):149-150.

26

EATING DISORDERS

Jessica A. Beauchene, MD, Shawn Hersevoort, MD, MPH, and
Jennifer A. Hersevoort, MD

- Eating disorders are highly prevalent and often characterized by severe disturbances in eating behavior and distress or excessive concern about body shape or weight.
- They require close attention as they often occur with severe medical or psychiatric comorbidities.
- Although the symptoms of eating disorders revolve around eating, they are more about coping with feelings than they are about food.
- Denial of symptoms and reluctance to seek help make treatment especially challenging.
- When assessing and treating a patient with an eating disorder, it is essential to form a strong therapeutic alliance.
- Patients with eating disorders are best cared for by an interdisciplinary team consisting of a mental health clinician, dietitian, and general medical clinician.
- Refeeding is the cornerstone of treatment of anorexia nervosa as there are no medications that are consistently effective.
- Any psychotherapy needs to include elements of psychoeducation, nutritional management, cognitive and behavioral strategies, and motivational enhancement.
- Recovery often takes years of hard work, with many patients dropping out too soon and relapsing.

INTRODUCTION

Eating disorders (EDOs) are highly prevalent and severe disturbances in eating behavior including excessive concern about body weight or shape. They require close attention as they often occur with severe medical or psychiatric comorbidities. Frequent denial of symptoms and reluctance to seek treatment make both diagnosis and treatment especially challenging. They are most often found in adolescents and young women, with anorexia nervosa having the highest lethality among all psychiatric disorders.[1] Assessment can be difficult as patients tend to conceal their symptoms because of denial, shame, and guilt. It is therefore essential to form a strong and rapid alliance with patients. These disorders include anorexia nervosa, bulimia nervosa, binge-eating disorder (BED), avoidant/restrictive food intake disorder (ARFID), pica, and rumination disorder. We will primarily focus on the first three disorders.

CLINICAL SIGNIFICANCE

EDOs are both common and chronic, with prevalence nearly 3% in adolescents and young adults.[2] They are far more common in females than in males, although they can occur in any age, sex, race, or ethnicity. Clinical populations reflect a 10:1 female to male ratio for anorexia and bulimia nervosa, but much more balanced in BED.[3] The 12-month prevalence of anorexia nervosa among young females is 0.4% and that of bulimia nervosa is 1% to 1.5%. Onset peaks in older adolescence and young adulthood, although rare cases can be seen as young as 5 years old. The 12-month prevalence of BED is 1.6% and 0.8%, respectively, among adult females and males in the United States.[3] Lifetime prevalence is around 3%. The average age of onset for BED is comparatively older, during the mid-20s. It is difficult to determine the prevalence of EDOs in the general population compared with primary care for a variety of reasons. These include a lack of systematic research, stigma, confidentiality, and lack of proper screening and diagnosis. Studies have shown that less than half are identified in a primary care setting. An even smaller number may present to mental health services.[1] Although these patients disproportionately exhibit symptoms related to psychological, general medical, gastroenterological, and gynecological complaints, it is often difficult to trace these back to an EDO without patient assistance. Many primary care providers lack the training or experience in recognizing and providing treatment and are only alerted to the problem once significant health issues have arisen.[4] For this reason it is important to have a policy of screening at-risk populations and patients with commonly associated symptoms (*Box 26-1, Table 26-1*).

BOX 26-1   SCOFF: VALIDATED SCREENING QUESTIONS FOR EATING DISORDERS IN PRIMARY CARE SETTINGS

- Do you make yourself **s**ick because you feel uncomfortably full?
- Do you worry that you have lost **c**ontrol over how much you eat?
- Have you recently lost more than **o**ne stone (14 pounds or 6.3 kg) in a 3-month period?
- Do you believe yourself to be **f**at when others say you are too thin?
- Would you say that **f**ood dominates your life?

Two positive answers are highly predictive of either anorexia nervosa or bulimia nervosa

---

From Morgan JF, Reid F, Lacey H. The SCOFF questionnaire: assessment of a new screening tool for eating disorders. *BMJ.* 1999;319:1467-1468.

Despite a lack of systematic study on the economic burden of EDOs in the United States, they are clearly expensive. These disorders are frequent, long-lasting, and often severe. The patients experience a tremendous decrease in quality of life. EDO patients have been found to have greater annual health care costs (by $1,869), lower employment rates (0.67 odds ratio), and lower yearly earnings when employed ($2,093).[5] Many must be seen on a weekly basis by a team of specialists, including a primary care provider, a psychiatrist, and a nutritionist.[6] Patients in residential treatment often require at least 3 months of treatment, at a distant facility costing around $30,000 monthly. After leaving a specialized program, patients may need years of follow-up care. As a general guideline, a third of patients recover fully, a third partially, and a third are chronically ill. Among patients with anorexia nervosa, approximately 50% have good outcomes, 25% intermediate, and 25% poor.[7] Patients with anorexia nervosa have a mortality rate of up to 20%, primarily from cardiac arrest or suicide. Little long-term follow-up data exist for bulimia nervosa. Short-term success is from 50% to 70%, with relapse rates between 30% and 50% after 6 months. These patients have an overall better prognosis as compared with those with anorexia nervosa, although they still see a two- to eight-time increase in all-cause mortality compared with the general population.[8] There are less data regarding the prognosis of BED; however, in one follow-up study at 5 years, 10% of patients maintained the diagnosis, 18% to 20% demonstrated partial remission, and 70% were in full remission.[14]

EDOs are associated with numerous comorbidities. These include substance-related, anxiety, obsessive–compulsive, mood, and personality disorders, as well as obesity, diabetes mellitus, thyroid, and malabsorptive disorders. Unipolar depression and bipolar disorder predispose patients to EDOs and are frequently co-occurring disorders. Major depression ranges from 50% to 75% in this population, most frequently in bulimia nervosa. Abuse of illegal substances and chemical dependence are also common. Up to 37% of diagnosed patients with anorexia or bulimia nervosa admit to abusing, or having a dependence on, alcohol or illegal substances.[9] Anxiety is ever-present in these patients, making it very difficult to decide if it is a component of the disorder or a frequent comorbid condition. EDO patients, especially those with anorexia nervosa, demonstrate frequent obsessive–compulsive symptoms or personality traits. Many are rigid, strict, organized, responsible, intransigent, and intolerant. Approximately 30% of EDO cases present with personality disorders, especially borderline and histrionic.[10] Sexual assault, highest in this demographic, is another risk factor. Complex trauma may or may not lead to a posttraumatic diagnosis in children, but it will predispose patients to a host of other psychiatric disorders. Adverse childhood experiences such as abuse and other social stressors associated with poverty lead to similar increases through risk-taking behaviors and poor health behaviors from social modeling. Another at-risk minority group is the LGBTQ (lesbian, gay, bisexual, transgender, queer) community.

Both types of diabetes mellitus are risk factors for EDOs, with bulimia nervosa seen three times as often in type 1, compared with type 2. This dangerous combination is sometimes referred to as *diabulimia*, where some patients intentionally limit their use of insulin to minimize weight gain. As with other forms of bulimia nervosa, this is particularly a problem in adolescent girls. Patients with this illness combination are at particularly elevated risk of developing retinopathy and other complications, including death. Obesity is a risk factor for developing anorexia nervosa or bulimia nervosa and is a frequent long-term consequence of BED. Up to 30% of patients seeking weight loss treatment, and 78% of obese veterans, demonstrate binge eating.[11] Malabsorption syndromes and gluten and lactose-intolerance are risk factors for anorexia nervosa. Thyroid diseases, both hyper- and hypothyroidism, are relevant in the onset, course, prognosis, and treatment of EDOs.

Pregnancy can present as an opportunity for recovery, or as a period of vulnerability for onset, persistence, or relapse of EDO symptoms. EDO patients are more likely to be depressed during pregnancy and postpartum. Medically, several risks are present in anorexia nervosa, including inadequate or excessive gestational weight gain, increased risk for antepartum hemorrhage, and lower birth weight. Bulimia nervosa is associated with increased risk for excessive weight gain and increased miscarriage. BED is the most likely to persist during pregnancy or recur in the first 3 years postpartum.[12] For all these reasons, a sober discussion of the risks of becoming pregnant is required for all women with a history of an EDO.

TABLE 26-1 Symptoms, Signs, Laboratory and ECG Findings, and Medical Complications in Eating Disorders

	ANOREXIA NERVOSA	BULIMIA NERVOSA	BINGE-EATING DISORDER
Symptoms	Generalized weakness and lassitude Difficulty concentrating Palpitations Abdominal pain and bloating Cold sensitivity Amenorrhea or menstrual irregularities Loss of libido Anxiety Depression	Abdominal bloating Constipation Sore throat Dyspepsia Menstrual irregularities Anxiety Depression	Anxiety Depression Dyspepsia and bloating

Clinical signs	Low BMI and body weight
	Orthostatic hypotension
	Skin cool to touch
	Lanugo
	Constipation
	Jaundice-like skin color
	Secondary amenorrhea
	Arrested development of secondary
	  sex characteristics
		Bloating/abdominal pain
		Orthostatic hypotension
		Loss of gag reflex
		Diarrhea or constipation
		Loss of tooth enamel and discoloration
		  of teeth
		Gum disease and dental caries
		Tender or swollen parotid and
		  submandibular glands
		Knuckle calluses
		Edema
		Acne
			High BMI and
			  consequences

ECG	Low voltage
	Bradycardia
	Prolonged QT interval
	Prolonged PR interval
	ST-T–wave abnormalities
		Low voltage
		Bradycardia
		Sinus tachycardia
		Prolonged QT interval
		U waves
			ST-T–waves changes
			  suggestive of
			  atherosclerotic changes

Laboratory	Dehydration Hypoglycemia Hyponatremia Hypophosphatemia Sick euthyroid syndrome	Dehydration Hypochloremia Hypokalemia Metabolic alkalosis Elevated serum amylase	Hypercholesterolemia Transaminitis Dyslipidemia
Medical complications	Gastroparesis Decreased cardiac mass Reduced cardiac chamber volumes Mitral valve prolapse Pericardial effusion Superior mesenteric artery syndrome Osteoporosis and fractures Infections Increased neonatal complications	GERD Esophageal rupture Postbinge pancreatitis Aspiration pneumonitis Pneumothorax or rib fracture Diabetes mellitus	Coronary heart disease Cholecystitis, cholelithiasis Gastric dilation/rupture Degenerative joint disease Diabetes mellitus Obstructive sleep apnea Nonalcoholic steatohepatitis

Adapted from Leung M, Harris T, Pomeroy C. Eating disorders. In: McCarron R, Xiong G, Bourgeois J, eds. Lippincott's Primary Care Psychiatry. Philadelphia: Lippincott Williams & Wilkins; 2009:147-163.

BMI, body mass index (kg/m²); ECG, electrocardiogram; GERD, gastroesophageal reflux disease.

DIAGNOSIS

DIAGNOSTIC CONSIDERATIONS

The EDOs include anorexia nervosa, bulimia nervosa, BED, ARFID, other specified feeding and eating disorder, and unspecified feeding and eating disorder. Pica, the eating of nonfood items, and rumination disorder, recurrent regurgitation of food, will not be discussed. In the transition from the *Diagnostic and Statistical Manual*-IV-TR (*DSM*-IV-TR) to the newest version, *DSM*-5, several changes were made. BED and ARFID were added as new diagnoses. ARFID is characterized as a failure to meet nutritional needs for reasons other than weight control, often associated with developmental disability or anxiety in children. In adults, the term *orthorexia* is sometimes used to describe weight loss due to a restricted diet believed by the patient to be healthy or necessary for personal reasons. Vegans are particularly vulnerable to this condition, although patients with delusions or paranoia over food are also at risk. The *other specified feeding or eating disorder* category was also introduced to describe clinically significant disorders that did not meet full criteria for other named disorders. These include *atypical anorexia* (limited weight loss), *bulimia nervosa of low frequency or limited duration, BED of low frequency or limited duration, purging disorder* (without binging), and *night eating syndrome.*[3] The *unspecified* category is used when information is limited, conflicting, or difficult to confirm. While determining diagnosis, it is helpful to both calculate a healthy target weight and correctly describe the unhealthy extremes (*Figure 26-1*). Terms such as *skinny, fat,* or *fluffy* are neither accurate nor useful.

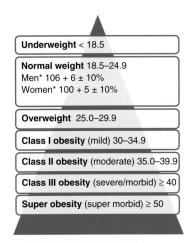

BMI, body mass index (kg/m²)

* Ideal body weight calculation for men and women

Men: 106 pounds (per 5 feet) + 6 pounds/inch (per inch over 5 feet) ± 10%

Women: 100 pounds (per 5 feet) + 5 pounds/inch (per inch over 5 feet) ± 10%

FIGURE 26-1 Classification of body weight based on BMI.

The three primary EDOs, anorexia nervosa, bulimia nervosa, and BED, each demonstrate different abnormalities in body weight, eating behavior, and distortions of thought and emotion. The particular combination determines which disorder is present (*Figure 26-2*). The SCOFF rating scale is an easy method for screening. The five questions screen for weight loss, attitude about food, sense of control over food, and self-evaluation of body image (*Box 26-1*). Positive answers to two of the questions are reported to yield 100% sensitivity and 87% specificity for detecting anorexia nervosa or bulimia nervosa.[13] Target groups for screening should include patients who are overweight, those with weight concerns without being overweight, and young people with low body mass index (BMI) compared with age-based reference values. Other adults who should be screened include women with menstrual disorders or amenorrhea, patients with gastrointestinal symptoms, or those with signs of repeated vomiting or starvation, such as Russell sign. Children with delayed or stunted growth should be screened, as well as children, adolescents, and young adults who perform sports that entail a high risk of developing an EDO. These include gymnastics, dance, swimming, wrestling, bodybuilding, and other highly competitive activities.[14]

Anorexia Nervosa

The core features of anorexia nervosa are low body weight due to reduced intake, intense fear of, or behaviors aimed at, preventing weight gain, and distorted perception of body weight and shape (*Figure 26-2*). Preoccupation with food and rituals related to meals are usually present. Other features include perfectionism, cognitive and behavioral rigidity, feelings of ineffectiveness, inhibited expression of emotion, social withdrawal, and restlessness or hyperactivity. Poor insight and resistance to treatment are also very common.[14] Symptoms are often egosyntonic (*in self-harmony*) and are therefore

Abnormal Eating Behaviors			Body Weight	Binge Eating	Compensation	Cognition	Frequency	Severity Marker
Body weight low*	Yes →	Anorexia nervosa	Low*	Maybe	Yes	"I am fat"	No requirement	BMI
↓ No								
Binge and compensate*	Yes →	Bulimia nervosa	Normal or high	Yes*	Yes*	"I am ugly"	Weekly binge/compensate for ≥3 months	Number of compensations
↓ No								
Binge only*	Yes →	Binge-eating disorder	Normal or high	Yes*	No	"I am ashamed"	Weekly binge for ≥3 months	Number of binges

BMI, body mass index
* Defining symptoms of each disorder

FIGURE 26-2 Diagnosing eating disorders.

not seen as problematic to patients. The presenting complaint may be anxiety, depression, or physical discomfort. This may include pain with eating, bloating, constipation, or subjective complaints of inability to "keep food down" (*Table 26-1*). Patients may attempt to hide their bodies by wearing bulky clothing, inflating their weight by hiding objects in their clothes, or drinking large amounts of water. Changes to *DSM*-5 include the elimination of amenorrhea and the weight requirement for a diagnosis, and two new subtypes. *Restricting type* involves restricted intake or excessive exercise to limit or decrease body weight. *Binge-eating/purging type* involves binge eating with compensatory weight control behaviors such as self-induced vomiting, exercising, and misuse of diet pills, diuretics, or laxatives.[3]

Anorexia nervosa is associated with numerous medical complications that are directly attributable to caloric restriction and weight loss. These include constipation, functional hypothalamic amenorrhea, antenatal and postpartum problems, osteoporosis, gastroparesis, bradycardia, mitral valve prolapse, myocardial atrophy, and pericardial effusion (*Table 26-1*).

Bulimia Nervosa

The diagnosis of bulimia nervosa requires both binge-eating and compensatory behaviors. This involves eating large amounts of food, over a short period. During these episodes, patients feel that they can neither control nor stop the eating behaviors. In addition, patients must use inappropriate compensatory behaviors to prevent weight gain, including self-induced vomiting; misuse of laxatives, diuretics, or enemas; and excessive exercise, fasting, or strict diets. Symptoms must be present at least weekly for 3 months or more (*Figure 26-2*). Changes to *DSM*-5 include a reduced requirement for frequency of binging and compensatory behavior from twice a week to once weekly. Additionally, illness subtypes were eliminated.

The most common medical symptoms in bulimia nervosa are lethargy, irregular menses, abdominal pain and bloating, and constipation. Complications include dehydration, hypokalemia, menstrual irregularities, Mallory–Weiss syndrome, dental caries, and erosion of dental enamel (*Table 26-1*).

Binge-Eating Disorder

BED is defined by the same binge-eating episodes seen in bulimia nervosa (*Figure 26-2*). Unlike in the other disorders, these patients do not take part in compensatory weight control measures. This, more often than not, leads to weight gain and frequently obesity. *DSM*-5 was the first version to include BED as a formal diagnosis, with only limited mention in previous versions. On inclusion, it became the most frequently seen disorder in the class.

Patients with BED may present with anxiety, depression, or bloating and are more likely than the general population to have comorbid general medical disorders such as chronic pain, diabetes, and hypertension. They tend to have a higher BMI and are more likely to be obese. They often describe somatic symptoms and dissatisfaction with health; however, there is little evidence of medical complications that can be directly attributed to binge-eating symptoms.

DIFFERENTIAL DIAGNOSIS

There are many medical illnesses that may present similarly to an EDO, but typically not with intentional weight loss or fear of gaining weight (*Table 26-2*). The disorders themselves can be difficult to differentiate. Anorexia nervosa and bulimia nervosa may have many of the same behaviors and symptoms; however, anorexia nervosa presents with abnormally low body weight, with a typical BMI <18.5 kg/m^2. Those with bulimia nervosa usually have normal or increased BMI. The two disorders are closely related and, for many, the diagnosis will change from one to the other over time. BED does not

TABLE 26-2 Differential Diagnosis of Eating Disorders

SYMPTOM	DIFFERENTIAL
Amenorrhea	Pregnancy Polycystic ovarian syndrome Hypothalamic dysfunction Prolactinoma Outflow tract abnormalities Congenital adrenal deficiency
Diarrhea	Laxative abuse Inflammatory bowel disease Malabsorption (e.g., celiac disease) Inflammatory bowel disease Superior mesenteric artery disorder
Intractable nausea and vomiting	Brain tumor Diabetes mellitus Disordered gastrointestinal dysmotility Hyperemesis gravidarum Pancreatitis
Endocrinologic abnormalities	Hyperthyroidism/hypothyroidism Adrenal insufficiency Hypopituitarism Diabetes mellitus
Severe wasting	Malignancy Tuberculosis Human immunodeficiency virus
Psychiatric	Depression Anxiety Body dysmorphic disorder Schizophrenia
Excessive eating	Temporal lobe or limbic seizures Lesions of the hypothalamus or frontal lobe Prader–Willi syndrome Kleine–Levin syndrome

Adapted from Leung M, Harris T, Pomeroy C. Eating disorders. In: McCarron R, Xiong G, Bourgeois J, eds. Lippincott's Primary Care Psychiatry. Philadelphia: Lippincott Williams & Wilkins; 2009:147-163.

have the inappropriate compensatory behaviors that occur in the others. ARFID is defined as failure to meet nutrition needs for reasons other than weight control. These include lack of interest in food, aversion to certain sensory characteristics, or concern about adverse consequences such as choking/vomiting, rather than a fear of gaining weight.

EDOs may also present as depression, anxiety, body dysmorphic disorder, or even schizophrenia. Although changes in appetite and eating behaviors may occur in these disorders, many of the other symptoms are usually absent. These include inappropriate compensatory behaviors, feelings of loss of control while eating, and preoccupation with weight and body shape. Body dysmorphic disorder differs from other disorders in that it is usually a preoccupation with a specific body part, rather than the overall body. Patients with schizophrenia may avoid eating because of delusions regarding food, or fear of being poisoned, rather than a concern over weight. Comorbid anxiety, depression, impulse control, substance use, and personality disorders are common in patients with anorexia nervosa. Patients with bulimia nervosa frequently struggle with unipolar major depression, specific phobia, posttraumatic stress, social anxiety, attention deficit hyperactivity, alcohol use, oppositional defiant, conduct, illicit drug use, and personality disorders. Associated with BED are bipolar, depressive, anxiety, and substance use disorders.[3]

BIOPSYCHOSOCIAL TREATMENT
OVERVIEW OF TREATMENT

Behavioral treatments and psychotherapy (*Table 26-3*) are the major focus of treatment, although medications can be helpful under certain circumstances (*Table 26-4*). Overall treatment goals focus on medical stabilization and normalization of eating behavior and weight through a balanced meal plan. Cessation of binging, purging, and other unhealthy behaviors are sought. Therapeutic exploration of underlying issues is undertaken, and skills related to affect regulation and interpersonal relationships are developed and fostered. Finally, a system of comprehensive social and vocational rehabilitation is developed.[15]

Preparation for treatment includes detailed psychiatric and medical assessments, physical examination, labs, collaborative team building, and determination of appropriate level of care. The primary factors that determine level of care are severity of weight loss, malnutrition, and medical stability. These levels, from least to most intensive, include outpatient, intensive outpatient, partial hospitalization, residential treatment, and inpatient hospitalization. The location should be determined based on medical status and weight, suicidality, motivation, co-occurring disorders, needs for structure, ability to control compulsive eating, purging behaviors, environmental stress, and availability of treatment.[16] Patients who are currently stable should

TABLE 26-3 Psychotherapy for Eating Disorders

AN	**Primary**	Adults: individual CBT, IPT, psychodynamic, or combination Children and adolescents: family therapy
	Secondary	Supportive clinical management, MI, and group (CBT, IPT, supportive, dynamic)
	Special	Family and couples therapy when family or marital problems are present
	Timing	Individual for at least 1 year
BN	**Primary**	CBT
	Secondary	IPT, psychodynamic, behavioral therapy
	Special	Family and couples therapy for adolescents, older patients with ongoing relationship conflict
	Timing	18-20 sessions over 5-6 months
BED	**Primary**	CBT individually, in groups, or in self-help formats
	Secondary	IPT and DBT
	Special	Behavioral weight loss therapy for patients primarily interested in losing weight
	Timing	10-20 sessions over 3-6 months

AN, anorexia nervosa; BED, binge-eating disorder; BN, bulimia nervosa; CBT, cognitive-behavioral therapy; DBT, dialectical behavioral therapy; IPT, interpersonal psychotherapy; MI, motivational interviewing.

be seen for frequent visits to monitor weight and medical stability. At this level of care, the primary care provider has a central role (*Table 26-5*). Patients who are not medically stable should be hospitalized for medical stabilization. Criteria for hospitalization include unstable vital signs, cardiac dysrhythmia (other than normal sinus bradycardia), weight less than 70% of ideal, serious medical complications, moderate to severe refeeding syndrome, or poor response to outpatient treatment (*Table 26-6*).

Anorexia Nervosa

In anorexia nervosa, refeeding is the cornerstone of treatment. This involves nutritional rehabilitation and psychotherapy. Psychotherapy is minimally effective if nutritional status is poor because of *starvation brain*, the reversible gray matter, and overall brain volume reduction associated with low body weight. Nutritional rehabilitation includes prescribing and supervising meals, and preventing binge eating and purging. Hospitalization may be necessary for treatment-resistant patients. Refeeding that is too rapid or aggressive can lead to potentially fatal *refeeding syndrome* as a result of fluid and electrolyte shifts leading to hypophosphatemia and volume overload. There are several approaches to refeeding, some slow and steady, with

TABLE 26-4	Pharmacologic Treatment of Eating Disorders		
	RECOMMENDED	**RECOMMENDED FOR COMORBIDITIES**	**NOT RECOMMENDED**
AN	Olanzapine	SSRI or SNRI (depression/anxiety) Buspirone (persistent anxiety) Hydroxyzine (episodic anxiety) Mirtazapine (mood/anxiety/insomnia) Quetiapine or risperidone (bipolar/psychosis)	Bupropion (seizure/weight loss) Stimulant (seizure/weight loss) BZD (dependence) TCA/MAOI (side effects)
BN	Fluoxetine SSRIs Topiramate	SSRI or SNRI (depression/anxiety) Buspirone (persistent anxiety) Hydroxyzine (episodic anxiety) Lamotrigine or oxcarbazepine (bipolar) Aripiprazole or lurasidone (bipolar/psychosis)	Bupropion or stimulant (seizure) Paroxetine or mirtazapine (weight gain) Quetiapine or olanzapine (weight gain) Lithium or divalproex (side effects) BZD (dependence) TCA (effective but side effects) MAOI (side effects)
BED	Lisdexamfetamine SSRIs Topiramate Bupropion	SSRI or SNRI (depression/anxiety) Buspirone (persistent anxiety) Hydroxyzine (episodic anxiety) Lamotrigine or oxcarbazepine (bipolar) Aripiprazole or lurasidone (bipolar/psychosis) Bupropion/naltrexone (weight loss)	Paroxetine or mirtazapine (weight gain) Quetiapine or olanzapine (weight gain) Lithium or divalproex (side effects) BZD (dependence) TCA (effective but side effects) MAOI (side effects)

AN, anorexia nervosa; , BED, binge-eating disorder; BN, bulimia nervosa; BZD, benzodiazepine; MAOI, monoamine oxidase inhibitor; SGA, second-generation antipsychotic; SNRI, selective norepinephrine and serotonin reuptake inhibitor; SSRI, selective serotonin reuptake inhibitor; TCA, tricyclic antidepressant.

TABLE 26-5	Primary Care Responsibilities in the Treatment of Eating Disorders
Psychosocial assessment	Develop and maintain therapeutic alliance with patient and family Screen for and monitor other comorbid psychiatric conditions including suicidality[a] Recognize and work with anxiety over treatment Elicit ongoing attitudes about body weight and shape, food, and eating Monitor meal patterns and other behaviors (e.g., diet, exercise, binge/purging, and rituals)
Medical evaluation and treatment	Weekly height and *blind* weight to follow body mass index Weekly vital signs: temperature, heart rate,[a] supine and standing blood pressure[a] Ongoing examination: skin, oropharyngeal, abdominal, neurologic Progressive correction of malnutrition and weight restoration (while avoiding refeeding syndrome)
Laboratory values	Comprehensive metabolic panel plus phosphorous and magnesium[a] Complete blood count with differential Iron studies Thyroid-stimulating hormone 25-Hydroxyvitamin D Urinalysis, urine toxicology, and pregnancy Electrocardiogram[a]
Education	Educate patients and relatives about physical health risks Detect and begin correcting maladaptive ideas about weight and health Educate about nutrition to normalize altered dietary behavior
Coordination	Assemble and coordinate the interdisciplinary team: primary care, dietitian, and mental health Monitor ongoing level of care needs Recognize, prevent, and manage recurrences collaboratively Assist team in developing a recurrence prevention plan once treatment goals are successful

[a] *Potentially critical or dangerous.*

less acute risk, and others more rapid and aggressive. Treatment rate must balance the need for reaching treatment goals before patients are tempted to leave treatment, but not so rapid as to create additional dangers.

Bulimia Nervosa

The standard treatment for bulimia nervosa includes nutritional rehabilitation, psychotherapy, and pharmacotherapy. Typically, the treatment is in the outpatient

TABLE 26-6 Indications for Hospitalization in Anorexia Nervosa

Weight	<75% ideal body weight or ongoing weight loss
Vascular	Arrhythmia, bradycardia (<50 bpm), hypotension (SBP <90), hypothermia (<96°F), orthostatic changes, syncope
Chemistry	Dehydration, intractable vomiting, electrolyte abnormalities, malnutrition
Psychiatric	Refusal to eat, suicidal ideation, or psychosis
Other	Cardiac failure, pancreatitis, seizure

bpm, beats per minute; SBP, systolic blood pressure.

or partial hospitalization setting, but hospitalization may be necessary for suicidal ideation or uncontrolled purging. Nutritional counseling is used to control binge eating and inappropriate compensatory behavior. Patients with bulimia are typically not as secretive about their behaviors while in treatment; however, psychotherapy is frequently stormy and may be prolonged. In the case of laxative misuse, patients must be advised on how to decrease gradually. Patients who vomit habitually should have regular dental check-ups and be provided with education on dental hygiene.

Binge-Eating Disorder

For patients with BED, psychotherapy is usually the most effective treatment, although there may be a role for behavioral weight loss therapy or pharmacotherapy.

PSYCHOPHARMACOLOGY (*TABLE 26-4*)

Recommended pharmacologic treatments of EDOs are summarized in *Table 26-4*.

Anorexia Nervosa

This disorder is unique in its resistance to pharmacologic intervention. There are no FDA-approved medications for treatment, and studies have not identified any that are consistently effective. One medication, olanzapine, has shown some utility (grade B evidence) in patients with high anxiety and agitation, and who are having difficulty meeting weight goals. It appears to reduce anxiety and cognitive rigidity, as well as improve weight gain. It is of particular benefit if the patient has a comorbid diagnosis for which the medication is indicated, such as bipolar disorder, schizophrenia, or treatment-resistant depression.[17] Quetiapine and risperidone also demonstrate benefit for depression, anxiety, and core eating pathology, but there is insufficient evidence regarding weight gain (grade C evidence).[18]

If comorbid conditions such as depression, anxiety, obsessive–compulsive, or posttraumatic stress disorder (PTSD) are present, antidepressants and other agents should be considered. The selective serotonin reuptake inhibitors (SSRIs) are usually first line. These include fluoxetine, sertraline, citalopram, escitalopram, fluvoxamine, and paroxetine. The antidepressant mirtazapine can also be used to help increase appetite and improve sleep. The medication buspirone may be helpful alone, or as an adjunct to antidepressants for the treatment of anxiety. For acute anxiety, the antihistamine hydroxyzine or antiepileptic gabapentin can be used as needed. Benzodiazepines (BZDs) should be avoided in most circumstances as patients may become dependent on them to cope with their feelings about, or fear of, food and weight gain. Medications that reduce appetite or cause weight loss should be avoided including amphetamines such as methylphenidate or the antidepressant bupropion. Additional risks for these agents include cardiac arrhythmia and seizure in patients who are underweight and/or prone to electrolyte abnormalities. Overall, malnourished, depressed patients are more prone to side effects and medical risks. Tricyclic antidepressants (TCAs), such as amitriptyline or nortriptyline, and monoamine oxidase inhibitors (MAOIs), such as phenelzine or tranylcypromine, should generally be avoided because of increased cardiac, hepatic, and seizure risks, as well as lethality in overdose.[17]

Bulimia Nervosa

In contrast to anorexia nervosa, starting an SSRI is indicated in bulimia nervosa. Antidepressant medications have been shown repeatedly to reduce the frequency of binge eating and vomiting, as well as prevent relapse, independent of other symptoms. Antidepressants alone may result in up to a 22% rate of abstinence from binging and purging.[19] The SSRI fluoxetine, most effective at 60 to 80 mg daily, is currently the only FDA-approved medication. If ineffective or not tolerated, another SSRI, such as sertraline, should be considered. If ineffective, it should be determined whether or not patient is taking the medication soon before vomiting. Some TCAs, such as imipramine, may have utility, but consistently cause far greater side effects than benefits. The use of buspirone or as needed hydroxyzine or gabapentin can be helpful. The American Psychiatric Association (APA) reported in 2012 that fluoxetine demonstrated grade A evidence for efficacy with a *good* risk–benefit ratio. TCAs and topiramate also demonstrated grade A evidence, but with *moderate* risk–benefit.[18]

Bupropion is contraindicated because of the seizure risk associated with electrolyte abnormalities common to purging. If a mood-stabilizing agent is needed, lithium and divalproex should be used with caution despite their effectiveness. Divalproex is usually associated with significant weight gain, which could increase distress and reduce treatment adherence. Lithium can be associated with arrhythmia, kidney disease, gait disturbance, nausea, and vomiting. Additionally, lithium levels can shift markedly with the rapid volume changes that may accompany binging or purging. Better choices may be antiepileptic medications such as lamotrigine or oxcarbazepine, or less likely to result in weight gain antipsychotics, such as aripiprazole or lurasidone. If an antipsychotic medication is needed, olanzapine and quetiapine should probably be avoided because of the high likelihood of weight gain. BZD and MAOIs are not recommended because of tolerability and safety concerns. Effective pharmacologic treatment should be maintained for at least 9 to 12 months before considering a taper.

Binge-Eating Disorder

Similar to bulimia nervosa, SSRIs are indicated in the treatment of BED. They have repeatedly demonstrated reduction in binge eating as well as associated depression and anxiety. Of note, they have not generally been associated with substantial weight loss, possibly because of weight gain side effects. SSRIs have the fewest adverse effects with the most evidence for efficacy. They are most likely to be more effective when used at the high end of the recommended dosage range compared with the treatment of depression. The stimulant lisdexamfetamine has recently been FDA approved for use in BED. It has been shown to both reduce the frequency of binge behaviors and suppress appetite. The anticonvulsant topiramate has also shown benefit in both binge-eating and sleep-related EDOs.

Bupropion, contraindicated in anorexia and bulimia nervosa, can be used in patients with BED, provided they do not suffer from serious comorbid anxiety or have elevated seizure risk from epilepsy or alcohol use. A new medication comprising both bupropion and naltrexone has been FDA approved for weight loss in combination with diet and exercise. There is some preliminary evidence that it may also be helpful in BED. The APA reported in 2012 that sertraline, citalopram, and escitalopram demonstrated grade A evidence for efficacy (with *good* risk-benefit), imipramine and topiramate, grade A (with *moderate* risk-benefit), and fluoxetine and fluvoxamine, grade D for inconsistent results.[18]

Psychopharmacology Pearls

- There are no FDA-approved medications for the treatment of anorexia nervosa.
- Consider fluoxetine, or another SSRI, for the treatment of bulimia nervosa.
- Bupropion is contraindicated in the treatment of anorexia and bulimia nervosa, but not BED.
- Treat comorbid psychiatric disorders (depression, anxiety, PTSD, bipolar) with standard therapies.
- Generally, avoid use of BZDs, TCAs, and MAOIs.

PSYCHOLOGICAL APPROACHES (*TABLE 26-3*)

Psychological approaches and their timing are summarized in *Table 26-3*.

Anorexia Nervosa

Cognitive-behavioral (CBT), interpersonal, psychodynamic, or a combination of psychotherapies has shown the best evidence for use in adults with anorexia nervosa. Other options include supportive clinical management and motivational interviewing for behavioral change. Child or adolescent patients appear to benefit most often from family therapy. Family and couples therapy is useful when family or marital problems are contributing to the maintenance of the disorder at any age. Group psychotherapy typically has a cognitive-behavioral, interpersonal, and/or psychodynamic focus. Care must be taken to help patients avoid competition to be the thinnest or sickest in the group, and to cope with demoralization from observation of the difficult chronic course of the illness in others.[20] For patients who have not improved through outpatient therapy, more intensive treatments such as combined individual and family therapy or day or inpatient care should be considered. The duration of psychological treatment should be at least 6 months when performed on an outpatient basis, and 12 months for individuals who have been under inpatient management. Individual therapy may be required for many years because of the nature of the illness and the need for ongoing support during recovery.

Bulimia Nervosa

CBT is the psychotherapy of choice. It is a highly detailed, manualized treatment that includes 18 to 20 sessions over 5 to 6 months. It is specifically directed at EDO symptoms and underlying maladaptive cognitions. It is useful in reducing binge eating symptoms and improving attitudes about body shape, weight, and restrictive dieting. Interpersonal and psychodynamically oriented psychotherapy may also be helpful. Behavioral techniques such as planned meals and self-monitoring further help with reduction of problem behaviors. Group psychotherapy may be based on cognitive-behavioral, interpersonal, psychodynamic, and/or supportive models. It can help the patient better cope with shame surrounding the disorder, and to provide peer-based feedback and support. Family and couples therapy should be considered, especially for adolescents who live with parents, older patients with ongoing conflicted interaction with parents, or adult patients with marital discord.[20]

Binge-Eating Disorder

CBT has been shown more effective than other psychotherapies for BED. It has also been studied more often and has the advantage of being adaptable for use in multiple self-help and group formats. Interpersonal psychotherapy or behavioral weight loss therapy are other alternatives. For overweight or obese patients with BED who are primarily interested in losing weight, behavioral weight loss therapy is suggested rather than psychotherapy or pharmacotherapy. Interpersonal and dialectical behavior therapies also show efficacy in treating behavioral and psychological symptoms, particularly when personality disorders are present. Other diets, behavior therapies, psychodynamic psychotherapy, and non–weight-directed psychosocial treatments are less well studied, but may be of benefit in some patients.[21]

OTHER TREATMENT CONSIDERATIONS

Several small or nonblinded studies have shown promise for exercise/strength training, mindfulness mediation, spirituality-focused group therapy, eye movement desensitization and reprocessing, yoga, and body awareness therapy. Gastric bypass surgery, although sometimes helpful in weight loss in BED, does not address the psychological aspects of the illness.[20] Noninvasive brain stimulation, including repetitive transcranial magnetic stimulation, has also shown promise for the treatment of obesity, anorexia nervosa, and bulimia nervosa.[16] Some benefits have been demonstrated for zonisamide and ondansetron in small studies. No benefits have been demonstrated from the use of acamprosate, lamotrigine, bright light, or warming therapies with heated baths, coats, or rooms.[18]

EDUCATION, PREVENTION, TREATMENT ADHERENCE

There are extensive EDO self-help materials and advocacy organizations. Many of these are described in both the 2006 and 2012 American Psychiatric Association (APA) practice guidelines.[18,20] Listed below are several of the best rated and most recent print and digital resources for the various disorders.

- *The Intuitive Eating Workbook: Ten Principles for Nourishing a Healthy Relationship with Food*, by Tribole and Elyse
- *8 Keys to Recovery from an Eating Disorder Workbook*, by Costin and Grabb
- *The Binge Code: 7 Unconventional Keys to End Binge Eating and Lose Excess Weight*, by Kerr
- *The Body Image Workbook for Teens: Activities to Help Girls Develop a Healthy Body Image in an Image-Obsessed World*, by Taylor

Like other mental disorders, EDOs have a complex and uncertain etiology. According to studies, a variety of biological and genetic vulnerability factors, psychological characteristics, and sociocultural aspects are involved. For those who enter treatment, there are obstacles to progress. Between 20% and 30% of patients drop out and relapse. Even those who continue in treatment can have lapses and slips, leaving them discouraged and demoralized. Wanting a quick and easy solution to their problems, patients may too often give up when they find that recovery can take months, or even years, of hard work. For many, the process can take 7 to 10 years or longer.[22] Messages that can help protect individuals from developing an EDO include following a healthy diet and eating at least one meal at home with the family as a child/adolescent, facilitating communication and improving self-esteem, avoiding conversations from turning to eating and image, and avoiding jokes about the body or weight.

Programs have been shown to be more effective when they are interactive, multisession, gender-specific, offered to people older than 15 years, and delivered by trained professionals. Those that incorporate contents related with body acceptance and induction-dissonance techniques, that assess effects using validated measures, that include psychoeducational contents, and that have shorter follow-up periods produce greater effects. Prevention programs have a greater effect on improving knowledge and a lesser effect on reducing incorrect behaviors and beliefs regarding eating.

WHEN TO REFER

- If the provider is unable or unwilling to provide the desired medical or psychiatric monitoring
- If the patient is not making progress with controlling weight or exercise recommendations
- If weight loss is ongoing or corrective weight gain is stagnant
- If the patient demonstrates bradycardia, hypothermia, or electrolyte disturbances
- When the patient needs more than weekly monitoring
- When family stress is not resolving

CASES AND QUESTIONS

CASE 1: A College Athlete with Abdominal Pain

A 19-year-old woman presents to a primary care clinic with a complaint of chronic, vague abdominal pain and constipation. She notes that low energy is interfering with her participation on the gymnastics team and her ability to maintain her nearly perfect grades. Review of systems is positive for occasional bloating and abdominal pain, cold intolerance, difficulty concentrating, and anxiety. She denies amenorrhea, although her menses are irregular. She is dressed in bulky clothing covering most of her body, uncharacteristic of the warm day outside. On examination, her height is 66 inches and she weighs 108 pounds (BMI

continued

17.43 kg/m²). Her vital signs include a temperature of 98.2°F, blood pressure of 94/66, heart rate of 54 beats per minute, and respirations of 18 per minute. On questioning about her weight, she is politely dismissive and states that she is far from the skinniest one on her team, or in her family. She denies concerns about being too thin, stating that she has always been this way and that peoples' concerns about her weight have always bothered her. She seems somewhat anxious yet superficially bright.

1. What is the most likely diagnosis?

   A. BED
   B. Major depressive disorder
   C. Anorexia nervosa
   D. Bulimia nervosa
   E. Thyroid disorder

   Correct answer: C. *This patient likely meets DSM-5 criteria for anorexia nervosa, including restriction of energy intake leading to significantly low body weight, intense fear of gaining weight, and undue influence of body weight on self-evaluation. Amenorrhea, although often present in anorexia, is no longer a requirement for the diagnosis. Other signs and symptoms include skin that is cool to the touch and the presence of lanugo.*

2. What should be the next step in workup?

   A. Referral to psychiatrist
   B. Basic labs and ECG
   C. Watchful waiting
   D. Bone density scan
   E. No intervention

   Correct answer: B. *This patient needs a thorough medical workup to screen for possible complications of anorexia nervosa, which should include complete blood count, electrolytes including phosphorous and magnesium, amylase, liver function tests, albumin, transferrin, thyroid panel, urine toxicology, and baseline ECG. Orthostatic vital signs should be checked, as her low heart rate and blood pressure likely reflect a hypometabolic state.*

3. What should be the primary goal of treatment?

   A. Repair of negative body image
   B. Restoration of weight
   C. Improved family function
   D. Improvement of depression and anxiety
   E. Correction of cognitive impairment

   Correct answer: B. *Early intervention is primarily focused on weight restoration and management of medical complications. The primary care physician should take a compassionate, nonjudgmental approach in an attempt to build rapport to ensure regular follow-up. A multidisciplinary approach is key to successful treatment, including a nutritionist who specializes in EDOs. She should have close medical follow-up, with regular blind weights and careful laboratory monitoring.*

CASE 2: An Overweight Woman with Anxiety

A 48-year-old woman presents to the primary care office to establish care after moving to be closer to her ailing mother. She reports that she is in good health, although is often fatigued, anxious, and down. She serves as the primary caretaker for her mother who recently had a stroke and finds this to be stressful and depressing. On examination, she is 65 inches tall and weighs 230 pounds (BMI 38.3 kg/m²). Her blood pressure is 155/90 mm Hg. Lab screening reveals hypercholesterolemia and elevated blood glucose. She reveals that the stress of her mother's condition has resulted in her increasingly turning to food for comfort. She has tried to decrease her intake but ends up hungrier than ever in the evening. During these times, she may eat an entire bag of chips, several bowls of cereal, and leftovers from that evening's meal. These episodes are happening on average twice a week and are increasing in frequency. She becomes tearful in the office and appears embarrassed and ashamed. She denies ever purging after the episodes and instead goes to sleep feeling uncomfortably full and disgusted with herself.

1. What is the most likely diagnosis?

   A. Bulimia nervosa
   B. BED
   C. Anorexia nervosa
   D. Major depressive disorder
   E. Body dysmorphic disorder

   Correct answer: B. *This patient is likely suffering from BED. She meets diagnostic criteria, with recurrent episodes of binge eating, resultant discomfort/disgust and embarrassment, and distress due to the binges. They have been occurring at least once a week over the past 3 months, and she denies compensatory behaviors, distinguishing her condition from bulimia.*

2. What comorbidities should be screened for?

   A. Substance abuse
   B. Depression
   C. Anxiety
   D. All of the above
   E. None of the above

   Correct answer: D. *A thorough psychiatric screening should be completed to identify comorbid depression, anxiety, and substance use disorders, which are common.*

3. What is the role of the primary care physician at this time?

   A. Refer to psychiatry
   B. Avoid talking about weight directly to avoid upsetting or embarrassing the patient
   C. Take a direct, nonconfrontational approach in partnering with patient
   D. Refer to a dietician
   E. None of the above

Correct answer: C. *A nonconfrontational, open approach can allow for direct communication and problem solving between patient and physician. Treatment should focus on decreasing the frequency of binge eating episodes, normalizing weight, and managing medical and psychiatric comorbidities. This patient would likely benefit from a multidisciplinary team, including a dietician or weight loss program as well as therapy to help her cope with her mother's ailing health and the stress of being a caretaker.*

CASE 3: A Constipated Young Woman and Her Boyfriend

A 24-year-old woman presents to her primary care physician, accompanied by her boyfriend. She complains of constipation and asks if she should continue trying to use laxatives, which were helpful in the past. She also notes a sore throat that is mildly bothersome but chronic in nature. Her boyfriend encourages the patient to disclose the true reason for the visit. While she appears irritated and embarrassed, she reports that her boyfriend is worried about her eating habits. She describes a lifelong history of difficulty with weight and food, beginning as a child when she was teased about being "chubby." She felt badly about her body and would often try to lose weight. She describes a chaotic childhood, with a stepfather who was abusive to herself and her sister. She currently exercises heavily and restricts in the first half of the day and then gives in to the urge to consume large amounts of food in the evening. She isolates in the bathroom when she does this, as she feels judged and embarrassed. She does this about once a week, although her boyfriend says he finds evidence more often than that. She denies purging, although her boyfriend thinks she is being untruthful. Physical examination reveals a blood pressure of 92/62 mm Hg, heart rate of 100 beats per minute, and BMI 23 kg/m^2.

1. What is the most likely diagnosis?

   A. BED
   B. Anorexia nervosa
   C. Body dysmorphic disorder
   D. Bulimia nervosa
   E. Orthorexia

   Correct answer: D. *She likely meets criteria for bulimia nervosa, with recurrent binges at least weekly for at least 3 months. There is suggestion of several forms of compensatory behaviors, including laxative use, exercise which may be excessive, and purging. Her self-evaluation appears unduly influenced by body weight. Other signs and symptoms to look for include sore throat, callused knuckles, dry mucous membranes, and enlarged parotids, all which highly suggest purging.*

2. What distinguishes this patient from one with anorexia nervosa?

   A. Evidence of purging
   B. Normal BMI
   C. Laxative abuse
   D. Episodes of binge eating
   E. Distorted body image

   Correct answer: B. *Binge eating, vomiting, laxative abuse, and distorted body image may all be present in both anorexia and bulimia nervosa; however, a diagnosis of anorexia requires a low body weight, whereas a diagnosis of bulimia does not. Individuals with bulimia nervosa often avoid detection, because of both secrecy/shame and the fact that BMI is often in a normal or high range.*

3. What of the following is not a recommended treatment for this patient?

   A. Fluoxetine
   B. Psychotherapy
   C. Bupropion
   D. Referral to dietician
   E. Referral to psychiatrist

   Correct answer: C. *Bupropion, while potentially helpful for comorbid depression, is contraindicated in patients with purging behaviors because of the increased risk of weight loss and seizure associated with electrolyte imbalance. Treatment should focus on normalizing eating behaviors and eliminating the binge–purge cycle. She may benefit from initiation of fluoxetine or other antidepressants. She should also be referred to a CBT therapist to help her identify disturbed eating patterns, examine dysfunctional thoughts, and build better coping mechanisms.*

4. What form of psychotherapy would be recommended for this patient?

   A. Supportive
   B. CBT
   C. Group
   D. Couples/family
   E. CBT and couples/family

   Correct answer: E. *Individual CBT is the treatment of choice for adults with bulimia nervosa. Family/couples therapy is additionally beneficial if there is evidence of family or marital discord.*

PRACTICAL RESOURCES

- National Eating Disorders Association: www.nationaleatingdisorders.org
  NEDA supports individuals and families affected by eating disorders and serves as a catalyst for prevention, cures, and access to quality care.
- National Association of Anorexia Nervosa and Associated Disorders: www.anad.org

continued

PRACTICAL RESOURCES—CONT'D

NAANAD, Inc. is a nonprofit organization working in the areas of support, awareness, advocacy, referral, education, and prevention.

- The Alliance for Eating Disorders Awareness: www.allianceforeatingdisorders.com
  The Alliance is a nonprofit organization dedicated to providing programs and activities aimed at outreach, education, and early intervention for all eating disorders.
- The Binge-Eating Disorder Association: www.bedaonline.com
  BEDA is a national organization focused on providing leadership, recognition, prevention, and treatment of BED and associated weight stigma. Through outreach, education and advocacy, BEDA facilitates increased awareness, proper diagnosis, and treatment of BED.
- Eating Disorder Hope: www.eatingdisorderhope.com
  Eating Disorder Hope™ offers education, support, and inspiration to eating disorder sufferers, their loved ones, and eating disorder treatment providers

ACKNOWLEDGMENT

We would like to acknowledge the authors of the original chapter, Margaret W. Leung, MD, MPH, Tracie Harris, MD, and Claire Pomeroy, MD, MBA as well as Sarah Stender, MD, who reviewed the chapter and made some very helpful additions.

REFERENCES

1. Smink FE, van Hoeken D, Hoek HW. Epidemiology of eating disorders: incidence, prevalence and mortality rates. *Curr Psychiatry Rep.* 2012;14:406-414.
2. Swanson S, Crow S, Le Grange D, Swendsen J, Merikangas K. Prevalence and correlates of eating disorders in adolescents. *Arch Gen Psychiatry.* 2011; Online Article E1–E10. doi:10.1001/archgenpsychiatry.2011.22.
3. American Psychiatric Association. Feeding and eating disorders. In: *Diagnostic and Statistical Manual of Mental Disorders.* 5th ed. Washington, DC; 2013. doi:10.1176/appi.books.9780890425596.dsm10.
4. Sim L, McAlpine D, Grothe K, Himes S, Cockerill R, Clark M. Identification and treatment of eating disorders in the primary care setting. *Mayo Clin Proc.* 2010;85:746-751. doi:10.4065/mcp.2010.0070.
5. Samnaliev M, Noh H, Sonneville K, Austin S. The economic burden of eating disorders and related mental health comorbidities: an exploratory analysis using the U.S. Medical Expenditures Panel Survey. *Prev Med Rep.* 2014;2:32-34. doi:10.1016/j.pmedr.2014.12.002.
6. Weissman R, Roselli F. Reducing the burden of suffering from eating disorders: unmet treatment needs, cost of illness, and the quest for cost-effectiveness. *Behav Res Ther.* 2017;88:49-64. doi:10.1016/j.brat.2016.09.006.
7. Klein D, Attia E. Anorexia nervosa in adults: clinical features, course of illness, assessment, and diagnosis. In: Yager J, ed. *UpToDate.* Waltham, MA; 2017. Accessed February 10, 2018.
8. Engel S, Steffen K, Mitchell J. Bulimia nervosa in adults: clinical features, course of illness, assessment, and diagnosis. In: Yager J, ed. *UpToDate.* Waltham, MA; 2017. Accessed February 10, 2018.
9. Franco K, Sieke E, Dickstein L, Falcone T. Eating Disorders. Cleveland Clinic Center for Continuing Education; 2017. http://www.clevelandclinicmeded.com/medicalpubs/diseasemanagement/psychiatry-psychology/eating-disorders/.
10. Sansone R, Levvit J, Sansone L. The prevalence of personality disorders among those with eating disorders. *Eat Disord.* 2005;13:7-21. doi:10.1080/10640260590893593.
11. Masheb R, Lutes L, Kim H, et al. High-frequency binge eating predicts weight gain among veterans receiving behavioral weight loss treatments. *Obesity.* 2015;23:54-61. doi:10.1002/oby.20931.
12. Crow S. Eating disorders in pregnancy. In: Yager J, Lockwood C, ed. *UpToDate.* Waltham, MA; 2017. Accessed February 10, 2018.
13. Morgan J, Reid F, Lacey JH. The SCOFF questionnaire: a new screening tool for eating disorders. *West J Med.* 2000;172:164-165.
14. Working group of the Clinical Practice Guideline for Eating Disorders. Clinical Practice Guideline for Eating Disorders. Madrid: Quality Plan for the National Health System of the Ministry of Health and Consumer Affairs. Catalan Agency for Health Technology Assessment and Research; 2009. Clinical Practice Guidelines in the NHS: CAHTA Number 2006/05-01.
15. Kaplan A, Halmi K. Eating disorders. In: Gabbard G, ed. *Treatment of Psychiatric Disorders.* 4th ed. Washington, DC: American Psychiatric Publishing; 2007:705-756.
16. Forman S. Eating disorders: overview of prevention and treatment. In: Yager J, ed. *UpToDate.* Waltham, MA; 2017. Accessed February 10, 2018.
17. Walsh T. Anorexia nervosa in adults: pharmocotherapy. In: Yager J, ed. *UpToDate.* Waltham, MA; 2017. Accessed February 18, 2018.
18. Yager J, Devlin M, Halmi K, et al. *Guideline Watch (August 2012): Practice Guideline for the Treatment of Patients with Eating Disorders.* 3rd ed. American Psychiatric Association; 2012.
19. Andersen AE, Yager J. Eating disorders. In: Sadock B, Sadock V, eds. *Kaplan and Sadock's Synopsis of Psychiatry.* 10th ed. Philadelphia: Lippincott Williams & Wilkins; 2007:727-739.
20. Yager J, Devlin M, Halmi K, et al. *American Psychiatric Association Practice Guideline for the Treatment of Patients with Eating Disorders.* 3rd ed. American Psychiatric Association; 2006.
21. Sysko R, Devlin M,. Binge eating disorder in adults. In: Yager J, ed. *UpToDate.* Waltham, MA; 2017. Accessed February 18, 2018.
22. Eddy K, Tabri N, Thomas J, et al. Recovery from anorexia nervosa and bulimia nervosa at 22-year follow-up. *J Clin Psychiatry.* 2017;78:184-189. doi:10.4088/JCP.15m10393.
23. Leung M, Harris T, Pomeroy C. Eating disorders. In: McCarron R, Xiong G, Bourgeois J, eds. *Lippincott's Primary Care Psychiatry.* Philadelphia: Lippincott Williams & Wilkins; 2009:147-163.

APPENDICES

PSYCHIATRIC MEDICATIONS

TABLE 5-4 Selective Serotonin Reuptake Inhibitors (SSRIs) and Serotonin Norepinephrine Reuptake Inhibitors (SNRIs) for Anxiety Disorders

SSRIs	STARTING DOSE (mg/day)	THERAPEUTIC DOSE (mg/day)	HALF-LIFE	DRUG INTERACTIONS
Fluoxetine (Prozac)	10	20-60	Long[a]	2D6 inhibitor
Sertraline (Zoloft)	25	50-200	Medium[a]	(–)
Citalopram (Celexa)	10	20-40	Short	(–)
Escitalopram (Lexapro)	5	10-30	Short	(–)
Paroxetine (Paxil)	10	20-60	Short	2D6 inhibitor
Paroxetine controlled release (Paxil CR)	12.5	12.5-25	Short	2D6 inhibitor
Fluvoxamine (Luvox)	50	150-300	Short	3A4 and 1A2 inhibitor
SNRIs				
Venlafaxine extended release (Effexor XR)	37.5	75-225	Short[a]	(–)
Duloxetine (Cymbalta)	30	60-120	Short	2D6 inhibitor

[a]Including active metabolites.

TABLE 8-4 First-Line Antidepressant Medications

CLASS	INITIAL DOSE (mg/day)[a]	THERAPEUTIC DOSE (mg/day)	PRACTICAL POINTERS FOR THE PCP[b]
Selective serotonin reuptake inhibitors (SSRIs)			
Sertraline (Zoloft)	50	50-200	Serotonin and dopamine reuptake inhibition Possible early and temporary diarrhea and dyspepsia Relatively low risk for drug interactions
Paroxetine Paroxetine CR (Paxil, Paxil CR)	20 12.5-20	20-60 25-75	High anticholinergic and antihistamine side effect profile Risk for sedation, weight gain, and dry mouth Short half-life with more risk for discontinuation syndrome High chance for drug interactions Unsafe during pregnancy—class D

TABLE 8-4 First-Line Antidepressant Medications (continued)

CLASS	INITIAL DOSE (mg/day)[a]	THERAPEUTIC DOSE (mg/day)	PRACTICAL POINTERS FOR THE PCP[b]
Fluoxetine (Prozac)	20	20-60	Long half-life and ideal for intermittently compliant patients Relatively inexpensive High chance for drug interactions
Fluvoxamine (Luvox)	50	50-300	Rarely used owing to high side effect profile
Citalopram (Celexa)	20	20-60	Structurally similar to escitalopram Low risk for drug interactions
Escitalopram (Lexapro)	10	10-20	Structurally similar to citalopram Low risk for drug interactions
Serotonin norepinephrine reuptake inhibitors (SNRIs)			
Venlafaxine XR (Effexor XR)	37.5	75-300	Structurally similar to desvenlafaxine (do not use concurrently) Dual action on serotonin and norepinephrine receptors *Not* consistently "activating" but usually does not cause sedation Sometimes used as an adjunct for chronic pain Not to be used in those with difficult-to-treat hypertension May increase blood pressure and heart rate, especially at higher dosing range (>150 mg/day) Non-XR formulation is rarely used due to side effect profile and twice-per-day dosing Short half-life with more risk for discontinuation syndrome Reduce dose with renal insufficiency
Desvenlafaxine (Pristiq)	50	50-100	Structurally similar to venlafaxine (do not use concurrently) Dual action on serotonin and norepinephrine receptors *Not* consistently "activating" but usually does not cause sedation Not to be used in those with difficult-to-treat hypertension Short half-life with more risk for discontinuation syndrome Reduce dose with renal insufficiency
Duloxetine (Cymbalta)	30	30-60	Dual action on serotonin and norepinephrine receptors *Not* consistently "activating" but usually does not cause sedation FDA approved for fibromyalgia and diabetic peripheral neuropathic pain Sometimes used for chronic neuropathic pain Short half-life with more risk for discontinuation syndrome Increased risk for drug interactions
Other			
Bupropion	75-150	300-450	
Bupropion SR (Wellbutrin SR)	100	300-400	Given twice per day Likely dual action on dopamine and norepinephrine receptors Contraindicated with seizure and eating disorders
Bupropion XL (Wellbutrin XL)	150	300-450	Increased risk for seizures in those with alcohol withdrawal Not used for anxiety disorders May worsen anxiety associated with depression No serotonin activity and no related sexual side effects XL formulation is supposed to have slower release and lower side effect profile (permits higher dosing and lower seizure risk) Less frequently used owing to side effect profile
Mirtazapine (Remeron)	15	15-45	Increases central serotonin and norepinephrine activity (possibly through presynaptic α_2-adrenergic receptor inhibition) Decreased frequency of sexual side effects Increased sedation and sleepiness at mainly *lower* doses Although not indicated for anxiety disorders, it may be helpful Remeron Soltab is orally dissolving for patients who cannot swallow

[a]*Initial dose should be decreased by half when treating an anxiety disorder or an elderly person.*
[b]*Drug interactions refer to commonly used medications that are principally metabolized by the P450 2D6 pathway.*
FDA, Food and Drug Administration; PCP, primary care physician.

TABLE 8-5 Side Effect Profiles of Antidepressant Classes

	SEXUAL DYSFUNCTION/ DECREASED LIBIDO	WEIGHT GAIN	SEDATION	CARDIAC
SSRIs	+++	+[a]	+/–[a]	0
SNRIs	+++	+/–	+/–	+ (↑ BP)
Mirtazapine	+	+++	++	+/–
Bupropion	0	0	0	+/– (↑ BP)

[a]Paroxetine and fluvoxamine are more likely to cause sedation and weight gain.
BP, blood pressure; SNRIs, serotonin norepinephrine reuptake inhibitors; SSRIs, selective serotonin reuptake inhibitors.

TABLE 9-1 Augmentation Options for Treatment-Resistant Depression

MEDICATION	THERAPEUTIC DOSE RANGE	SIDE EFFECTS
Atypical antipsychotics		
Aripiprazole	2-15 mg	Sedation, abnormal metabolic labs, weight gain, akathisia, increased prolactin, QTc prolongation
Quetiapine	150-300 mg	
Olanzapine (adjunctive to fluoxetine)	6-18 mg	
Risperidone	1-3 mg	
Ziprasidone	40-160 mg	
Brexpiprazole	2-3 mg	
Others		
Lithium	600-900 mg/0.6-0.9 mmol/L blood level	Ataxia, tremor, nausea, diarrhea, polyuria, renal dysfunction, hypothyroidism
T3	25-50 μg	
Modafinil	100-400 mg	Rare cutaneous reactions (TEN, SJS), cytochrome p450 interactions
SAM-e	800-1,600 mg	
Methylfolate	15-30 mg	
Omega-3 (EPA)	1-2 g	
Bupropion	150-450 mg	HTN, seizures (do not give in patients with epilepsy or other risk factors predisposing to seizure)
Mirtazapine	15-45 mg	Sedation, increase in cholesterol, weight gain
Lamotrigine	25-100 mg	Cutaneous reactions (TEN, SJS)
Pramipexole	1-5 mg	Sedation, nausea, dizziness, tremor, compulsive behavior
Lisdexamfetamine	20-70 mg	Dry mouth, anxiety, appetite suppression, increase in BP

TEN, toxic epidermal necrolysis; SJS, Stevens–Johnson syndrome; HTN, hypertension; BP, blood pressure.

TABLE 10-3 Common Medications Used in the Treatment of Bipolar Mania

TREATMENT OF ACUTE MANIA

MEDICATION	STARTING DOSE	TARGET DOSE	COMMON SIDE EFFECTS	RARE SIDE EFFECTS	PREGNANCY CATEGORY
Lithium	300 mg BID	600-1,200 mg (target level 0.6-1.2 mmol/L)	GI discomfort, tremor, weight gain	Renal toxicity, hypothyroidism, diabetes insipidus	D
Valproate	500-750 mg BID	1,200-3,000 mg (target level 50-100 mg/L)	GI discomfort, sedation, weight gain, tremor	Hepatic failure, pancytopenia, thrombocytopenia	D
Olanzapine	10 mg QHS	20 mg	Sedation, weight gain	Metabolic symptoms, NMS	C
Quetiapine	IR—300 mg QHS; increase by 100 mg Q1-2 days	600-800 mg	Sedation, weight gain, orthostasis	Metabolic symptoms, NMS	C
	XR—300 mg QHS; can double dose within 1-2 days	600 mg	Weight gain		
Aripiprazole	15 mg QHS	30 mg	Akathisia, restlessness		C
Risperidone	1 mg QHS or BID	6 mg	Weight gain, EPS, constipation	Prolactinemia, NMS	C
Asenapine	10 mg QHS	20 mg	Sedation, weight gain, dizziness, EPS	Metabolic symptoms, NMS	C
Haloperidol	5-10 mg QHS or BID	20 mg	Sedation, EPS, constipation	NMS, Parkinsonism	C

BID, dosed twice a day; EPS, extrapyramidal symptom; GI, gastrointestinal; IR, immediate release; NMS, neuroleptic malignant syndrome; QHS, dosed nightly; XR, extended release. Medications indicated for acute mania are typically sedating and, as such, dosed at nighttime to optimize sleep function.

TABLE 10-4 Common Medications Used in the Treatment of Bipolar Depression

TREATMENT OF ACUTE DEPRESSION

MEDICATION	STARTING DOSE	TARGET DOSE	COMMON SIDE EFFECTS	RARE SIDE EFFECTS	PREGNANCY CATEGORY
Lithium	300 mg BID	600-1,200 mg (target level 0.4-1.2 mmol/L)	GI discomfort, tremor, weight gain	Renal toxicity, hypothyroidism, diabetes insipidus	D
Lamotrigine	25 mg/day × 2 weeks, then double every 2 weeks	200 mg		Rash/SJS associated with rapid titration	C
Olanzapine/ fluoxetine	5/20 mg/day or 10/40 mg/ day	10/40 mg	Weight gain, sedation (from olanzapine)		C/C
Quetiapine	200-300 mg/night	300-600 mg	Sedation, weight gain, orthostasis	Metabolic symptoms	C
Lurasidone	20-40 mg/day	120 mg	Akathisia		B

BID, dosed twice a day; GI, gastrointestinal; SJS, Stevens–Johnson syndrome.

TABLE 11-9 First-Line Antipsychotic Medications for Schizophrenia[a]

	STARTING DOSE	TARGET RANGE[a] (mg/day)	PRIMARY CARE TITRATION SCHEDULE	EPS	ORTHOSTATIC HYPOTENSION	METABOLIC SYNDROME[b]	SEDATION	OTHER
Haloperidol (Haldol) (available in long-acting injectable formulations)	2-5 mg PO BID	20-40 mg/day	Increase up to 5 mg daily, as tolerated	+++	+	+/−	+	
Risperidone[c] (Risperdal) (available in long-acting injectable and ODT formulations)	1 mg BID or 2 mg QHS	4-6	Increase up to 2 mg daily, as tolerated	+++	++	++	++	Hyperprolactinemia
Olanzapine[c] (Zyprexa) (available in long-acting injectable and ODT formulations)	5-10 mg QHS	10-30	Increase 5 mg every 3-5 days, as tolerated	+	+	+++	+++	Not to be routinely used for the treatment of insomnia
Quetiapine[d] (Seroquel)	50-100 mg BID	300-800	Increase 50-100 mg every 2 days, as tolerated (monitor for orthostatic hypotension)	+/−	+++	++	+++	
Quetiapine (Seroquel XR)	300 mg QHS	400-800	Increase every 1-2 days, as tolerated	+/−	+++	++	+++	
Ziprasidone[e,f] (Geodon)	40 mg BID (must be taken with meals)[f]	40-160	Increase every other day to target dose, as tolerated	+	+	+	++	QTc prolongation
Aripiprazole[c] (Abilify) (available in long-acting injectable and ODT formulations)	10-15 mg QAM	10-30	Increase dose after 2 days, as tolerated	+/−	+	+	+	
Paliperidone[c,g] (Invega) (available in long-acting injectable formulation)	6 mg QAM	6-12	Increase by increments of 3 mg every 5 days, as tolerated	++	+	++	++	

TABLE 11-9 First-Line Antipsychotic Medications for Schizophrenia[a]   (continued)

	STARTING DOSE	TARGET RANGE[a] (mg/day)	PRIMARY CARE TITRATION SCHEDULE	EPS	ORTHOSTATIC HYPOTENSION	METABOLIC SYNDROME[b]	SEDATION	OTHER
Asenapine (Saphris) (available in ODT formulation)	5 mg BID	5-20	Increase by increments of 5 mg over one week	+	+	+	++	Dysgeusia
Iloperidone (Fanapt)	1 mg BID	6-24	Increase by 2 mg BID each day	+++	+	+	+++	
Lurasidone[f] (Latuda)	40 mg QAM	40-160	Increase by 20 mg per day	+++	+	+	+++	
Brexpiprazole (Rexulti)	1 mg PO QAM	1-4	Increase to 2 mg per day for three days, then increase to 4 mg per day	+	+	++	+++	
Cariprazine (Vraylar)	1.5 mg PO QAM	6-12	Increase by 1.5 mg per day	+++	+	+	++	

Monitoring

Initial:
Baseline weight and body mass index, waist circumference, vital signs, fasting glucose or Hgb A1C, and lipid profile
Consider doing a pregnancy test and drug toxicology
Neurologic examination (+/− brain imaging) should be performed if psychotic symptoms present after the age of 50 years
An ECG should be performed on patients who have cardiac disease
First 4 weeks: BMI, EPS, vital signs, prolactin (if clinical symptoms of hyperprolactinemia exist)
First 12 weeks: BMI, EPS, vital signs, fasting glucose of Hemoglobin A1C (Hg A1C), a lipid profile
Quarterly: BMI
Annually: BMI, EPS, fasting glucose of Hemoglobin A1C (Hg A1C)
Every 3-5 years: lipid panel
Special populations:
Medically compromised or elderly: Start antipsychotics at half the starting dose. Titrate over longer period, increase by half the recommended dose.
Pregnant/lactating: Most SGAs are categorized under class C. Consider lurasidone (Latuda), which is in Class B. Start at 20 mg BID, increase by 10-20 mg/day up to a maximum of 160 mg/day

[a]*Dosing information derived from Lehman AF, Lieberman JA, Dixon LB, et al; American Psychiatric Association. Practice guideline for the treatment of patients with schizophrenia, second edition. Am J Psychiatry. 2004;161(S2):1-56 and the authors' clinical expert opinion. These doses do not apply to geriatric or pediatric patients.*
[b]*Metabolic effects include hyperglycemia, weight gain, and hyperlipidemia.*
[c]*Patients may be able to transition to an intramuscular depot formulation of the drug.*
[d]*Because of its low potency, quetiapine is ideal for patients who are sensitive to dopamine blockade, particularly patients sensitive to EPS.*
[e]*Contraindications to the use of ziprasidone include persistent QTc >500 ms, recent acute myocardial infarction, and uncompensated heart failure.*
[f]*Should be taken with food, as it increases bioavailability.*
[g]*Paliperidone is the active metabolite of risperidone. Relative risks for metabolic syndrome and EPS are similar to risperidone.*
BMI, body mass index; ECG, electrocardiogram; EPS, extrapyramidal symptoms.

TABLE 12-8 Agents Approved for the Treatment of Dementia

NAME	FORMULATION	FDA APPROVAL	DOSE RANGE	ADVERSE EFFECTS	COMMENTS
Cholinesterase inhibitors					
Donepezil	Tablet, orally disintegrating tablet	Alzheimer disease, mild to severe	5-23 mg	Nausea, vomiting, muscle cramps, bradycardia, decreased appetite, vivid dreams; effects tend to decrease after 1-2 weeks	May be helpful in LBD and vascular dementia as well
Rivastigmine	Capsule, transdermal patch	Alzheimer disease, mild to moderate; Parkinson dementia	4.6-13.3 mg		
Galantamine	Tablet, extended release capsule, solution	Alzheimer disease, mild to moderate	8-24 mg		
NMDA receptor antagonist					
Memantine	Tablet, extended release capsule, solution	Alzheimer disease, moderate to severe	5-20 mg, in divided doses twice daily XR: 7-28 mg	Transient sedation, generally well tolerated	May be helpful in vascular dementia as well

TABLE 13-6 Medications for Maintenance Treatment of Alcohol Use Disorders

MEDICATION	DOSAGE AND ADVERSE EFFECTS	SIDE EFFECTS/CAUTION/COMMENTS
Naltrexone (Revia, Vivitrol) • FDA approved	50-100 mg daily, may start 25 mg daily for several days 380 mg IM q4 weeks (intramuscular) Side effects: nausea, headache, insomnia, decreased hedonic drive	• Must be opioid free (opiates, semisynthetics and synthetics) with negative urine opioid test, otherwise may induce full opioid withdrawal. Consider naloxone challenge • Contraindication: active opioid use, pregnancy • Caution in patients with depression, suicidal ideation, thrombocytopenia, acute hepatitis, or liver failure • Baseline evaluation: liver transaminases, opioid urine drug screen, pregnancy test • Pregnancy Category C
Acamprosate (Campral) • FDA approved	666 mg TID, preferably with meals Avoid if creatinine clearance less than 30 mL/minute Side effects: diarrhea, anxiety, asthenia, insomnia	• Pretreatment abstinence may improve response. May be continued despite alcohol relapse • Requires dose adjustment in renal failure • Caution in patients with depression, anxiety. Monitor for suicidal ideation • Baseline evaluation: renal function • Pregnancy Category C
Disulfiram (Antabuse) • FDA approved	250 mg/day, range 125-500 mg daily Side effects: metallic taste, headache, hepatotoxicity, peripheral neuropathy, psychosis, delirium Must avoid alcohol-containing medications and foods	• Must be abstinent from alcohol at least 12 hours and have zero blood alcohol • Toxic reaction of headache, vomiting, malaise, and generalized distress when used with alcohol • Drug interactions with isoniazid and metronidazole, phenytoin, warfarin, oral hypoglycemics • Baseline evaluation: liver transaminases, then monthly ×3, then periodically • Pregnancy Category C
Topiramate (Topamax, Qudexy) • Off-label	50 mg/day, titrate 25-50 mg daily each week to maximum 150 mg BID, to minimize side effects. Taper off if no response in 3 months Side effects: cognitive dysfunction, paresthesia, nervousness, fatigue, ataxia, abdominal pain, decreased effectiveness of oral contraceptives, increased risk of cleft lip/palate during first trimester	• May be continued despite alcohol relapse • Caution in patients with depression, seizure disorder, or pregnancy • Do not suddenly discontinue because of risk of rebound seizures • Baseline evaluation: renal function, pregnancy • Pregnancy Class C

TABLE 13-6 Medications for Maintenance Treatment of Alcohol Use Disorders   (continued)

MEDICATION	DOSAGE AND ADVERSE EFFECTS	SIDE EFFECTS/CAUTION/COMMENTS
Gabapentin (Neurontin, Horizant, Gralise) • Off-label	*Mild–moderate alcohol withdrawal:* 400 mg TID × 3 days, then 400 mg BID ×1 day, then 400 mg once ×1 day, with additional prn dosing *Maintenance.* Day 1, 300 mg, increase by 300 mg a day to 600 mg TID as tolerated Side effects: dizziness, sedation, nightmares, diarrhea	• Requires dose adjustment in renal failure • Caution in patients with depression and suicidal ideation • Abuse potential at supratherapeutic doses. Monitor usage/prescribing patterns • Baseline evaluation: renal function • Pregnancy Category C

Modified from Department of Veterans Affairs. Management of substance use disorder (SUD) (2015)—VA/DoD clinical practice guidelines; 2015. https://www.healthquality.va.gov/guidelines/mh/sud/. Accessed October 1, 2017.
BID, twice daily; IM, intramuscular; TID, three times daily.

TABLE 14-2 FDA-Approved Medications for Opioid Use Disorder

	METHADONE	BUPRENORPHINE	NALTREXONE PO/VIVITROL IM
Mechanism of action	• Synthetic μ-opioid receptor antagonist	• Partial opioid agonist with high affinity at μ-opioid receptor	• Long-acting opioid antagonist
Prescribing	• Federally regulated for treatment of opioid use disorder • Can only be prescribed at an opioid treatment program (OTP) • Withdrawal management, reduces cravings	• Can be prescribed in primary care setting • Prescribers need to have DATA 2000 waiver from the DEA (SAMHSA) • Withdrawal management, reduces cravings	• Can be prescribed in primary care setting • Naltrexone PO—administered daily • Vivitrol IM—extended release injectable Naltrexone, administered every 4 weeks • No effect on withdrawals, reduces cravings • No addictive potential
Dosing	• Administered daily as an oral dose • Individualized therapeutic dose is determined to maintain an asymptomatic state (no withdrawal symptoms, or signs/symptoms of overmedication)	• Sublingual absorption, with poor oral bioavailability • Owing to its unique pharmacologic properties, it can cause acute opioid withdrawal taken while on a full opioid agonist • Formulated as a combination pill with naloxone (Suboxone) as a deterrent for abuse—if taken correctly naloxone is not absorbed	• Most effective when utilized following detoxification from opioids—need 7 to 10 days abstinent from opioids • Naltrexone PO—can start 25 mg daily for 5 days, then increase to 50 mg daily for maintenance • Vivitrol IM—380 mg injected intramuscularly every 4 weeks
Common adverse effects	• Cardiac: prolonged QTc • GI: constipation, abdominal pain • Endocrine: hormonal dysregulation, sexual dysfunction	• Headaches • GI: constipation, nausea • Endocrine: hormonal dysregulation, sexual dysfunction	• Headache • Nausea/vomiting • Dysphoria • Myalgia • Insomnia

Adapted from Lee J, Kresina TF, Campopiano M., et al. Use of pharmacotherapies in the treatment of alcohol use disorders and opioid dependence in primary care. Biomed Res. 2015:1-11. Stine SM, Kosten TR. Pharmacologic interventions for opioid dependence. In: Ries RK, Fiellin DA, Miller SC, Saitz R, eds. The ASAM Principles of Addiction Medicine. 5th ed. Philadelphia, PA: Wolters Kluwer; 2014:735-777. American Society of Addiction Medicine. National practice guidelines for the use of medications in the treatment of addiction involving opioid use. American Society of Addiction Medicine. Published June 1, 2015. https://www.asam.org/docs/default-source/practice-support/guidelines-and-consensus-docs/asam-national-practice-guideline-supplement.pdf?sfvrsn=24. Accessed July 3, 2017.

TABLE 19-1 Cytochrome P450 Activities of Psychotropics and Commonly Used Medications in Primary care

	1A2	2B6	2C8	2C9	2C19	2D6	2E1	3A4,5,7
Strong inhibitors	Fluvoxamine		Gemfibrozil	Fluconazole		Bupropion		Indinavir
	Ciprofloxacin		Trimethoprim			Fluoxetine		Nelfinavir
						Paroxetine		Ritonavir
						Quinidine		Clarithromycin
								Itraconazole
								Ketoconazole
								Nefazodone
								Saquinavir
								Suboxone
								Telithromycin
Moderate inhibitors				Amiodarone		Duloxetine		Aprepitant
						Sertraline		Erythromycin
						Terbinafine		Fluconazole
								Grapefruit juice
								Verapamil
								Diltiazem
Weak inhibitors	Cimetidine					Amiodarone		Cimetidine
						Cimetidine		
Inducers	Carbamazepine	Artemisinin		Carbamazepine	Enzalutamide		Ethanol	Efavirenz
	Char-grilled meat	Carbamazepine		Nevirapine	Rifampin		Isoniazid	Nevirapine
	Rifampin	Efavirenz		Phenobarbital	Ritonavir			Carbamazepine
	Tobacco	Nevirapine		Rifampin	St. John's wort			Phenobarbital
		Phenobarbital		St. John's wort				Phenytoin
		Phenytoin						Rifabutin
		Rifampin						Rifampin
								St. John's wort
								Troglitazone
								Pioglitazone

Adapted from The Flockhart Table. ©2016 by The Trustees of Indiana University.[2]

TABLE 19-2 Monitoring Guidelines for Psychiatric Medications for Primary Care

	BASELINE VS/PE	FOLLOW-UP VS/PE	BASELINE LABORATORY TESTS	FOLLOW-UP LABORATORY TESTS	ECG	THERAPEUTIC DRUG MONITORING
Antidepressants						
All	Pulse, BP, weight/ BMI	Pulse, BP, weight/ BMI each visit	TSH	As clinically indicated	No	N/A
Mood stabilizers						
Lithium	Pulse, BP, weight/ BMI	Pulse, BP, weight/ BMI each visit	CBC, BMP, TSH, UPT	CBC, BMP +/– UPT q3-6 months, TSH q6-12 months	Recommended >40 years of age	Lithium level after increases; q3 months ×2; q6-12 months
Divalproex	Pulse, BP, weight/ BMI	Pulse, BP, weight/ BMI each visit	CBC, LFTs, TSH, UPT	CBC, LFTs +/– UPT q3 months ×3, then q12 months	No	Valproic acid level after increases; annually
Carbamazepine	Pulse, BP, weight/ BMI	Pulse, BP, weight/ BMI each visit	CBC, CMP, TSH, UPT	CBC, CMP q3 months ×3, then q12 months	No	Carbamazepine level after increases; q3 months ×2; q12 months
Lamotrigine	Pulse, BP, weight/ BMI	Pulse, BP, weight/ BMI each visit	TSH	As clinically indicated	No	N/A
Atypical antipsychotics						
All, including ziprasidone and clozapine	Pulse, BP, weight/ BMI, AIMS	Pulse, BP, weight/ BMI each visit, AIMS q6-12 months	Glucose or hemoglobin A1c, lipids	Glucose or hemoglobin A1c, lipids at 3 months, then q12 months	No	N/A
Ziprasidone					If risk factors, after increases	N/A
Clozapine		Refer to psychiatrist	CBC	Per REMS protocol		

AIMS, Abnormal Involuntary Movement Scale.

TABLE 24-6 Drugs Commonly Used "Off-label" for Insomnia

DRUG	PERTINENT SIDE EFFECTS	COMMENTS
Antidepressants		
Mirtazapine (Remeron)	Somnolence and increased appetite	May be beneficial if patient has comorbid depression and insomnia. Mirtazapine's sedating effect is inversely dose dependent. As the dose increases, the noradrenergic activity counteracts the sleep-inducing H_1 antihistaminic effect of mirtazapine
Trazodone (Desyrel)	Residual daytime sedation, headache, orthostatic hypotension, priapism, cardiac arrhythmias	One of the most commonly prescribed agents for the treatment of insomnia. May be beneficial if patient has comorbid depression and insomnia. May be an acceptable alternative for patients for whom BzRAs are contraindicated (severe hypercapnea or hypoxemia, or history of substance abuse or dependence). Usually dosed much lower (50-100 mg) than when used for depression
Tricyclic antidepressants (TCAs)	Delirium, decreased cognition and seizure threshold, orthostatic hypotension, tachycardia, ECG abnormalities	**Avoid** in hospitalized patients because of their anticholinergic, antihistaminic, and cardiovascular side effects. Not recommended as a treatment for insomnia or other sleep problems unless comorbid depression is present. As with other antidepressants, TCAs are usually used at significantly lower doses than for depression
Antihistamines		
Diphenhydramine (Benadryl)	Residual daytime sedation, weight gain, delirium, orthostatic hypotension, blurred vision, urinary retention	Antihistamines are one of the most commonly used over-the-counter agents for chronic insomnia. If possible, avoid in patients >60 years old
Hydroxyzine (Vistaril)	Residual daytime sedation, weight gain, delirium, orthostatic hypotension, blurred vision, urinary retention	Efficacy as an anxiolytic has not been established. Not FDA approved for insomnia. **Avoid** in patients >60 years old and those with closed-angle glaucoma, prostatic hypertrophy, severe asthma, and COPD
Antipsychotics		
Quetiapine (Seroquel)	Sedation, orthostatic hypotension, metabolic derangements (e.g., weight gain, dyslipidemia, and glucose dysregulation)	The most sedating of the atypical antipsychotics; it is frequently used as a sleep aid. Not recommended for insomnia or other sleep problems unless there is comorbid psychotic or bipolar disorder. Is dosed much lower (25-100 mg) when used for insomnia. Other less expensive sedative-hypnotic agents should be used first

BzRAs, benzodiazepine receptor agonists; COPD, chronic obstructive pulmonary disease; ECG, electrocardiogram; FDA, Food and Drug Administration; TCAs, tricyclic antidepressants (doxepin, amitriptyline, imipramine, nortriptyline, desipramine).

TABLE 1-2 The AMPS Screening Tool for Common Psychiatric Conditions

	SCREENING QUESTIONS	FOLLOW-UP QUESTIONS	DIAGNOSTIC AND TREATMENT INSTRUMENTS[a]
Anxiety	"Is anxiety or nervousness a problem for you?"	• "Please describe how your anxiety affects you on an everyday basis." • "What triggers your anxiety?" • "What makes your anxiety get better?"	Generalized Anxiety Disorders Scale (GAD-7)
Mood	**Depression[b]** 1. "Have you been feeling depressed, sad, or hopeless over the past 2 weeks?" 2. "What do you usually like to do for fun and have you stopped doing this over the past few weeks?" **Mania/hypomania** 1. "Have you ever felt the complete opposite of depressed, *when friends and family were worried about you because you were too happy*?" 2. "Have you ever had excessive amounts of energy running through your body, to the point where you did not need to sleep for days?"	• "What is your depression like on an everyday basis?" • "How does your depression affect your daily life?" • "When did this last happen, and please tell me what was going on at that time." • "How long did this last?" • "Were you using any drugs or alcohol at the time?" • "Did you require treatment or hospitalization?"	Patient Health Questionnaire (PHQ-9) Mood Disorder Questionnaire (MDQ)
Psychosis	1. "Do you hear or see things that other people do not hear or see?" 2. "Do you have thoughts that people are trying to follow, hurt, or spy on you?" 3. "Do you ever get messages from the television or radio?"	• "When did these symptoms start?" • "What triggers your symptoms?" • "What makes your symptoms get better?"	None recommended for the primary care setting
Substance use	1. "How much alcohol do you drink per day?" 2. "Have you been using any cocaine, methamphetamines, heroin, marijuana, PCP, LSD, ecstasy, or other drugs?"	If yes: • "How often do you use?" • "Do you think use of this substance is a problem in your life?" • "As a result of the use, did you experience any problems with relationships, work, finances, or the law?" • "Have you ever used any drugs by injection?" If no: • "Have you ever used any of these drugs in the past?"	• CAGE[c] • CAGE-AID (adapted to include drugs) • Alcohol Use Disorders Identification Test (AUDIT-C)

(continued)

TABLE 1-2 The AMPS Screening Tool for Common Psychiatric Conditions (continued)

	SCREENING QUESTIONS	FOLLOW-UP QUESTIONS	DIAGNOSTIC AND TREATMENT INSTRUMENTS[a]
Suicide[d]	1. "Do you ever wish you could go to sleep and not wake up?" 2. "Do you have any thoughts of wanting to hurt or kill yourself or somebody else?"	• "Have you ever tried to hurt or kill yourself in the past?" • "What is the chance you will try to hurt or kill yourself within the next 2-4 weeks?" • "Do you have guns or other items you could use to harm yourself?"	

[a]*These are suggested instruments that could be considered. More details about relevant instruments are available in the corresponding chapters.*
[b]*If either of these two questions is answered affirmatively, follow-up questions should be asked and a PHQ-9 should be administered.*
[c]*See Chapters 6 and 7 for details.*
[d]*Suggest asking about suicide if one of the AMPS questions is positive.*

TABLE 1-3 Key Features of the Mental Status Examination (MSE)

Appearance	• What is the status of the hygiene and grooming and are there any recent changes in appearance?
Attitude	• How does the patient relate to the clinician? • Is the patient cooperative, guarded, irritable, etc., during the interview?
Speech	• What are the rate, rhythm, and volume of speech?
Mood	• How does the patient describe his or her mood? • This should be reported as described by the patient.
Affect	• Does the patient's facial expressions have full range and reactivity? • How quickly does the affect change (lability)? • Is the affect congruent with the stated mood and is it appropriate to topics under discussion?
Thought process	• *How* is the patient thinking? • Does the patient change subjects quickly or is the train of thought difficult to follow?
Thought content	• *What* is the patient thinking? • What is the main theme or subject matter when the patient talks? • Does the patient have any delusions, obsessions, compulsions, suicidal, or homicidal thoughts?
Perceptions	• Does the patient have auditory, visual, or tactile hallucinations?
Cognition	• Is the patient alert? • Is the patient oriented to person, place, time, and the purpose of the interview?
Insight	• Does the patient recognize that there is an illness or disorder present? • Is there a clear understanding of the treatment plan and prognosis?
Judgment	• How will the patient secure food, clothing, and shelter in a safe environment? • Is the patient able to make decisions that support a safe and reasonable treatment plan?
Reliability	• Is the patient able to provide information that is consistent and accurate with other sources?

TABLE 4-1 High-Yield Questions

SECTION	QUESTION	RELEVANCE
History of present illness	1. People often understand their problems in their own way, which may be similar or different from how doctors explain the problem. How would you describe your problem to someone else? 2. Sometimes people use particular words or phrases to talk about their problems. Is there a specific term or expression that describes your problem?	Opens dialogue about patient's cultural beliefs and idioms.
Medical history	1. Often, people also look for help from people outside of medical clinics and hospitals. What kind of treatment from other sources have you sought for your problem? 2. How helpful have they been?	Ascertains cultural resources for healing and the perceived effectiveness of such healing practices.
Social history	1. Please tell me about the important people, positive and negative, in your life including your intimate or romantic partners. How have they affected or been affected by your problem? 2. Are there barriers that make it difficult for you to get the help you need, such as financial barriers, insurance issues, discrimination, language barriers, or cultural issues? 3. Are there considerations about your background, such as culture, race, ethnicity, sexual orientation, or gender identity that you feel I should know about to give you the best care possible?	These questions help patients elaborate on their cultural identity and sociocultural determinants that are relevant to their treatment and health.

TABLE 5-1 Generalized Anxiety Disorder 7-Item (GAD-7) Scale

HOW OFTEN DURING THE PAST 2 WEEKS HAVE YOU FELT BOTHERED BY:

1. Feeling nervous, anxious, or on edge?	0	1	2	3
2. Not being able to stop or control worrying?	0	1	2	3
3. Worrying too much about different things?	0	1	2	3
4. Trouble relaxing?	0	1	2	3
5. Being so restless that it is hard to sit still?	0	1	2	3
6. Becoming easily annoyed or irritable?	0	1	2	3
7. Feeling afraid as if something awful might happen?	0	1	2	3

Each question is answered on a scale of:
0 = not at all
1 = several days
2 = more than half the days
3 = nearly every day

A score of 8 or more should prompt further diagnostic evaluation for an anxiety disorder.

TABLE 7-1 Diagnostic Criteria for Trauma and Stressor-Related Disorders

Adjustment disorder	• Alteration in mood with marked distress and decreased functioning • Occurs within 6 months of stressor
Posttraumatic stress disorder (PTSD)	• Experience of a traumatic event • Reexperiencing (intrusive distressing memories, distressing dreaming, or flashbacks) • Avoidance/numbing (avoiding distressing memories or external reminders, lack of reaction/response to emotional triggers) • Negative cognition or mood (a distorted sense of blaming oneself or others, inability to remember events, decreased interest in activities) • Increased arousal and reactivity due to perceived persistent threat (irritability or aggressive behavior, hypervigilance, exaggerated startle, or sleep disturbances) • Symptoms lasting beyond 4 weeks from the traumatic event
Acute stress disorder	• Symptoms of PTSD within first 4 weeks after a traumatic event

TABLE 8-6 Examples of Dysfunctional Thoughts and Reconstruction Strategies

AUTOMATIC DYSFUNCTIONAL THOUGHTS	RECONSTRUCTED THOUGHTS
"*Nobody* likes me."	"That can't be true because my wife and kids love me."
"I'm a failure at *everything* I do."	"Maybe I'm just not good in this one area."
"I will *never* amount to *anything*."	"I already have a good job and I might get a promotion next year."
"I will *never* feel normal again."	"Depression can get better with medication and therapy."
"I have *always* been depressed."	"Not true—I was very happy when I got married and graduated from college!"

Patient Health Questionnaire (PHQ-9)
Nine-Symptom Depression Checklist

Name: _____   Date: _____

Over the *last 2 weeks*, how often have you been bothered by any of the following problems? (Please circle your answer.)

	Not at All	Several Days	More than Half the Days	Nearly Every Day
1. Little interest or pleasure in doing things	0	1	2	3
2. Feeling down, depressed, or hopeless	0	1	2	3
3. Trouble falling or staying asleep, or sleeping too much	0	1	2	3
4. Feeling tired or having little energy	0	1	2	3
5. Poor appetite or overeating	0	1	2	3
6. Feeling bad about yourself—or that you are a failure or have let yourself or your family down	0	1	2	3
7. Trouble concentrating on things, such as reading the newspaper or watching television	0	1	2	3
8. Moving or speaking so slowly that other people could have noticed. Or the opposite—being so fidgety or restless that you have been moving around a lot more than usual	0	1	2	3
9. Thoughts that you would be better off dead or of hurting yourself in some way	0	1	2	3

Add Columns, [____] + [____] + [____]

Total Score*, [____]   *Score is for healthcare provider

10. If you circled *any* problems, how *difficult* have these problems made it for you to do your work, take care of things at home, or get along with other people? (Please circle your answer.)	Not Difficult at All	Somewhat Difficult	Very Difficult	Extremely Difficult

A score of: 0–4 is considered non-depressed; 5–9 mild depression; 10–14 moderate depression; 15–19 moderately severe depression; and 20–27 severe depression.

FIGURE 8-2 Patient Health Questionnaire (PHQ-9) nine-symptom depression checklist. (PHQ is adapted from PRIME MD TODAY. PHQ Copyright ©1999 Pfizer Inc. All rights reserved. Reproduced with permission. PRIME MD TODAY is a trademark of Pfizer Inc.)

TABLE 13-3 Brief Screening Instruments

NIAAA SINGLE QUESTION SCREENING

Question	"How many times in the past year have you had X or more drinks in a day?" (X = 5 for men, 4 for women)
Scoring	More than 1 instance is a positive screen

AUDIT-C

Questions	POINTS				
	0	1	2	3	4
1. How often did you have a drink containing alcohol in the past year?	Never	Monthly or less	2-4 times a month	2-3 times a week	4 or more times a week
2. How many drinks did you have on a typical day when you were drinking in the past year?	None, or 1-2	3-4	5-6	7-9	10 or more
3. How often did you have five or more drinks on one occasion in the past year?	Never	Less than monthly	Monthly	Weekly	Daily or almost daily
Scoring	A score of ≥6 for men and ≥4 for women is considered positive and warrants further investigation.				

National Institute on Alcohol Abuse and Alcoholism. Helping Patients Who Drink Too Much: A Clinician's Guide; 2008. https://www.niaaa.nih.gov/guide. Accessed January 10, 2017. This questionnaire (the AUDIT) is reprinted with permission from the World Health Organization

TABLE 15-2 Feelings of Countertransference and Reactions to Avoid

PROVIDER'S FEELING	PERSONALITY DISORDER	POTENTIAL PROVIDER PITFALLS	SUGGESTED ACTION
Anger (patient is viewed as manipulative)	• Borderline • Antisocial • Narcissistic	Overreaction to provocation, retaliation (e.g., verbal/physical abuse of patient, substandard care, inappropriate comments in charting)	• Be aware of feelings and unconscious bias • Process with peers, such as in Balint groups • Strict adherence to evidence-based standard of care
Fear of patient (physical or legal threat)	• Antisocial • Paranoid	Immediate emotional or physical overresponse (out of proportion to threat)	• Maintain personal safety • Thorough documentation • Appropriate familiarity with clinic policy and procedure
Sympathy	• Borderline (sympathy by some providers associated with negative views by other providers may represent *splitting* by the patient) • Dependent	Overindulgence or desire to "rescue" the patient	• Regular, structured, and scheduled visits with the same provider that do not run over scheduled time • Splitting should be dealt with by interdisciplinary meetings to make sure all members of team are acting in accordance with treatment plan and not providing "special" treatment
Anger, self-doubt	• Narcissistic • Paranoid	Putting down the patient; questioning your own abilities in a nonrealistic way	• Examine your abilities in a realistic way • Seek peer support, process in Balint groups
Frustration	• Borderline • Avoidant • Dependent	Patients do not follow-through with treatment recommendations or rely heavily on providers	• Set clear expectations • Ally yourself with patient's family/friends to assist (as permitted by privacy restrictions) • Treat patient with a consistent team approach so that no single provider burns out
Attraction	• Histrionic • Borderline	Inappropriate relationship with patient	• Consider using a chaperone for examinations requiring examination of genitalia, even in gender-matched provider–patient situations • Do not see the patient after-hours or in social settings

Name: _____

Thought Record				
Date	**Situation** *What was happening at the time? What were you doing?*	**Thought(s)** *What was going through your mind?* **On a scale from 0 to 100%, how much do you believe what you were thinking?*	**Emotion(s)** *How were you feeling at the time? Sad? Angry? Another emotion?* **On a scale from 0 to 100, how intense was your emotion?*	**Behavior** *What did you do in response to, or to cope with, your emotion(s)? Did you yell at somebody or get into bed? Did you take a walk or drink alcohol?*

Name: _____

Thought Record							
Date	**Situation** *What was happening at the time? What were you doing?*	**Thought** *What was going through your mind?* **On a scale from 0 to 100%, how much do you believe what you were thinking?*	**Emotion(s)** *How were you feeling at the time? Sad? Angry? Another emotion?* **On a scale from 0 to 100, how intense was your emotion?*	**Physical Feeling(s)** *How did your body feel?* *For example, shaky, heart racing, tense, pain?*	**Behavior(s)** *What did you do in response to, or to cope with, your emotion(s)? For example, did you yell at somebody or get into bed? Did you take a walk or drink alcohol?*	**Alternative Thought(s)** *What is a more helpful or realistic way to think about the situation?*	**Alternative Behavior(s), Emotion(s), and Physical Feeling(s)** *What might be a more helpful way to respond or cope? Do you think you'd experience different emotions/physical feelings?*

FIGURE 16-2 Sample Thought Records.

Name: _____   Date: _____

Hourly Pleasant Activity Schedule (indicate planned activity and then record your mood or sense of accomplishment during/after the activity on a scale from 0 to 10, with 0 = worst possible mood/sense of accomplishment and 10 = best possible mood/sense of accomplishment)

	Monday		Tuesday		Wednesday		Thursday		Friday		Saturday		Sunday	
(Example)	*Go to library*	7			*Call a friend*	8	*Go for a walk*	6			*Watch TV*	5		
7am-8am														
8am-9am														
9am-10am														
10am-11am														
11am-12pm														
12pm-1pm														
1pm-2pm														
2pm-3pm														
3pm-4pm														
4pm-5pm														
5pm-6pm														
6pm-7pm														
7pm-8pm														
8pm-9pm														
9pm-10pm														

FIGURE 16-4 Hourly pleasant activity schedule.

Name: _____ Date: _____

Pleasant Activity Schedule (indicate planned activity and then record your mood or sense of accomplishment during/after the activity on a scale from 0 to 10, with 0 = worst possible mood/sense of accomplishment and 10 = best possible mood/sense of accomplishment)							
	Monday	Tuesday	Wednesday	Thursday	Friday	Saturday	Sunday
Morning							
Midday							
Evening							

FIGURE 16-5 Pleasant activity schedule.

TABLE 16-2 Common Cognitive Distortions/Types of Unhelpful Thinking

DISTORTION	DESCRIPTION	EXAMPLE
All-or-nothing thinking	When you see things in black and white terms; as "either/or."	"I can't do anything when I'm in pain."
Mind reading	When you think you know what someone else is thinking (and usually assume something negative).	"He's thinking I look terrible."
Discounting or ignoring the positive	When you focus on the negative aspects of something and assume the positive aspects don't count.	"It doesn't matter that I used to take my medication every day; I'm a failure because I haven't taken any medication over the past week."
Catastrophizing or magnifying	When you think something is much worse than it actually is; you blow things out of proportion.	"If I have a panic attack at work I'll lose control and everyone will think I'm crazy."
Fortune-telling	When you think you can predict the future.	"If someone offers me a cigarette I won't be able to refuse it."
Overgeneralization	When you perceive an overly negative pattern in something but base this on a single or rare event.	"I always seem to mess up my diet."
Emotional reasoning	When you draw conclusions based on how you're feeling.	"I feel anxious when my partner says she's going to be home late so she must be cheating on me."
Regret focus	When you focus on mistakes you made in the past, rather than on what you can do now.	"I should have never let myself gain so much weight."

Modified from Burns DD. The Feeling Good Handbook: Using the New Mood Therapy in Everyday Life. New York, NY: William Morrow & Co.; 1989. Leahy RL. Cognitive Therapy Techniques: A Practitioner's Guide. New York, NY: Guilford Press; 2003.

BOX 16-2   QUESTIONS TO HELP PATIENTS EXAMINE THE ACCURACY OR HELPFULNESS OF THEIR THINKING

Is there any evidence that my thought is true? (What is the evidence?)

Is there any evidence that my thought is not true? (What is the evidence?)

What would I say to a friend who had the same thought?

Is there another way to think about this situation?

If I was a lawyer and had to make a case for the opposite of my thought, what would I say?

If my thought is true, what's the worst that can happen?

If my thought is true, what do I need to do to solve my problem?

TABLE 18-1 Motivational Interviewing Principles

MI PRINCIPLE	RATIONALE	SKILLS/TOOLS	AS COMPARED WITH ...
Express empathy	• Demonstrate acceptance and understanding of patient ambivalence	• Reflective listening • Open-ended questions • Summary	• Providing data and statistics to convince patient of need for change
Support self-efficacy	• Build patient's confidence in their ability to change	• Affirmations • Reflect change talk • Identify patient's strengths	• Getting too far ahead of patient (misalignment with stage of change) • Focusing on what's going wrong rather than patient's attempts to change
Roll with resistance	• Refrain from confronting or arguing about patient's behavior • Use as opportunity to learn about patient's experience	• Reflective listening • Open-ended questions	• Engaging in power struggle • Arguing with patient about why they should change • Giving ultimatums
Develop discrepancy	• Evoke/illuminate discrepancy between patient behavior and patient's beliefs/values	• Use decisional balance • Use change rulers • Reflective listening • Open-ended questions • Summary	• Arguing for healthy behavior based on provider's values • Pointing out inconsistencies in patient behavior

TABLE 19-4 Risk Factors for Drug-Induced QT Prolongation

UNMODIFIABLE	MODIFIABLE
Female gender	Hypokalemia/hypomagnesaemia
Age >65	Bradycardia (including recent conversion from AF)
Congenital long QT syndrome	Use of other QT prolonging medication
Family history of sudden death	Use of medications that inhibit metabolism of QT prolonging medication
History of drug-induced QT prolongation	Starvation or obesity
Structural heart disease/LV dysfunction	Overdose or rapid IV administration of QT prolonging medication
Renal or hepatic insufficiency	

Modified from New Zealand Medicines and Medical Devices Safety Authority. Drug-induced QT prolongation and Torsades de Pointes – the facts. Prescriber Update. 2010;31(4):27-29. Reprinted by permission of Medsafe.

INDEX

Note: Page numbers followed by "f" indicate figures and "t" indicate tables.